COLOR ATLAS AND SYNOPSIS OF ECHOCARDIOGRAPHY

NOTICE

COLOR ATLAS AND SYNOPSIS OF ECHOCARDIOGRAPHY

EDITOR

David A. Orsinelli, MD, FACC, FASE

Professor, Internal Medicine

Division of Cardiovascular Medicine

The Ohio State University Wexner Medical Center

Columbus, Ohio

SERIES EDITOR

William T. Abraham, MD, FACP, FACC, FAHA, FESC

Professor of Medicine, Physiology, and Cell Biology

Chair of Excellence in Cardiovascular Medicine

Director, Division of Cardiovascular Medicine

Deputy Director, Davis Heart and Lung Research Institute

The Ohio State University

Columbus, Ohio

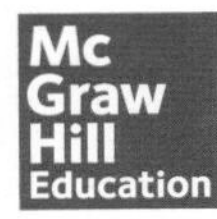

New York Chicago San Francisco Athens London Madrid Mexico City
Milan New Delhi Singapore Sydney Toronto

Color Atlas and Synopsis of Echocardiography, 1ed.

1 2 3 4 5 6 7 8 9 0 CTP/CTP 18 17 16 15

Set ISBN 978-0-07-174736-3; Set MHID 0-07-174736-2;
Book ISBN 978-0-07-174676-2; Book MHID 007174676-5
DVD ISBN 978-0-07-174735-6; DVD MHID 0-07-174735-4
EBook ISBN 978-0-07182954-0; EBook MHID 0-07-182954-7

This book was set in Perpetua by Cenveo® Publisher Services.
The editors were Christine Diedrich and Christie Naglieri.
The production supervisor was Richard Ruzycka.
Project management was provided by Kritika Kaushik, Cenveo Publisher Services.
The cover designer was Thomas De Pierro.
CTPS was the printer and binder.

Library of Congress Cataloging-in-Publication Data

Color atlas and synopsis of echocardiography/editor, David A. Orsinelli.
p. ; cm.
Includes bibliographical references.
ISBN 978-0-07-174736-3 (hardcover : alk. paper)—
ISBN 0-07-174736-2 (hardcover : alk. paper)
I. Orsinelli, David A., editor.
[DNLM: 1. Echocardiography—methods—Atlases.
2. Cardiovascular Diseases—diagnosis—Atlases. WG 17]
RC683.5.U5
616.1′207543—dc23

2014014805

DEDICATION

I would like to dedicate this atlas to my wonderful wife, Maryellen H. Orsinelli, RN, RDCS, FASE, without whose love, support, and understanding this book would not have been possible. Her patience and acceptance of my time away from home to work on this project is deeply appreciated. I would also like to dedicate this book to my parents, Dr. and Mrs. David (Linda) Orsinelli. Without their love and support, my career would not have been possible. They emphasized the importance of education and instilled in me the values of hard work, dedication, and a commitment to excellence. I truly owe my career to them.

David A. Orsinelli, MD, FACC, FASE

CONTENTS

Gerard P. Aurigemma, MD, FAHA, FASE,FACC
Professor of Medicine and Radiology
Department of Medicine, Division of Cardiology
University of Massachusetts Medical School
Worcester, Massachusetts

Rebecca Baumann, MD
Fellow, Department of Medicine, Division of Cardiology
University of Massachusetts Medical School
Worcester, Massachusetts

Peter M. Bittenbender, MD*
Cardiologist, Summa Health System
Akron General Medical Center
Akron, Ohio

Vincent Brinkman, MD
Assistant Professor, Internal Medicine
The Ohio State University Wexner Medical Center
Division of Cardiovascular Medicine
Columbus, Ohio

Brigid MacKenna-Carlson, MD
Assistant Professor of Medicine
Department of Medicine
University of Massachusetts Medical School
Worcester, Massachusetts

Karen Dugan, MD
Internal Medicine Resident
University of Chicago Medical Center
Chicago, Illinois

Sitaramesh Emani, MD
Assistant Professor of Medicine
Advanced Heart Failure & Cardiac Transplant
The Ohio State University Wexner Medical Center
Columbus, Ohio

Jason Evanchan, DO*
Cardiologist
Aultman Hospital-Cardiovascular Consultants
Canton, Ohio

Jarrod Ferrara, MD
Fellow, Cardiovascular Medicine
University of Massachusetts Medical School
Worcester, Massachusetts

Anthony Garcia, MD
Fellow, Department of Medicine, Division of Cardiology
University of Massachusetts Medical School
Worcester, Massachusetts

Demet Menekse Gerede, MD
Echocardiography Laboratory
Cleveland Clinic Foundation
Cleveland, Ohio

Richard A. Grimm, DO, FACC
Staff Cardiologist
Director, Echocardiography Laboratory
Cardiovascular Medicine, Heart & Vascular Institute, Cleveland Clinic
Cleveland, Ohio

Nkechinyere Ijioma, MBBS*
Fellow, Interventional Cardiology
The Mayo Clinic
Division of Cardiovascular Diseases
Rochester, Minnesota

Saurabh Jha, MD, MS
Fellow, Cardiovascular Imaging
Division of Cardiovascular Medicine
Cleveland Clinic Foundation
Cleveland, Ohio

John A. Larry, MD
Associate Professor of Internal Medicine
Cardiovascular Section Director, OSU Hospital East
Ohio State University Hospital East
Columbus, Ohio

Gina G. Mentzer, MD, HFSA, FAHA*
Cardiologist
Heart Failure, Transplant & Mechanical Circulatory Support
Medical Director, AIMS for HF program
(Advanced Integrated Medicine and Surgery for Heart Failure program)
Women's Heart Program
Nebraska Heart Institute & Heart Hospital
Lincoln, Nebraska

Chad M. Miller, MD
Associate Professor of Neurosurgery and Neurology
The Ohio State University Wexner Medical Center
Columbus, Ohio

David A. Orsinelli, MD, FACC, FASE
Professor, Internal Medicine
The Ohio State University Wexner Medical Center
Division of Cardiovascular Medicine
Columbus, Ohio

Gaurav R. Parikh, MD, FAHA, FASE, FACC
Fellow, Department of Medicine, Division of Cardiology
University of Massachusetts Medical School
Worcester, Massachusetts

Kyle Pfahl, MD*
Fellow, Interventional Cardiology
William Beaumont Hospital
Royal Oak, Michigan

Kavita Sharma, MD
Assistant Professor, Internal Medicine
The Ohio State University Wexner Medical Center
Division of Cardiovascular Medicine
Columbus, Ohio

CONTRIBUTORS

Andrew Slivka, MD
Professor of Neurology
The Ohio State University Wexner Medical Center
Columbus, Ohio

Sakima A. Smith, MD*
Assistant Professor of Medicine
The Ohio State University Wexner Medical Center
Division of Cardiovascular Medicine
Columbus, Ohio

Gbemiga Sofowora, MBChB, FACC
Clinical Assistant Professor, Internal Medicine
The Ohio State University Wexner Medical Center
Division of Cardiovascular Medicine
Columbus, Ohio

Dennis A. Tighe, MD, FACC, FACP, FASE
Associate Director, Noninvasive Cardiology
UMass-Memorial Medical Center
Professor of Medicine
University of Massachusetts Medical School
Worcester, Massachusetts

Teerapat Yingchoncharoen, MD
Fellow, Heart Failure/Transplantation
Heart and Vascular Institute
The Cleveland Clinic Foundation
Cleveland, Ohio

*Current affiliation. At the time of contribution to this atlas, the author was fellow in the Division of Cardiovascular Medicine at The Ohio State University Wexner Medical Center in Columbus, Ohio

PREFACE

Patients with cardiovascular disease are encountered in virtually every field of medicine, from the family practitioner and general internist to the surgeon and even the obstetrician. While other "advanced imaging" modalities such as cardiac MRI and CT are able to noninvasively evaluate cardiac structure and function and provide complimentary and additional information for the clinician, no modality other than echocardiography can provide a rapid noninvasive evaluation of the heart and great vessels. Echocardiography is available in virtually any clinical setting, from the emergency department to the ICU, the operating room and the stress lab, at the bedside and in the office.

Thus, almost every patient with known or suspected cardiac disease will be evaluated with an echocardiogram, usually as the first line-imaging tool. Echocardiography has become by far the most frequently ordered and performed cardiovascular test after the electrocardiogram. As its use has expanded, the indications and "appropriateness" in clinical cardiology have come under increasing scrutiny. In this atlas, we will explore the utility of echocardiography in clinical medicine using a case-based format. We will highlight, when available, current clinical guidelines and appropriate use criteria that should guide the utilization of echocardiography. References are intended to direct the interested reader to core references and guideline statements, including references to recently published appropriate use criteria.

Chapter 1 provides a brief review of the various echocardiographic methods commonly used in day-to-day practice.

Coronary artery disease (CAD) remains the leading cause of death in the developed world. Chapter 2 explores the role of echo in the diagnosis and management of patients with known or suspected CAD.

Echocardiography is instrumental in the management of patients with valvular heart disease, and in fact is the diagnostic test of choice in evaluating the patient with a heart murmur and with previously diagnosed valvular heart disease. It was the development and acceptance of Doppler echocardiography as a method to quantify valvular heart disease that led to the widespread acceptance and increasing utilization of echocardiography. Chapter 3 provides many examples of the use of echocardiography in patients with valvular heart disease.

Assessment of ventricular function is one of the most frequently asked questions for the echocardiographer. After a complete history and physical, a comprehensive echocardiogram should be the initial diagnostic test in the management of the heart failure patient, according to the most recent heart failure guidelines. In Chapters 4 and 5, contributors from the University of Massachusetts provide insight into the echocardiographic assessment of the patient with new onset dyspnea, known or suspected heart failure, and a variety of cardiomyopathies.

One of the initial descriptions of the use of echocardiography in the United States was a seminal paper by Dr. Harvey Feigenbaum in 1965 describing the use of cardiac ultrasound to detect pericardial fluid. Echocardiography remains the principal imaging method to assess pericardial disease, especially in the acute setting, and is the imaging method of choice to diagnose the presence of pericardial effusions. Chapter 6 explores the use of echocardiography in pericardial disease.

In Chapter 7, various diseases of the aorta are discussed, and in Chapter 8, our colleagues in neurology give us their perspective on the use of echocardiography in the patient with a stroke or TIA.

Contributors from the Cleveland Clinic, in Chapters 9 and 10, explore the use of echocardiography to evaluate intracardiac masses and address the use of echocardiography in patients with atrial fibrillation, a rapidly expanding patient population.

Chapters 11 and 12 briefly review the use of echocardiography in patients with pulmonary hypertension and pulmonary embolism as well as selected systemic diseases that can affect the heart.

Finally, in Chapter 13, the expanding role of echocardiography, especially transesophageal echo, in interventional procedures, is discussed.

This atlas is not intended to replace or duplicate the many comprehensive textbooks in the field of echocardiography. Rather, the goal of this atlas is to highlight the current role of echocardiography in clinical cardiology and to provide the interested reader up to date references in the field. It is my hope that this atlas will be of interest to medical students who are increasingly being exposed to various ultrasound modalities in their training, house officers and fellows, as well as primary care physicians and the cardiologist.

David A. Orsinelli, MD, FACC, FASE

ACKNOWLEDGMENTS

I would first like to acknowledge the many contributing authors for the time and effort they put into this project. This atlas would not have been possible without their hard work. They all have put in countless hours on their own time to provide the cases for this book.

I would also like to acknowledge my many mentors and teachers who have inspired me throughout my career, especially the faculty in the Echo Lab at the University of Massachusetts who first instilled in me the interest in echocardiography. It was during my fellowship that my interest in echocardiography, which has been the focus and my passion during my career in cardiology, was developed. Special thanks to Dr. Gerry Aurigemma, my fellowship program director and Echo Lab director, mentor, friend, and colleague who continues to be a resource for me.

Thanks also to the staff at McGraw Hill for their patience and understanding in this process from concept development to completion. Finally, I would like to thank Dr. Bill Abraham, the series editor, for inviting me to edit this atlas and contribute to this series.

David A. Orsinelli, MD, FACC, FASE

ABBREVIATIONS

AMI: Acute Myocardial Infarction
ACC: American College of Cardiology
AHA: American Heart Association
ACEi: Angiotensin Converting Enzyme inhibitor
AR: Aortic Regurgitation
AS: Aortic Stenosis
AV: Aortic Valve
AVR: Aortic Valve Replacement
AF: Atrial Fibrillation
Afl: Atrial Flutter
AV: Atrial Ventricular
AICD: Automatic Implantable Cardioverter Defibrillator
BAV: Balloon Aortic Valvuloplasty
BMV: Balloon Mitral Valvuloplasty
BPM: Beats per Minute
BP: Blood Pressure
BMI: Body Mass Index
BNP: Brain Natiuretic Peptide
CCT: Cardiac Computed Tomography
CRT: Cardiac Resynchronization Therapy
CMP: Cardiomyopathy
CV: Cardioversion
CVA: Cerebral Vascular Accident
CXR: Chest X-Ray
cbc: Complete blood count
CHF: Congestive Heart Failure
COPD: Chronic Obstructive Pulmonary Disease
CT: Computed Tomography
CAD: Coronary Artery Disease
DE-CMR: Delayed Enhancement Cardiac MRI
DCM: Dilated Cardiomyopathy
DES: Drug Eluting Stent
EF: Ejection Fraction
ECG: Electrocardiogram
EP: Electrophysiologic
ED: Emergency Department
EMB: Endomyocardial biopsy
HR: Heart Rate
HTN: Hypertension
HCM: Hypertrophic Cardiomyopathy
ICD: Implantable Cardiac Defibrillator
IVC: Inferior Vena Cava
INR: International Normalized Ratio
IABP: Intraaortic Balloon Pump
IV: Intravenous
IVDA: Intravenous Drug Abuse
LA: Left Atrium
LAA: Left Atrial Appendage
LAD: Left Anterior Descending
LV: Left Ventricle
L: Liter
LVAD: Left Ventricular Assist Device
LVH: Left Ventricular Hypertrophy
MRA: Magnetic Resonance Angiography
MRI: Magnetic Resonance Imaging
MR: Mitral regurgitation
MS: Mitral Stenosis
MVP: Mitral Valve Prolapse
MV: Mitral Valve
MI: Myocardial Infarction
NYHA: New York Heart Association
NSAIDS: Nonsteroidal Anti-inflammatory Drugs
O_2: Oxygen
PLAX: Parasternal long axis
PND: Paroxysmal Nocturnal Dyspnea
PCI: Percutaneous Coronary Intervention
PET-CT: Positron Emmision Tomography-Computed Tomography
PA: Pulmonary Artery
PASP: Pulmonary Artery Systolic Pressure
PH: Pulmonary Hypertension
PR: Pulmonary Regurgitation
PS: Pulmonary Stenosis
PV: Pulmonary Valve
RWT: Relative Wall Thickness
RA: Right Atrium
RCA: Right Coronary Artery
RV: Right Ventricle
RVSP: Right Ventricular Systolic Pressure
SVG: Saphenous Vein Graft
STS: Society of Thoracic Surgeons
SEC: Spontaneous Echocardiographic Contrast
SVC: Superior Vena Cava
SBP: Systolic Blood Pressure
TAVR: Transcatheter Aortic Valve Replacement
3D: Three-Dimensional
TEE: Transesophageal Echocardiography
TIA: Transient Ischemic Attack
TTE: Transthoracic Echocardiography
TR: Tricuspid Regurgitation
TS: Tricuspid Stenosis
TV: Tricuspid Valve
2-D: Two-Dimensional
VSD: Ventricular Septal Defect
VT: Ventricular Tachycardia

1 AN ATLAS TO EXPLORE THE CURRENT USE OF ECHOCARDIOGRAPHY IN CLINICAL MEDICINE

David A. Orsinelli, MD, FACC, FASE

INTRODUCTION

As a clinical tool in cardiovascular medicine, there are few if any techniques that can rival the role of echocardiography. It is a noninvasive (or semi-invasive in the case of transesophageal echocardiography) diagnostic test with no known untoward side effects (including the lack of radiation) that allows for a comprehensive assessment of cardiac anatomy and physiology. It can provide insight into the diagnosis of patients with suspected cardiac disease, help guide management, and provide important prognostic information. Unlike competing imaging methods, echocardiography is portable and can be performed in virtually any clinical setting, including the outpatient clinic, an inpatient echocardiography laboratory, the patient's bedside, the critical care environment, the emergency department, and the operating room.

Since cardiac disease is so ubiquitous and echocardiography plays such an integral role in its diagnosis and management, most clinicians (not only cardiologists) need to understand the role of echocardiography and its strengths and weaknesses, as well as its limitations. Echocardiography can play a significant role in the diagnosis and management of a broad spectrum of patients. Such patients could include the outpatient presenting to a primary care physician with new physical exam findings such as a murmur or symptoms such as dyspnea, the established cardiac patient with new symptoms, or the hemodynamically unstable ICU patient. The clinical application of echocardiography and guidelines for its use in a variety of clinical situations are addressed in the ACC/AHA/ASE guideline report most recently updated in 2003.[1]

Due to its many advantages and capabilities, the utilization of echocardiography in clinical medicine in general and in cardiovascular practice in particular has exploded since its initial description nearly 60 years ago.[2] Echocardiography has become by far the most frequently ordered and performed cardiovascular test after the electrocardiogram. It would be quite unusual for a patient with cardiovascular disease not to have had an echocardiogram.

While echocardiography has many advantages, one would be remiss to ignore its limitations. Challenges with image quality and acquisition due to patient characteristics such as underlying lung disease (eg, COPD) and body habitus, as well as difficulty in appropriately positioning patients, especially in critical care settings may lead to suboptimal images.

Echocardiography is very "user-dependent," not only in the acquisition of images, but also in its interpretation. Quality improvement in echocardiography has thus become an important aspect of the field. Many professional organizations, including the American Society of Echocardiography (ASE) and the American College of Cardiology (ACC), have formulated guidelines for training in the performance and interpretation of echocardiograms.[3,4] The Intersocietal Commission for the Accreditation of Echocardiography Laboratories (ICAEL) was formed in 1996 to address the need for standardization and quality improvement of echocardiographic laboratories. Now known as the Intersocietal Accreditation Commission (IAC)—Echocardiography, its goal is, "Improving health care through accreditation."[5] Echocardiography labs that are accredited by IAC-Echocardiography must be staffed by sonographers and physicians who meet standards for training and ongoing education in the field, demonstrate a commitment to quality, follow established guidelines, and have in place a quality improvement process.

BRIEF HISTORICAL REVIEW

Starting in the 1940s, there were many early efforts to utilize ultrasound in medicine in general and cardiology in particular as a diagnostic tool. It was the collaborative efforts of Dr. Inge Edler, a cardiologist, and Dr. Hellmuth Hertz, a physicist, to employ ultrasound to examine the heart that are generally acknowledged as the beginning of echocardiography.[6] Their initial work was published in 1954.[7]

After this initial publication and the subsequent publication in 1965 in the United States by Feigenbaum demonstrating the use of ultrasound to detect pericardial effusion,[8] the field of echocardiography rapidly developed. The seminal publications by Holen and Hatle in the late 1970s,[9,10] in which Doppler echocardiography was demonstrated to be a reliable noninvasive technique to accurately assess valve function, led to more widespread acceptance and utilization of echocardiography. The development of two-dimensional imaging, including the first real-time scanner[6,11] that enabled clinicians to view the heart in real-time, also demonstrated the potential of this technique. Thus, after an initial period of skepticism in the 1960s and 1970s, the use of echocardiography as a clinical tool in cardiovascular medicine exploded.[6] Over the past 3 to 4 decades, improvements in transducer technology, advances in computers, and the development of additional techniques such as transesophageal echocardiography, intracardiac echocardiography, tissue Doppler techniques, and strain imaging, to name a few, have led to even more applications for echocardiography. In spite of the rapid development of other advanced imaging techniques, such as cardiovascular computed tomography (CT) and cardiovascular magnetic resonance imaging (MRI), echocardiography remains the mainstay of the noninvasive evaluation of patients with known or suspected cardiovascular disease.

There are many excellent, comprehensive textbooks on echocardiography.[12,13] This Atlas is not intended to replace or duplicate those books. Rather, we will highlight the current role of echocardiography in clinical medicine using a case-based format with an evidence-based approach to its role in clinical cardiology. When available, references to current clinical guidelines and the recently revised appropriate use criteria for echocardiography[14] will be incorporated into the discussions.

REVIEW OF TECHNIQUES AND METHODOLGIES

A variety of echocardiographic techniques and methodologies currently exist (Figure 1-1-1).Our challenge as echocardiographers is to apply the correct "tools" to the clinical situation. As a clinician requesting an echocardiogram, the challenge and responsibility is to provide relevant clinical information and the specific questions being asked from the study so that appropriate techniques can be employed and the clinical questions can be addressed. Standard echocardiography textbooks can provide the interested reader a more comprehensive review of these modalities.

M-MODE ECHOCARDIOGRAPHY

M-mode echocardiography, first displayed on strip chart recordings in the early 1970s, provides a one-dimensional, "ice-pick" view of the heart (Figure 1-1-2). While initially obtained with a "blind" dedicated M-mode transducer, M-mode echocardiograms are now obtained with 2-dimensional guidance, thus reducing the errors generated by oblique, off-axis images. Since the heart is a 3-dimensional structure, a single linear assessment of the heart has obvious limitations. However, M-mode echo still has a role to play in current day echocardiography.[15]

M-mode echocardiography provides excellent spatial and temporal resolution (far exceeding the temporal resolution of 2-dimensional imaging), which allows for more precise timing of events and an

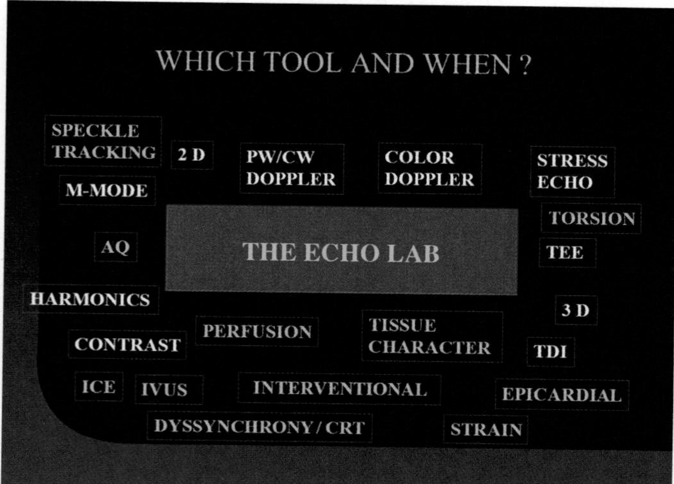

FIGURE 1-1-1 "Tools" available in a modern echocardiography laboratory.

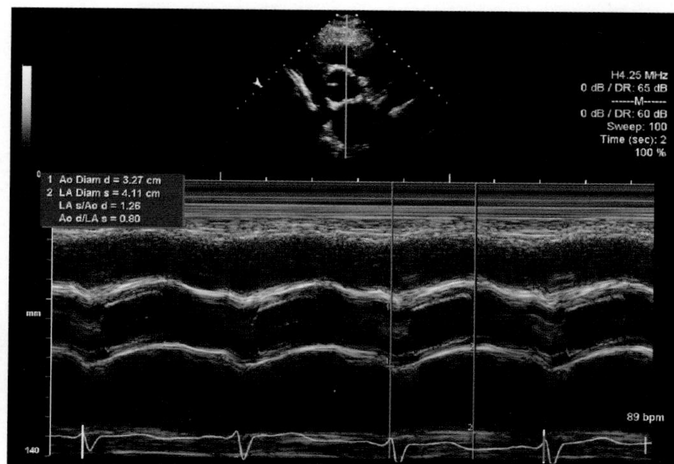

FIGURE 1-1-2 Normal 2-D guided M-mode of the aortic valve and left atrium.

assessment of the motion of rapidly moving cardiac structures such as valves. There remain many clinically useful roles. For example, M-mode assessment of the free wall of the right atrium or right ventricle may help to determine the presence of diastolic chamber collapse, a sign of cardiac tamponade (Figure 1-1-3). The assessment of right ventricular function using M-mode to assess TAPSE (tricuspid annular plane systolic excursion) is a useful marker of right ventricular function.[16]

While 2-dimensional (2-D) and 3-dimensional (3-D) imaging clearly provide a more comprehensive assessment of cardiac chambers, linear dimensions of cardiac structures remain an important quantitative measure. For example, current guidelines for the management of valvular heart disease[17] still employ linear dimensions in the decision-making algorithms for the management of patients with aortic and mitral regurgitation.

TWO-DIMENSIONAL ECHOCARDIOGRAPHY

Two-dimensional echocardiography (2DE), which provides real-time dynamic images of cardiac structure and function, is the mainstay

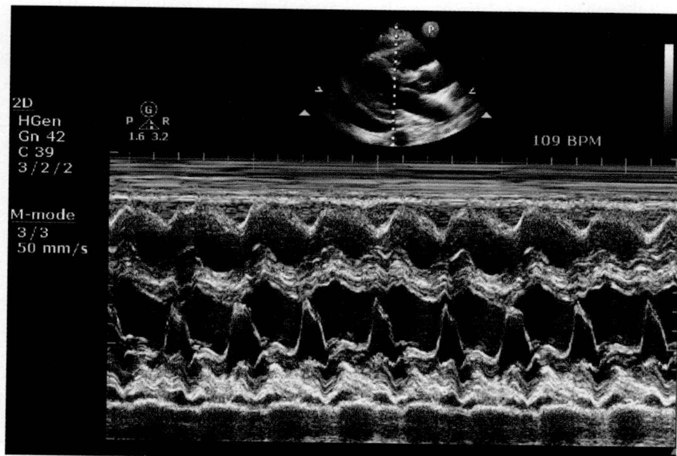

FIGURE 1-1-3 M-mode echocardiogram demonstrating right ventricular diastolic collapse in a patient with cardiac tamponade.

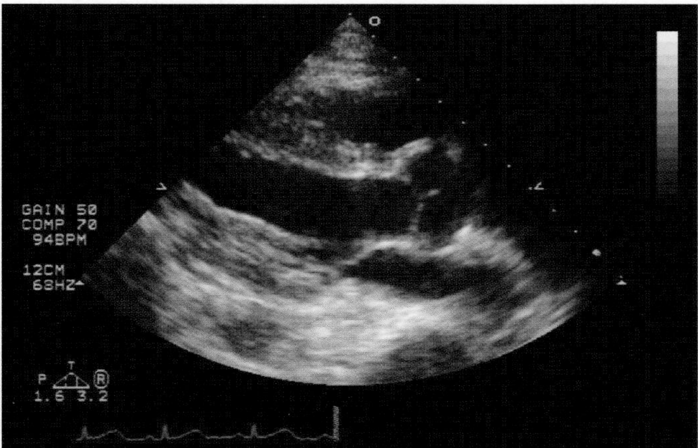

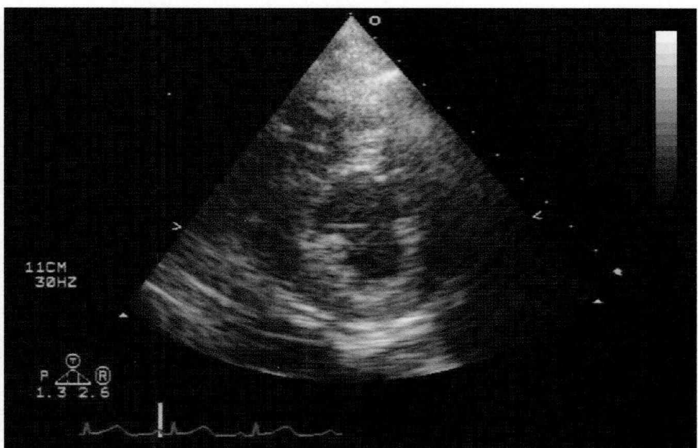

FIGURE 1-1-4 Two-dimensional image of the left ventricle demonstrating a normal left ventricle in the parasternal long axis view (L) and short axis (R) views ►(see Videos 1-1-4).

of current clinical echocardiography. Initially introduced in the 1970s, image quality has dramatically improved over the years due to improvements in transducer technology, image processing algorithms, and advances in computer technology that allow for more rapid processing.

Current 2DE systems provide a robust platform for the evaluation of cardiac structure and function, including the assessment of left and right ventricular structure and function, cardiac chamber dimensions, the assessment of valvular heart disease, and the evaluation of the great vessels and the pericardium. Two-dimensional imaging forms the back-bone of the modern day echocardiography laboratory (Figure 1-1-4).

DOPPLER ECHOCARDIOGRAPHY

Based on the Doppler principal of frequency shifts of the ultrasound signal generated by moving targets in relationship to the transducer, Doppler echocardiography utilizes red blood cells as the moving ultrasound reflector to provide an evaluation of blood flow, allowing an assessment of valvular function (regurgitation and stenosis) and the assessment of intracardiac shunts. Recent advances in the use of the Doppler technique now also allow for the assessment of tissue velocity data (see Tissue Doppler Imaging).

Both spectral (pulsed wave and continuous-wave) and color flow Doppler techniques are utilized to assess valvular function. For example, continuous-wave Doppler can be used to define aortic valve gradients (Figure 1-1-5) in order to evaluate the presence and severity of aortic stenosis. Color flow Doppler can be employed to assess valvular regurgitation (Figure 1-1-6) and intracardiac shunts (Figure 1-1-7).

COLOR DOPPLER M-MODE

By combining the benefits of M-mode and color Doppler imaging, this technique results in an image with high temporal and spatial resolution. Color M-mode has been employed in the assessment of left ventricular filling to assess diastolic function and can be used to better define the width of the aortic regurgitation (AR) signal to aid in quantification of the severity of AR (Figure 1-1-8).

TISSUE DOPPLER IMAGING (TDI)

By changing various system settings and filters to better detect tissue velocity information as opposed to blood flow, the Doppler technique has been used to assess tissue (myocardial) velocities (Figure 1-1-9).[18] In recent years, tissue Doppler imaging (TDI) has emerged as an important adjunctive imaging modality. By extracting the tissue velocity information, computation of myocardial strain and strain rate is possible. Utilizing this technique has further advanced our understanding of systolic and diastolic function, played a role in evaluating the timing of cardiac motion in the evaluation of patients with left ventricle (LV) dyssynchrony, and provides insight into myocardial mechanics.[19]

SPECKLE TRACKING ECHOCARDIOGRAPHY (STE)

Utilizing speckles that are present in grayscale B-mode images, speckle tracking echocardiography (STE) is a new technique employed to assess myocardial function.[20] Unlike the TDI technique, STE is angle-independent. By processing data from 2-D images offline, this technique allows for the derivation of myocardial

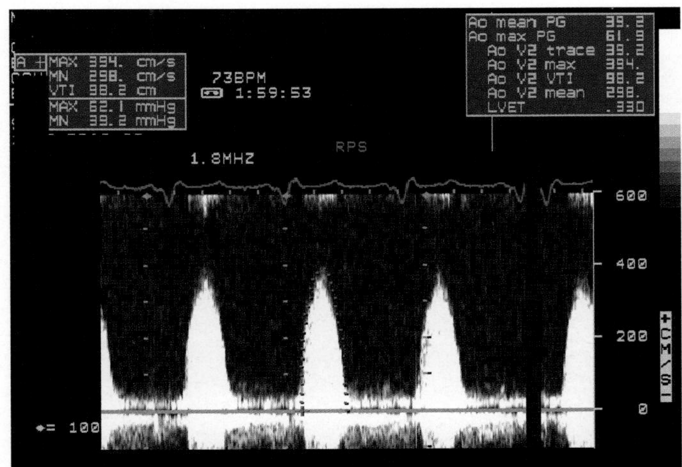

FIGURE 1-1-5 Continuous-wave Doppler demonstrating an elevated aortic valve gradient in a young patient with severe aortic stenosis due to a bicuspid aortic valve.

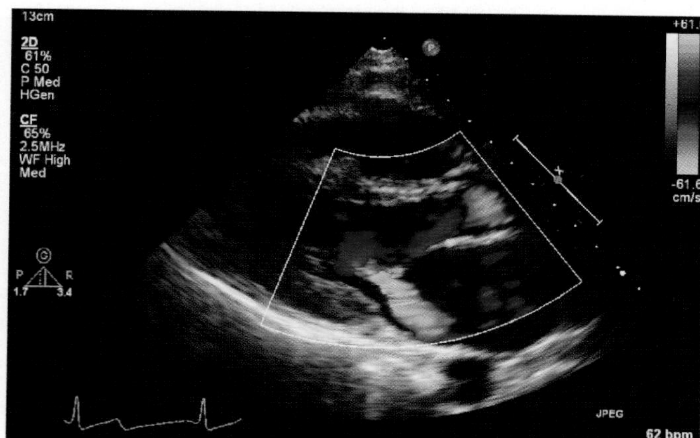

FIGURE 1-1-6 Color Doppler demonstrating mitral and aortic regurgitation in a patient with rheumatic valve disease ►(see Video 1-1-6).

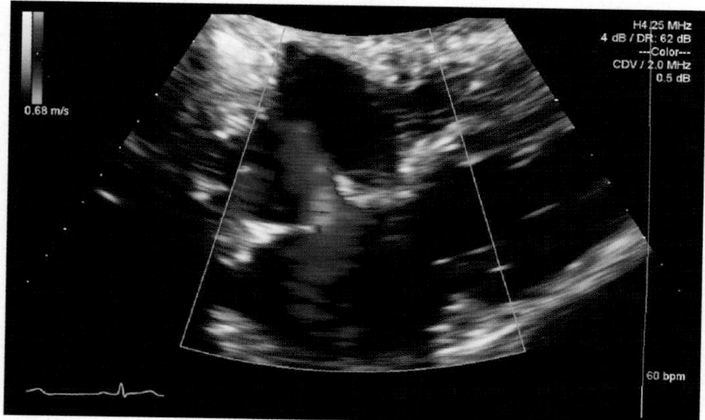

FIGURE 1-1-7 Subcostal view demonstrating a secundum atrial septal defect ►(see Video 1-1-7).

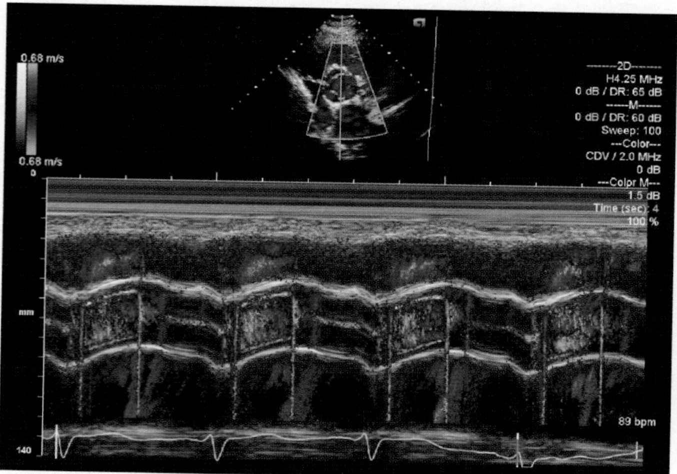

FIGURE 1-1-8 Color M-mode demonstrating aortic regurgitation (AR).

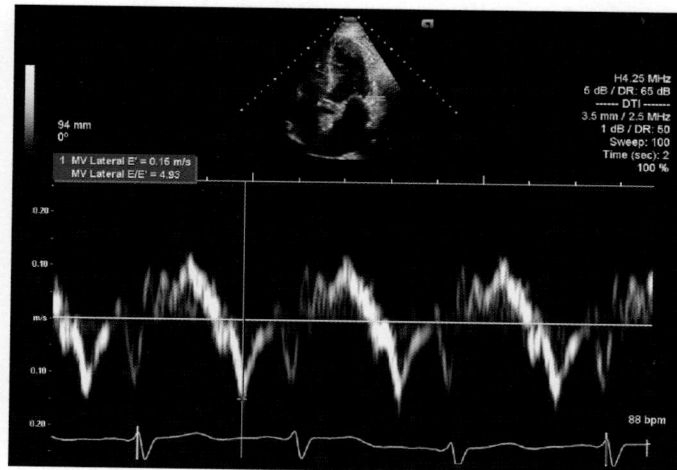

FIGURE 1-1-9 Tissue Doppler imaging of the lateral mitral valve annulus.

velocity, strain, and strain rate. This information can be used to assess systolic and diastolic function, evaluate patients with LV dyssynchrony, and provide further insight into myocardial mechanics. While it is currently used largely a research tool, STE is finding its way into clinical echocardiography.

THREE-DIMENSIONAL ECHOCARDIOGRAPHY (3DE)

Initial 3-D echocardiograms were generated by reconstructing a series of 2-D echocardiographic data sets. Significant technological advances over the past decade now allow for real-time image acquisition and image display in current 3DE systems (for both transthoracic and transesophageal probes) (Figure 1-1-10). This 3-D capability has further expanded the use of echocardiography in a variety of settings. While clearly not as commonly employed as standard 2-D imaging, 3-D imaging has been demonstrated to provide more accurate assessment of chamber volumes and mass, and regional LV function and dyssynchrony. It also provides more comprehensive views of valvular structure and quantitation of valvular regurgitation, as well as playing a role in stress imaging.[21] As clinicians become more

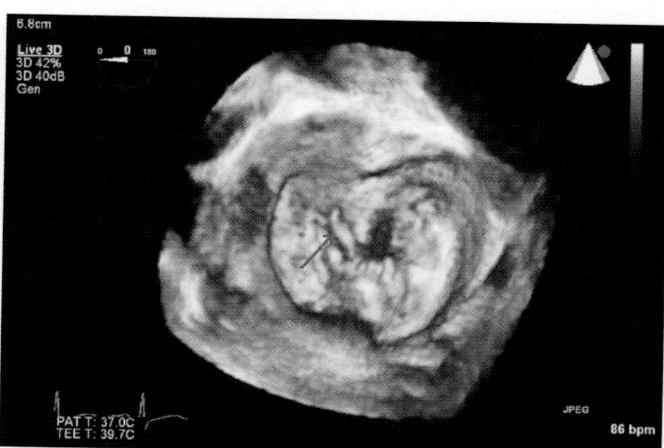

FIGURE 1-1-10 Three-dimensional TEE image of the mitral valve demonstrating a torn (arrow) chord and flail P_2 segment ►(see Video 1-1-10).

familiar with this new imaging capability, the role of 3-D imaging will continue to expand.

STRESS ECHOCARDIOGRAPHY

Stress echocardiography is predicated on the principal that myocardial ischemia results in regional left ventricular dysfunction. By imaging the heart prior to and during or after stress, both resting regional wall motion abnormalities (due to prior myocardial infarction or hibernating myocardium) and transient stress provoked wall motion abnormalities (due to myocardial ischemia) can be detected. Stress echo improves diagnostic sensitivity and specificity compared to a nonimaging stress test. Other than standard contraindications and risks for stress testing, there are no contraindications to the procedure.

Stress echocardiography was initially reported in 1979 using M-mode imaging to detect transient regional dysfunction.[22] Subsequently, 2-D imaging was employed, which allows for a comprehensive assessment of all segments of the LV.[23] The development of digital echocardiographic image acquisition, which enabled side-by-side comparison of rest and stress images, furthered the clinical application of stress echo using both exercise (treadmill and supine bicycle) and pharmacologic stress agents.

Stress echocardiography now plays a significant role in the evaluation and management of patients with known or suspected coronary artery disease, offering an alternative to nuclear perfusion imaging. Stress echocardiography has many advantages over nuclear imaging (lack of radiation, lower cost, faster turnaround time, immediate results, greater specificity, the ability to assess valves and the pericardium), but it also has several limitations (more subjective, issues with image quality, operator dependence, lower sensitivity). Overall accuracy is comparable to stress perfusion imaging.[24] In addition, stress echocardiography can be utilized in the assessment of patients with valvular heart disease and pulmonary hypertension to assess exercise capacity and the hemodynamic response to exercise.

The clinical application of stress echocardiography will be highlighted in the sections on coronary artery disease and valvular heart disease.

TRANSESOPHAGEAL ECHOCARDIOGRAPHY (TEE)

First described by Side and Gossling in 1971[25] who used a continuous-wave Doppler transducer to measure blood flow in the aorta, transesophageal echocardiography (TEE) (Figure 1-1-11) rapidly evolved from an M-mode only imaging modality to current multi-plane transducers with the full spectrum of imaging and Doppler modalities.

The clinical use of TEE has developed in both the intraoperative setting as a monitoring tool and as a diagnostic imaging modality in the awake /sedated patient. As TEE probe capabilities have evolved, its clinical applications have expanded. There are currently many clinical scenarios in which TEE is useful either as an adjunct to a transthoracic (TTE) study or as the primary echocardiographic study (Table 1-1-1). TEE does provide several advantages over TTE, including excellent image quality in virtually all patients and the ability to assess posterior cardiac structures. It is invaluable in the assessment of mitral valve disease and in the assessment of the left atrium, as well as having an important role in the assessment of prosthetic valves. Intraoperative TEE remains an important monitoring tool in a variety of settings.

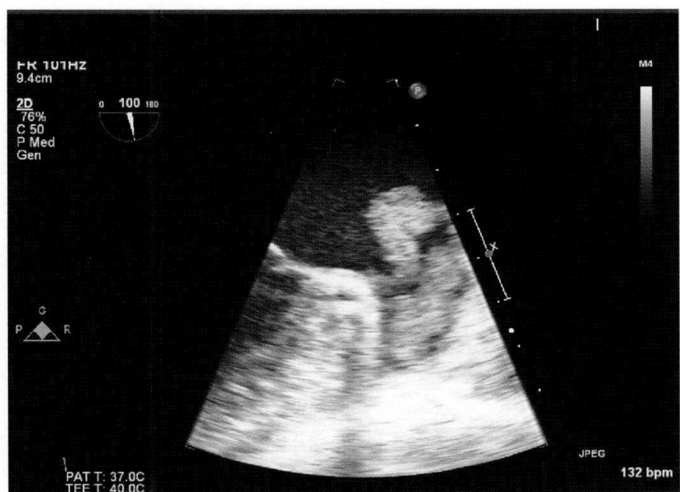

FIGURE 1-1-11 Transesophageal echocardiogram demonstrating a left atrial thrombus in a patient prior to planned cardioversion ►(see Video 1-1-11).

TEE is a semi-invasive procedure that unlike standard transthoracic imaging does have attendant risks and potential complications as well as contraindications (Table 1-1-2).

CONTRAST ECHOCARDIOGRAPHY

Contrast echocardiography involves the use of an intravenously administered agent that has different acoustic properties from the heart and blood, due to the presence of a gas (air, perfluorocarbon) in the microbubble.

Agitated saline, in which air microbubbles are generated, is used to detect intracardiac and intrapulmonary shunts. Since these microbubbles are filtered out in the lungs, detection of saline contrast in the left heart chambers is evidence of such shunting.

New perfluorocarbon-based agents (surrounded by a lipid or albumin sphere) are small enough to pass through the lungs and provide excellent opacification of the left heart. These transpulmonic contrast agents are invaluable tools in the echocardiography laboratory. Use of these agents in a variety of settings has been demonstrated to improve image quality (Figure 1-1-12). This results in improved diagnostic accuracy for standard 2-D imaging and has been shown to improve the accuracy of stress echocardiography. Additional uses of contrast include the enhancement of Doppler signals and the use of contrast to evaluate myocardial perfusion (still largely a research application).[26]

TABLE 1-1-1 Indications for TEE

Indications for TEE
Assessment for potential cardiac sources of embolism
Inadequate TTE to answer clinical question
Endocarditis and its complications
Valvular heart disease (native and prosthetic)
Congenital heart disease
Prior to cardioversion/ablation procedures for atrial dysrhythmias
Aortic pathology (dissection, intramural hematoma)
Intra-operative monitoring

TABLE 1-1-2 Contraindications and Complications for TEE

Contraindications
Esophageal Pathology (strictures, malignancy)
Active upper GI bleeding
Inability to cooperate
Hemodynamic/respiratory instability
Potential Complications
Esophageal injury
Aspiration/pneumonia
Respiratory depression
Adverse reaction to medications
Complications related to IV insertion
Sore throat
Hemodynamic instability (hypotension, hypertension, dysrhythmias)

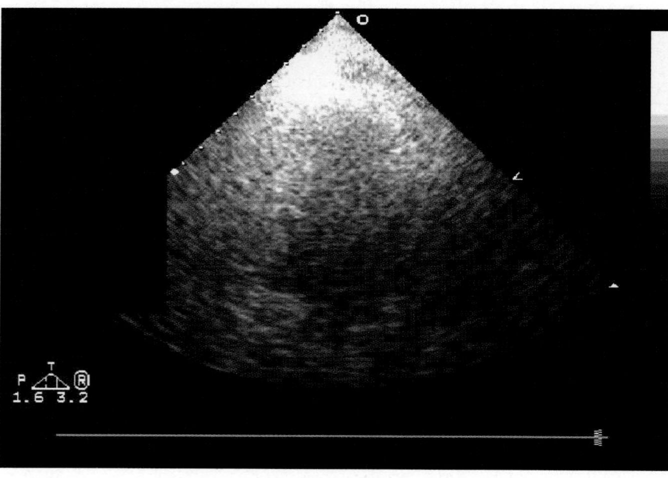

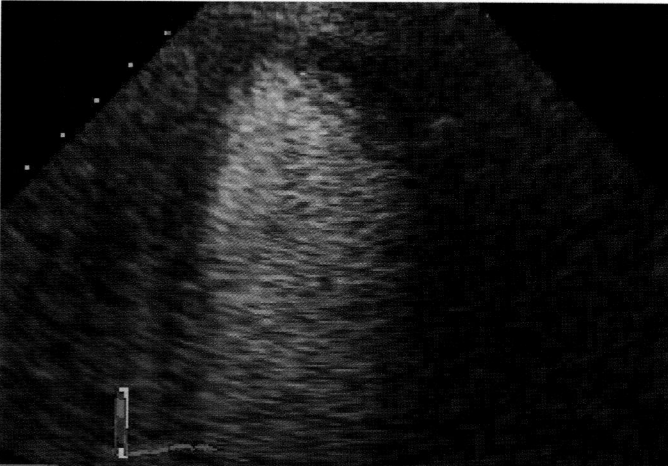

FIGURE 1-1-12 Contrast echocardiogram demonstrating improved endocardial border definition in a patient with suboptimal images. Baseline (noncontrast) images (top panel) and contrast enhanced images (bottom panel) ►(see Videos 1-1-12).

While quite safe, rare complications and side effects can occur as a result of contrast echocardiography, including anaphylactoid reactions, headache, and back or flank pain. In 2007, the United States Food and Drug Administration (FDA) released a "Black Box" warning for the use of these agents, which unfortunately lead to a dramatic decrease in their utilization. Over time, with additional safety data available[27] and a better understanding of the safety concerns and monitoring requirements, echocardiographers became more comfortable using these agents. Contrast utilization (appropriately) increased, and today its use is an essential element in day-to-day echocardiography.

Recently, the FDA has further refined the "Black Box" warning. Current contraindications include known hypersensitivity to the agent, known or suspected intracardiac shunting, intra-arterial injection, and pregnancy.

HAND-CARRIED ULTRASOUND (HCU)

As technology has evolved, miniaturization of ultrasound systems has led to the development of extremely portable systems with most, if not all, imaging modalities, as well as much smaller hand-carried ultrasound devices with varying capabilities and imaging modalities (Figure 1-1-13). These hand-carried ultrasound (HCU) systems have the potential to provide "point of care" imaging of the heart in a variety of clinical settings (office, intensive care units, emergency departments). HCU can provide a focused evaluation of the heart and serve as an extension of the physical examination.[28] The use of HCU

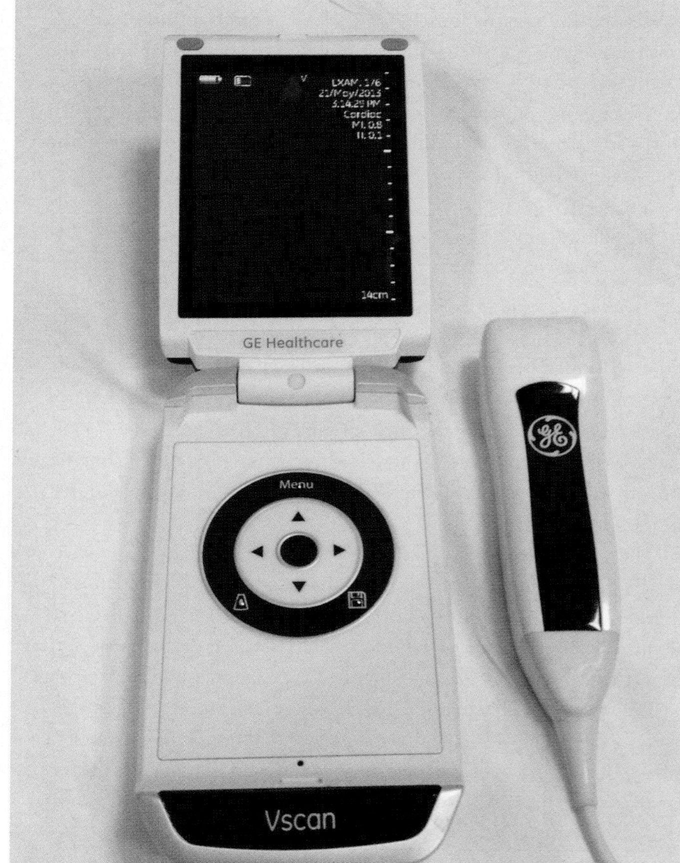

FIGURE 1-1-13 Photo of a current generation HCU.

has tremendous potential, but it also raises concerns regarding quality (both of the images and the interpretation of the data) and the need for appropriate training and utilization of these devices. The exact role of these devices and the appropriate dissemination of this technology outside of the purview of cardiologists continues to develop. Clearly, appropriate training and utilization of this technology will be required to improve patient care.[29]

CLINICAL APPLICATIONS AND COMPARISONS TO OTHER TECHNIQUES

Echocardiography is unsurpassed as an imagining modality in its clinical utility. Its versatility is a significant strength. Unlike cardiac catheterization, it is noninvasive with few, if any, risks, it does not employ potentially nephrotoxic contrast agents, and it does not expose the patient to radiation. In the stress-testing arena, its lack of radiation and rapid turnaround time are distinct advantages compared to nuclear perfusion imaging. Compared to other advanced noninvasive imaging techniques, such as cardiovascular computed tomography (CT) and cardiovascular magnetic resonance imaging (MRI), echocardiography is portable, does not employ radiation or iodinated contrast (CT), and is not limited in patients with renal failure (MRI). Echocardiography thus remains the mainstay of the noninvasive evaluation of patients with known or suspected cardiovascular disease. In the following chapters, we will explore the use of echocardiography in a variety of clinical scenarios, highlighting many of the techniques outlined above.

VIDEO LEGENDS

1. Video 1-1-4 L: Two-dimensional image of the left ventricle demonstrating a normal left ventricle in the parasternal long axis view
2. Video 1-1-4 R: Two-dimensional image of the left ventricle demonstrating a normal left ventricle in the parasternal short axis view.
3. Video 1-1-6: Color Doppler demonstrating mitral and aortic regurgitation in a patient with rheumatic valve disease
4. Video 1-1-7: Subcostal view demonstrating a secundum atrial septal defect
5. Video 1-1-10: Three dimensional TEE image of the mitral valve demonstrating a torn (arrow) chord and flail P2 segment
6. Video 1-1-11: Transesophageal echocardiogram demonstrating a left atrial thrombus in a patient prior to planned cardioversion.
7. Video 1-1-12 L:Contrast echocardiogram demonstrating improved endocardial border definition in a patient with sub-optimal images. Baseline (non-contrast) images are of poor quality.
8. Video 1-1-12 R: Contrast echocardiogram demonstrating improved endocardial border definition in a patient with sub-optimal images. Contrast enhanced images demonstrate improved endocardial border definition.

REFERENCES

1. Cheitlin MD, Armstrong WF, Aurigemma GP, et al. ACC/AHA/ASE 2003 guideline update for the clinical application of echocardiography- summary article A report of the American College of Cardiology/American Heart Association Task Force on practice guidelines. (ACC/AHA/ASE 2003 Committee to Update the 1997 Guidelines for the Clinical Application of Echocardiography). *J Am Coll Cardiol*. 2003;42:954-970.
2. Pearlman AS, Ryan T, Picard MH, Douglas PS. Evolving trends in the use of echocardiography. *J Am Coll Cardiol*. 2007;49:2283-2291.
3. Bellar GA, Bonow RO, Fuster V, et al. ACCF 2008 Recommendations for training in adult cardiovascular medicine core cardiology training (COCATS 3) (Revision of the 2002 COCATS Training Statement). *J Am Coll Cardiol*. 2008;51:333-414.
4. Ehler D, Carney DK, Dempsey AL, et al. Guidelines for cardiac sonographer education: recommendations of the American Society of Echocardiography Sonographer Training and Education Committee. *J Am Soc Echocardiogr*. 2001;14:77-84.
5. http://www.icael.org
6. Feigenbaum H. Evolution of echocardiography. *Circulation*. 1996;93(7):1321-1327.
7. Edler I, Hertz CH. Use of ultrasonic reflectoscope for the continuous recording of movements of heart walls. *Kungl Fysiogr Sallsk Lung Forth*. 1954;24:40.
8. Feigenbaum H, Waldhausen JA, Hyde LP. Ultrasound diagnosis of pericardial effusion. *JAMA*. 1965;191:711-714.
9. Holen J, Simonsen S. Determination of pressure gradient in mitral stenosis with Doppler echocardiography. *Br Heart J*. 1979;41:529-535.
10. Hatle L, Angelsen B, Tromsdal A. Noninvasive assessment of aortic stenosis by Doppler ultrasound. *Br Heart J*. 1979;43:284-292.
11. Born N, Lancee CT, Honkoop J, Hugenholtz PC. Ultrasonic viewer for cross-sectional analysis of moving cardiac structures. *Biomed Eng*. 1971;6:500.
12. Armstrong WF, Ryan T. *Feigenbaum's Echocardiography*. 7th ed. Philadelphia, PA: Lippincott Williams and Wilkins; 2010.
13. Otto CM. *Textbook of Clinical Echocardiography*. 4th ed. Philadelphia, PA: Saunders Elsevier; 2009.
14. Douglas PS, Garcia MJ, Haines DE, et al. ACCF/ASE/AHA/ASNC/HFSA/HRS/SCAI/SCCM/SCCT/SCMR 2011 appropriate use criteria for echocardiography: a report of the American College of Cardiology Foundation Appropriate Use Criteria Task Force, American Society of Echocardiography, American Heart Association, American Society of Nuclear Cardiology, Heart Failure Society of America, Heart Rhythm Society, Society of Cardiovascular Angiography and Interventions, Society of Critical Care Medicine, Society of Cardiovascular Computed Tomography, and Society of Cardiovascular Magnetic Resonance. *J Am Coll Cardiol*. 2011;57(9):1126-1166. doi: 10.1016/j.jacc.2010.11.002.
15. Feigenbaum H. Role of M-mode techniques in today's echocardiography. *J Am Soc Echocardiogr*. 2010; Mar; 23(3):240-257.
16. Rudski LG, Lai WW, Afilalo J, Hua L, et al. Guidelines for the echocardiographic assessment of the right heart in adults: a

report from the American Society of Echocardiography. *J Am Soc Echocardiogr*. 2010;23:685-713.

17. Nishimura RA, Otto CM, Bonow RO, et al. 2014 AHA/ACC guideline for the management of patients with valvular heart disease:executive summary; A report of the American College of Cardiology/American Heart Association Task Force on Practice Guidelines. *J Am Coll Cardiol.* 2014;63:2348-2388.
18. Sutherland GR, Bijnens B, McDicken WN. Tissue Doppler myocardial imaging: historical perspective and technological considerations. *Echocardiography*. 1999;16:445-457.
19. Mor-Avi V, Lang RM, Badano LP, et al. Current and evolving techniques for the quantitative evaluation of cardiac mechanics: ASE/EAE consensus statement on methodology and indications. *J Am Soc Echocardiogr*. 2011;24:277-313.
20. Gorcsan J, Tanaka H. Echocardiographic assessment of myocardial strain. *J Am Coll Cardiol*. 2011;58:1401-1413.
21. Lang RM, Badano LP, Tsang W, et al. EAE/ASE Recommendations for image acquisition and display using three-dimensional echocardiography. *J Am Soc Echocardiogr*. 2012;25:3-46.
22. Mason SJ, Weiss JL, Weisfeldt ML, Garrison JB, Fortuin NJ. Exercise echocardiography: detection of wall motion abnormalities during ischemia. *Circulation*. 1979;59:50-59.
23. Wann LS, Faris JV, Childress RH, Dillon JC, Weyman AE, Feigenbaum H. Exercise cross-sectional echocardiography in ischemic heart disease. *Circulation*. 1979;60:1300-1308.
24. Marwick TH. Stress echocardiography. *Heart*. 2003;89:113-118.
25. Side CD, Gossling RG. Non surgical assessment of cardiac function. *Nature*. 1971;232:335-336.
26. Mulvagh SL, Rakowski H, Vannan MA, et al. American Society of Echocardiography consensus statement on the clinical applications of ultrasonic contrast agents in echocardiography. *J Am Soc Echocardiogr*. 2008;21(11):1179-1201.
27. Wei K, Mulvagh SL, Carson L, et al. The safety of Definity and Optison for ultrasound image enhancement: a retrospective analysis of 78,383 administered contrast doses. *J Am Soc Echocardiogr*. 2008;21(11):1202-1206.
28. Zoghbi, WA. Echocardiography at the point of care: an ultrasound future. *J Am Soc Echocardiogr*. 2011;24:132-134.
29. Seward JB, Douglas PS, Erbel R, et al. Hand-carried ultrasound (HUC) device: recommendations regarding new technology. A report from the Echocardiography Task Force on New Technology of the Nomenclature and Standards Committee in the American Society of Echocardiography. *J Am Soc Echocardiogr*. 2002;15:369-373.

2 ECHOCARDIOGRAPHY IN THE EVALUATION AND MANAGEMENT OF THE PATIENT WITH KNOWN OR SUSPECTED CORONARY ARTERY DISEASE

John A. Larry, MD

INTRODUCTION

Coronary artery disease (CAD) and its sequelae affect millions of individuals. In addition, many patients present with symptoms that may be due to ischemic heart disease. Echocardiography has assumed a central role in the evaluation and management of patients with known or suspected CAD. By virtue of its ability to noninvasively assess cardiac structure and function, echocardiography can provide anatomic information that is useful in the evaluation of these patients.

In patients with ongoing chest pain, an echo in the acute setting can provide evidence against myocardial ischemia as the etiology of the symptoms if there are no regional wall motion abnormalities and may provide clues to other potential diagnoses such as a pericardial process, acute pulmonary embolism, or aortic pathology.

In the postmyocardial infarction (MI) setting, echocardiography plays a critical role in the evaluation and management of the patient, including an assessment of ejection fraction (EF) postmyocardial infarction (MI), which is essential to provide prognostic information as well as to help guide medical management and assess these patients for potential device therapy such as implantable cardiac defibrillators (ICD).

In the acute setting, for patients who develop hemodynamic instability or evidence of acute heart failure, echocardiography is invaluable to assess the EF. In addition, echocardiography is essential for evaluating the patient for post-MI mechanical complications such as acute mitral regurgitation (MR) or ventricular septal defects (VSD), free wall rupture, or RV infarction.

The advent of stress echocardiography in the mid to late 1980s provided an alternative to stress nuclear (perfusion) imaging as a noninvasive means of evaluating and risk stratifying patients with chest pain syndromes. With improvement in digital image acquisition and displays, stress echo now provides a robust method of evaluating such patients, with results comparable to nuclear techniques. Exercise stress echo using treadmill, or less commonly bicycle stress, and pharmacologic stress echo, most often employing dobutamine in the US, are frequently used tests to evaluate patients with known or suspected CAD.

In this chapter, Dr. Larry will explore the use of echocardiography in the patient with chest pain and suspected or known CAD (stress testing) and in the assessment of the post-MI patient, including patients with mechanical complications of an acute MI.

SECTION 1

Negative Stress ECHO

CLINICAL CASE PRESENTATION

A 45 year old man with hypertension that has not been well controlled presents for evaluation. He was seen in the office and mentioned 3 separate episodes of non-radiating chest discomfort, lasting 30 minutes, located in the left chest, accompanied by mild dyspnea during the third episode.

His exam revealed blood pressure of 135/88 mm Hg, pulse of 75 beats/min, and a respiratory rate of 16 breaths/min. The jugular venous pressure (JVP) was normal; carotid upstrokes were normal; no bruits were appreciated. The lungs were clear to auscultation and percussion, the abdomen benign, and the extremities free of edema, with normal distal pulses.

An ECG revealed normal sinus rhythm (NSR) and nonspecific ST-T wave abnormalities. He was sent to the chest pain unit in the local emergency department. Serial troponin levels were negative.

DIFFERENTIAL DIAGNOSIS

The differential diagnosis of acute/sub-acute chest pain is extensive and includes life-threatening causes as well as less serious etiologies, such as musculoskeletal pain. Listed below are the acute and potentially life-threatening causes that must be excluded:

- Acute coronary syndrome
- Acute aortic dissection
- Pericarditis with effusion/tamponade
- Pulmonary embolism
- Pneumothorax
- Esophageal perforation

CLINICAL FEATURES

Individuals with chest pain raise clinical concern for the potential of one of a handful of serious, potentially life-threatening etiologies of chest pain.

After clinical, radiographic, and laboratory exclusion of other etiologies, the possibility of unstable angina remains.

- Noninvasive evaluation of those patients with an intermediate probability of ischemic heart disease can be exceptionally useful.
- In patients with positive studies, one's level of concern for high-grade coronary disease increases and may warrant an invasive evaluation.
- In the situation of a negative study, the probability of an ischemic etiology causing the patient's symptoms is reduced to a low level, and their prognosis from a cardiac perspective is excellent.

ECHOCARDIOGRAPHIC EVALUATION

Due to his intermediate probability of myocardial ischemia and an ECG with baseline abnormalities that would render a stress ECG indeterminate, he underwent a treadmill stress echo, commensurate with current appropriateness guidelines.[1] He exercised 9.5 minutes of the Bruce protocol, stopping due to leg fatigue. He achieved 88% maximum predicted HR. He exhibited no chest pain. The stress ECG demonstrated 1 mm ST depression of indeterminate significance due to the baseline ECG abnormality. The baseline echo demonstrated normal wall motion and ejection fraction (EF). Poststress imaging revealed no wall motion abnormalities and an appropriate increase in EF (Figures 2-1-1 and 2-1-2).

DIAGNOSIS

Non-ischemic chest pain

MANAGEMENT

Not only does the negative stress echo study in this situation carry a high negative predictive value, but the study has very favorable prognostic implications. Thus, for most such patients, no further cardiac evaluation is warranted.

- In a study by McCulley, et al, those at intermediate or high pretest probability of coronary disease with a normal test had cardiac event-free survival rates of 99.2%, 97.8%, and 97.4% at 1, 2, and 3 years of follow-up.[2]
- Furthermore, the exercise time on the treadmill carries additional prognostic significance. Those with a workload of more than 7 METS had event-free survival rates of 99.4% at 1 year and 98.7% at 2 years.
- A meta-analysis published by Metz, et al, found the negative predictive value for MI and cardiac death was 98.8% (95% confidence interval [CI] 98.5 to 99.0) over 36 months of follow-up for myocardial perfusion imaging, and 98.4% (95% CI 97.9 to 98.9) over 33 months for echocardiography.[3]
- Such patients do, however, warrant appropriate treatment of their modifiable risk factors.

FOLLOW-UP

The patient was advised to maintain follow up of his hypertension and cardiac risk factors for long-term risk reduction of cardiac events and discharged home. Further evaluation of non–life-threatening, noncardiac etiologies of chest pain can be pursued as an outpatient.

VIDEO LEGENDS

1. Video 2-1-1 A: Baseline long axis view demonstrating normal wall motion.
2. Video 2-1-1 B: Immediate poststress long axis view demonstrating normal wall motion and an improvement in EF.
3. Video 2-1-1 C: Baseline short axis view demonstrating normal wall motion.

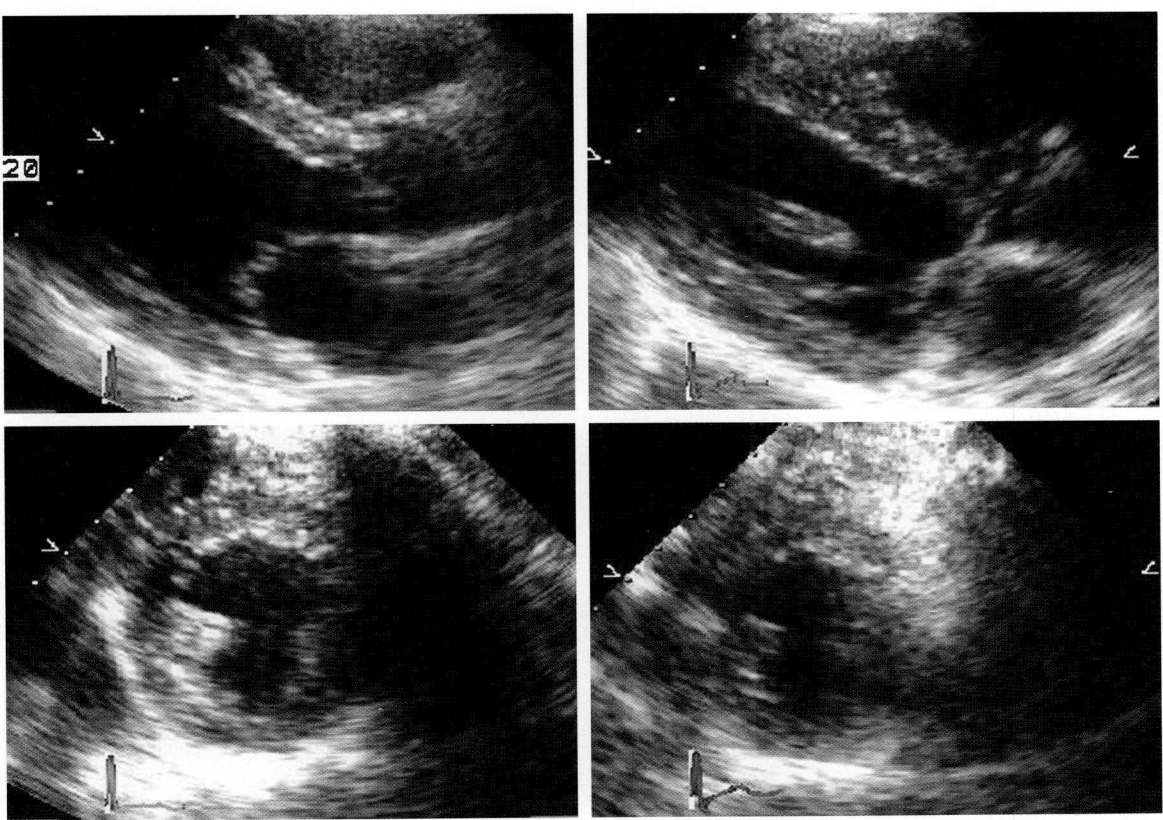

FIGURE 2-1-1 Baseline (left) and poststress (right) of the parasternal images from our patient which demonstrate normal global/regional function at rest and poststress ► (see Video 2-1-1).

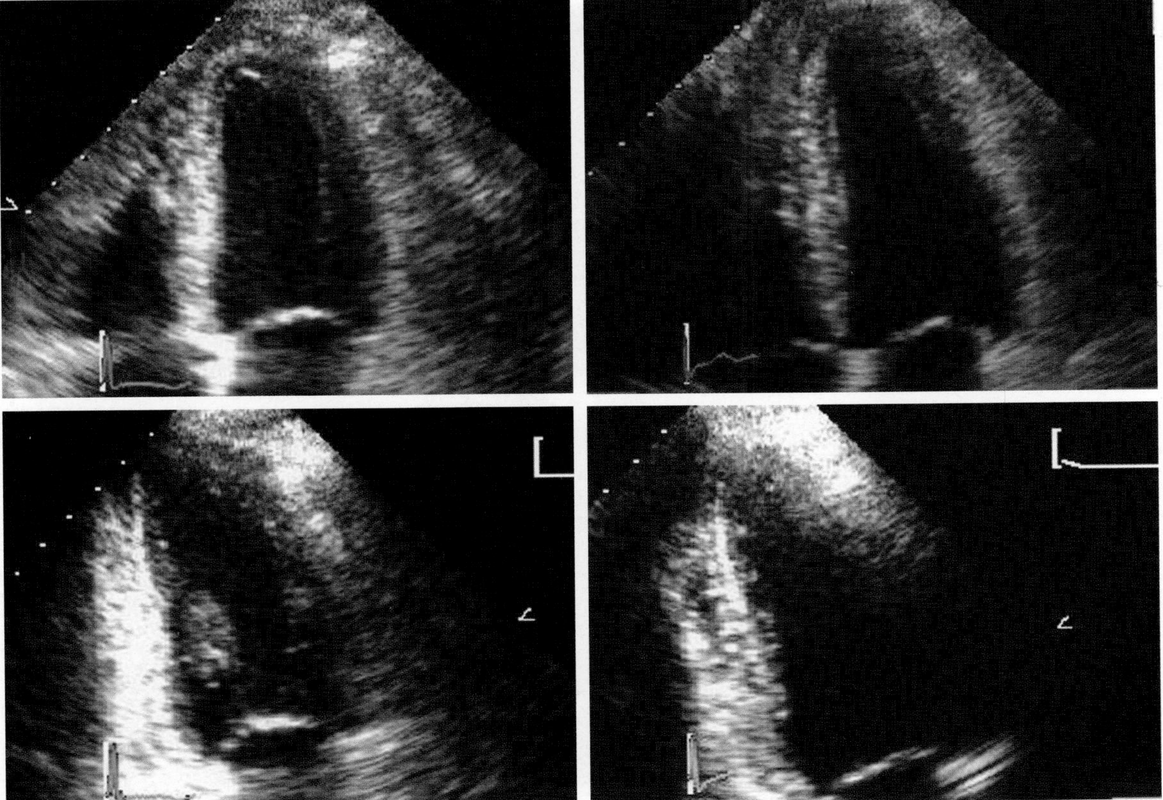

FIGURE 2-1-2 Baseline (left) and poststress (right) of the apical images from our patient which demonstrate normal global/regional function at rest and poststress ► (see Video 2-1-2).

4. Video 2-1-1 D: Immediate poststressshort axis view demonstrating normal wall motion and an improvement in EF.
5. Video 2-1-2 A: Baseline apical 4 chamber view demonstrating normal wall motion.
6. Video 2-1-2 B: Immediate poststress apical 4 chamber view demonstrating normal wall motion and an improvement in EF.
7. Video 2-1-2 C: Baseline apical 2 chamber view demonstrating normal wall motion.
8. Video 2-1-2 D: Immediate poststress apical 2 chamber view demonstrating normal wall motion and an improvement in EF.

REFERENCES

1. Douglas PS, Garcia MJ, Haines DE, et al. ACCF/ASE/AHA/ASNC/HFSA/HRS/SCAI/SCCM/SCCT/SCMR 2011 appropriate use criteria for echocardiography: a report of the American College of Cardiology Foundation Appropriate Use Criteria Task Force, American Society of Echocardiography, American Heart Association, American Society of Nuclear Cardiology, Heart Failure Society of America, Heart Rhythm Society, Society for Cardiovascular Angiography and Interventions, Society of Critical Care Medicine, Society of Cardiovascular Computed Tomography, and Society for Cardiovascular Magnetic Resonance. *J Am Coll Cardiol*. 2011;57(9):1126-1166. doi:10.1016/j.jacc.2010.11.002.
2. McCully RB, Roger VL, Mahoney DW, et al. Outcome after normal exercise echocardiography and predictors of subsequent cardiac events: follow up of 1,325 patients. *J Am Coll Cardiol*. 1998;31:144-149.
3. Metz, LD, Beattie M, Hom R, et al. The prognostic value of normal exercise myocardial perfusion imaging and exercise echocardiography: a meta-analysis. *J Am Coll Cardiol*. 2007;49(2):227-237.

SECTION 2

Abnormal Stress ECHO

CLINICAL CASE PRESENTATION

The patient is a 51-year-old man with no past cardiac history. He has a past history of Type 2 diabetes and hypertension, both of which have been well managed. He is a manual laborer who presented with complaints of generalized fatigue for a few weeks and exertional dyspnea for 1 week. His exam was benign, and an ECG showed evidence of left ventricular hypertrophy (LVH) with secondary ST-T abnormality. His chest x-ray (CXR) was unremarkable, as was basic laboratory assessment.

DIFFERENTIAL DIAGNOSIS

The differential diagnosis of new onset fatigue and dyspnea is extensive and includes:

- Myocardial ischemia
- LV systolic dysfunction
- Hypertension-induced diastolic dysfunction
- Pericardial effusion with hemodynamic effect
- Pulmonary hypertension
- Pulmonary embolism
- Parenchymal lung disease

ECHOCARDIOGRAPHIC EVALUATION

His symptoms of exertional dyspnea and fatigue raised an intermediate probability of an ischemic etiology.

- Due to his intermediate probability of an ischemic etiology for his symptoms, a treadmill stress echo was ordered.
- With the resting ECG displaying LVH with secondary ST-T abnormality, pursuing stress testing with echo imaging was appropriate, as the baseline ECG abnormalities decrease the predictive value of postexercise ST changes.

Stress Test Results

- His resting echo images were normal. He exercised 7 minutes on the Bruce protocol, stopping due to chest discomfort (angina) and dyspnea.
- He exhibited nearly 1 mm ST depression from baseline.
- The postexercise images revealed LV dilation, with severe hypokinesis or akinesis of the anterior, lateral, and apical segments. The left ventricular ejection fraction (LVEF) dropped from 55% to 35% (Figures 2-2-1 and 2-2-2)

Stress Echo Evaluation and Interpretation

- The echocardiographic criteria for the detection of myocardial ischemia is the development of new or worsening regional contractile function (regional wall motion abnormality) during stress.
- A region of myocardium that exhibits normal contractile function at baseline that becomes hypokinetic or akinetic poststress, or a region of myocardium that is hypokinetic at baseline that becomes akinetic poststress, constitutes an abnormal response.
- The worse the LVEF and the greater the number of LV segments that are abnormal poststress, the worse the prognosis.[2]
- Our patient's study displayed several high-risk features, including LV dilation, multiple wall motion abnormalities, and a significant drop in LVEF postexercise. This group of individuals with these high-risk features derives the greatest benefit from further evaluation with coronary angiography and revascularization.

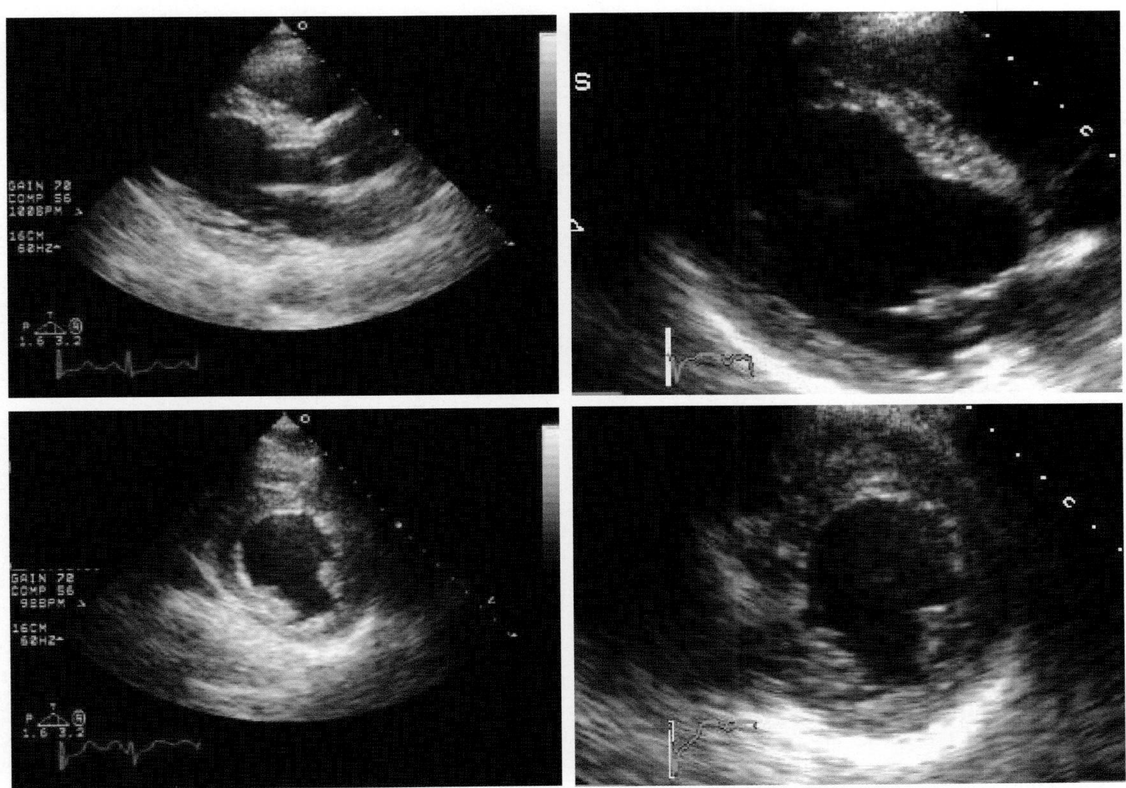

FIGURE 2-2-1 Baseline (left) and poststress (right) of the parasternal images from our patient, which demonstrate normal global/regional function at rest with multiple new wall motion abnormalities as described in the text poststress. Note also the LV cavity dilation ► (see Video 2-2-1).

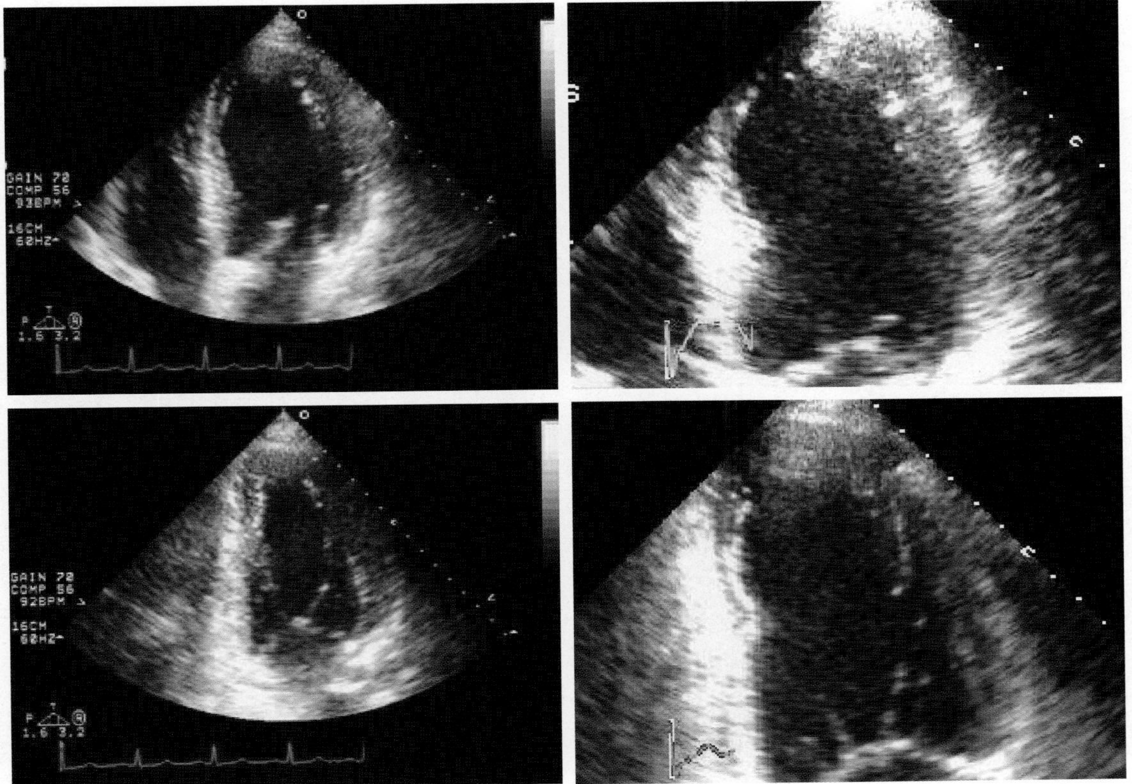

FIGURE 2-2-2 Baseline (left) and poststress (right) of the apical images from our patient which demonstrate normal global/regional function at rest with multiple new wall motion abnormalities as described in the text poststress ► (see Video 2-2-2).

DIAGNOSIS

Myocardial ischemia with high-risk features

MANAGEMENT

- Due to the abnormal stress echo with high-risk features, cardiac catheterization with coronary angiography was recommended.
- This study demonstrated a chronic total occlusion of the left anterior descending (LAD) artery with the distal vessel filling via collaterals, and a 90% stenosis of the obtuse marginal (Figure 2-2-3).
- Surgical revascularization was performed, and he had an unremarkable postoperative course and recovery.

FOLLOW-UP

Post revascularization (surgical or percutaneous) management should include pharmacologic therapy and treatment of modifiable risk factors:

- This patient's pharmacologic therapy consisted of aspirin, a thienopyridine, β-blocker, statin agent, and an ACE inhibitor.
- He was referred to cardiac rehabilitation for a graded exercise program and dietary education, with periodic lipid assessment to ensure he achieves and maintains NCEP ATP III goals.

VIDEO LEGENDS

1. Video 2-2-1 A: Baseline long axis view demonstrating normal wall motion.
2. Video 2-2-1 B: Immediate poststress long axis view demonstrating new anteroseptal wall motion abnormalities with LV dilation
3. Video 2-2-1 C: Baseline short axis view demonstrating normal wall motion.
4. Video 2-2-1 D: Immediate poststress short axis view demonstrating new anterior and septal wall motion abnormalities.
5. Video 2-2-2 A: Baseline apical 4 chamber view demonstrating normal wall motion.
6. Video 2-2-2 B: Immediate poststress apical 4 chamber view demonstrating new apical wall motion abnormalities.
7. Video 2-2-2 C: Baseline apical 2 chamber view demonstrating normal wall motion.
8. Video 2-2-2 D: Immediate poststress apical 2 chamber view demonstrating new anterior and apical wall motion abnormalities. The apex appears dyskinetic.

REFERENCES

1. Douglas PS, Garcia MJ, Haines DE, et al. ACCF/ASE/AHA/ASNC/HFSA/HRS/SCAI/SCCM/SCCT/SCMR 2011 appropriate use criteria for echocardiography: a report of the American College of Cardiology Foundation Appropriate Use Criteria Task Force, American Society of Echocardiography, American Heart Association, American Society of Nuclear Cardiology, Heart Failure Society of America, Heart Rhythm Society, Society for Cardiovascular Angiography and Interventions, Society of Critical Care Medicine, Society of Cardiovascular Computed Tomography, and Society for Cardiovascular Magnetic Resonance. *J Am Coll Cardiol*. 2011;57(9):1126-1166. doi: 10.1016/j.jacc.2010.11.002.
2. Yao S, Qureshi E, Sherrid M, Chaudhry F. Practical applications in stress echocardiography: risk stratification and prognosis in patients with known or suspected ischemic heart disease. *J Am Coll Cardiol*. 2003;42(6):1084-1090.

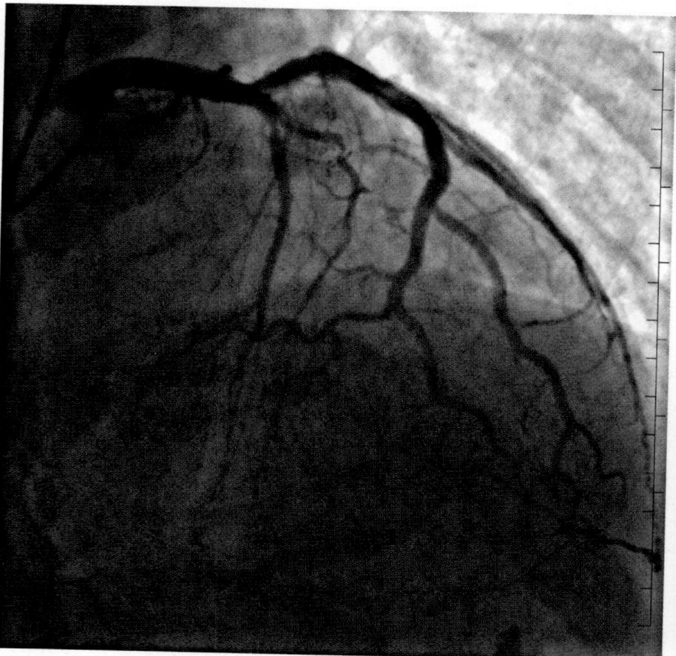

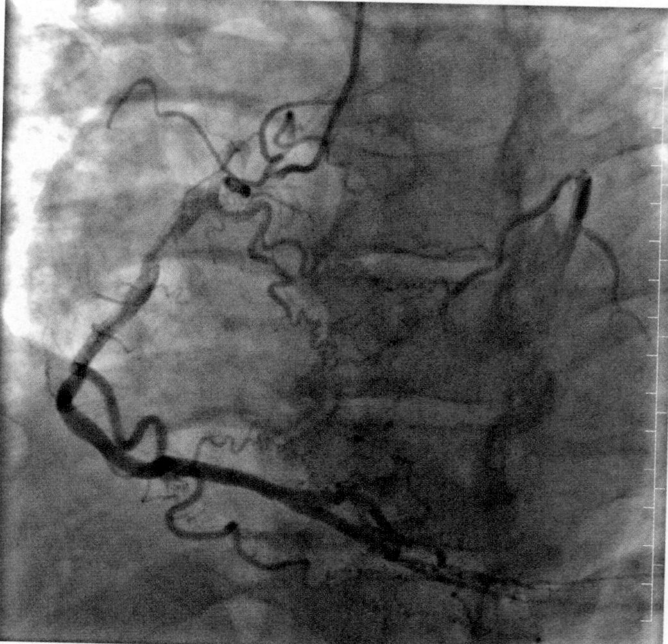

FIGURE 2-2-3 Representative still images from the patient's coronary angiogram. The panel on the left demonstrates the left coronary artery anatomy. The LAD is not seen as it is totally occluded. The right coronary angiogram seen on the right panel demonstrates collateral flow from the RCA to the LAD.

SECTION 3

Chest Pain in a Young Female with Previous PCI Procedures

CLINICAL CASE PRESENTATION

A 41-year-old woman with systemic lupus erythematosus (SLE), hypertension, and CAD status postpercutaneous revascularization of the LAD and right coronary artery (RCA), identified when she presented with unstable angina 2 years ago, presents with increasing frequency of chest pain. Over the past year, she has noted episodes of substernal, nonradiating chest discomfort without associated symptoms, lasting no more than 5 minutes in duration. The discomfort has been occurring more frequently in the past couple of weeks. She also notes episodes of exertional dyspnea in addition to brief spells of lightheadedness and fatigue. Her past history is otherwise notable for chronic back pain for which she takes narcotic therapy.

She is afebrile, her blood pressure is 109/69 mm Hg, her pulse is 63 beats/min, and her respiratory rate is 12 breaths/min. The JVP is normal; no carotid bruits are appreciated. The lungs were clear to auscultation and percussion. The PMI was non-displaced. S_1 and S_2 were normal; no murmurs, gallops, or rubs were evident. Her abdomen was benign, and the extremities were free of edema with normal distal pulses.

An ECG revealed sinus bradycardia and was normal.

DIFFERENTIAL DIAGNOSIS

The differential diagnosis of chest pain in this patient is extensive.

- One must first exclude recurrent myocardial ischemia in this patient with known CAD.
- If recurrent myocardial ischemia is excluded, pursuit of other nonischemic cardiac causes (such as pericardial involvement from her SLE) or other noncardiac causes would be appropriate.

ECHOCARDIOGRAPHIC EVALUATION

- Her clinical situation does not raise concern for other serious etiologies of chest pain, and her clinical probability of the symptoms being due to myocardial ischemia is intermediate.
- Her ECG did not suggest a pericardial process (see Chapter 6).
- A stress test with imaging is a reasonable first step in her evaluation.
- As she cannot walk any significant distance due to her chronic back pain, she underwent a dobutamine stress echo.
    - Pharmacologicess testing is an accepted alternative to physical stress testing in individuals who are unable to exercise.
- Dobutamine was infused intravenously in a graded fashion to a peak dose of 40 mcg/kg/min.
    - She had no symptoms, but exhibited 1.5 mm ST depression on ECG and displayed multiple wall motion abnormalities at peak infusion, involving the inferior, inferolateral, apex, and septal walls.
    - Her LVEF dropped from 55% at baseline to 35% at peak infusion. Figures 2-3-1 to 2-3-4 demonstrate each view at baseline, low dose, intermediate dose, and peak dobutamine infusion in a quad screen format, which facilitates interpretation. This study reflected adverse prognostic features, as discussed in the previous case.[1,2]

DIAGNOSIS

Myocardial ischemia with high-risk stress echo features

MANAGEMENT

Due to the marked abnormalities noted on this study, cardiac catheterization with coronary angiography was recommended and performed.

- The LAD stent was patent with no significant lesions throughout the course of the vessel.
- The proximal RCA stents were patent, but distal to the stents a 95% lesion was identified. A new drug-eluting stent was placed (Figure 2-3-5).
- Her hospital course was unremarkable, and she has remained free of chest pain in the early post discharge period.

FOLLOW-UP

Post revascularization management should include pharmacologic therapy and treatment of modifiable risk factors:

- Her pharmacologic therapy at the time of discharge consisted of aspirin, a thienopyridine, β-blocker, statin agent, and an ACE inhibitor.
- She was referred to cardiac rehabilitation for a graded exercise program and dietary education, with periodic lipid assessment to ensure she achieves and maintains NCEP ATP III goals.

VIDEO LEGENDS

1. Video 2-3-1 A: Baseline parasternal long axis view demonstrating normal wall motion and EF
2. Video 2-3-1 B: Low dose parasternal long axis view demonstrating normal wall motion
3. Video 2-3-1 C: Intermediate dose parasternal long axis view demonstrating normal wall motion
4. Video 2-3-1 D: Peak infusion parasternal long axis view demonstrating mild inferolateral hypokinesis
5. Video 2-3-2 A: Baseline parasternal short axis view demonstrating normal wall motion and EF

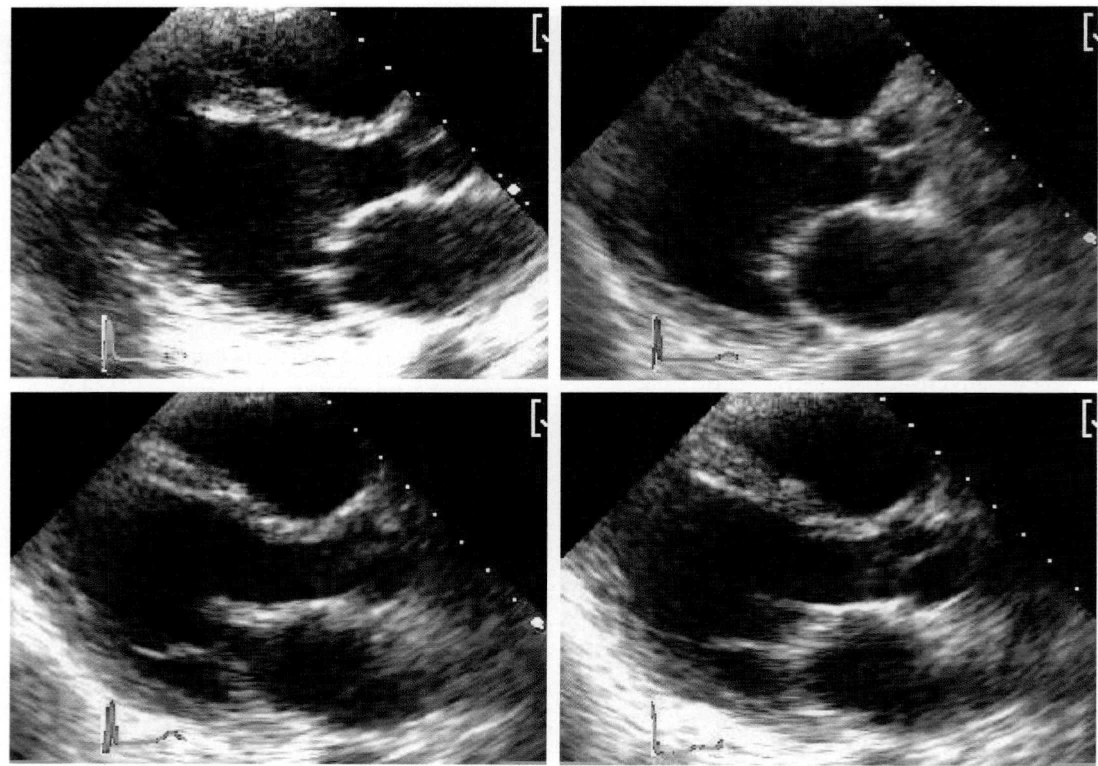

FIGURE 2-3-1 Parasternal long axis view at baseline (upper left), low dose (upper right), intermediate dose (lower left), and peak dobutamine infusion (lower right). The accompanying videos demonstrate normal wall motion at rest with new wall motion abnormalities at peak infusion as described in the text ► (see Video 2-3-1).

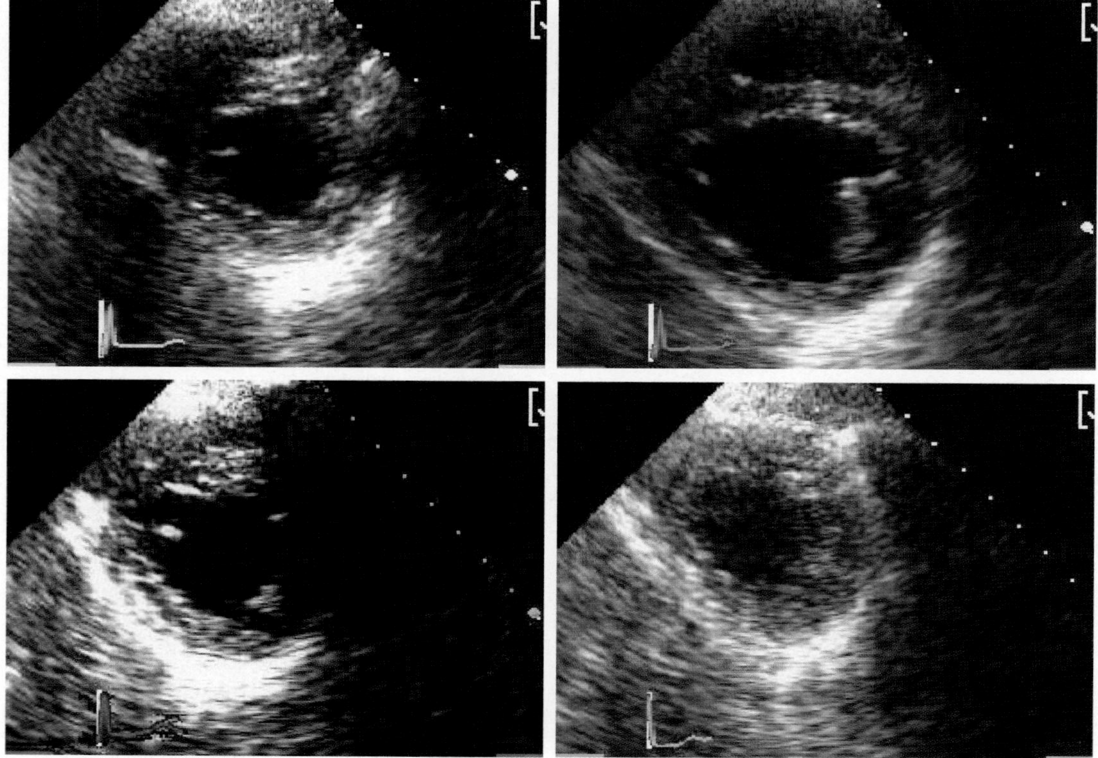

FIGURE 2-3-2 Parasternal short axis at baseline (upper left), low dose (upper right), intermediate dose (lower left), and peak dobutamine infusion (lower right). The accompanying videos demonstrate normal wall motion at rest with new wall motion abnormalities at peak infusion as described in the text ► (see Video 2-3-2).

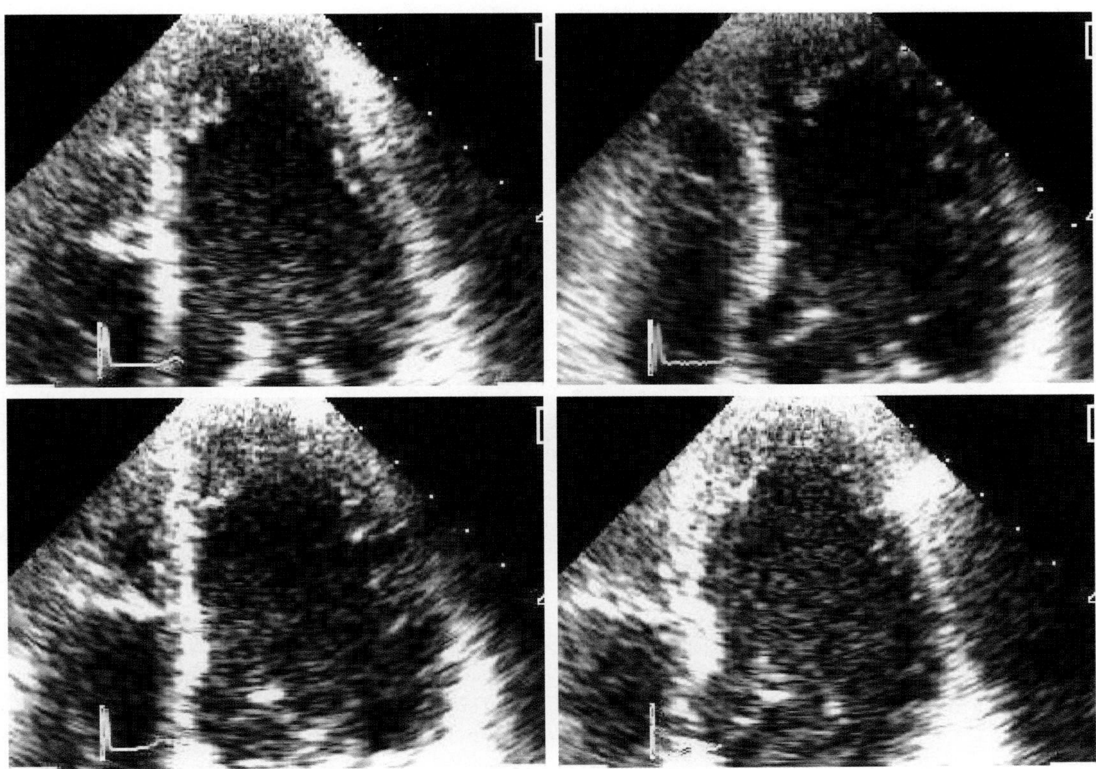

FIGURE 2-3-3 Apical 4 chamber view at baseline (upper left), low dose (upper right), intermediate dose (lower left), and peak dobutamine infusion (lower right), The accompanying videos demonstrate normal wall motion at rest with new wall motion abnormalities at peak infusion as described in the text ► (see Video 2-3-3).

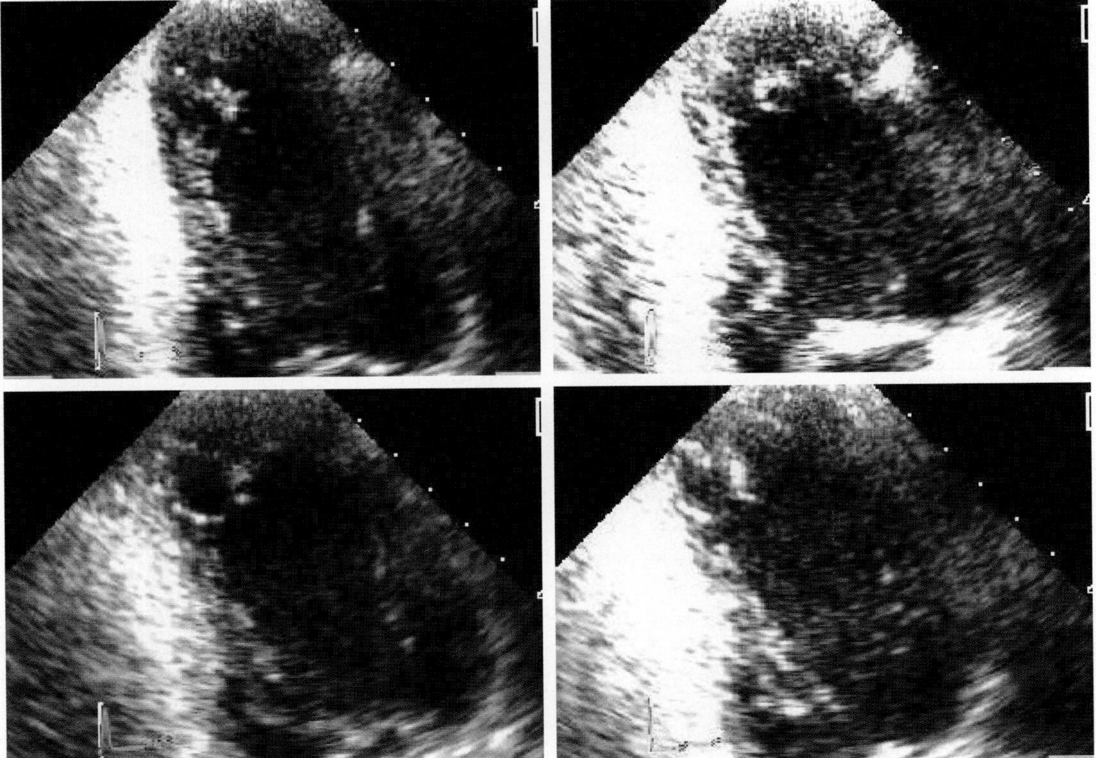

FIGURE 2-3-4 Apical 2 chamber view at baseline (upper left), low dose (upper right), intermediate dose (lower left), and peak dobutamine infusion (lower right). The accompanying videos demonstrate normal wall motion at rest with new wall motion abnormalities at peak infusion as described in the text ► (see Video 2-3-4).

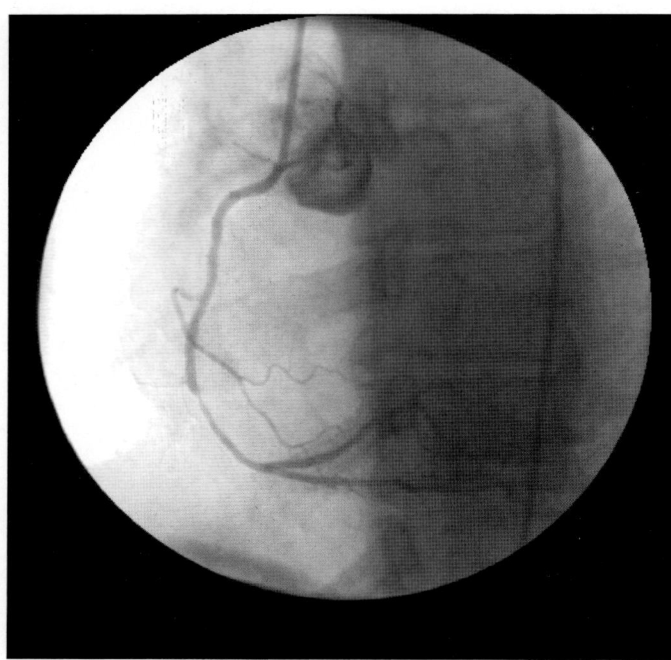

FIGURE 2-3-5 RCA angiogram from this patient. The proximal RCA stents were patent, but distal to the stents, a 95% lesion is seen.

6. Video 2-3-2 B: Low dose parasternal short axis view demonstrating normal wall motion
7. Video 2-3-2 C: Intermediate dose short axis view demonstrating a subtle inferior wall motion abnormality
8. Video 2-3-2 D: Peak infusion short axis view demonstrating inferior and inferoapical wall motion abnormalities. This SAX image is more apical than at the other stages.
9. Video 2-3-3 A: Baseline apical 4 chamber view demonstrating normal wall motion and EF
10. Video 2-3-3 B: Low dose apical 4 chamber view demonstrates basal inferior septal hypokinesis
11. Video 2-3-3 C: Intermediate dose apical 4 chamber view demonstrates akinesis of the inferior septum
12. Video 2-3-3 D: Peak infusion apical four chamber view demonstrates akinesis of the inferior septum and an apical wall motion abnormality
13. Video 2-3-4 A: Baseline apical 2 chamber view demonstrating normal wall motion and EF
14. Video 2-3-4 B: Low dose apical 2 chamber view demonstrating inferior hypokinesis
15. Video 2-3-4 C: Intermediate dose apical 2 chamber view demonstrating inferior hypokinesis
16. Video 2-3-4 D: Peak infusion apical 2 chamber view demonstrating inferior akinesis

REFERENCES

1. Yao S, Qureshi E, Sherrid M, Chaudhry F. Practical applications in stress echocardiography: risk stratification and prognosis in patients with known or suspected ischemic heart disease. *J Am Coll Cardiol*. 2003;42(6):1084-1090.
2. Marwick TH, Case C, Sawada S, et al. Prediction of mortality using dobutamine echocardiography. *J Am Coll Cardiol*. 2001;37:754-760.

SECTION 4

Post-MI LV Systolic Dysfunction

CLINICAL CASE PRESENTATION

A 52-year-old man with a 30-year history of diabetes status post–kidney-pancreas transplant presented to the ED with general malaise, recent fever, and left-sided chest discomfort associated with numbness and tingling of the left fingers.

He was afebrile, his blood pressure was 122/53 mm Hg, his pulse was 59 beats/min, and his respiratory rate was 18 breaths/min. His JVP was normal, lungs were clear, and cardiac exam reportedly free of murmurs or gallops. No LE edema was evident.

An ECG revealed NSR, with ST elevation in the anterior leads. Cardiac catheterization revealed acute occlusion of the LAD and high-grade stenosis of a diagonal branch with a chronically occluded RCA that filled distally via collaterals. Percutaneous coronary intervention (PCI) of the LAD with stent implantation was performed as well as PCI of the diagonal vessel. A ventriculogram was deferred given the renal transplant history. A transthoracic echo demonstrated an EF of 30% to 35% with anterior, lateral, and apical wall motion abnormalities.

His hospital course was uneventful, and he was discharged on aspirin, a thienopyridine, metoprolol succinate, statin, and ACE inhibitor therapy. He was referred to cardiac rehab.

ECHOCARDIOGRAPHIC EVALUATION

He did well clinically. At 3 months post-MI, a follow-up echocardiogram was obtained to reassess left ventricular function. This was performed to risk stratify the patient and to determine if he was a candidate for an ICD. As seen in Figure 2-4-1 and Figure 2-4-2 and the accompanying videos, despite optimal medical therapy, his LVEF was now ~25%.

DIAGNOSIS

Ischemic cardiomyopathy with severe LV systolic dysfunction post-anterior MI

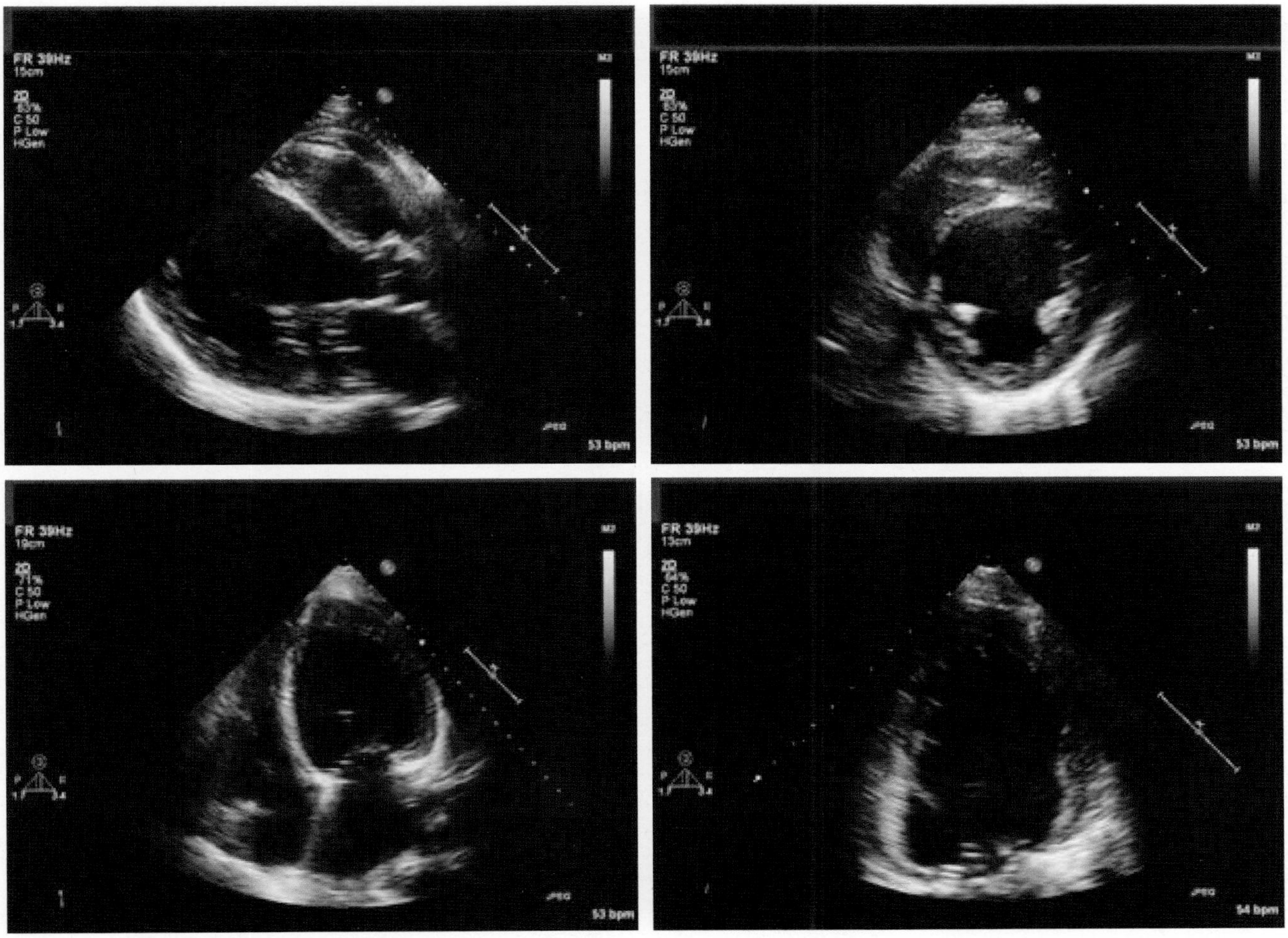

FIGURE 2-4-1 Quad screen view of the LV in the parasternal long axis (upper left), short axis (upper right), and apical 4 chamber (lower left) and apical 2 chamber (lower right) views ▶ (see Video 2-4-1).

MANAGEMENT

Post-MI therapy is directed at treatment of risk factors and the prevention of LV remodeling.

- Following myocardial infarction, stretched, infarcted tissue leads to increased left ventricular volume, which can lead to volume and pressure load on noninfarcted zones, causing myocyte hypertrophy that is both concentric and eccentric. Changes in neurohormonal levels, LV hemodynamics, and the presence of hypertension can all impact the remodeling process. If this process continues, there is decline in regional contractility of noninfarcted tissue, increase in end systolic volume index, and decrease in overall LV ejection fraction.[1]

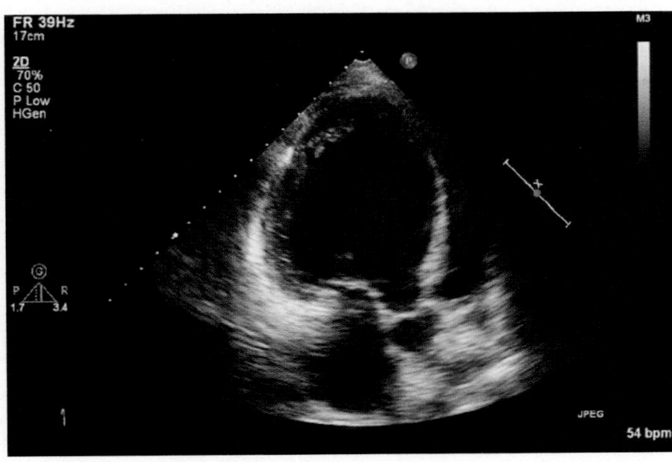

FIGURE 2-4-2 Apical 3 chamber view of this patient ▶(see Video 2-4-2).

- Reassessment of LVEF post-MI with echocardiography is warranted, especially in these patients with evidence of LV dysfunction in the acute setting.
- LV function remains a strong predictor of outcome postmyocardial infarction. Those individuals with the greatest degree of LV systolic dysfunction post-MI have the highest risk of congestive heart failure and ventricular arrhythmia, the latter of which often manifests as sudden cardiac death.
- The MADIT-2 trial evaluated 1232 patients with prior MI and EF less than 30% who did not have serious ventricular arrhythmias at the time of enrollment (2).
    - Subjects were randomized to implantable cardiac defibrillator (ICD) implantation or continued optimal medical therapy. During an average follow-up of 20 months, the mortality rate was

19.8% in the standard therapy arm, as opposed to 14.2% in the ICD arm, a relative risk reduction of 31%.
- As a consequence of this trial, current ACC/AHA guidelines[3] list ICD implantation as a class IA indication for patients post-MI with EF less than 30% on optimal medical therapy. The EF should be reassessed approximately 6 weeks post-MI/revascularization.

FOLLOW-UP

- As a result of the findings on echocardiography, our patient was referred for ICD implantation for primary prevention of sudden cardiac death, which was performed uneventfully.
- He was maintained on aggressive medical therapy (β-blocker, ACE inhibitor, and aldactone) designed to prevent worsening LV dysfunction and recurrent acute coronary syndromes (aspirin and statin therapy), in addition to continued heart-healthy dietary habits and physical activity.
- His defibrillator was monitored longitudinally in the arrhythmia device follow-up clinic. Three years later, he received an appropriate ICD shock for ventricular tachycardia. Repeat echo revealed stable, but severe, LV dysfunction. He has had no further events and clinically is doing well with medical therapy.

VIDEO LEGENDS

1. Video 2-4-1 A: Parasternal long axis view demonstrating a dilated LV with septal akinesis
2. Video 2-4-1 B: Parasternal short axis view demonstrating a dilated LV with septal akinesis
3. Video 2-4-1 C: Apical 4 chamber view demonstrating septal hypokinesis and apical akinesis
4. Video 2-4-1 D: Apical 2 chamber view demonstrating anteroapical and inferior wall motion abnormalities
5. Video 2-4-2: Apical 3 chamber view demonstrating septal and apical wall motion abnormalities

REFERENCES

1. McKay RG, Pfeffer MA, Pasternak RC, et al. Left ventricular remodeling after myocardial infarction: a corollary to infarct expansion. *Circulation*. 1986;74:693.
2. Moss AJ, Zareba W, Hall WJ, et al. Prophylactic implantation of a defibrillator in patients with myocardial infarction and reduced ejection fraction. *N Engl J Med*. 2002;346:877–883.
3. Epstein AE, DiMarco JP, Ellenbogen KA, et al. ACC/AHA/HRS 2008 Guidelines for Device-Based Therapy of Cardiac Rhythm Abnormalities: a report of the American College of Cardiology/American Heart Association Task Force on Practice Guidelines (Writing Committee to Revise the ACC/AHA/NASPE 2002 Guideline Update for Implantation of Cardiac Pacemakers and Antiarrhythmia Devices) *J Am Coll Cardiol*. 2008;51(21):e1-62.

SECTION 5

Post-MI with Shock and Respiratory Failure

CLINICAL CASE PRESENTATION

A 51-year-old man with no past cardiac history presented to the ED with a 90-minute history of left-sided chest discomfort associated with general malaise. His past history was unremarkable, and there was no family history of premature CAD.

He was married and worked as a mechanic, and had a 35-pack-year smoking history. He consumed 8 beers per day but denied illicit drug use. The review of systems was unremarkable.

On examination, he was an age-appropriate man initially in no acute distress. The initial vitals were: blood pressure 116/59 mm Hg, pulse 114 beats/min, respiratory rate 15 breaths/min, and temp 97.9° F (36.6° C). The skin was free of xanthelasma. The HEENT exam was unremarkable. The JVP was not elevated. The carotid upstrokes were normal; no bruits were auscultated. His PMI was non-displaced. S_1 and S_2 were normal. A soft systolic murmur was reported; no gallops were noted. The abdomen was benign without aneurysm or bruits. The extremities were free of edema with normal distal pulses and no peripheral bruits. No neurologic deficits were noted.

His initial CXR revealed normal heart size, clear lungs, no pleural fluid, and no mediastinal or hilar abnormality identified.

The initial ECG showed sinus tachycardia with nonspecific ST abnormality (Figure 2-5-1).

His initial troponin level returned at 2.4 ng/ml (normal less than 0.11 ng/ml).

While in the ED, he developed hypotension with a BP of 86/53 mm Hg and tachypnea with respiratory rates recorded between 25 and 31 breaths/min.

DIFFERENTIAL DIAGNOSIS

The patient presents with an acute non-ST elevation myocardial infarction complicated by hypotension and respiratory failure

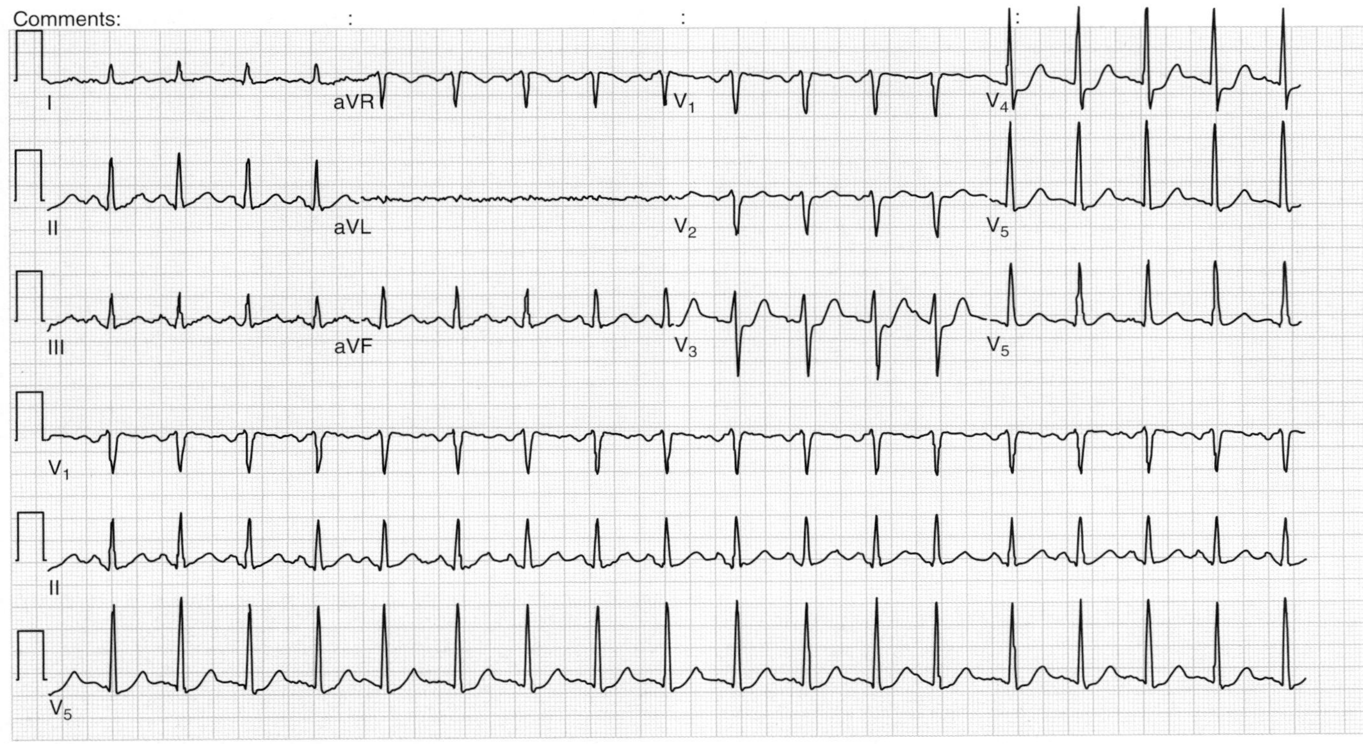

FIGURE 2-5-1 Initial ECG demonstrating sinus tachycardia and nonspecific ST changes.

(cardiogenic shock). Possible causes of his hemodynamic instability include:

- LV dysfunction with or without RV dysfunction
- Acute MR
- Acute VSD or free wall rupture

MANAGEMENT AND DIAGNOSTIC TESTING

He was started on aspirin, clopidogrel, and IV unfractionated Heparin, but due to hypotension, a β-blocker, nitroglycerin, or an ACE inhibitor were not administered. Arrangements were made for urgent catheterization with further recommendations pending the catheterization results.

In the catheterization lab, he required urgent intubation for respiratory distress/failure. Coronary angiography demonstrated a near total occlusion of an obtuse marginal branch of the circumflex artery (Figure 2-5-2). Left ventricular angiography revealed preserved systolic function and severe MR.

ECHOCARDIOGRAPHIC EVALUATION

An urgent echo was obtained. This demonstrated a hyperdynamic LV with evidence of severe MR due to papillary muscle rupture (Figures 2-5-3 to 2-5-7). The TTE images were suboptimal; however, intra-operative TEE confirmed the findings (Figures 2-5-8 and 2-5-9).

DIAGNOSIS

Acute MR due to papillary muscle rupture:

- An uncommon, but hemodynamically and clinically devastating complication of myocardial infarction, is rupture of the papillary muscle, which results in acute severe MR.
- As the LA compliance cannot accommodate the acute increase in regurgitant flow, acute pulmonary edema, respiratory failure, hypotension and/or shock are clinical consequences.[1,2]

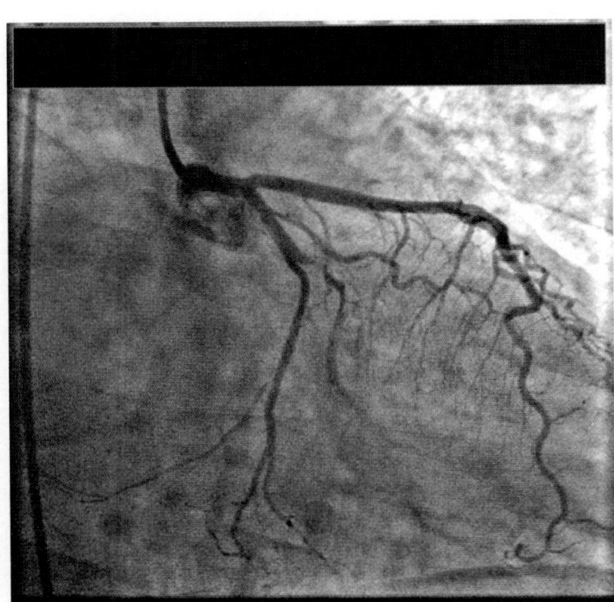

FIGURE 2-5-2 Catheterization film demonstrating a subtotal occlusion of an obtuse marginal branch of the circumflex artery.

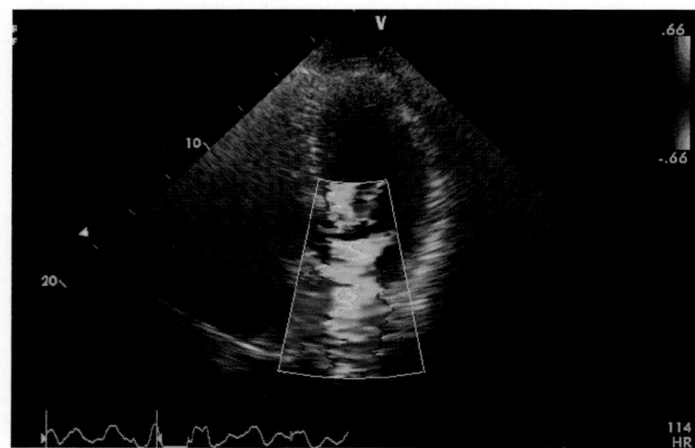

FIGURE 2-5-3 TTE image: Color Doppler demonstrating severe MR.

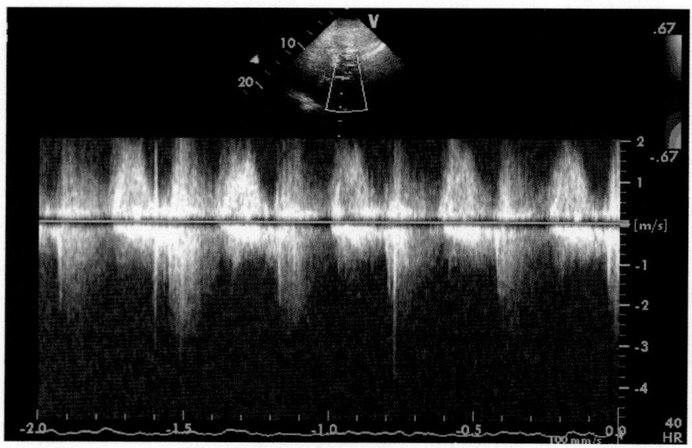

FIGURE 2-5-4 Continuous wave Doppler demonstrating severe MR. The velocity is low due to the patient's hypotension coupled with a high LA pressure.

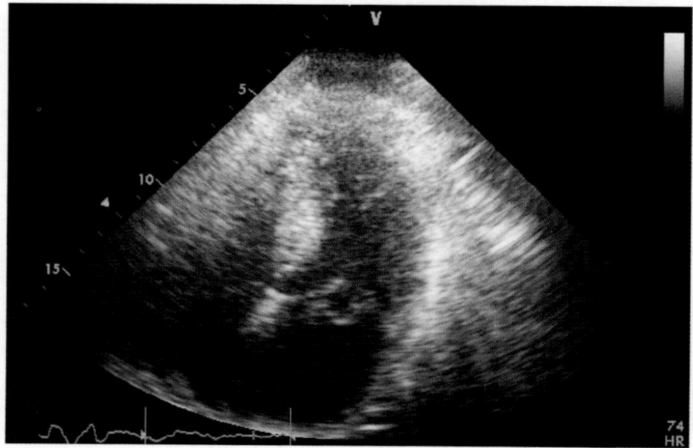

FIGURE 2-5-5 Apical 4 chamber view demonstrating a flail posterior leaflet ▶ (see Video 2-5-5).

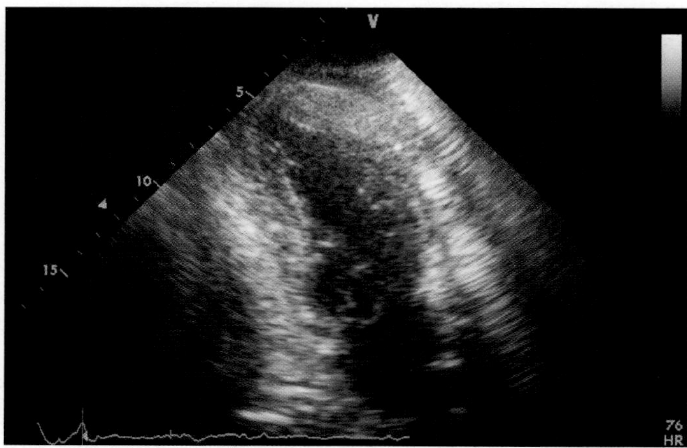

FIGURE 2-5-6 Apical 2 chamber view demonstrating the flail MV ▶ (see Video 2-5-6).

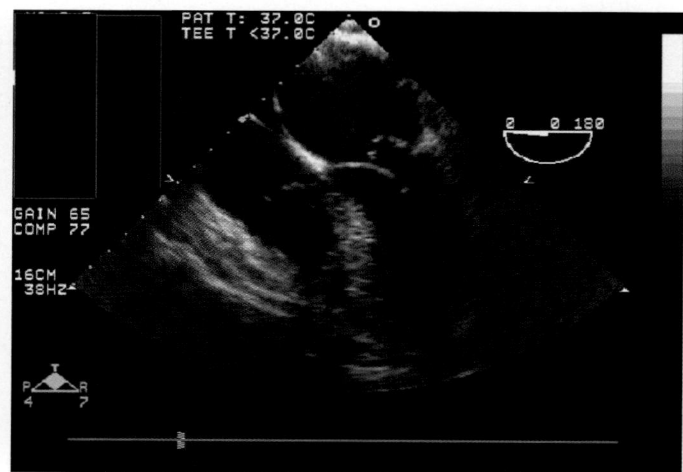

FIGURE 2-5-7 Intraoperative TEE image demonstrating the posterior flail leaflet.

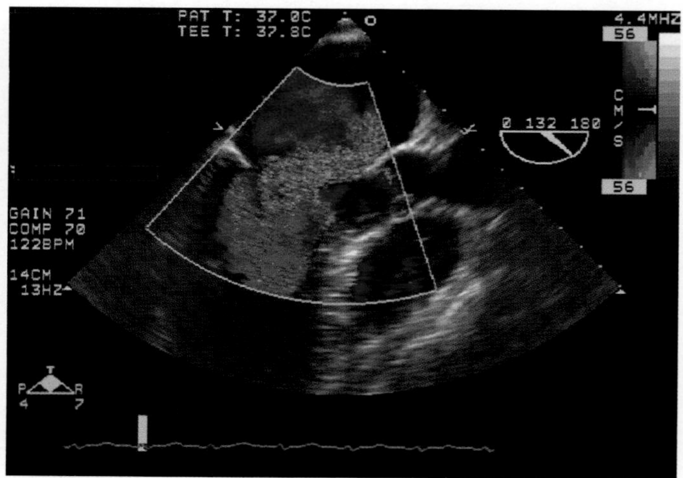

FIGURE 2-5-8 Intraoperative TEE with color Doppler demonstrating severe MR ▶ (see Video 2-5-8).

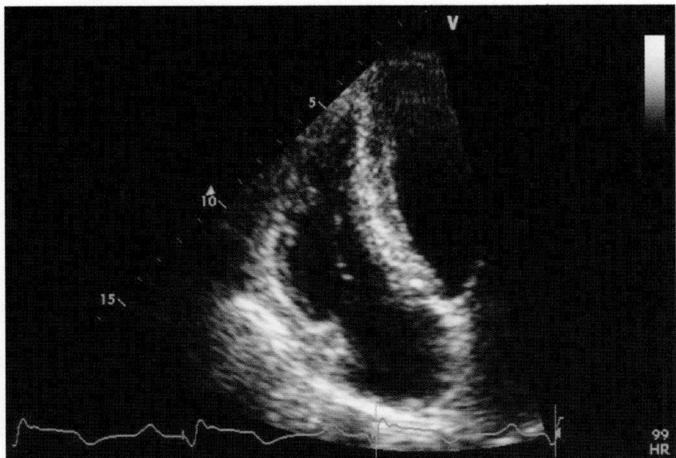

FIGURE 2-5-9 From a different patient. An apical 4 chamber view demonstrating an RV MI, another cause of acute hypotension in a patient with an MI ► (see Video 2-5-9).

- This entity is felt to be responsible for ~5% of deaths following myocardial infarction.[1]
- The posteromedial papillary muscle is the most common to rupture, due to its single blood supply.
- The diagnosis can be made by echocardiography.
  - Echocardiographic features include severe MR and flail segments of the valve with a portion of the papillary muscle attached to the chordae prolapsing into the LA.
- Urgent recognition of this entity, followed by temporary support with an IABP and urgent surgical intervention,[2] are required to manage this postmyocardial infarction complication. Typically, valve replacement is pursued, although there are published case reports regarding surgical repair.[3,4]

SUBSEQUENT MANAGEMENT

An intra-aortic balloon pump was placed. He was immediately taken to the operating suite and underwent emergency median sternotomy. Intra-operatively, the posterior medial papillary muscle was noted to be infarcted, with disruption of the superior portion of the papillary muscle with the attached chordae in the P_2 and P_3 regions of the valve. Replacement of the mitral valve was performed with a mechanical valve, in addition to closure of an incidentally identified PFO. His postoperative course was unremarkable.

FOLLOW-UP

He was discharged on aspirin, warfarin, β-blocker, statin, and an ACE inhibitor. Due to the prosthetic valve, he was advised of the importance of antibiotic prophylaxis prior to dental procedures, for the prevention of bacterial endocarditis. Cardiac rehabilitation and serial follow-up of his CAD and prosthetic valve were arranged.

VIDEO LEGENDS

1. Video 2-5-5: Apical 4 chamber view demonstrating a flail posterior leaflet
2. Video 2-5-6: Apical 2 chamber view demonstrating the flail MV
3. Video 2-5-8: Intra-operative TEE demonstrating severe MR
4. Video 2-5-9: An apical four chamber view demonstrating an RV MI, another cause of acute hypotension in a patient with an MI

REFERENCES

1. Nishimura RA, Schaff HV, Shub C, Gersh BJ, Edwards WD, Tajik AJ. Papillary muscle rupture complicating acute myocardial infarction: analysis of 17 patients. *Am J Cardiol*. 1983;51:373-377.
2. Clements SD Jr, Story WE, Hurst JW, Craver JM, Jones EL. Ruptured papillary muscle, a complication of myocardial infarction: clinical presentation, diagnosis, and treatment. *Clin Cardiol*. 1985;8:93-103.
3. Tavakoli R, Weber A, Vogt P, Brunner HP, Pretre R, Turina M. Surgical management of acute mitral valve regurgitation due to post-infarction papillary muscle rupture. *J Heart Valve Dis*. 2002;11:20-25.
4. Fasol R, Lakew F, Wetter S. Mitral repair in patients with a ruptured papillary muscle. *Am Heart J*. 2000;139:549-554.

SECTION 6

Post-MI Ventricular Septal Defect

CLINICAL CASE PRESENTATION

A 69-year-old white female presented with 4 to 5 days of waxing and waning chest burning, which she described as severe heartburn, associated with nausea and vomiting. As the discomfort became persistent, and the pain moved into her left shoulder, she asked her husband to call EMS. In the ED, her ECG revealed inferior ST elevation. She proceeded directly to the catheterization lab, and on initial evaluation it was found that her blood pressure was 60/42 mm Hg and her heart rate was 98 beat/min. She was started on dopamine, and an intra-aortic balloon pump (IABP) was placed. She was found to have 100% proximal RCA occlusion, and underwent aspiration thrombectomy and PCI with 2 DES to the proximal RCA. She was also noted to have an 80% mid-LAD lesion, which was not intervened upon at that time.

Postintervention, she was anxious, tachypneic, and in distress with clinical evidence of cardiogenic shock. Her vitals revealed a blood pressure of 92/54 mm Hg, a heart rate of 112 beats/min, and her oxygen saturation was 100% on 100% a non-rebreather face mask. She was continued on a dopamine drip at a rate of 10 mcg/kg/min, and IABP support was continued. She had inspiratory rales bilaterally. She was tachycardic with normal S_1 and S_2; a grade III/VI holosystolic murmur best heard at the left lower sternal border was noted. Her abdominal exam was benign, the right femoral sheath site was free of hematoma or bruit, and a left femoral venous central venous catheter was intact. The extremities were cool to the touch, and she had palpable but diminished distal pulses.

DIFFERENTIAL DIAGNOSIS

Acute inferior ST elevation MI and 2-vessel CAD status post PCI of the RCA, with cardiogenic shock and a new murmur. Possible diagnosis:

- Acute MR due to papillary muscle rupture.
- Acute ventricular septal rupture/defect.

ECHOCARDIOGRAPHIC EVALUATION

An urgent TTE was obtained (Figures 2-6-1 to 2-6-5). This study demonstrated moderate segmental LV systolic dysfunction with a large VSD present. One can readily appreciate the defect in the mid portion of the inferior septum with left to right flow across the defect, especially in the subcostal view. In addition, there is RV hypokinesis.

MANAGEMENT

Urgent surgical consultation was obtained.

- She was taken to the OR early in her course, where pericardial patch closure of the VSD and a saphenous vein graft (SVG) to the LAD was performed.
- Postsurgical intervention, she exhibited persistent cardiogenic shock, with development of renal failure, continued respiratory insufficiency, liver failure, and increased lactic acidosis.
- 6 days postoperatively, she expired.

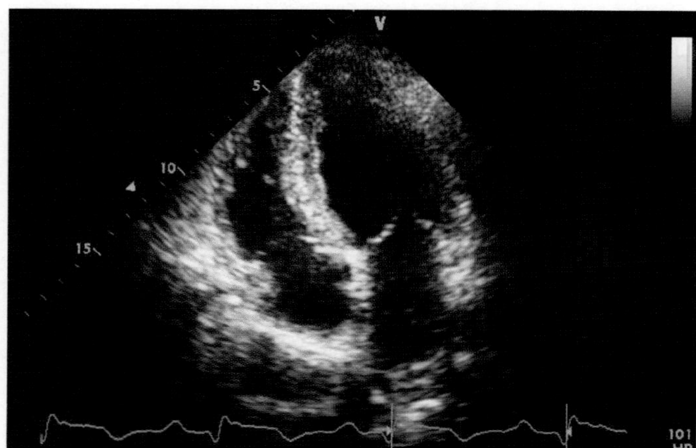

FIGURE 2-6-1 Apical 4 chamber view demonstrating an inferior septal wall motion abnormality and RV hypokinesis. The VSD is not seen in this still frame. ► (see Videos 2-6-1)

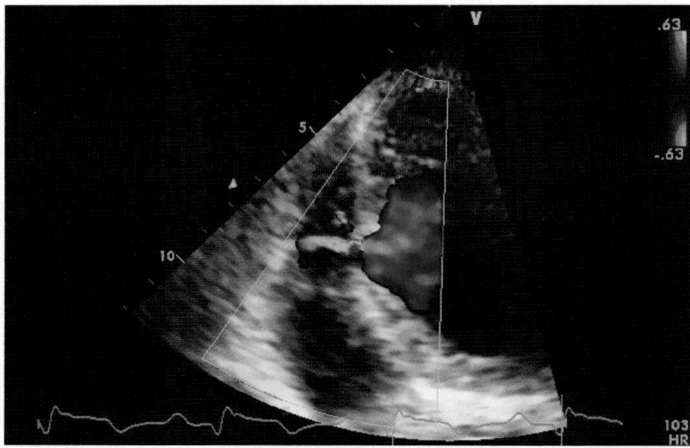

FIGURE 2-6-2 The VSD is seen in this apical 4 chamber view (posterior tilt) with color Doppler ► (see Video 2-6-2).

DISCUSSION

Post-MI ventricular septal rupture is a rare complication of acute MI that carries a very high mortality rate.

- In those who do not undergo surgical intervention, survival is very low. In one published series, even with surgical intervention, the mortality was 36%[1] but increases to over 80% in those with cardiogenic shock at the time of surgery.
- In the STS database, the mortality rate was 43%. Post surgical VSD repair, 75% of those patients died or exhibited significant morbidity, with postoperative dialysis being the most common complication.[2] While those who undergo operative intervention earlier post-MI have a higher mortality, there is a selection bias toward less sick patients who can delay surgery. There is interest in percutaneous closure of these defects, and work in this area continues.

VIDEO LEGENDS

1. Video 2-6-1 A: Apical 4 chamber view demonstrating an inferior septal wall motion abnormality and RV hypokinesis. The VSD is not seen in this view.
2. Video 2-6-1 B: Apical 4 chamber view demonstrating an inferior septal wall motion abnormality and RV hypokinesis. The VSD is now seen.
3. Video 2-6-2: The VSD is seen in this apical 4 chamber view (posterior tilt) with color Doppler
4. Video 2-6-3 L: Apical 2 chamber view without color Doppler demonstrating an inferior wall motion abnormality.
5. Video 2-6-3 R: Apical 2 chamber view with color Doppler demonstrating an inferior wall motion abnormality and minimal MR
6. Video 2-6-3 C: Apical 3 chamber view demonstrating an inferolateral wall motion abnormality
7. Video 2-6-4: Subcostal view demonstrating a large inferior septal defect
8. Video 2-6-5: Subcostal view with color Doppler demonstrating the VSD with left to right flow
9. Video 2-6-6: TEE images from a different patient demonstrating an inferior septal VSD due to an acute inferior MI

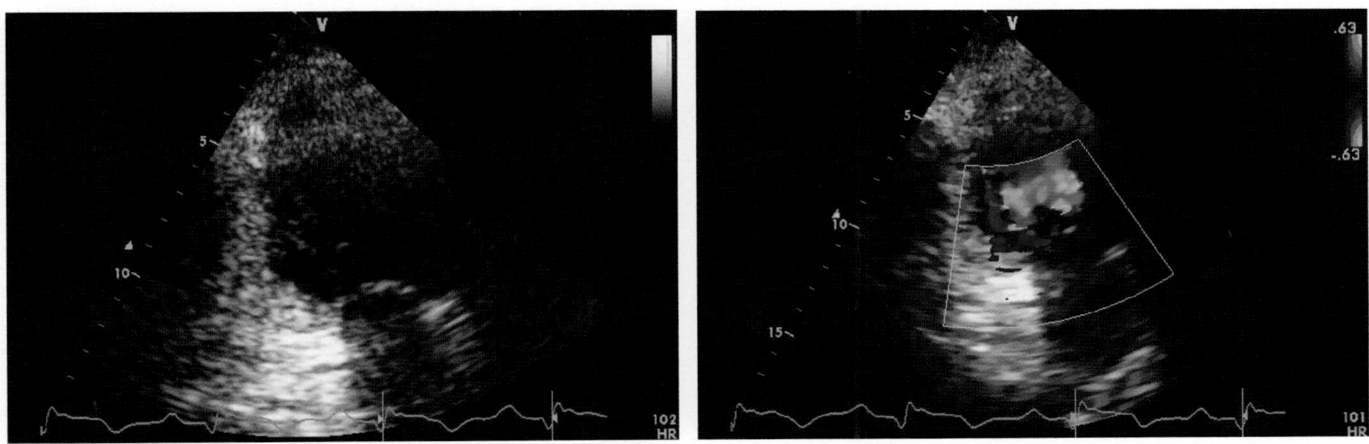

FIGURE 2-6-3 Apical 2 chamber view without (L) and with (R) color Doppler demonstrating an inferior wall motion abnormality and minimal MR ► (see Videos 2-6-3).

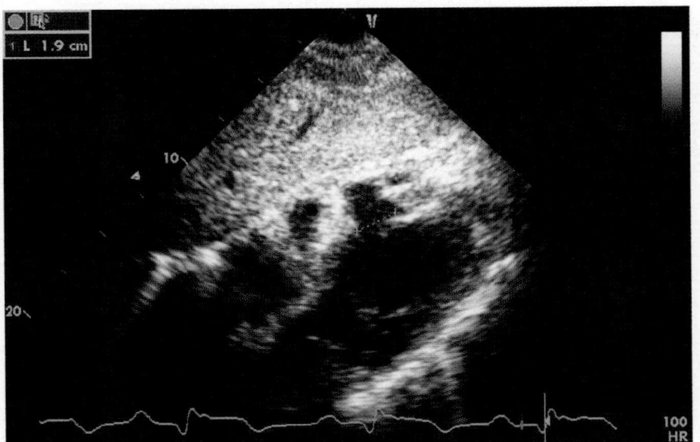

FIGURE 2-6-4 Subcostal view demonstrating a large inferior septal defect ► (see Video 2-6-4).

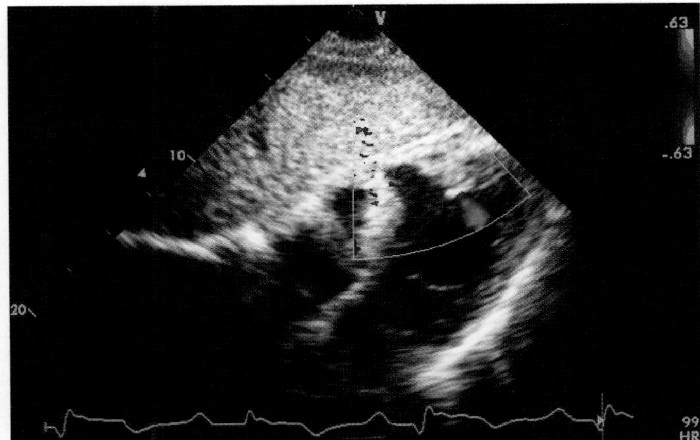

FIGURE 2-6-5 Subcostal view with color Doppler demonstrating the VSD with left to right flow ► (see Video 2-6-5).

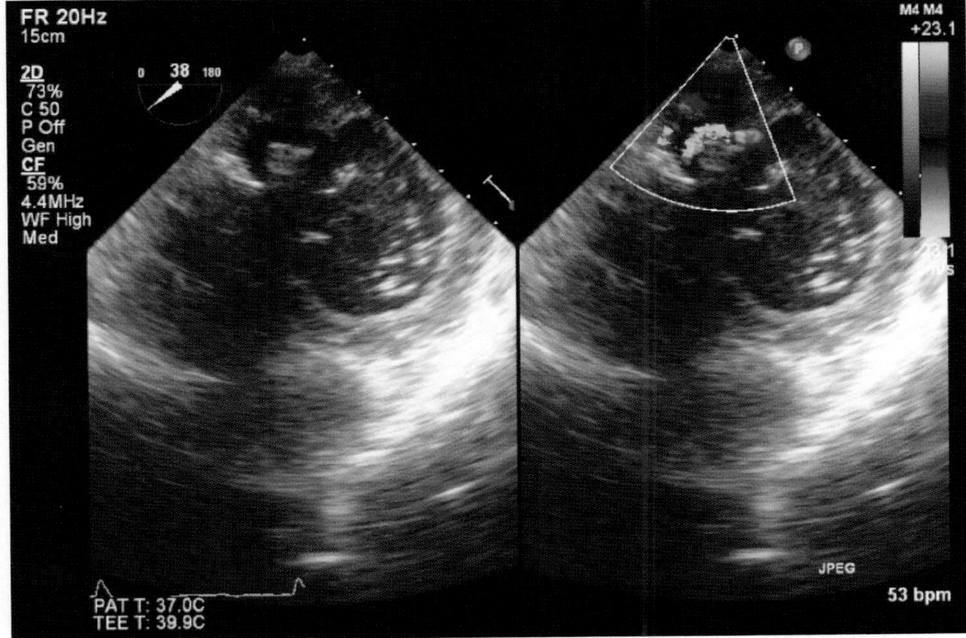

FIGURE 2-6-6 TEE images from a different patient demonstrating an inferior septal VSD due to an acute inferior MI. This defect involves the more basal inferior septum ► (see Video 2-6-6).

REFERENCES

1. Mantovani V, Mariscalco G, Leva C, Blanzola C, Sala A. Surgical repair of post-infarction ventricular septal defect: 19 years of experience. *Int J Cardiol*. 2006:4;108(2):202-206.

2. Arnaoutakis GJ, Zhao Y, George TJ, Sciortino CM, McCarthy PM, Conte JV. Surgical repair of ventricular septal defect after myocardial infarction: outcomes from the Society of Thoracic Surgeons National Database. *Ann Thorac Surg*. 2012;94(2):436-443.

3 ECHOCARDIOGRAPHIC ASSESSMENT OF VALVULAR HEART DISEASE

Kavita Sharma, MD, Gina G. Mentzer, MD, and David A. Orsinelli, MD, FACC, FASE

INTRODUCTION

Echocardiography is the principal imaging method employed to assess patients with known or suspected valvular heart disease, including those with prosthetic valves. It has largely supplanted the use of invasive cardiac catheterization in the evaluation and management of these patients.[1-3] The publications by Holen and Hatle in the late 1970s[4,5] in which Doppler echocardiography was demonstrated to be a reliable noninvasive technique to accurately assess valve function resulted in more widespread acceptance and utilization of echocardiography. Important early publications also validated the use of echocardiography and the Doppler technique in the assessment of cardiovascular hemodynamics.

While other imaging techniques, such as cardiac CT and MRI, have provided additional tools to evaluate cardiac valves, they currently play a secondary role in the assessment of valve structure and function in most settings. MRI may play a larger role in the assessment of ventricular size and function in the future.

The use of echocardiography is a Class 1 indication for the evaluation of many clinical scenarios in which valvular heart disease is suspected.[2] In the recently revised appropriate use criteria for echocardiography,[3] echocardiography is deemed appropriate in a variety of clinical scenarios in patients with known or suspected valvular heart disease. The 2014 guideline for the management of patients with valvular heart disease provides an excellent resource for the role of echocardiography in evaluating and managing these patients.[1]

In this chapter, we will explore the use of echocardiography in a variety of clinical settings in patients with valvular heart disease, including native valve disease, endocarditis, and patients with prosthetic heart valves.

SECTION 1

Asymptomatic Severe Aortic Stenosis

David A. Orsinelli, MD, FACC, FASE

CLINICAL CASE PRESENTATION

The patient is an 82-year-old man with a longstanding history of a heart murmur. He was initially seen in consultation at the request of his primary care physician 11 years ago for an evaluation of a heart murmur. At that time, he was completely asymptomatic and categorically denied any angina, dyspnea, heart failure symptoms, or syncope. An echocardiogram was obtained which demonstrated severe aortic stenosis. In view of his lack of symptoms, the patient was managed expectantly. Over the ensuing 11 years, he was seen frequently for follow-up and underwent periodic echocardiography (Figures 3-1-1 to 3-1-5). He continued to deny any symptoms and was quite physically active, frequently working out at his local fitness center with no limitations. His echocardiogram (Table 3-1-1) demonstrated progressive worsening of his aortic stenosis with significant increases in the calculated aortic valve gradients. His physical examination was consistent with severe aortic stenosis. He demonstrated delayed carotid upstrokes with diminished volume, a harsh, late peaking systolic ejection murmur that radiated to the carotids and across the precordium, and an absent aortic component of the second heart sound. His lungs were clear, and he had no lower extremity edema. A brain naturetic peptide (BNP) was obtained, which was elevated at 306. In order to further risk stratify him, he underwent a stress test during which time he remained asymptomatic; however, he developed significant ST depression and ventricular ectopy (Figure 3-1-6). His blood pressure response was hypotensive. Given the findings on his stress test, surgery was recommended, but the patient declined, stating that he felt fine. Shortly thereafter, however, he began to notice a questionable decrease in his functional capacity. Whether or not he truly developed new symptoms, or simply began to recognize symptoms that he had ignored or not recognized but which became evident after the concerns raised on the stress test, is not clear. He contacted his physician. Further diagnostic testing, including cardiac catheterization, was undertaken, and he subsequently underwent aortic valve replacement with a 27 mm pericardial valve. He had an uneventful surgical course. Postoperatively, in retrospect, he stated that he was somewhat limited and in fact felt that his exercise capacity had improved.

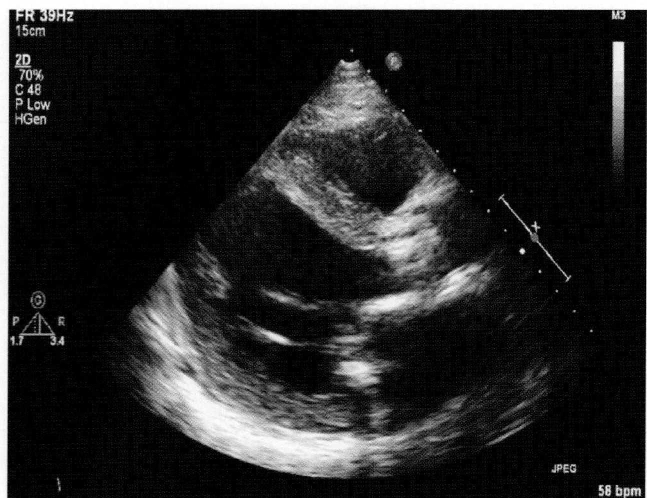

FIGURE 3-1-1 Parasternal long axis view demonstrating LVH, a heavily calcified, immobile AV as well as mitral valve thickening and annular calcification ▶ (see Video 3-1-1).

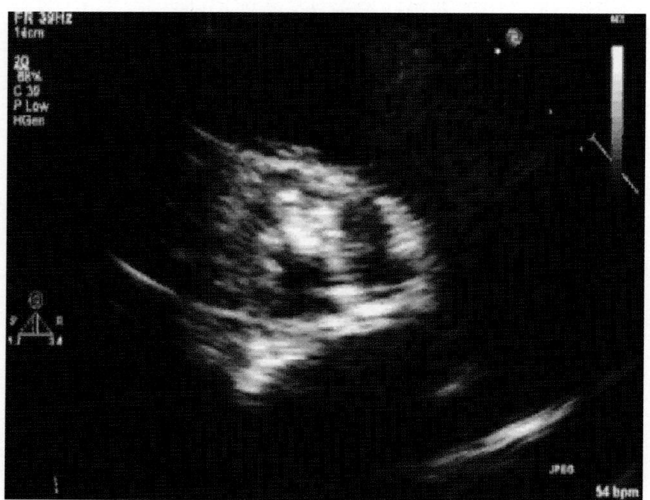

FIGURE 3-1-2 Parasternal short axis view of the heavily calcified aortic valve ▶ (see Video 3-1-2).

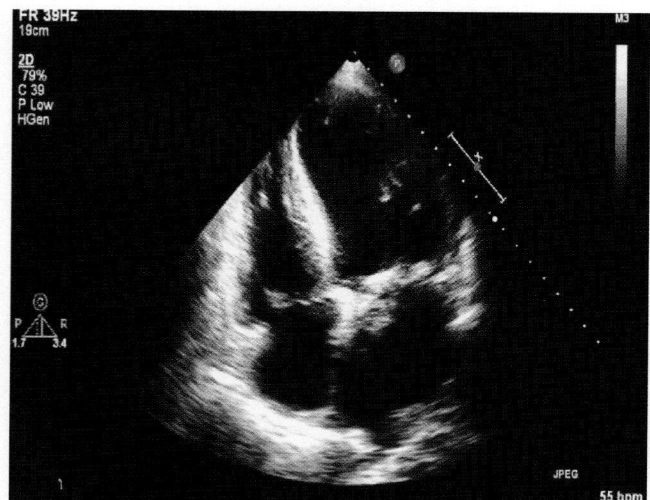

FIGURE 3-1-3 Apical 4 chamber view demonstrating LVH and preserved LV ejection fraction ▶ (see Video 3-1-3).

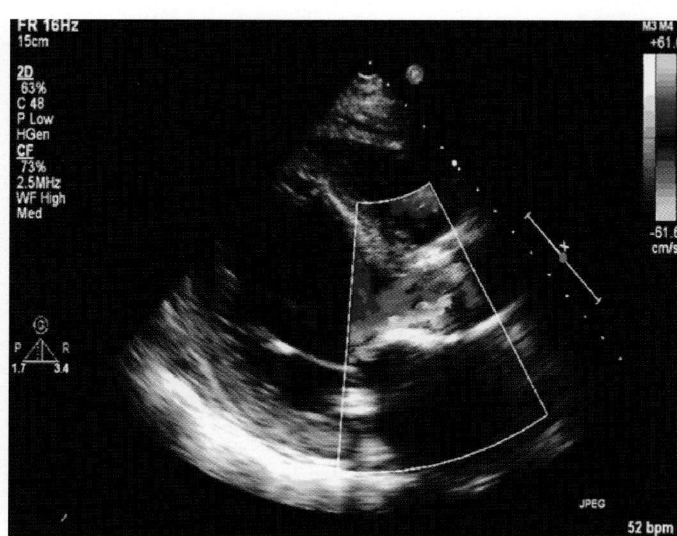

FIGURE 3-1-4 Parasternal long axis view with color Doppler demonstrating mild aortic regurgitation as well as mitral insufficiency ▶ (see Video 3-1-4).

CLINICAL FEATURES AND NATURAL HISTORY[1]

- Most patients with mild to moderate aortic stenosis (AS) are asymptomatic.
- As the severity of the stenosis progresses, patients may experience angina, syncope, or congestive heart failure. Once symptoms develop, the prognosis is poor. After the onset of symptoms, average survival is 5 years (angina), 3 years (syncope), and 2 years after the onset of congestive heart failure.[6]
- The most feared complication of aortic stenosis is sudden cardiac death. Patients with symptomatic AS are at high risk for sudden cardiac death, while sudden death occurs quite rarely and infrequently in patients with asymptomatic aortic stenosis.
- The rate of progression varies among individuals. Thus, careful monitoring of the patient is warranted.

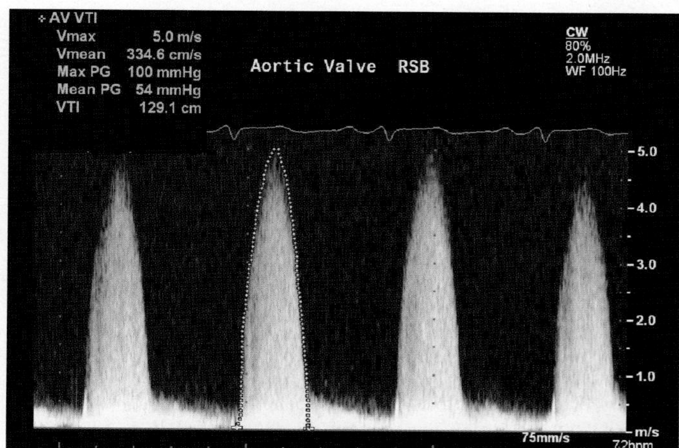

FIGURE 3-1-5 Continuous-wave Doppler demonstrating markedly elevated peak and mean aortic valve gradients. These velocity measurements were obtained from the right parasternal window.

TABLE 3-1-1 Serial Echocardiographic Data Over an 11-year Period

DATE	EF (%)	AV vel	PEAK GRAD	MEAN GRAD	AVA	AR	EST RVSP
Initial	65	4.4	79	49	0.9	2+	30
1 year	65	4.6	84	51	1.0	1+	30
3 year	60	5.3	115	69	0.5	2+	39
6 year	65	5.4	118	76	0.5	2+	49
10 year	60	5.5	121	68	0.6	2+	57
11 year	60	5.6	125	81	0.6	2+	69

EF = ejection fraction; AV vel = peak aortic valve velocity (m/s); GRAD = gradient (mm Hg); AVA = aortic valve area by continuity equation (cm^2); AR = aortic regurgitation; EST RVSP = estimated right ventricular systolic pressure (mm Hg).

EPIDEMIOLOGY

- Aortic stenosis is the most common form of valvular heart disease in adults, with a reported prevalence of 2% to 9% in the elderly.[1,7,8]
- The precursor of AS, aortic sclerosis, was detected in 29% of subjects over the age of 65 in an echocardiographic study.[10]

PATHOPHYSIOLOGY AND ETIOLOGY

- Obstruction to left ventricular outflow and the resultant increase in LV pressure leads to LVH and potentially LV systolic dysfunction.
- Increased oxygen demand can lead to angina.
- Systolic and diastolic dysfunction may result in symptoms of congestive heart failure.
- Fixed cardiac output and dysrhythmias can lead to syncope and sudden cardiac death.
- The most common causes of AS include calcification of a congenitally bicuspid AV (~50% of surgically replaced valves in the US and Europe), calcification of a trileaflet valve and rheumatic valve disease.[1,10,11]
- The underlying etiology of aortic stenosis is a function of age.[1,11] Congenital abnormalities of the aortic valve predominate in children, adolescents, and young adults.

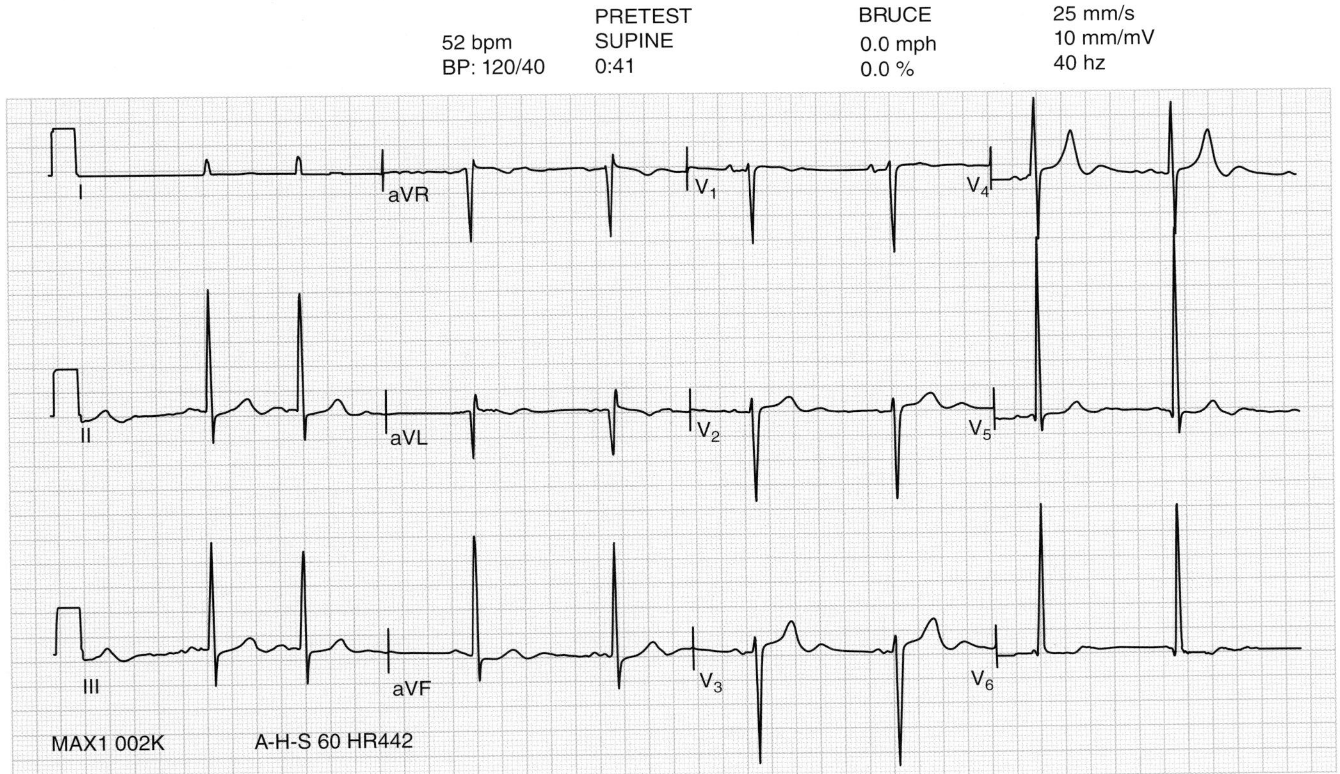

FIGURE 3-1-6 Baseline ECG from the patient described in the case presentation.

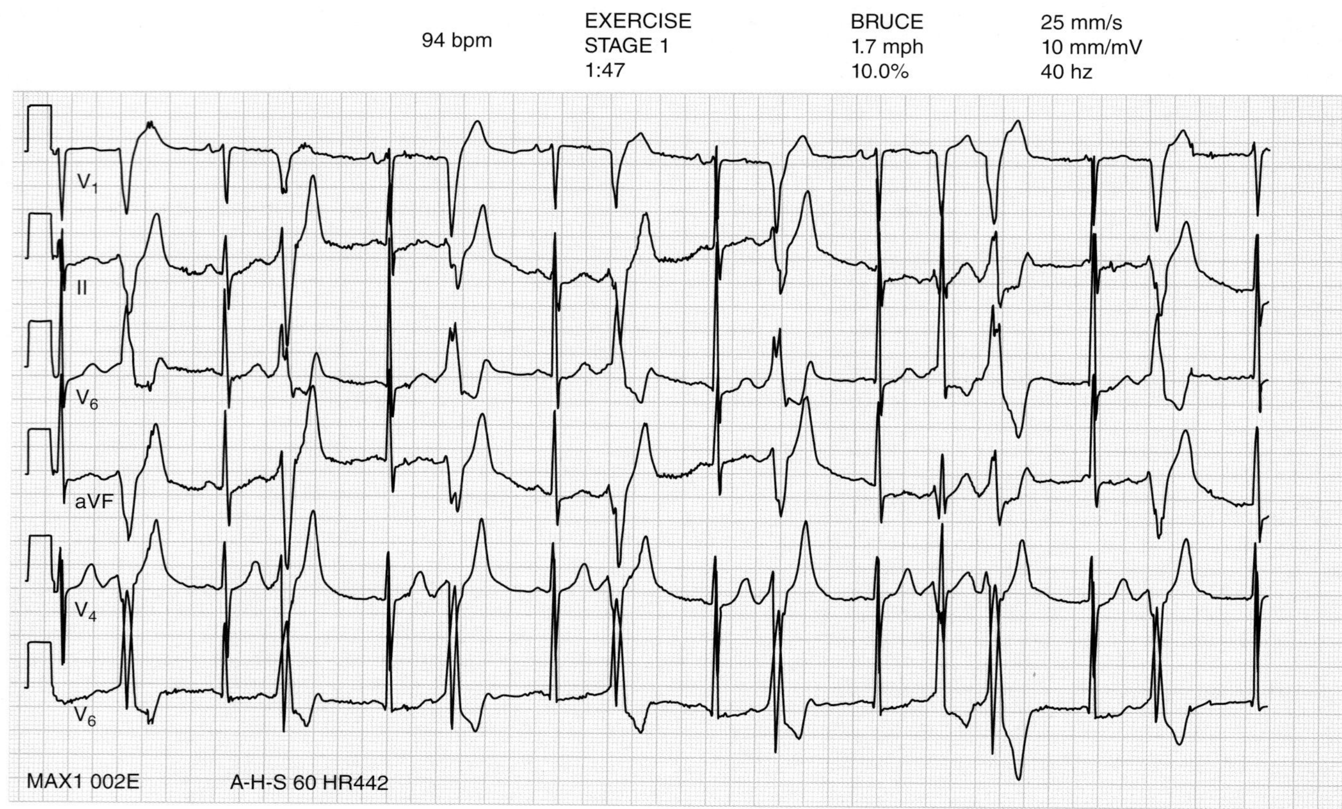

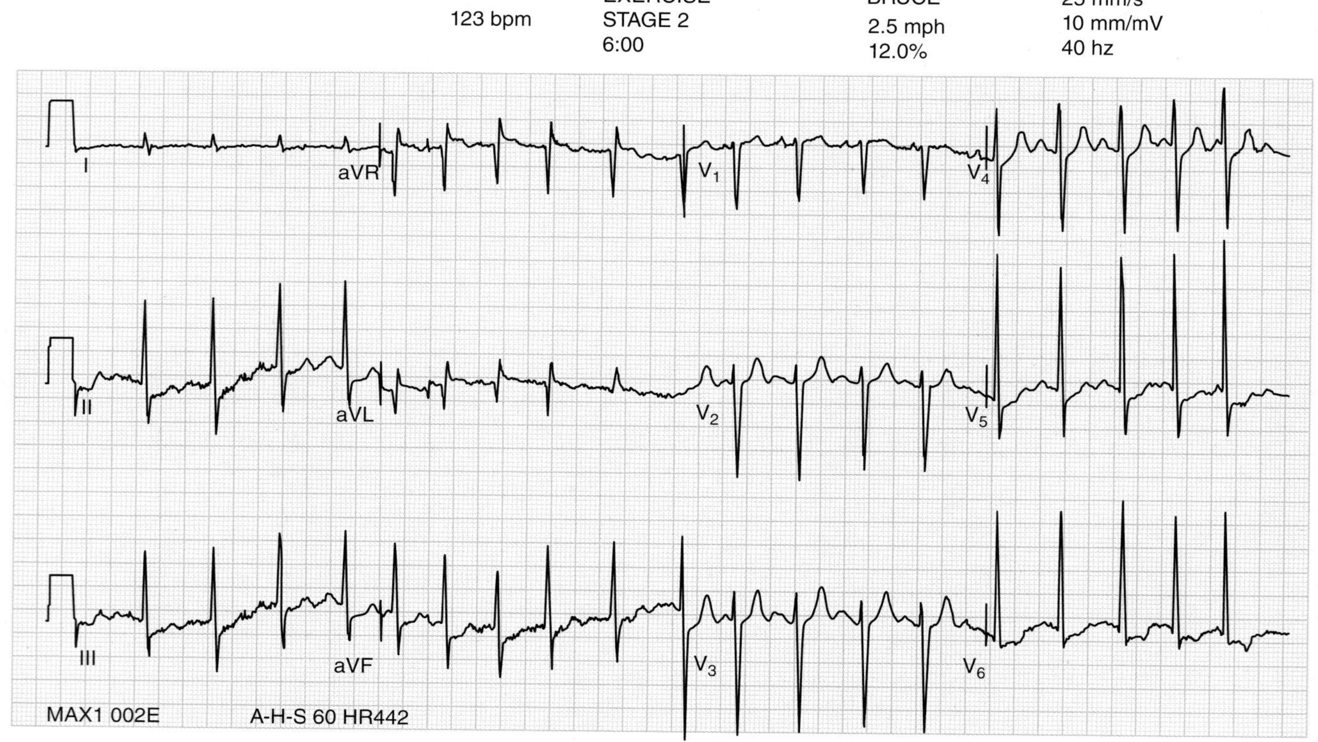

FIGURE 3-1-6 Rhythm strip (upper panel) and peak stress ECG (bottom panel) from the case presentation.

- Acquired AS, due to calcification of a congenitally abnormal valve an initially normal trileaflet AV, predominates in older patients.
- The calcification process is an active disease process (rather than a "wear and tear" process). It is characterized by active inflammation, lipid accumulation, and calcification.[1]
- Rheumatic valvular aortic stenosis is becoming much less frequent in the developed world. Most patients have concomitant mitral valve disease.

ECHOCARDIOGRAPHY

Echocardiography remains the standard diagnostic tool to assess for the presence and severity of aortic stenosis (Figures 3-1-7 to 3-1-11). A transthoracic echo with a comprehensive Doppler examination is appropriate.[1,3] Echocardiography can evaluate left ventricular size, structure, and function, including evidence of left ventricular hypertrophy and systolic and diastolic function. In addition to evaluating the aortic valve (including determination of peak and mean gradient as well as calculated valve area) and the presence of aortic regurgitation, concomitant valvular heart disease can also be detected. The proximal portion of the aorta can frequently be imaged quite well.

- There are many potential measures of AS that can be obtained by echocardiography.[10] They all have potential limitations and advantages (Table 3-1-2). Current standards recommend that several measures be obtained in all patients (A), with other parameters reasonable (R) if additional data is needed. Many other parameters that can be assessed are not currently recommended for clinical use.
  - AS jet velocity (A). It is critical to interrogate the Doppler signal from multiple windows, using data from highest velocities measured.
    - Peak velocity.
    - Character of the continuous-wave Doppler signal, including its shape, acceleration time.
  - Calculation of mean gradient from the Doppler signal (A).
  - Calculation of the AV area using the continuity equation (A).

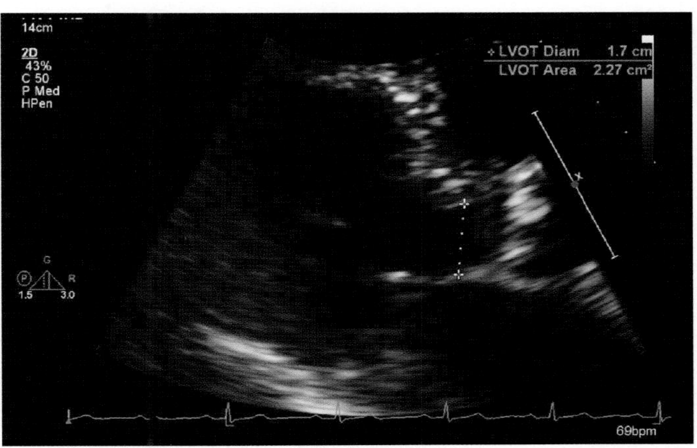

FIGURE 3-1-8 Parasternal long axis image demonstrating the LVOTd measurement.

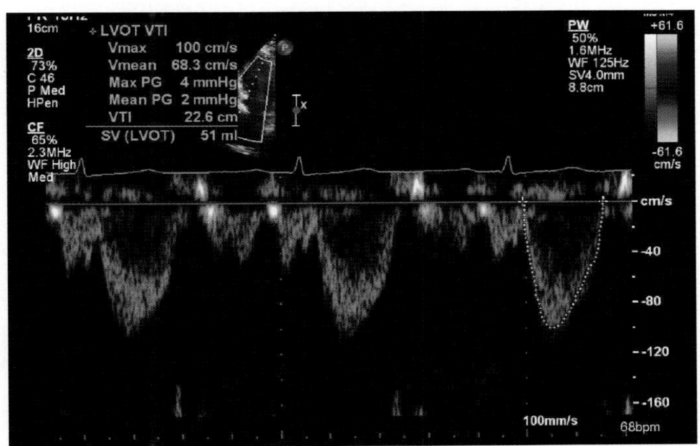

FIGURE 3-1-9 Pulsed wave Doppler of the LVOT velocity (V_1) and VTI.

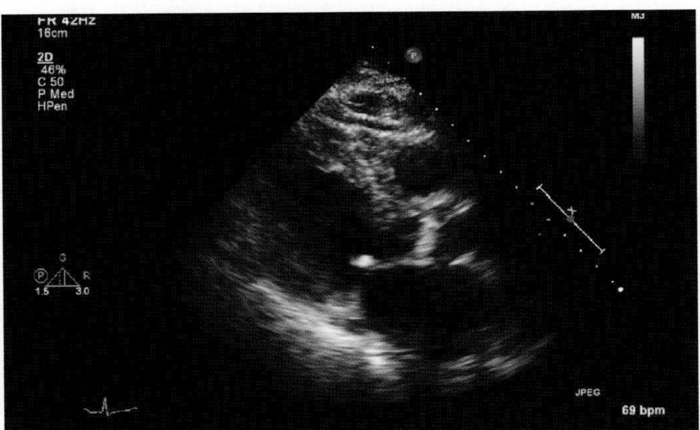

FIGURE 3-1-7 Parasternal long axis view of a different patient demonstrating a heavily calcified, restricted AV ▶ (see Video 3-1-7). Figures 3-1-8 to 3-1-10 demonstrate the measurements obtained in this patient to calculate the AVA by the continuity equation.

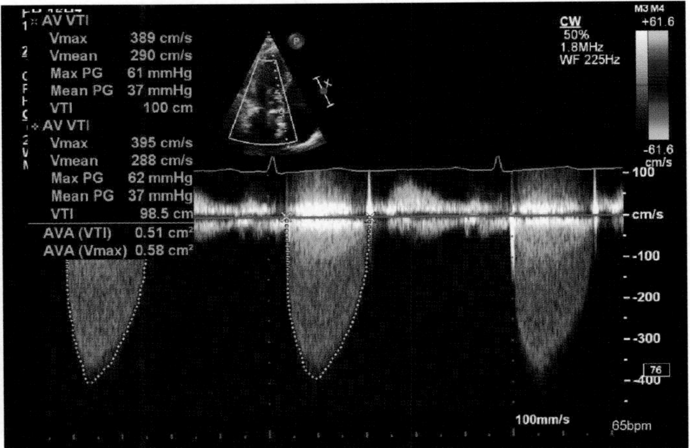

FIGURE 3-1-10 Continuous-wave Doppler of the peak AV velocity (V_2). In this patient, using the continuity equation, the calculated AVA is 0.51 cm sq using the VTI method and 0.58 using the Vmax data.

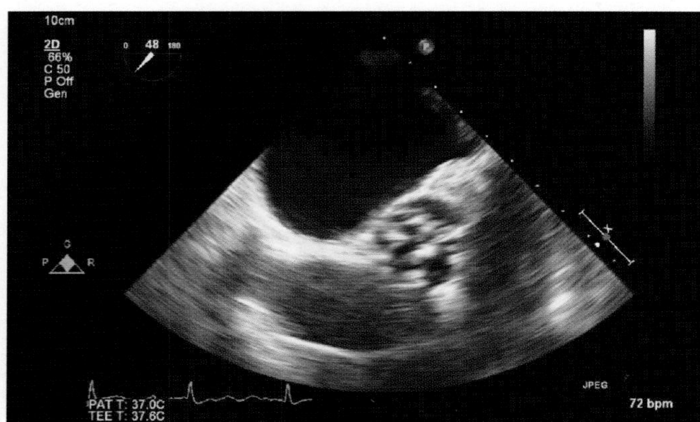

FIGURE 3-1-11 Intraoperative TEE prior to a TAVR demonstrating severe AS ▶ (see Video 3-1-11).

    - Careful attention to accurately measuring the LVOT diameter and sample volume placement for the LVOT velocity.
    - The preferred method is to use the LVOT and AV time velocity integrals; however, it is acceptable to substitute the respective peak velocities.
  - Calculation of the dimensionless index, the ratio of the LVOT velocity and the AV velocity (R). A ratio ≤0.25 suggests severe AS.
  - Planimetry of the AV orifice (R).

- The frequency of serial echocardiograms depends upon the initial study data, the severity of the AS, and the patient's symptoms.[1]
  - For patients with mild aortic stenosis, an echocardiogram is recommended every 3 to 5 years.
  - For patients with moderate aortic stenosis, the recommendation is for echocardiography every 1 to 2 years.
  - For patients with severe aortic stenosis, an annual echocardiogram is appropriate.
- New or changing symptoms or a significant change in physical exam findings should prompt an echocardiogram.
- Transesophageal echocardiography plays a limited role in the diagnosis and management of patients with aortic stenosis. In selected patients with discordant clinical, echocardiographic, and catheterization data, TEE may be useful to better define the AV anatomy.
  - TEE is used for intraprocedural monitoring of patients undergoing aortic valve replacement (AVR), both surgical and with transcatheter AVR. It also has a role in the management of patients with suspected AV endocarditis and prosthetic valve dysfunction.

OTHER DIAGNOSTIC TESTING AND PROCEDURES[1,10]

- Cardiac catheterization should be performed in most cases only to evaluate the patient for concomitant coronary artery disease in anticipation of surgery. In patients with equivocal

TABLE 3-1-2 Selected Echocardiographic Parameters for the Evaluation of Aortic Stenosis

Parameter	Advantages	Disadvantages
AS jet velocity	Direct measure.	Requires careful alignment of ultrasound beam.
	Strongest predictor of outcome.	Flow dependent.
Mean gradient	Averaged from velocity curve.	Accuracy depends on accurate velocity data.
	Values comparable to invasive measures.	Flow dependent.
Continuity equation (VTI)	Measures effective orifice area.	Measurement error more likely.
	Relatively flow independent.	Requires LVOTd measurement as well as LVOT and AV velocity measurements.
	Feasible in most patients.	
Simplified continuity equation	Uses more easily measured velocities.	Similar to above.
		Assumes LVOT and AV velocity curves are similar in shape.
Velocity ratio	Doppler-only.	Limited longitudinal data.
	No need to measure LVOT.	Ignores LVOT size variability.
	Less variability than continuity equation.	
Planimetry	Useful if Doppler data not available.	Difficult with severe valve calcification.
		Anatomic and effective valve areas may be different.

Adapted with permisison from Baumgartner H, Hung J, Bermejo J, Chambers JB, Evangelista A, Griffin BP et. al. Echocardiographic assessment of valve stenosis: EAE/ASE recommendations for clinical practice. *J Am Soc Echocardiogr.* 2009;22(1):1-23.[10]

echocardiographic findings or discrepancies between clinical examination findings and the echocardiogram, cardiac catheterization with hemodynamic assessment to determine aortic valve gradient and valve area may be warranted.

- In patients with congenital aortic valve pathology (eg, bicuspid valves) or in patients with suspected aortopathy, further imaging of the aorta may be warranted using either cardiac magnetic resonance angiography or CT scanning.
- Exercise testing in asymptomatic patients may be useful to identify symptoms and risk stratify the patient. The identification of a limited functional capacity, the development of symptoms, an abnormal blood pressure response, or significant dysrhythmias may prompt more serious consideration for AVR in the asymptomatic patient. Stress testing (other than a dobutamine stress test to assess low gradient AS) is contraindicated in the patient with symptomatic AS.

DIFFERENTIAL DIAGNOSIS

- While the symptoms of aortic stenosis may be caused by a variety of cardiac diseases, including ischemic heart disease (angina), cardiomyopathies of a variety of etiologies (dyspnea/CHF), and syncope (dysrhythmias, HCM), once the diagnosis of AS is made, symptoms are usually attributed to the aortic valve disease.
- In patients with concomitant cardiac diseases such as coronary artery disease, other valvular heart disease, or other co-morbidities (eg, COPD), it may be difficult to ascribe symptoms entirely to the valve.
- On rare occasions, it may be difficult to determine the exact location of a stenosis (eg, a subaortic membrane, hypertrophic cardiomyopathy, supravalvar AS). Careful echocardiographic assessment, along with data from other imaging modalities, is warranted.

DIAGNOSIS

- The diagnosis of AS is made by a combination history, physical examination, and echocardiography.
- The severity of AS is based primarily on echocardiographic data (Table 3-1-3).
- Patients with a low cardiac output may have severe AS with a lower mean gradient (low-output or low-gradient AS). Dobutamine echocardiography may be used to better define the AV pathology and assess for contractile reserve in the patient with a low EF.
- On rare occasions, cardiac catheterization with hemodynamic assessment is needed to determine the severity of AS.
- Cardiac MRI and cardiac CT play a limited role in the diagnostic assessment of AS.
- All patients should have an ECG and chest x-ray as part of the initial diagnostic evaluation.

MANAGEMENT[1]

- The management of patients with severe symptomatic aortic stenosis is relatively straightforward. Assuming a patient is a candidate for surgery, surgical replacement of the aortic valve is warranted expeditiously. For patients who are felt to be either high risk or in whom surgery is contraindicated, percutaneous aortic valve replacement is becoming an option. At the present time, two transcatheter valves are available for clinical use in the United States for inoperable ("extreme risk") and high risk patients with severe symptomatic AS. Both the Medtronic CoreValve and the Edwards SAPIEN Valve have received FDA approval in the United States for use in selected individuals. Transcatheter valve technology is rapidly developing and newer devices, as well as expanded indications for current valves, are undergoing active clinical investigation.
- The management of patients with asymptomatic aortic stenosis remains somewhat controversial. Some authors advocate elective aortic valve replacement to prevent sudden cardiac death. Others recommend a watchful waiting approach. The role of BNP testing and stress testing remains somewhat controversial as well, though stress testing is being utilized more frequently. Annual echocardiography is warranted, as is careful clinical observation and follow-up.
- The only effective treatment for AS is valve replacement surgery (or for selected individuals, transcatheter-based AV replacement).
  - AVR should be recommended in symptomatic patients, patients undergoing other cardiac surgical procedures such as coronary artery bypass grafting, and asymptomatic patients with an LV ejection fraction <50%.
  - AVR should be considered in the asymptomatic patient with an abnormal stress test, patients with severe valve calcification, and in individuals who demonstrate rapid progression of the

TABLE 3-1-3 Classification of the Severity of Aortic Stenosis

Parameter	Mild AS	Moderate AS	Severe AS
Jet velocity	2.0-2.9 m/sec	3-3.9 m/sec	≥4.0 m/sec
Mean gradient (mm Hg)	<20	20-39 mm Hg	≥40 mm Hg
Valve area (cm^2)	>1.5 cm^2	1.0-1.5 cm^2	≤1 cm^2
Valve area index (cm^2/m^2)			≤0.6

Adapted with permisison from Bonow RO, Carabello BA. Chattterjee K, de Leon AC Jr, Faxon DP, Freed MD, et.al. 2008 focused update incorporated in to the ACC/AHA 2006 guidelines for the management of patients with valvular heart disease: a report of the American College of Cardiology/American Heart Association Task Force on Practice Guidelines (writing committee to develop guidelines for the management of patients with valvular heart disease). *J Am Coll Cardiol.* 2008;52(13):e1-e142.[1]

valve stenosis, as well as individuals who may experience a delay between symptom onset and surgery.

- There currently is no role for "medical therapy" in the management of patients with AS, other than to manage symptoms in patients who are not candidates or who refuse surgery.
- While there was some initial data suggesting that statin therapy could delay the progression of AS, current evidence suggests that statins do not prevent progression of AS.[12,13]
- Antibiotic prophylaxis to prevent infective endocarditis is no longer recommended for patients with native valve AS.[1,14]
    - Patients with rheumatic valve disease should be given appropriate prophylaxis to prevent recurrent rheumatic fever.

FOLLOW-UP[1]

- In patients with severe, asymptomatic aortic stenosis and in whom surgery is deferred, very careful clinical follow-up is warranted. Such patients should be seen frequently and extensively questioned as to the development of symptoms including angina, dyspnea, or heart failure and syncope. Careful attention to subtle changes in their functional capacity should be elicited as well. The development of any symptoms related to their valvular heart disease is an indication for proceeding to valve replacement.
- Patients with severe AS should undergo an echocardiogram on an annual basis to define changes in left ventricular function as well as progression of their aortic valve disease. Echocardiographic findings that should prompt consideration of valve replacement (even with no symptoms) include rapid progression of the valvular stenosis and deterioration of LV function.
- Postoperatively, patients who have undergone aortic valve replacement warrant continued clinical follow-up on an annual basis, surveillance for symptoms, management of anticoagulation, and endocarditis prophylaxis for dental procedures in accordance with the recently revised AHA guidelines.[1,14]
- All patients should undergo a baseline echocardiogram post AVR. This serves to establish the normal (expected) parameters for the individual patient's valve as well as the baseline LV function and concomitant cardiac abnormalities.
    - Routine serial or annual echocardiography is not warranted in the absence of symptoms.[1,3]
    - In patients with a biological valve, annual echocardiograms may be considered after 10 years.[1]
    - In selected patients with a mechanical or bioprosthetic valve, earlier echocardiography (≥3 years) may be appropriate.[3]
    - In patients with a prosthetic valve, more frequent echocardiography may be appropriate if the patient has other cardiac disease that would warrant more frequent assessment by echocardiography.
- Echocardiography should be performed if patients develop symptoms possibly related to their prosthetic valve or changes in their physical examination.

VIDEO LEGENDS

1. Video 3-1-1: Parasternal Long axis view demonstrating LVH, a heavily calcified, immobile AV as well as mitral valve thickening and annular calcification
2. Video 3-1-2: Parasternal short axis view of the heavily calcified aortic valve
3. Video 3-1-3: Apical 4-chamber view demonstrating LVH and preserved LV ejection fraction
4. Video 3-1-4: Parasternal long axis view with color Doppler demonstrating mild aortic regurgitation as well as mitral insufficiency
5. Video 3-1-7: Parasternal long axis view of a different patient demonstrating a heavily calcified, restricted AV
6. Video 3-1-11: Intraoperative TEE prior to a TAVR demonstrating severe AS

REFERENCES

1. Nishimura RA, Otto CM, Bonow RO, et al. 2014 AHA/ACC guideline for the management of patients with valvular heart disease:executive summary; a report of the American College of Cardiology/American Heart Association Task Force on Practice Guidelines. *J Am Coll Cardiol.* 2014;63:2348-2388.
2. Cheitlin MD, Armstrong WF, Aurigemma GP, et al. ACC/AHA/ASE 2003 guideline update for the clinical application of echocardiography- summary article A report of the American College of Cardiology/American Heart Association Task Force on practice guidelines. (ACC/AHA/ASE 2003 Committee to Update the 1997 Guidelines for the Clinical Application of Echocardiography). *J Am Coll Cardiol.* 2003;42:954-970.
3. Douglas PS, Garcia MJ, Haines DE, et al. ACCF/ASE/AHA/ASNC/HFSA/HRS/SCAI/SCCM/SCCT/SCMR 2011 appropriate US criteria for echocardiography: a report of the American College of Cardiology Foundation Appropriate Use Criteria Task Force, American Society of Echocardiography, American Heart Association, American Society of Nuclear Cardiology, Heart Failure Society of America, Heart Rhythm Society, Society of Cardiovascular Angiography and Interventions, Society of Critical Care Medicine, Society of Cardiovascular Computed Tomography, and Society of Cardiovascular Magnetic Resonance. *J Am Coll Cardiol.* 2011;57(9):1126-1166. doi: 10.1016/j.jacc.2010.11.002.
4. Holen J, Simonsen S. Determination of pressure gradient in mitral stenosis with Doppler echocardiography. *Br Heart J.* 1979;41:529-535.
5. Hatle L, Angelsen B, Tromsdal A. Noninvasive assessment of aortic stenosis by Doppler ultrasound. *Br Heart J.* 1979;43:284-292.
6. Ross J Jr, Braunwald E. Aortic stenosis. *Circulation.* 1968;38:61-67.
7. Freeman RV, Otto CM. Spectrum of calcific aortic valve disease: pathogenesis, disease progression, and treatment strategies. *Circulation.* 2005;111:3316-3326.
8. Lindroos M, Kupari M, Heikkila, Tilvis R. Prevalence of aortic valve abnormalities in the elderly: an echocardiographic study of a random population sample. *J Am Coll Cardiol.* 1993;21:1220-1225.

9. Otto CM, Lind BK, Kitzman DW, Gersh BJ, Siscovick DS. Association of aortic-valve sclerosis with cardiovascular mortality and morbidity in the elderly. *N Engl J Med*. 1999;341:142-147.

10. Baumgartner H, Hung J, Bermejo J, et al. Echocardiographic assessment of valve stenosis: EAE/ASE recommendations for clinical practice. *J Am Soc Echocardiogr*. 2009;22:1-23.

11. Roberts WC, Ko JM. Frequency by decades of unicuspid, bicuspid, and tricuspid aortic valves in adults having isolated aortic valve replacement for aortic stenosis, with or without associated aortic regurgitation. *Circulation*. 2005;111:920-925.

12. Rosenhek R, Rader F, Loho N, et al. Statins but not angiotensin-converting enzyme inhibitors delay progression of aortic stenosis. *Circulation*. 2004;110:1291-1295.

13. Chan KL, Teo K, Dumesnil JG, Ni A, Tam J, ASTRONOMER Investigators. Effect of lipid lowering with rosuvastatin on progression of aortic stenosis: results of the aortic stenosis progression observation: measuring effects of rosuvastatin (ASTRONOMER) trial. *Circulation*. 2010;121:306-314.

14. Wilson W, Taubert KA, Gewitz M, et al. Prevention of infective endocarditis: Guidelines from the American Heart Association: a guideline from the American Heart Association Rheumatic Fever, Endocarditis, and Kawasaki Disease Committee, Council on Cardiovascular Disease in the Young, and the Council on Clinical Cardiology, Council on Cardiovascular Surgery and Anesthesia, and the Quality of Care and Outcomes Research Interdisciplinary Working Group. *Circulation*. 2007;116:1736-1754.

SECTION 2

Low-Output, Low-Gradient Aortic Stenosis

Kavita Sharma, MD

PATIENT STORY (CLINICAL CASE PRESENTATION)

A 53-year-old white male with a history of hypertension and obesity presented with a chief complaint of dyspnea on exertion and leg swelling. His symptoms began two years ago. He has had no medication changes. He reported a history of a heart murmur but had not sought medical attention or follow-up in several years.

His physical examination demonstrates jugular venous distension, a normal S_1, with a soft A_2 component of S_2, an S_3 gallop, and a faint 2/6 late-peaking systolic murmur heard best at the right upper sternal border. There were bilateral crackles at the bases of the lungs, a distended abdomen, and 2+ bilateral pitting edema below the knees. His electrocardiogram demonstrated normal sinus rhythm and an isolated premature atrial contraction. An echocardiogram revealed a severely dilated left ventricle, with severe global left ventricular dysfunction, a left ventricular ejection fraction of 10%, and a calcified, restricted aortic valve with a mean aortic gradient of 22 mm Hg (Figures 3-2-1 to 3-2-6). He underwent cardiac catheterization, which demonstrated no obstructive coronary artery disease, a mean aortic gradient of 26 mm Hg, and a calculated aortic valve area of 1.0 cm^2.

To further clarify the severity of the aortic stenosis (AS) in the setting of low cardiac output and to test for contractile reserve, the patient underwent dobutamine stress echocardiography. With dobutamine infusion (Table 3-2-1), the calculated aortic valve area remained essentially unchanged, the mean gradient increased to 36 mm Hg, and contractile reserve was present, as demonstrated by an increase in the LVOT VTI and an improvement in EF. The patient was referred for surgery and had successful mechanical aortic valve replacement. Postoperatively, he reported an improvement in his symptoms. Postoperative echocardiogram demonstrated improved left ventricular function (Figure 3-2-7).

PATHOPHYSIOLOGY AND ETIOLOGY

- Severe AS is defined as an aortic valve area less than or equal to 1.0 cm^2, mean aortic gradient greater than or equal to 40 mm Hg, or a jet velocity greater than or equal to 4.0 M per second.[1]
- Severe AS may be present with a lower transvalvular gradient and velocity if the cardiac output is low.[1]
- The most common causes of AS are calcification of a normal trileaflet aortic valve or a congenital bicuspid valve.[1] The obstruction generally develops gradually, and the left ventricle adapts with increasing hypertrophy.[2] If the hypertrophy is inadequate to compensate for the increasing pressure, a decrease in ejection fraction occurs.[3]
- Alternatively, a depressed ejection fraction may represent a cardiomyopathy. It can be difficult to determine whether the low ejection fraction is secondary to the cardiomyopathy or due to the valve stenosis.[4] In either situation, the low cardiac output and low gradient

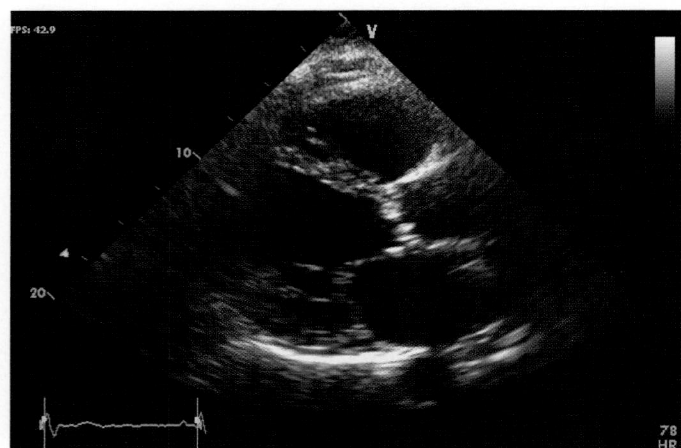

FIGURE 3-2-1 Parasternal long axis view demonstrating a calcified, restricted AV and a dilated LV with severely depressed LV function ► (see Video 3-2-1).

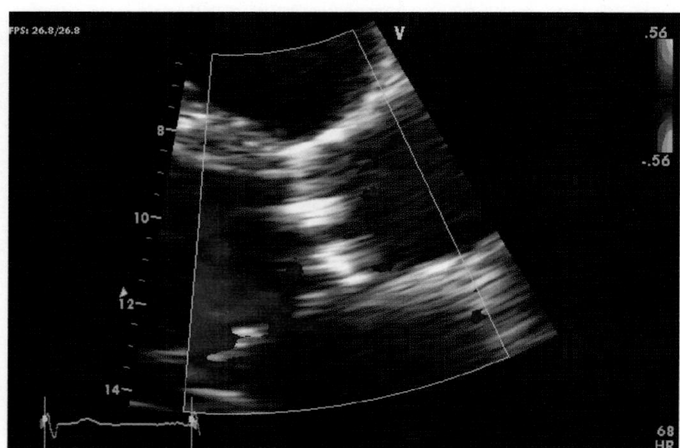

FIGURE 3-2-2 Parasternal long axis, focused on the aortic valve, demonstrating a calcified, restricted aortic valve. Color Doppler demonstrates no aortic regurgitation ► (see Video 3-2-2).

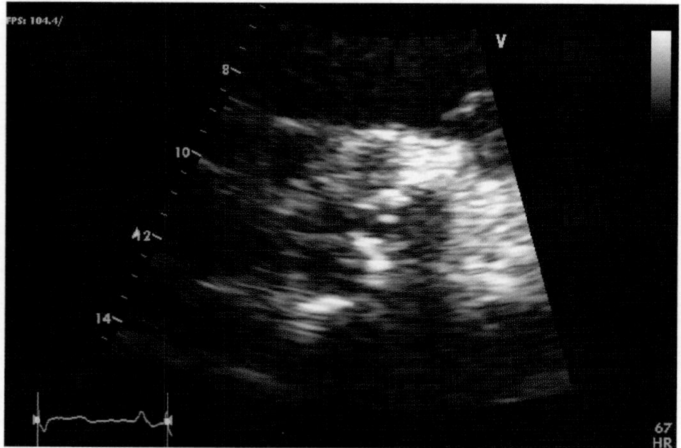

FIGURE 3-2-3 Parasternal short axis of the aortic valve, demonstrating calcified, restricted leaflets ► (see Video 3-2-3).

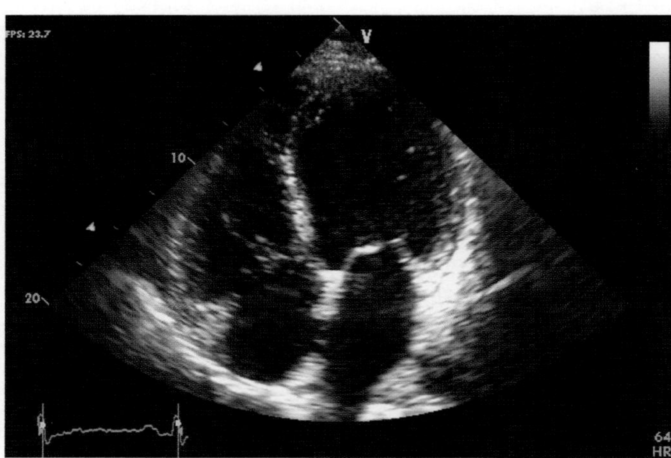

3-2-4 Apical 4 chamber view demonstrating severely decreased LV function as well as RV dysfunction ► (see Video 3-2-4).

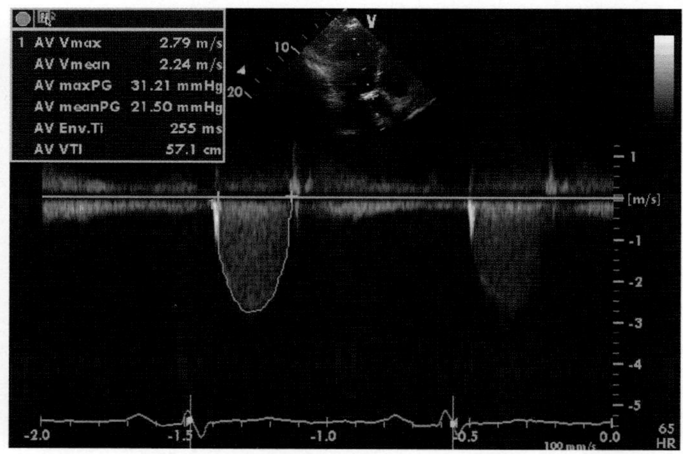

FIGURE 3-2-5 Continuous-wave Doppler across the aortic valve demonstrating a mean gradient of 22 mm Hg.

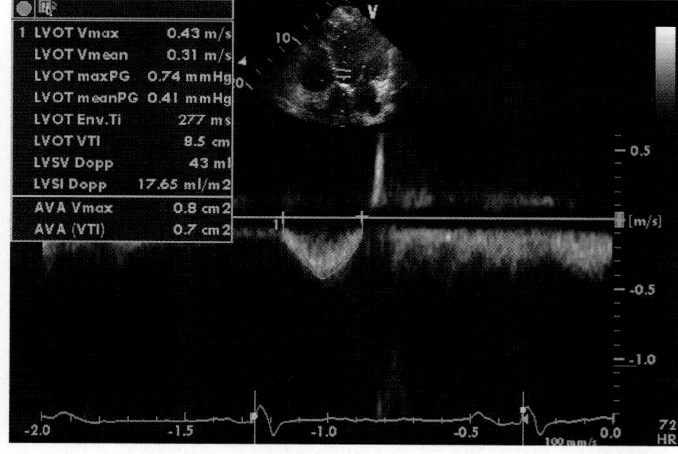

FIGURE 3-2-6 Pulse wave Doppler at the LVOT, measuring the LVOT TVI, used in determining the dimensionless index and calculating the AV area. In this patient, the LVOT VTI is quite low, consistent with low stroke volume.

TABLE 3-2-1 Dobutamine Stress Echo Results

	Baseline	5 mcg/kg	10 mcg/kg	20 mcg/kg
Mean AV gradient (mm Hg)	21	26	34	36
AV peak gradient (mm Hg)	31	33	54	65
LVOT TVI (cm)	9	10	10	14
AV TVI (cm)	57	62	64	75
AV area (cm sq)	0.6	0.6	0.6	0.7

AV: Aortic Valve; LVOT: Left ventricular outflow tract; VTI: Velocity time Integral; AV area based on VTI method with a measured LVOT diameter = 2.2 cm

contribute to a calculated effective valve area that can meet criteria for severe AS.[1]

- Aortic valve replacement for severe AS in the setting of a normal ejection fraction carries a risk of mortality of less than 1%.[5] The risk increases in the setting of a low ejection fraction.[5] If the low ejection fraction is caused by a depressed contractility (primary myopathic process) as opposed to severe AS, surgery will be less beneficial.[6]

EPIDEMIOLOGY

- AS is the most common valvular abnormality in the United States. However, of those patients with AS, only 5% are comprised of the subset of patients with low ejection fraction and a low aortic valve gradient.[5]

ECHOCARDIOGRAPHY

- Echocardiography, including Doppler echocardiography, is employed to assess the presence/severity of AS (see Section I: Asymptomatic Severe Aortic Stenosis).
- A complete transthoracic echocardiogram should be performed in patients with low-gradient, low-output AS, similar to those with AS and a normal ejection fraction. The extent of valve calcification and the status of the other valves should be assessed.
- In cases of low-gradient, low-output AS in the setting of impaired ejection fraction, Dobutamine echocardiography can be utilized. It is a class IIa indication in the ACC/AHA Guidelines for the Management of Patients with Valvular Heart Disease.[1]
- Dobutamine echocardiography may distinguish between truly severely stenotic AS and resultant low ejection fraction from only mild to moderate AS with a concurrently depressed ejection fraction (due to a cardiomyopathy).
  - Dobutamine echocardiography can determine whether contractile reserve, defined as the appearance of increased contractility with dobutamine infusion, is present. The presence or absence of contractile reserve provides important prognostic information with regard to operative mortality.
  - Baseline echocardiographic images are obtained, and include the left ventricular outflow tract (LVOT) diameter, the LVOT time velocity integral (TVI), the LVOT velocity, the aortic valve (AV) TVI, the AV velocity, and the AV mean gradient.
  - The left ventricular ejection fraction (LVEF) is obtained at baseline.
  - Dobutamine infusion is begun at 2.5 to 5 micrograms/kg/min and is sequentially increased in 5 micrograms/kg/min increments (every 3-5 minutes) to a maximum of 20 micrograms/kg/min. The hemodynamic information and reassessment of the LVEF are obtained at each stage.
  - If, with dobutamine infusion, the aortic valve area increases, the gradient remains the same, and there is an increase in stroke volume, then severe AS is unlikely.[1,5] If, however, with dobutamine infusion, the aortic valve area remains the same, with increased gradient and an increase in stroke volume, then severe AS is likely.
  - In those patients with severe AS, dobutamine infusion will increase the LVOT velocity and the AV velocity proportionally; therefore, the ratio between LVOT velocity and the AV velocity will remain stable throughout the infusion. In those patients with milder AS, the LVOT velocity will increase more with dobutamine than the aortic valve velocity (due to the increase in the aortic valve area). Therefore the ratio between the LVOT velocity and the AV velocity will increase.
  - If the stroke volume increases by more than 20%, then contractile reserve is present. Patients who fail to demonstrate contractile

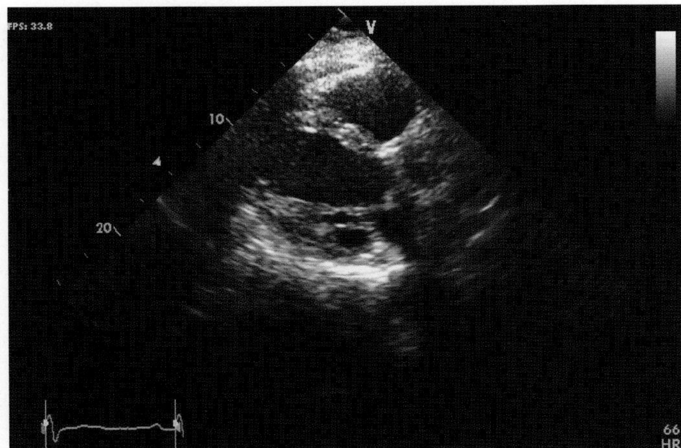

FIGURE 3-2-7 Postoperative parasternal long axis, demonstrating improvement in LV function and the presence of a bio-prosthetic AV ► (see Video 3-2-7).

reserve have a very poor prognosis with surgery as compared to those patients with contractile reserve (32%-33% versus 5%-8%).[7-10]

OTHER DIAGNOSTIC TESTING AND PROCEDURES

- Echocardiography without dobutamine and cardiac catheterization hemodynamic assessments without dobutamine are often performed in the patient with low-gradient, low-output AS. Both have inherent flaws in their ability to define the severity of AS in the setting of low cardiac output.
- In echocardiography, the continuity equation is used to estimate aortic valve area; however, it relies on the LVOT TVI and AV TVI, both of which are based on the cardiac output.
- In cardiac catheterization hemodynamic assessments, the calculated valve area is proportional to the stroke volume. Furthermore, the constant in the Gorlin formula varies with transvalvular flow.[11,12]
- As an alternative to dobutamine echocardiography, a dobutamine challenge may be performed in the cardiac catheterization laboratory, and a similar assessment of the aortic valve area, gradient, and the cardiac output may be obtained.[1,8]
- Prior to undergoing open-heart surgery, coronary angiography should be performed to assess for the presence of concomitant coronary artery disease and the need for coronary bypass grafting at the time of surgery.

MANAGEMENT

- Aortic valve replacement is (either surgical AVR or transcatheter aortic valve replacement [TAVR], depending on surgical risk) indicated for symptomatic patients with severe AS and for patients with severe AS and an ejection fraction less than 50%.[1]
- Those patients with low output severe AS and contractile reserve have a better outcome with aortic valve replacement than medical therapy and should undergo replacement.[1,5]
- In those patients with low output severe AS and no evidence of contractile reserve, the choice is a difficult one; either face an operative mortality of 32% to 33% or an abysmal prognosis without surgery.[13]

FOLLOW-UP AND PATIENT EDUCATION

- In patients who are not candidates for surgery, careful clinical follow-up and treatment of congestive heart failure is appropriate. Their prognosis is poor.
- Patients who undergo AVR should be followed clinically and undergo follow-up echocardiography as detailed elsewhere in this chapter. Endocarditis prophylaxis is indicated in patients post-AVR.

SUMMARY

- In patients with severe symptomatic AS, AVR is the preferred treatment. In the setting of severe AS and a low ejection fraction, AVR is also recommended.
- In those patients with low-gradient, low-output AS, further investigation is required. Dobutamine echocardiography can differentiate those patients with truly severely stenotic AS from those with a cardiomyopathy and only mild to moderate AS. Additionally, assessment of contractile reserve can be performed with dobutamine echocardiography, further risk-stratifying patients for surgery.

VIDEO LEGENDS

1. Video 3-2-1: Parasternal long axis view demonstrating a calcified, restricted AV and a dilated LV with severely depressed LV function
2. Video 3-2-2: Parasternal long axis, focused on the aortic valve, demonstrating a calcified, restricted aortic valve. No aortic regurgitation is seen with color Doppler.
3. Video 3-2-3: Parasternal short axis of the aortic valve, demonstrating calcified, restricted leaflets
4. Video 3-2-4: Apical four-chamber view demonstrating severely decreased LV function as well as RV dysfunction
5. Video 3-2-7: Post-operative parasternal long axis, demonstrating improvement in LV function and the presence of a bio-prosthetic AV

REFERENCES

1. Nishimura RA, Otto CM, Bonow RO, et al. 2014 AHA/ACC guideline for the management of patients with valvular heart disease:executive summary; a report of the American College of Cardiology/American Heart Association Task Force on Practice Guidelines. *J Am Coll Cardiol.* 2014;63:2348-2388.
2. Spann JF, Bove AA, Natarajan G, Kreulen T. Ventricular performance, pump function and compensatory mechanisms in patients with aortic stenosis. *Circulation.* 1980;62:576-582.
3. Krayenbuehl HP, Hess OM, Ritter M, Monrad ES, Hoppeler H. Left ventricular systolic function in aortic stenosis. *Eur Heart J.* 1988;9 Suppl E:19-23.
4. Huber D, Grimm J, Koch R, Krayenbuehl HP. Determinants of ejection performance in aortic stenosis. *Circulation.* 1981;64:126-134.
5. Martinez MW, Nishimura RA. Approach to the patient with aortic stenosis and low ejection fraction. *Curr Cardiol Rep.* 2006;8:90-95.
6. Carabello BA, Green LH, Grossman W, Cohn LH, Koster JK, Collins JJ Jr. Hemodynamic determinants of prognosis of aortic valve replacement in critical aortic stenosis and advanced congestive heart failure. *Circulation.* 1980;62:42-48.
7. Monin JL, Monchi M, Gest V, Duval-Moulin AM, Dubois-Rande JL, Gueret P. Aortic stenosis with severe left ventricular dysfunction and low transvalvular pressure gradients: risk stratification by low-dose dobutamine echocardiography. *J Am Coll Cardiol.* 2001;37:2101-2107.
8. Nishimura RA, Grantham JA, Connolly HM, Schaff HV, Higano ST, Holmes DR Jr. Low-output, low-gradient aortic stenosis in patients with depressed left ventricular systolic function: the clinical utility of the dobutamine challenge in the catheterization laboratory. *Circulation.* 2002;106:809-813.
9. Monin JL, Quere JP, Monchi M, et al. Low-gradient aortic stenosis: operative risk stratification and predictors for

long-term outcome: a multicenter study using dobutamine stress hemodynamics. *Circulation*. 2003;108:319-324.

10. Quere JP, Monin JL, Levy F, et al. Influence of preoperative left ventricular contractile reserve on postoperative ejection fraction in low-gradient aortic stenosis. *Circulation*. 2006;113:1738-1744.
11. Burwash IG, Thomas DD, Sadahiro M, et al. Dependence of Gorlin formula and continuity equation valve areas on transvalvular volume flow rate in valvular aortic stenosis. *Circulation*. 1994;89:827-835.
12. Cannon SR, Richards KL, Crawford M. Hydraulic estimation of stenotic orifice area: a correction of the Gorlin formula. *Circulation*. 1985;71:1170-1178.
13. Lange RA, Hillis LD. Dobutamine stress echocardiography in patients with low-gradient aortic stenosis. *Circulation*. 2006;113:1718-1720.

SECTION 3

Aortic Valve Stenosis: Bicuspid Aortic Valve

Gina G. Mentzer, MD

CLINICAL CASE PRESENTATION

A 31-year-old man with a history of hypertension and obesity presented to an outpatient clinic appointment at The Ohio State University's Wexner Medical Center with complaints of chest heaviness upon exercise and dizziness going up three flights of stairs. He denied any episodes of syncope. He has noticed this over the past 3 months and limited his exercise routine. He denies orthopnea, lower extremity edema, or paroxysmal nocturnal dyspnea (PND). He has been told during his high school physical exam that he had a heart murmur but did not have any further follow-up or cardiac evaluation.

On exam, he was an overweight man. His blood pressure (BP) was 160/100 mm Hg. His cardiac exam revealed an early medium-pitched, systolic ejection click and a 3/6 systolic ejection murmur in the upper right sternal border. In addition, a faint, high-pitched early diastolic decrescendo murmur was heard along the left sternal border. Simultaneous palpation of his radial and femoral arteries demonstrated a delay in the femoral arterial pulse. His exam was felt to be consistent with a bicuspid aortic valve (AV) with aortic stenosis (AS) and aortic regurgitation (AR) as well as coarctation of the aorta. This was confirmed with echocardiography (Figures 3-3-1 to 3-3-4). He also underwent an MRA of his aorta (Figure 3-3-5), which demonstrated a mildly dilated ascending aorta as well as evidence of aortic coarctation. He was felt to have mild to moderate AS. He underwent percutaneous treatment of his coarctation with a stent with an improvement in his BP as well as his symptoms. He will be followed with serial examinations and echocardiography for his AV disease, as well as serial MRA of his aorta.

CLINICAL FEATURES OF AORTIC STENOSIS

- Most patients are asymptomatic until the stenosis becomes severe. They are often detected when a murmur is appreciated on physical examination.
  - In asymptomatic patients, confirmation of the etiology of the murmur and the severity of the valvular heart disease with echocardiography is warranted.
  - In athletes (as was the case in our patient), when a murmur is detected on examination for sports participation, further investigation is warranted.
- Dyspnea on exertion is the most prevalent presenting feature.
- Approximately 50% of patients develop symptoms of heart failure (HF), including dyspnea, orthopnea, paroxysmal nocturnal dyspnea, fatigue, cough, and weight gain.
- Around 35% develop angina pectoris, especially with exertion.
- Although more rare, 15% develop exertional dizziness or syncope that can be quite limiting.
- Features of heart failure including elevated jugular venous distention (JVD), hepatomegaly, and an S_3 gallop that may be appreciated on physical examination.
- Physical exam may demonstrate a pulsus parvus et tardus, crescendo-decrescendo harsh, systolic ejection murmur at the upper right sternal border that radiates into carotids bilaterally and may be associated with an early systolic ejection click.

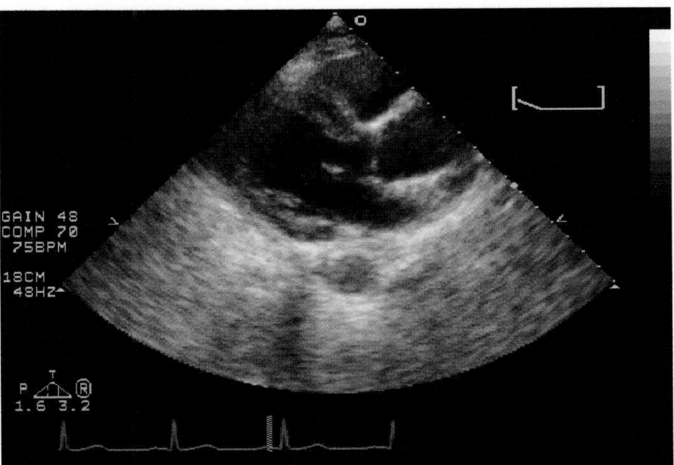

FIGURE 3-3-1 Parasternal long axis view demonstrates a mildly thickened AV with mild aortic root dilation ► (see Video 3-3-1).

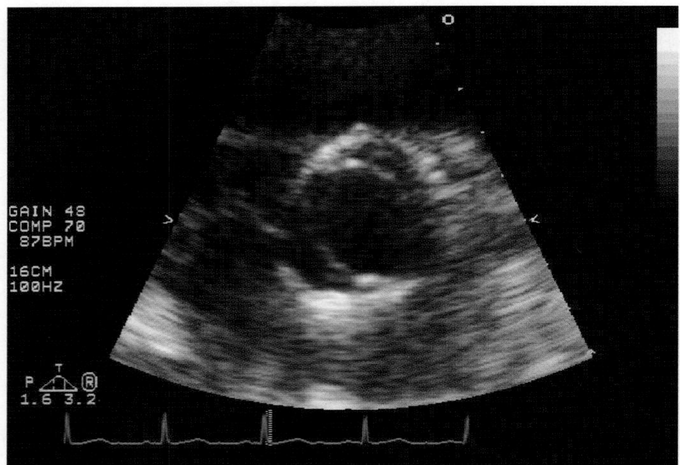

FIGURE 3-3-2 Zoomed parasternal short axis view of the bicuspid AV ► (see Video 3-3-2).

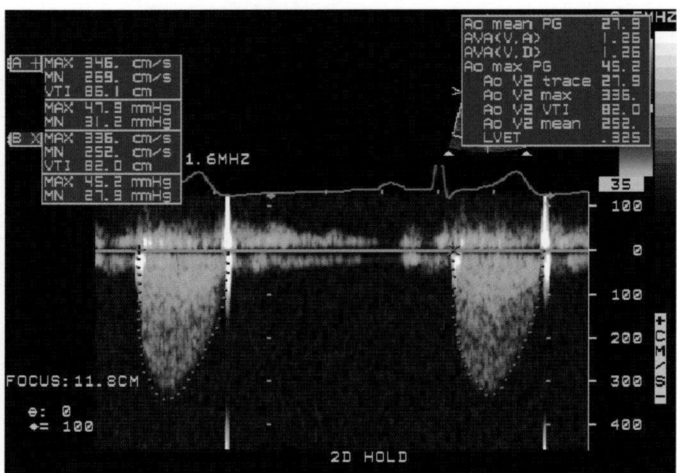

FIGURE 3-3-4 Continuous-wave Doppler demonstrating the peak and mean gradients across the AV in our patient. The average peak (46 mm Hg) and mean (29 mm Hg) gradients as well as the calculated AVA (1.26 cm sq) are noted.

EPIDEMIOLOGY

- Bicuspid AV is present in as many as 1% to 2% of the population, but it is often underestimated and undetected as it can remain silent during infancy, childhood, and adolescence. In many cases, it is an incidental finding unless significant stenosis is present or infective endocarditis occurs. It is most commonly found in men age 50 or younger and affects males in a 2:1 or greater preponderance.
- In developed countries, a bicuspid AV is the etiology of severe AS in approximately 50% of young adults with AS.
- Most cases are sporadic with familial clusters identified in 10% to 17% in first-degree relatives of probands. Bicuspid AV is associated with aortopathy (see Chapter 7, Section V: Aortopathy in Bicuspid Aortic Valve Disease). First degree relatives of probands should be screened for AV and aortic pathology. Recent evidence suggests autosomal dominant inheritance with variable penetrance.[1]

PATHOPHYSIOLOGY AND ETIOLOGY

- It is related to abnormal embryologic development and associated with syndromes such as coarctation of the aorta (>50% with a bicuspid AV), Williams syndrome (11.6% with supravalvular aortic stenosis), and Turner syndrome (30% have bicuspid AV).[2-4]
- Findings are typically one complete line of coaptation. Most have a fusion of the raphe between the right and left coronary cusps (86%) and of the raphe between the left and non-coronary cusps (3%).[5]
- With aging, the valve can have sclerosis, calcification, and degeneration with symptoms of critical AS and heart failure. One-third

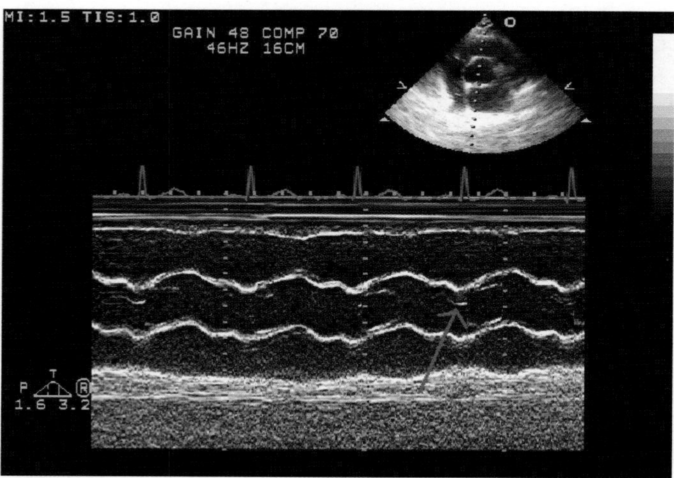

FIGURE 3-3-3 M-mode of the AV demonstrates an eccentric diastolic closure line of the AV leaflets consistent with a bicuspid AV.

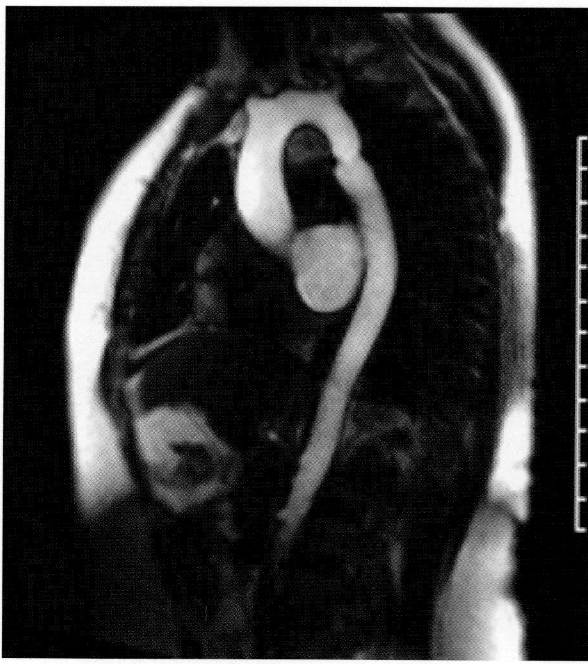

FIGURE 3-3-5 MRA of the aorta in the patient with a bicuspid valve, demonstrating a dilated ascending aorta and coarctation of the aorta.

of patients over the age of 20 have complications including aortic regurgitation (AR) if they present with AS symptoms at a younger age.[6]

ECHOCARDIOGRAPHY

A complete echocardiographic evaluation is suggested as a class I recommendation by the American College of Cardiology and American Heart Association (ACC/AHA).[7] This assessment utilizes a combination of short-axis (SAX) and long-axis (LAX) images to identify the number of leaflets as well as leaflet mobility, thickness, and calcification. Two-dimensional imaging and Doppler echocardiography are utilized to determine the level of obstruction, left ventricular (LV) function, and associated lesions.

Using transthoracic echocardiogram (TTE), the following structural parameters are assessed:

- Diagnosis is most often reliable in the parasternal SAX when the two cusps are seen in systole with only two commissures framing an elliptical systolic orifice (Figure 3-3-2).
- Parasternal long-axis (PLAX) demonstrates a thickened AV with systolic doming of the leaflets. In some cases, dilatation of the ascending aorta may be seen. There may be associated aortic regurgitation as well.
- M-mode in the parasternal long axis view demonstrates an eccentric diastolic closure line of the AV leaflets (Figure 3-3-3).
- Standard hemodynamic valvular measurements include AS jet velocity, mean transaortic gradient, and valve area by the continuity equation.[8]
- Evaluate LV size, function, and wall thickness.
- Evaluate for coexisting lesions such as AR, coarctation of the aorta, ventricular septal defect (VSD), patent ductus arteriosus, aortic aneurysm, aortic dissection, infective endocarditis, and Shone's complex.
- 3-D echocardiography may enhance visualization.

Transesophageal Echocardiogram (TEE)

- TEE can be used when improved visualization/clarification of valve anatomy is needed (Figures 3-3-6 and 3-3-7).

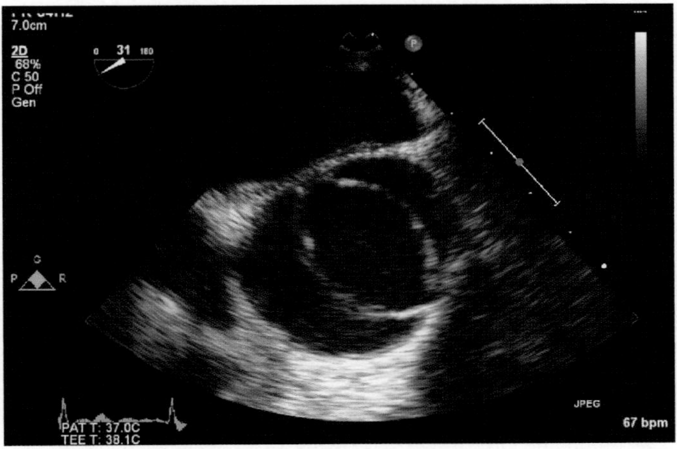

FIGURE 3-3-6 TEE short axis view of a bicuspid AV ▶ (see Video 3-3-6).

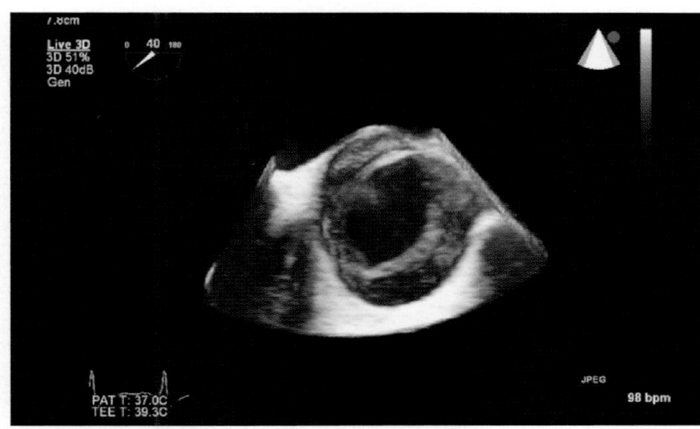

FIGURE 3-3-7 Three-dimensional TEE from a different patient demonstrating fusion of the right and left AV cusps ▶ (see Video 3-3-7).

- TEE may also provide a better assessment of the aortic anatomy, though CT angiography or MRA of the aorta is more often employed as these modalities can provide an assessment of the entire aorta.
- TEE is indicated in cases of suspected endocarditis if the TTE images do not provide adequate information.

OTHER DIAGNOSTIC TESTING AND PROCEDURES

- Common ECG findings include left ventricular hypertrophy, left atrial enlargement, and atrial fibrillation.
- Computed tomography (CT), Magnetic Resonance Imaging (MRI), and Angiography (MRA) can be utilized for improved visualization of the valve (Figure 3-3-8) and, more importantly, the aorta.
- Invasive cardiac catheterization is recommended if echocardiography is nondiagnostic or discrepant with clinical findings to define the hemodynamic severity of the AS.

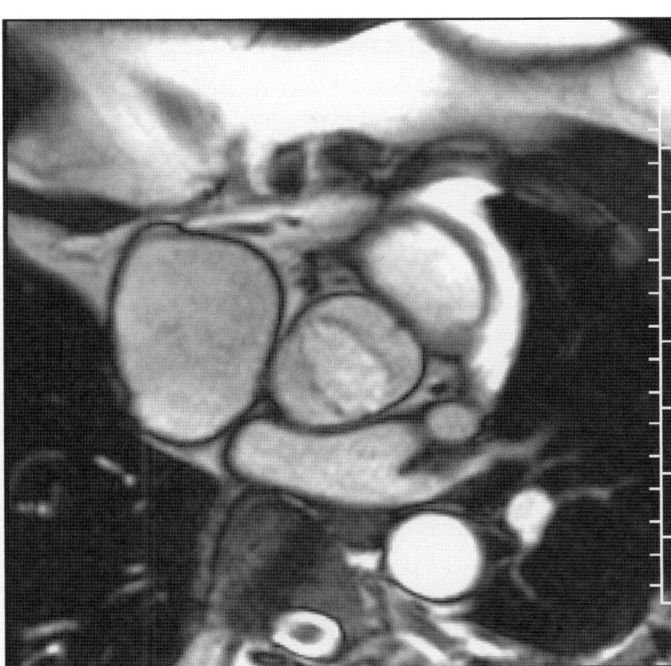

FIGURE 3-3-8 MRI of a bicuspid valve in a short axis view.

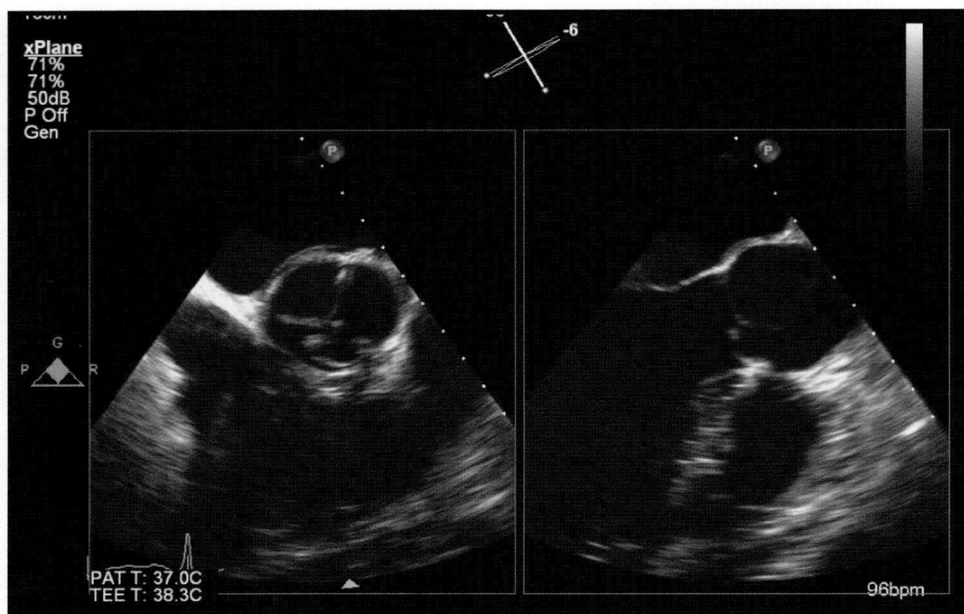

FIGURE 3-3-9 TEE X-plane view of a bicuspid AV ▶ (see Video 3-3-9) in another patient demonstrating prolapse of the fused right and left cusps. The patient had severe, eccentric AR.

DIAGNOSIS

- The presence of a congenital bicuspid AV is determined from clinical examination and history as well as direct visualization by echocardiography of the fused raphe on short axis imaging of the valve and the M-mode appearance.
- The classification of aortic stenosis severity is described in detail in Section 1 of this chapter.

Current European and US guidelines summarize these features in more detail for the interested reader.[7,9,10]

DIFFERENTIAL DIAGNOSIS

The differential diagnosis includes calcific aortic stenosis of a trileaflet valve, rheumatic heart disease, subaortic or supravalvular aortic stenosis, mitral valve prolapse, ventricular septal defect, and Ebstein anomaly.

MANAGEMENT

Medical Therapy

- Asymptomatic patients should be monitored for symptoms and progression of the underlying valve stenosis and aortic pathology.
- It is reasonable to give a β-adrenergic blocking agent to patients with bicuspid valves and dilated aortic roots (diameter greater than 40 mm) who are not candidates for surgical correction and who do not have moderate to severe AR.[7]

Imaging Surveillance

- Patients with bicuspid AV, jet velocity greater than 4.0 m/sec, or severe AR should have an annual TTE. For a jet velocity of 3.0 to 4.0 m/sec, or moderate AR, TTE should be done every 1 to 2 years. For a jet velocity of less than 3.0 m/sec and mild AR, surveillance with TTE should be done every 3 to 5 years.
- Patients with dilatation of the aortic root or ascending aorta (diameter greater than 4.0 cm) should undergo serial evaluation of aortic root/ascending aorta size and morphology by TTE, MRI, or CT on a yearly basis, or if symptoms suggest a clinical change.[7]
- Evaluation for aortopathy including coarctation should be done by CT or MRI (Figures 3-3-8).

Surgical Intervention

- AV replacement and/or aortic root repair or replacement is warranted based on the hemodynamic severity of the valve disease and the presence of significant aortic pathology.
- Criteria for bicuspid AV replacement are similar to those for other causes of severe AS. Patients with severe AS and symptoms (angina, syncope, CHF) warrant AV replacement (AVR).
- In the asymptomatic patient with severe AS due to a bicuspid AV, consider valve replacement if one or more of the following features is present: LVEF less than 50%, moderate-to-severe AR, abnormal exercise test shows poor functional capacity, abnormal blood pressure response, or symptoms of chest pain.[7] Please see Section I: Asymptomatic Severe Aortic Stenosis for further discussion.
- Average survival after onset of symptoms in patients with severe AS is 2 to 3 years with a high risk of sudden death; therefore, surgery to replace the AV is recommended if symptoms are present.
- In patients with bicuspid AV undergoing AVR due to severe AS or AR, repair of the aortic root or replacement of the ascending aorta is indicated if the diameter of the aortic root or ascending aorta is greater than 4.5 cm.[7,10]
- Surgery to repair the aortic root or replace the ascending aorta is recommended in patients with bicuspid AV if the diameter of the aortic root or ascending aorta is greater than 5.0 or 5.5 cm or if

TABLE 3-3-1 Classification of Aortic Stenosis (AS) Severity in Those with Normal LV Function as Determined by the ESC and AHA/ACC Guidelines [8-10]

TTE parameter	Aortic sclerosis	Mild AS	Moderate AS	Severe AS
Aortic jet velocity (m/s)	≤2.5	2.6-2.9	3.0-4.0	>4.0
Mean gradient (mm Hg)		<20	20-40	>40
Aortic valve area (AVA) (cm^2)		>1.5	1.0-1.5	<1.0
Indexed AVA (cm^2/m^2)		>0.85	0.60-0.85	<0.6
Velocity ratio		>0.50	0.25-0.50	<0.25

This table demonstrates the classification of aortic stenosis (AS) severity in patients with normal LV function as determined by the ESC and AHA/ACC guidelines.

the rate of increase in diameter is 0.5 cm per year or more.[7,10] The presence of significant aortic pathology in patients without hemodynamically significant valve pathology can make decision making complicated in terms of whether or not to pursue valve replacement (in a patient who otherwise would not warrant AVR) at the time of aortic surgery. This decision is made on a case-by-case basis with input from the surgeon, cardiologist, and patient.

PATIENT EDUCATION

- First-degree family members (especially males) should be screened by their physician, including a thorough physical examination, an ECG, and an echo to assess the AV and aorta.
- Prophylactic antibiotics for dental, gastrointestinal, and gynecologic procedures are no longer indicated. The risk of endocarditis is 10% to 30% over a lifetime. If a previous history of endocarditis exists, then prophylactic antibiotics are recommended.[10]
- Anomalous coronary arteries such as a left dominant coronary arterial system are commonly associated with a bicuspid AV. In rare cases, the left coronary artery may arise from the pulmonary artery.[5]
- Screen for familial hypercholesterolemia or early CAD. A cardiac diet and more aggressive primary prevention for cardiovascular events are recommended to delay sclerosis and calcification.
- There are no activity limitations for patients with a normally functioning bicuspid AV with normal aorta dimensions after thorough clinical evaluation. With AV insufficiency and aortic root diameter greater than 45 mm, patients should avoid strenuous isometric activity, such as weight lifting, rope climbing, and pull-ups and can participate only in low-intensity competitive sports.
- Risk of aortic root dissection is 5%, unless the individual has Marfan syndrome, then the risk is 40%.[11]

FOLLOW-UP

The patient was found to have a bicuspid aortic valve and aortic coarctation. Following repair of the coarctation, he will need periodic[3] surveillance of his aorta with MRA (or CTA). He will also require serial follow-up of his aortic valve with echocardiography.

VIDEO LEGENDS

1. Video 3-3-1: Parasternal long axis view demonstrates a mildly thickened AV with mild aortic root dilation
2. Video 3-3-2: Zoomed parasternal short axis view of the bicuspid AV
3. Video 3-3-6: TEE short axis view of a bicuspid AV
4. Video 3-3-7: 3 D TEE from a different patient demonstrating fusion of the right and left AV cusps
5. Video 3-3-9: TEE X-plane view of a bicuspid AV in another patient demonstrating prolapse of the fused right and left cusps. The patient had severe, eccentric AR.

REFERENCES

1. Cripe L, Andelfinger G, Martin LJ, Shooner K, Benson DW. Bicuspid aortic valve is heritable. *J Am Coll Cardiol.* 2004;44(1):138-143.
2. Duran AC, Frescura C, Sans-Coma V, Angelini A, Basso C, Thiene G. Bicuspid aortic valves in hearts with other congenital heart disease. *J Heart Valve Dis.* 1995;4(6):581-590.
3. Hallidie-Smith KA, Karas S. Cardiac anomalies in Williams-Beuren syndrome. *Arch Dis Child.* 1988;63(7):809-813.
4. Sachdev V, Matura LA, Sidenko S, et al. Aortic valve disease in turner syndrome. *J Am Coll Cardiol.* 2008;51(19):1904-1909.
5. Libby P, Bonow RO, Mann DL, Zipes DP, Braunwald E, eds. *Braunwald's Heart Disease: A Ttextbook of Cardiovascular Medicine.* Eighth 8th ed. Philadelphia, PA: Saunders Elsevier; 2008; No. 1-2.
6. Ward C. Clinical significance of the bicuspid aortic valve. *Heart.* 2000;83(1):81-85.
7. Bonow RO. Bicuspid aortic valves and dilated aortas: A critical review of the ACC/AHA practice guidelines recommendations. *Am J Cardiol.* 2008;102(1):111-114.
8. Baumgartner H, Hung J, Bermejo J, et al. Echocardiographic assessment of valve stenosis: EAE/ASE recommendations for clinical practice. *Eur J Echocardiogr.* 2009;10(1):1-25.

9. Vahanian A, Baumgartner H, Bax J, et al. Guidelines on the management of valvular heart disease: The task force on the management of valvular heart disease of the European Society of Cardiology. *Eur Heart J*. 2007;28(2):230-268.
10. Nishimura RA, Carabello BA, Faxon DP, et al. ACC/AHA 2008 guideline update on valvular heart disease: Focused update on infective endocarditis: A report of the American College of Cardiology/American Heart Association Task Force on Practice Guidelines endorsed by the Society of Cardiovascular Anesthesiologists, Society for Cardiovascular Angiography and Interventions, and Society of Thoracic Surgeons. *J Am Coll Cardiol*. 2008;52(8):676-685.
11. Michelena HI, Khanna AD, Mahoney D, et al. Incidence of aortic complications in patients with bicuspid aortic valves. *JAMA*. 2011;306(10):1104-1112.

SECTION 4

Acute Aortic Regurgitation

Jason Evanchan, DO and Kavita Sharma, MD

CLINICAL CASE PRESENTATION

A 48-year-old man with a history of hypertension underwent the Ross Procedure in 1998 (autograft of his pulmonary valve to the aortic valve, with allograft of his pulmonic valve) for treatment of aortic insufficiency of unclear etiology. He had done well postoperatively, working as a construction worker. For 3 weeks prior to presentation, however, he developed progressive weakness and shortness of breath. On the day prior to admission, his breathing worsened to the point that he was having labored breathing at rest. He had mild chest pressure, orthopnea, and a 5-pound weight gain.

On presentation to the emergency department, his blood pressure was 135/62 mm Hg, his heart rate was 105 beats/min, and his oxygen saturations were adequate but required 2 L nasal cannula. His cardiac and pulmonary exam exhibited a short decrescendo diastolic murmur heard best over the left sternal border. He had bibasilar crackles and elevated jugular venous pressures to the angle of the jaw at 45°. He had bilateral lower extremity edema.

A chest x-ray showed pulmonary edema. Transthoracic echocardiogram demonstrated a moderately enlarged left ventricle, with an EF of 50%. He had moderate pulmonic stenosis (homograft) and severe aortic regurgitation (Figures 3-4-1 to 3-4-5).

He went to the operating room and underwent aortic valve replacement (AVR) with a Capentier-Edwards Perimount Magna valve. He also had a pericardial patch enlargement of the pulmonary valve annulus and right ventricular outflow tract with a pulmonary valve replacement with a Carpentier-Edwards Perimount Magna valve. He has done well postoperatively and has returned to work.

CLINICAL FEATURES

- Patients with acute severe aortic regurgitation (AR) present with signs of CHF, including shortness of breath, orthopnea, paroxysmal nocturnal dyspnea, and edema.[1]
- Patients can have myocardial ischemia and chest pain secondary to supply demand mismatch, as well as decreased coronary perfusion pressure from the low aortic diastolic pressure.
- Findings associated with the underlying cause of the acute AR can often be elicited.

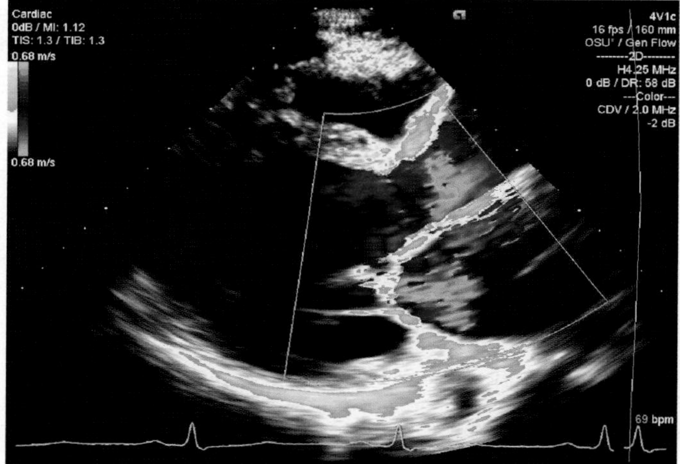

FIGURE 3-4-1 Parasternal long axis view with color Doppler demonstrating severe AR. MR is also noted ► (see Video 3-4-1).

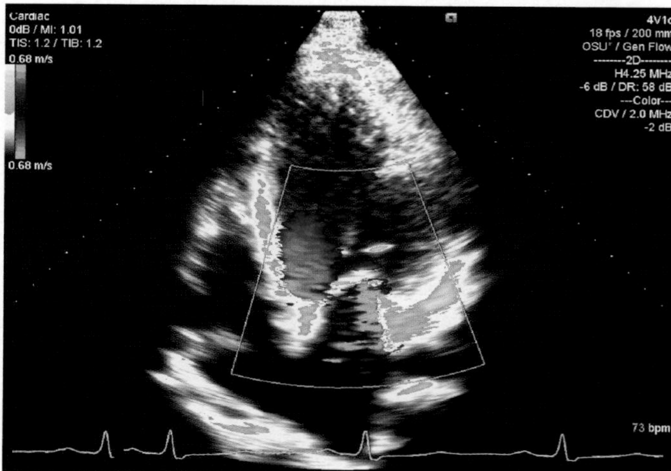

FIGURE 3-4-2 Apical 4 chamber with color Doppler demonstrating the color Doppler jet in the LV and a hyperdynamic LV ► (see Video 3-4-2).

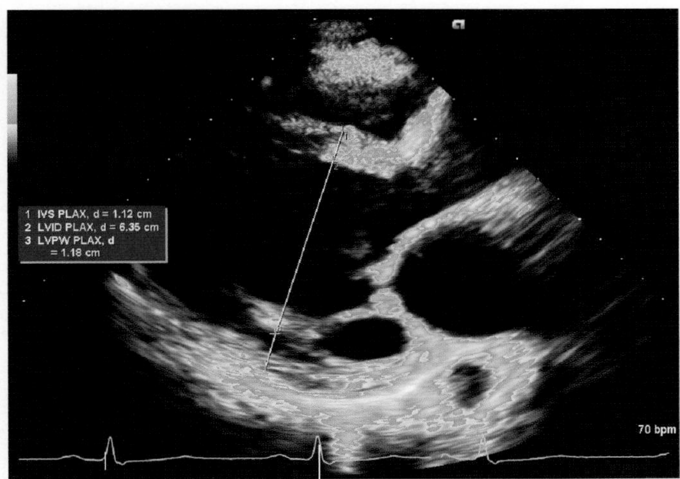

FIGURE 3-4-3 Parasternal long axis view demonstrating a dilated LV.

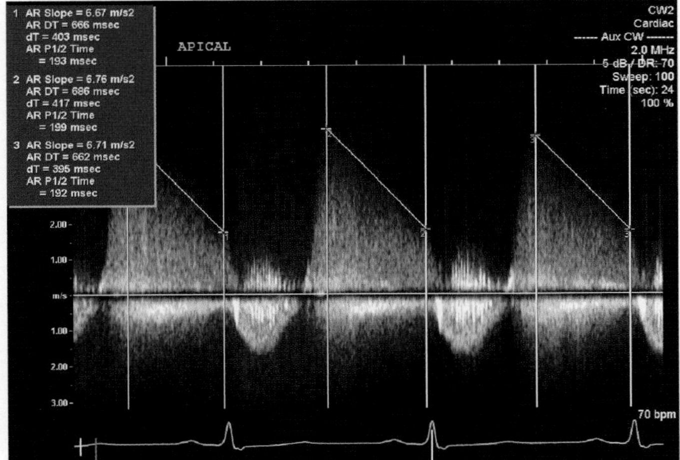

FIGURE 3-4-4 Continuous-wave Doppler demonstrating a pressure half-time of 195 msec consistent with severe AR.

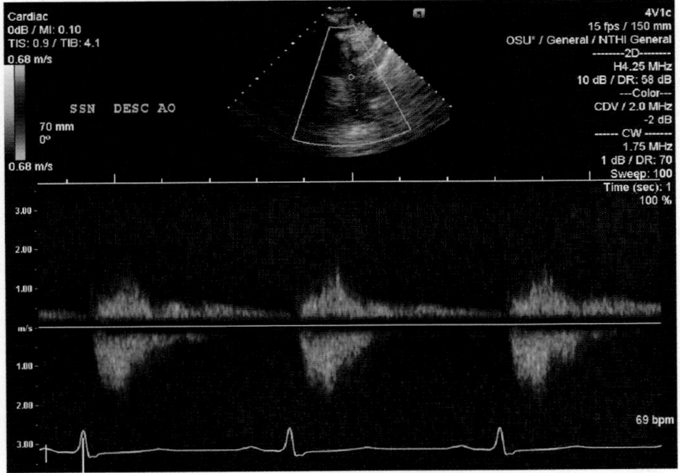

FIGURE 3-4-5 Spectral Doppler of the descending aorta demonstrating holosystolic flow reversal.

EPIDEMIOLOGY

- Trace aortic regurgitation (AR) or greater was seen in 13.0% of men and 8.5% of women in the Framingham Heart Study.[1] Severe aortic regurgitation is much less common.

PATHOPHYSIOLOGY AND ETIOLOGY

- Acute AR can be caused by abnormalities of the aortic valve leaflets, or secondary to the problems with the aortic root/ascending aorta.[1,2]
- The most common causes of acute AR are infective endocarditis, aortic dissection, trauma, and acute dysfunction of a prosthetic valve.[1]
- In acute, severe AR there is a sudden, large regurgitant volume into a normal sized ventricle. The ventricle is not able to compensate, and there is an abrupt increase in LVEDP and left atrial pressure.[3]
- There is a decrease in effective forward stroke volume. Although tachycardia develops, it is often insufficient to maintain forward cardiac output, and cardiogenic shock and pulmonary edema ensue.[2]
- The LVEDP increases, and with rapidly decreasing aortic diastolic pressure the coronary perfusion pressure drops. With the increased demand secondary to tachycardia, signs and symptoms of myocardial ischemia can develop.[2]

ECHOCARDIOGRAPHY (SEE TABLE 3-4-1)

- Echocardiography, using 2-D echocardiography with color flow and comprehensive spectral Doppler evaluation, is essential in the assessment of aortic regurgitation.[4]
- Echocardiography is indicated to confirm the diagnosis based on physical exam, to assess the cause of AR, to assess the severity of AR, and assess (and follow over time) LV dimension, mass, and LV function (all Class I, LOE B recommendations).[1,5]
- Two-dimensional echo is used to assess the valve anatomy (eg, bicuspid valve, presence of vegetations) and structural deformities. The aortic root and proximal ascending aorta can be well visualized, and the diagnosis of an ascending thoracic aortic aneurysm as the cause of the AR can often be made. Additionally, the adaptive changes of the ventricle can be measured and followed. This becomes important in the decision and the timing of surgery in chronic AR patients.
- The severity of AR is assessed using color flow and spectral Doppler.
- Using color flow Doppler imaging, a regurgitant jet that is 65% of the LV outflow tract diameter is considered severe aortic regurgitation.[4]
- The rate of deceleration of the regurgitant diastolic flow reflects the rate of equalization of pressure between the aortic and the LV diastolic pressures (Figure 3-4-4). This can be measured with Doppler as the "pressure half time." In general, the more severe the AR, the more rapid the deceleration of the regurgitant jet and the shorter the "pressure half time." A pressure half time of <200 ms is suggestive of severe AR.[4]
- It is normal to have a small amount of early diastolic blood flow reversal in the descending and abdominal aorta. As AR progresses, however, the duration and the velocity of that flow increases. In severe AR, holodiastolic flow reversal can be seen using spectral Doppler (Figure 3-4-5).

TABLE 3-4-1 Selected Echocardiographic Parameters for the Evaluation of Aortic Regurgitation

Parameter	Advantages	Disadvantages
Left ventricular size	Enlargement sensitive for chronic significant AR, important for outcomes. Normal size virtually excludes significant chronic AR.	Enlargement seen in other conditions. May be normal in acute significant AR.
Aortic cusp alterations	Simple, usually abnormal in severe AR; flail valve denotes severe AR.	Poor accuracy; may grossly underestimate or overestimate the defect.
Jet width or jet cross-sectional area in LVOT-color flow	Simple, very sensitive, quick screen for AR.	Expands unpredictably below the orifice. Inaccurate for eccentric jets.
Vena contracta width	Simple, quantitative, good at identifying mild or severe AR.	Not useful for multiple AR jets. Small values, thus small error leads to large percentage error.
Proximal isovelocity surface area (PISA)	Quantitative. Provides both lesion severity (effective regurgitant orifice area) and volume overload (regurgitant volume).	Feasibility is limited by aortic valve calcifications. Not valid for multiple jets, less accurate in eccentric jets. Provides peak flow and maximal effective regurgitant orifice area. Underestimation is possible with aortic aneurysm. Limited experience.
Flow quantitation-pulsed wave	Quantitative. Valid in multiple jets and eccentric jets. Provides both lesion severity (effective regurgitant orifice area and regurgitant fraction) and volume overload (regurgitant volume).	Not valid for combined MR and AR, unless pulmonic site is used.
Jet profile continuous-wave	Simple. Faint or incomplete jet compatible with mild AR.	Qualitative. Overlap between moderate and severe AR. Complementary data only.
Jet deceleration rate (pressure half time)- continuous-wave	Simple.	Qualitative. Affected by changes in left ventricular and aortic diastolic pressures.
Diastolic flow reversal in descending aorta-pulsed wave	Simple.	Depends on rigidity of aorta. Brief velocity reversal is normal.

AR = aortic regurgitation

Adapted with permission from Zoghbi WA, Enriquez-Sarano M, Foster E, et al. Recommendations for evaluation of the severity of native valvular regurgitation with two-dimensional and Doppler echocardiography. *J Am Soc Echocardiogr.* 2003;16(7):777-802.[4]

- Echocardiography can quantify the regurgitant volume, regurgitant fraction, and the regurgitant orifice area. While this can be time consuming, it is helpful in differentiating degrees of moderate AR (2 plus to 3 plus), and in borderline cases.
- Transesphageal echocardiography (TEE) is particularly useful in assessing the anatomy of the valve and the aorta.[4]

OTHER DIAGNOSTIC MODALITIES

- If aortic dissection is suspected TEE, MRA (limited in unstable patients) and CTA are extremely valuable.[1]
- Cardiac catheterization is rarely needed in acute, severe AR and can delay surgery unnecessarily.[1]

MANAGEMENT

- Medical therapy for acute, severe AR is supportive only, and death without urgent surgical intervention is common.[1]
- β-blockers with aortic dissection should be used with caution.
- While awaiting surgery, medical therapy with vasodilators, such as nitroprusside, and inotropes can be used as temporizing measures to bridge to surgery.[3]
- Invasive hemodynamic monitoring may be useful to guide therapy (Figure 3-4-6).
- Intra-aortic balloon pumps are contraindicated, as they can worsen the AR.[1]

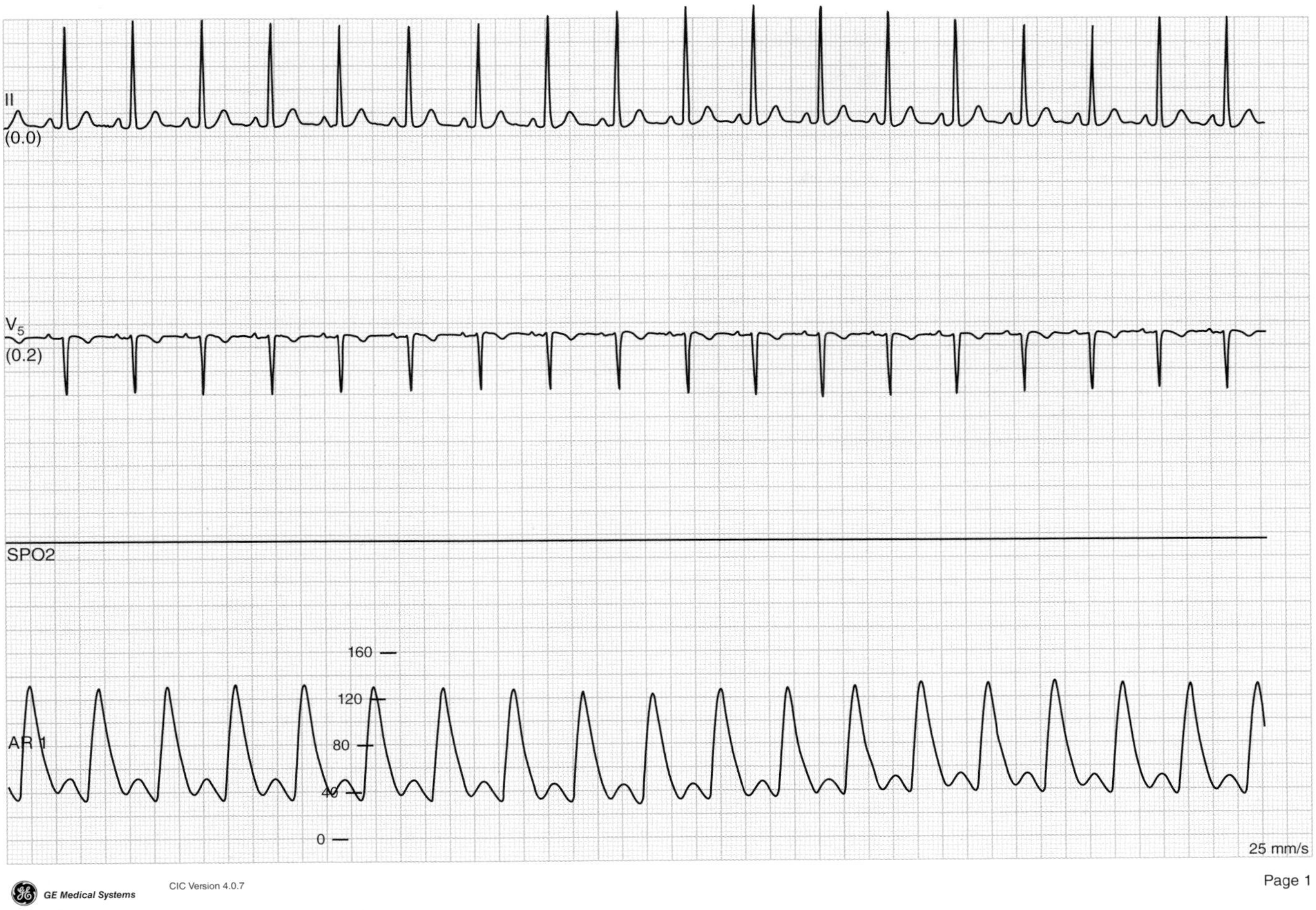

FIGURE 3-4-6 Arterial line tracing from a different patient with acute AR due to endocarditis demonstrating tachycardia and a wide pulse pressure.

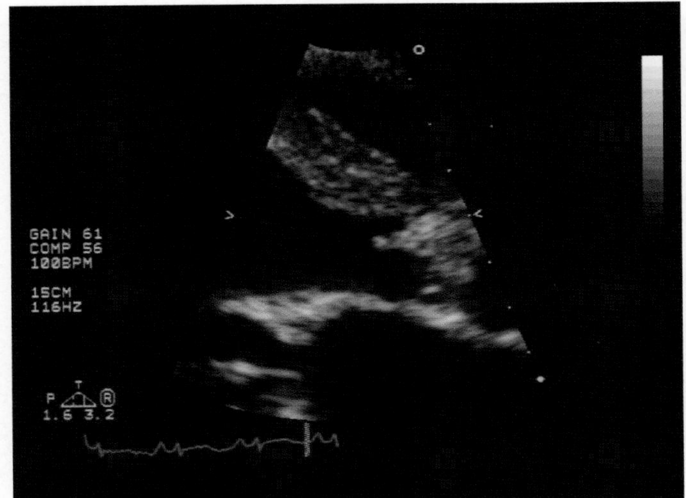

FIGURE 3-4-7 Parasternal long axis view from a different patient demonstrating a large aortic valve vegetation that resulted in severe acute AR ► (see Video 3-4-7).

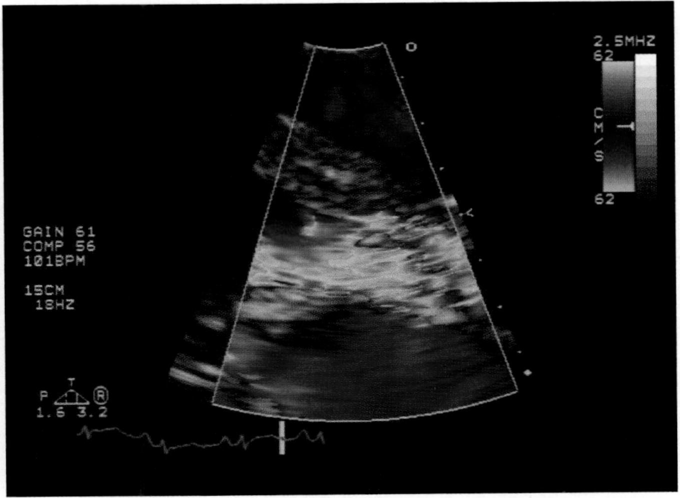

FIGURE 3-4-8 Parasternal long axis view with color Doppler from the patient seen in Figure 3-4-7 demonstrating severe acute AR ► (see Video 3-4-8).

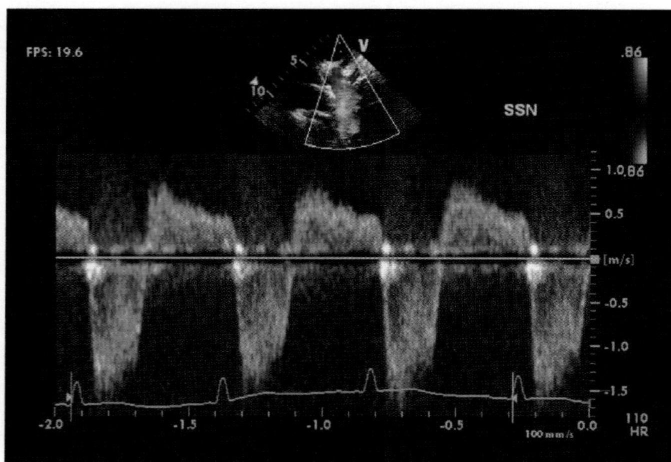

FIGURE 3-4-9 Pulsed Doppler of the descending aorta from the patient in Figures 3-4-7 and 3-4-8 with severe acute AR demonstrating impressive holodiastolic flow reversal. The antegrade (systolic) VTI was 26 cm. The retrograde (diastolic) VTI was 18 cm, consistent with a regurgitant fraction well over 60%.

FOLLOW-UP

- Patients with acute aortic regurgitation require urgent surgical attention.

SUMMARY

- The most common causes of acute AR are infective endocarditis, aortic dissection, trauma, and acute dysfunction of a prosthetic valve.
- Echocardiography is valuable in the diagnosis.
- Surgery is essential to patient survival in acute severe aortic regurgitation.

PATIENT EDUCATION AND MANAGEMENT

- Following AVR, patient follow-up and serial echocardiography is warranted as detailed in other sections of this chapter[1,5].

FIGURE LEGENDS

1. Video 3-4-1: Parasternal long axis view with color Doppler demonstrating severe AR. MR is also noted.
2. Video 3-4-2: Apical four chamber with color Doppler demonstrating the color Doppler jet in the LV and a hyperdynamic LV.
3. Video 3-4-7: Parasternal long axis view from a different patient demonstrating a large aortic valve vegetation that resulted in severe acute AR.
4. Video 3-4-8: Parasternal long axis view with color Doppler from the patient in fig 7 (video 3) demonstrating severe acute AR.

REFERENCES

1. Bonow RO, Carabello BA, Chatterjee K, et al. 2008 focused update incorporated into the ACC/AHA 2006 guidelines for the management of patients with valvular heart disease: A report of the American College of Cardiology/American Heart Association Task Force on Practice Guidelines (Writing Committee to revise the 1998 guidelines for the management of patients with valvular heart disease). Endorsed by the Society of Cardiovascular Anesthesiologists, Society for Cardiovascular Angiography and Interventions, and Society of Thoracic Surgeons. *J Am Coll Cardiol*. 2008;52:e1-142.
2. Roberts WC, Ko JM, Jones WH 3rd. Causes of pure aortic regurgitation in patients having isolated aortic valve replacement at a single US tertiary hospital (1993 to 2005). *Circulation*. 2006;114:422-429.
3. Stout KK, Verrier ED. Acute valvular regurgitation. *Circulation*. 2009;119(25):3232-3241.
4. Zoghbi WA, Enriquez-Sarano M, Foster E, et al. Recommendations for evaluation of the severity of native valvular regurgitation with two-dimensional and Doppler echocardiography. *J Am Soc Echocardiogr*. 2003;16:777-802.
5. Nishimura RA, Otto CM, Bonow RO, et al. 2014 AHA/ACC guideline for the management of patients with valvular heart disease:executive summary; a report of the American College of Cardiology/American Heart Association Task Force on Practice Guidelines. *J Am Coll Cardiol*. 2014;63:2348-2388.

SECTION 5

Chronic Aortic Regurgitation

Jason Evanchan, DO and Kavita Sharma, MD

CLINICAL CASE PRESENTATION

The patient is a 52-year-old woman with a past history of gastric ulcer, autoimmune hepatitis with cirrhosis, hypertension, and chronic aortic regurgitation (AR). She has a bicuspid aortic valve and moderate dilation of the aortic root. Her most recent echocardiogram was obtained 18 months ago and demonstrated moderate to severe AR, with a normal left ventricular (LV) chamber size, and an ejection fraction of 60%. She was lost to follow-up until recently. She presents with a 3 to 4 week history of progressive dyspnea on exertion, lower extremity edema, and a cough. She has some left-sided chest pressure, orthopnea, and lightheadedness. She has endorsed noncompliance with both medications and diet.

On examination, her blood pressure was 125/52 mm Hg and her pulse was 95 beats/min. Cardiovascular auscultation revealed a pan-diastolic grade 3/6 blowing, decrescendo murmur. It was best appreciated in the left upper sternal border with the patient sitting

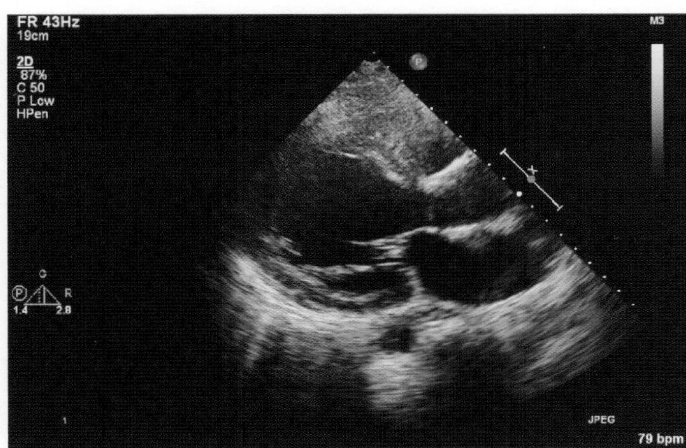

FIGURE 3-5-1 Parasternal long axis demonstrating a dilated LV with mild LV dysfunction ► (see Video 3-5-1).

forward in full expiration. There was a systolic flow murmur heard best over the aortic valve. There was elevated jugular venous distension at 10 cm and bilateral crackles in both lower lung fields. There were bounding "water hammer" pulses in bilateral upper and lower extremities, with brisk carotid upstrokes. She had bilateral lower extremity 1 plus pitting edema.

Transthoracic echocardiogram revealed that the LV was dilated with a left ventricular end diastolic dimension of just over 6 cm. The ejection fraction was decreased at 45%. The aortic valve was bicuspid, with severe aortic regurgitation (Figures 3-5-1 to 3-5-5).

She underwent left heart catheterization in preparation for surgery that revealed no coronary artery disease. At surgery, she was found to have a leaflet perforation of the noncoronary leaflet, but there was no evidence of endocarditis. She underwent an aortic valve replacement with a bioprosthetic valve, and a mitral valve repair for concomitant mitral insufficiency.

CLINICAL FEATURES/NATURAL HISTORY

- Patients with mild to moderate AR rarely have symptoms related to their AR. Patients with severe AR can be asymptomatic for years to decades.

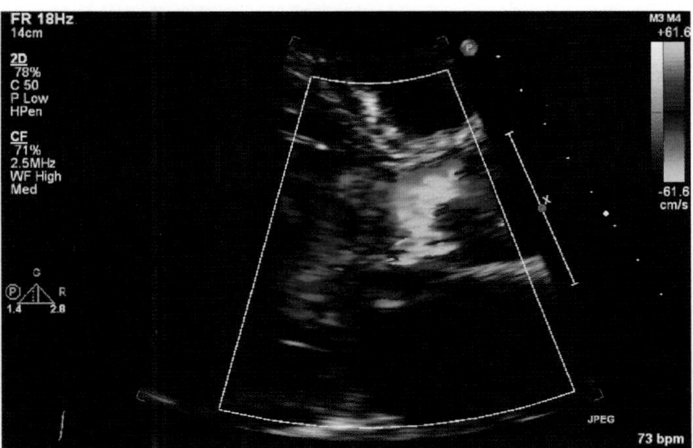

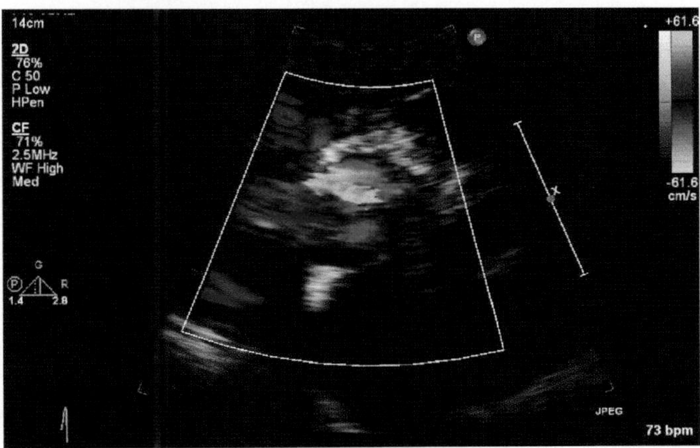

FIGURE 3-5-3 Parasternal long axis (upper panel) and short axis (lower panel), focused on the aortic valve, with color flow Doppler, demonstrating the AR jet ► (see Video 3-5-3).

- Symptoms related to pulmonary congestion, such as dyspnea on exertion, orthopnea, and paroxysmal nocturnal dyspnea occur gradually. Patients often gradually curtail their activities and may not initially appreciate their decreased functional/exercise capacity.

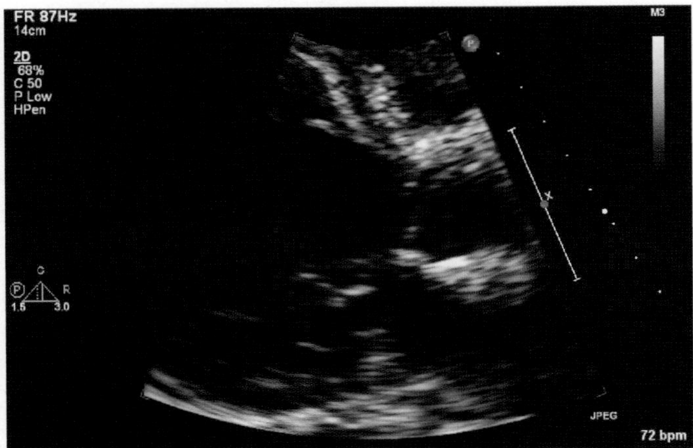

FIGURE 3-5-2 Parasternal long axis, focused on the aortic valve, demonstrating mild leaflet prolapse, which is not uncommonly seen in patients with a bicuspid valve ► (see Video 3-5-2).

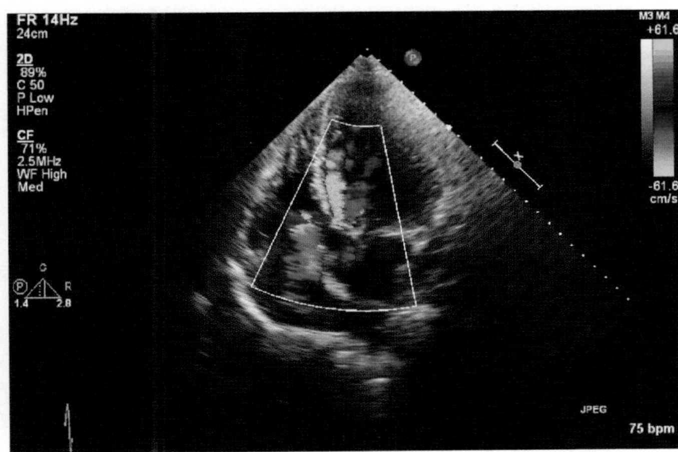

FIGURE 3-5-4 Apical 5 chamber view with color Doppler demonstrating the AR jet ► (see Video 3-5-4).

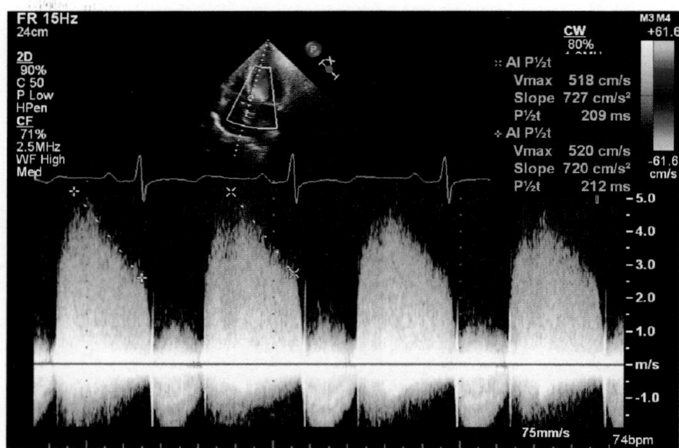

FIGURE 3-5-5 Continuous-wave Doppler demonstrating a dense spectral Doppler signal. The pressure half-time of the aortic regurgitation is approximately 200 msec.

- Patients with chronic AR can have symptomatic premature ventricular contractions related to the increased left ventricular volume after a premature beat.
- Angina occurs late in the course and can be from latent coronary artery disease, left ventricular hypertrophy with subendocardial ischemia, and supply demand mismatch.
- Unfortunately, by the time clinical symptoms develop there is usually considerable LV dilation and LV dysfunction present.
- Important prognostic indicators include the severity of AR, the presence of symptoms, and the LV size and ejection fraction.
- In asymptomatic patients, survival free of aortic valve replacement is directly proportional to the degree of AR. In patients with severe AR, 62% required an aortic valve replacement (AVR) by 5 years, compared to only 2% with mild, and 23% of moderate AR patients.[6]
- Asymptomatic patients with normal LV function have a fairly good prognosis. When LV dysfunction occurs, however, they quickly develop symptoms and prognosis worsens.[2]
- When patients become symptomatic, there is a rapid decline in functional status with worsening prognosis. Patients with chronic severe AR and New York Heart Association (NYHA) Class III or IV symptoms had a survival of only 28% at 4 years if managed conservatively. This is compared to a 75% 10-year survival in patients in NYHA Class I, which is similar to age-matched normal population.[7]

EPIDEMIOLOGY

- Trace aortic regurgitation (AR) or greater was seen in 13.0% of men and 8.5% of women in the Framingham Heart Study.[1] Severe aortic regurgitation is much less common.

PATHOPHYSIOLOGY/ETIOLOGY

- Aortic regurgitation can develop from primary leaflet abnormalities or secondary to aortic pathology.
- Primary leaflet abnormalities cause incomplete coaptation of the leaflets from altered leaflet structure, decreased leaflet mobility or tethering, from leaflet perforation or leaflet prolapse. AR is caused by leaflet abnormalities 43% of the time.[3] The most common causes are rheumatic heart disease, infective endocarditis, and congenital aortic regurgitation from a bicuspid aortic valve.
- Aortic root and ascending aortic abnormalities can lead to AR roughly 57% of the time.[3] Dilation of the aortic root and aortic annulus causes the leaflets to separate, with resultant AR. An age-related idiopathic ascending aortic aneurysm, often associated with hypertension, is the most common cause of aortic root enlargement. Other potential causes, such as Marfan syndrome may also be present (see Chapter 7).
- The diastolic regurgitation from the aorta to the LV presents a volume load to the LV and results in an increase in the left ventricular end diastolic volume (LVEDV).
- The increased LVEDV initially results in an increased forward stroke volume. With this, patients often get an increase in systolic pressure. Because of the diastolic regurgitation, the diastolic pressure declines, resulting in an increased pulse pressure.
- Chronic increased wall tension leads to a compensatory, eccentric more than concentric, hypertrophy of the left ventricle.[2]
- Ischemia can develop from a supply-demand mismatch. Increased myocardial demand develops from elevated systolic pressure and increased LV mass, and decreased supply is a result of decreased diastolic blood pressure and thus decreased coronary perfusion pressure.
- During the chronic, compensatory phase, the LV is able to adapt to these changes without a significant increase in LV end-diastolic pressure.
- With severe chronic AR, progressive LV dilation with interstitial fibrosis develops over time. This results in decreased compliance, an increase in LVEDP, a decrease in the ejection fraction and cardiac output, and progressive symptoms.

ECHOCARDIOGRAPHY (SEE TABLE 3-4-1) IN SECTION 4

- Echocardiography, using 2-D echocardiography with color flow and comprehensive spectral Doppler evaluation, is essential in the assessment of aortic regurgitation.[5]
- Echocardiography is indicated to confirm the diagnosis based on physical exam, to assess the cause of AR, to assess the severity of AR, and assess (and follow over time) LV dimension, mass, and LV function (all Class I, LOE B recommendations).[2]
- Two-dimensional echo is used to assess the valve anatomy (eg, bicuspid valve) and structural deformities. The aortic root and proximal ascending aorta can be well visualized, and the diagnosis of a thoracic, ascending aorta aneurysm as the cause of the AR can often be made. Additionally, the adaptive changes of the ventricle can be measured and followed. This becomes important in the decision and the timing of surgery in chronic AR patients.
- The severity of AR is assessed primary using color flow and spectral Doppler.

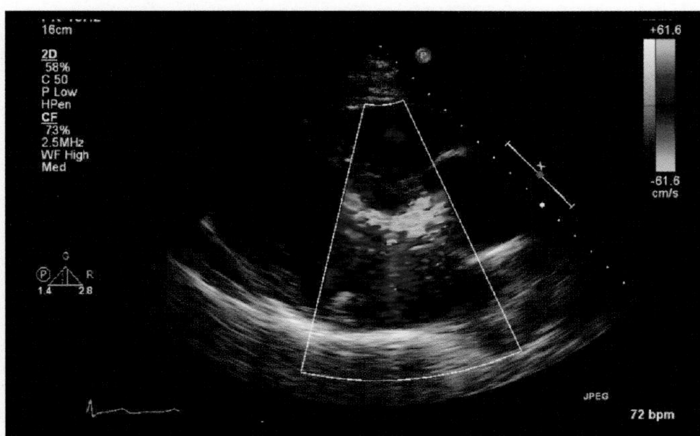

FIGURE 3-5-6 Parasternal long axis view from another patient demonstrating severe AR due to a dilated aortic root with a trileaflet AV ► (see Video 3-5-6).

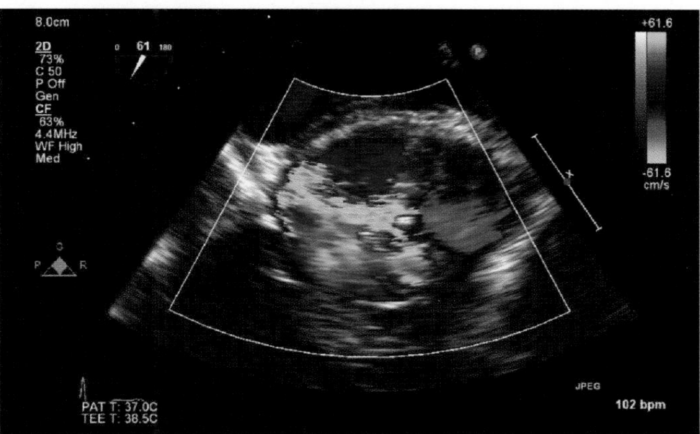

FIGURE 3-5-8 TEE short axis view from another patient (lost to follow-up for many years) with a bicuspid AV and AR who presented with CHF symptoms. His TTE demonstrated a dilated, mildly hypokinetic LV. TEE (performed due to suboptimal TTE images) demonstrated severe AR ► (see Video 3-5-8). He was referred for surgical AVR.

- Using color flow imaging, a regurgitant jet that is 65% of the LV outflow tract diameter is considered severe aortic regurgitation.[5]
- The rate of deceleration of the regurgitant diastolic flow reflects the rate of equalization of pressure between the aortic and the LV diastolic pressures (Figure 3-5-5). This can be measured with Doppler as the pressure half time. In general, the more severe the AR, the more rapid the deceleration of the regurgitant jet and the shorter the pressure half time. A pressure half time of <200 ms is suggestive of severe AR.[5]
- It is normal to have a small amount of diastolic blood flow reversal in the descending aorta. As AR progresses, however, the duration and the velocity of that flow increase. In severe AR, holodiastolic flow reversal can be seen using spectral Doppler.
- Echocardiography can be employed to quantify the regurgitant volume, regurgitant fraction, and the regurgitant orifice area. While this can be time consuming, it is helpful in differentiating degrees of moderate AR (2 plus to 3 plus), and in borderline cases.
- Transesphageal echocardiography (TEE) is rarely needed to evaluate the severity of the AR. If there are poor acoustic windows on the surface echo, however, TEE may be required. TEE is particularly useful in assessing the anatomy of the valve and the aorta.[5]

OTHER DIAGNOSTIC MODALITIES

- Cardiac MRI is indicated to assess LV volume and LV function in patients who have suboptimal echocardiogram images (Class I, LOB).[2] Additionally, with suboptimal TTE images, MRI can be used to estimate severity of AR, although there is less evidence to support this (Class IIa, LOB).[2]
- Because of the gradual, progressive nature of symptom development, patients often do not appreciate their decline in exercise capacity. In this population, exercise stress testing can be useful (Class IIa, LOB).[2]
- Cardiac catheterization is rarely indicated in the diagnosis of AR. It can be used, however, to assess severity of AR, or to assess aortic root size when noninvasive tests are inconclusive or discordant with clinical findings (Class I, LOB). Additionally, coronary angiograms are often needed prior to AV replacement in patients greater

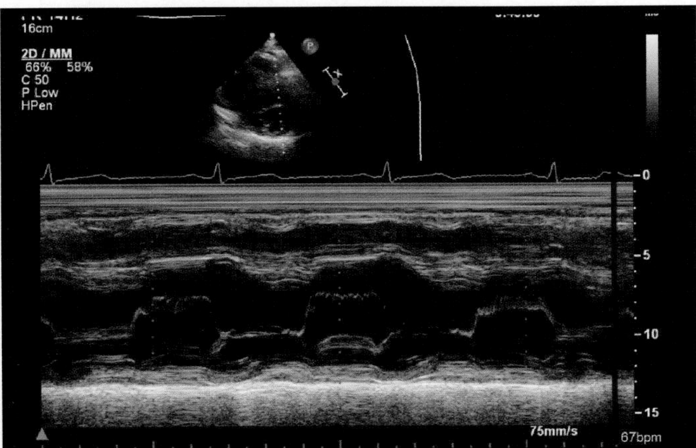

FIGURE 3-5-7 M-mode of the mitral valve demonstrating diastolic fluttering of the anterior MV leaflet due to the AR jet impinging on the valve.

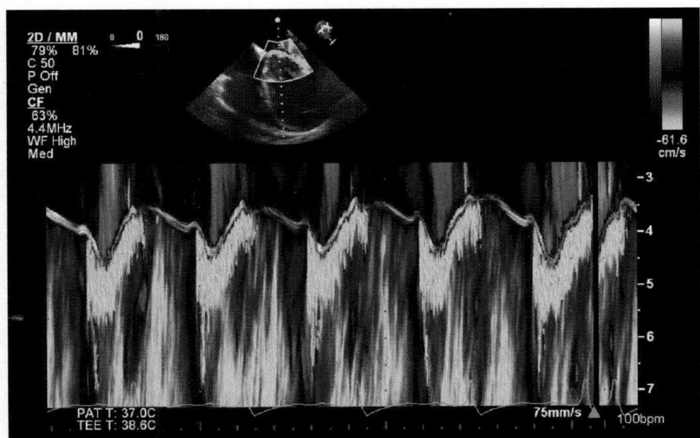

FIGURES 3-5-9 Color M-mode from the patient in Figure 3-5-8 demonstrating the AR jet impinging on the anterior MV leaflet and early closure of the MV.

than 50 years old, or if latent coronary disease is suspected based on symptoms or risk factors.

MANAGEMENT

- There is no good medical therapy for chronic, severe aortic regurgitation, and the only effective treatment is aortic valve replacement.
- Aortic valve replacement (AVR) is indicated for severe AR in patients who are symptomatic[2] (Class I, LOE B). If it is not clear if the patient is having symptoms, then an exercise stress test can be considered.
- Surgery is also indicated for asymptomatic patients with chronic severe AR who have LV systolic dysfunction (EF <50%), or who are undergoing CABG or other cardiac or aortic surgery[2] (Class I, LOE B Valve Guidelines).
- Surgery can be considered in patients with severely dilated left ventricles (LV end systolic dimensions >5.5 cm, or LV end diastolic dimensions >7.5 cm)[2] (Class IIa).
- Because of the benign prognosis, surgery is NOT indicated for asymptomatic patients with mild, moderate, or severe AR and normal LV systolic function and normal to only mildly dilated LV dimensions[2] (Class III, LOE B).
- When deciding if and when to pursue an aortic valve replacement, multiple other factors need to be considered: if the valve is bicuspid, if the aorta is dilated, if the patient has Marfan syndrome, etc. Please refer to the individual sections in this atlas or the guidelines for further details.
- Vasodilator therapy can be used for severe AR as a bridge to more definitive therapy, but surgery should not be delayed or deferred while medical management of a vasodilator is tried (Class I, LOE B).

FOLLOW-UP

- Patients with chronic, severe AR should have frequent assessments for the development of symptoms. At any point, if symptoms develop (subjectively or with decreased exercise capacity on stress testing), they should be referred for an aortic valve replacement.
- They should also be periodically assessed via echo for LV function and chamber dimensions. The frequency of assessment depends on symptom development, or the rate of change of LV dimensions on previous studies.
    - For example, if the patient is clinically stable and the LV dimensions are normal and stable, one can repeat the TTE in 12 months. If the LV dimensions appear to be increasing, then the frequency of echocardiograms can range from every 6 months, to as frequently as every 3 months.
- Regardless of the interval between echocardiograms, patients with severe chronic aortic regurgitation should be frequently assessed for the presence of symptoms.
- After aortic valve replacement, baseline echocardiography is recommended, along with follow-up for endocarditis prophylaxis, anticoagulation, and follow-up echocardiography after a change in symptoms.

SUMMARY

- Chronic aortic regurgitation can be caused by abnormalities of the aortic valve itself, or secondary to aortic pathology.
- Severe, chronic AR can be well tolerated for years, but patients often develop gradual onset decreased exercise tolerance and symptoms of heart failure.
- Echocardiography is the mainstay in the diagnosis and in the follow-up for chronic AR.
- The frequency of follow-up echocardiography depends on the severity of the AR, the LV dimensions, and EF.
- Important prognostic factors in chronic severe AR include the presence of symptoms, decreased ejection fraction, and LV chamber dilation.
- When treatment for AR is indicated, there are no good medical treatments for AR. Aortic valve surgery is the only viable option.

FIGURE LEGENDS

1. Video 3-5-1: Parasternal long axis demonstrating a dilated LV with mild LV dysfunction
2. Video 3-5-2: Parasternal long axis, focused on the aortic valve, demonstrating mild leaflet prolapse which is not uncommonly seen in patients with a bicuspid valve
3. Video 3-5-3 L: Parasternal long axis, focused on the aortic valve, with color flow Doppler, demonstrating the AR jet
4. Video 3-5-3 R: Parasternal short axis, focused on the aortic valve, with color flow Doppler, demonstrating the AR jet
5. Video 3-5-4: Apical five chamber view with color Doppler demonstrating the AR jet
6. Video 3-5-6: Parasternal long axis view from another patient demonstrating severe AR due to a dilated aortic root with a trileaflet AV
7. Video 3-5-8: TEE short axis view from a patient (lost to follow-up for many years) with a bicuspid AV and AR who presented with CHF symptoms. TEE (performed due to suboptimal TTE images) demonstrates severe AR

REFERENCES

1. Singh JP, Evans JC, Levy D, et al. Prevalence and clinical determinants of mitral, tricuspid, and aortic regurgitation (the Framingham Heart Study). *Am J Cardiol.* 1999;83(6):897-902.
2. Bonow RO, Carabello BA, Chatterjee K, et al. 2008 focused update incorporated into the ACC/AHA 2006 guidelines for the management of patients with valvular heart disease: a report of the American College of Cardiology/American Heart Association Task Force on Practice Guidelines (Writing committee to develop guidelines for the management of patients with valvular heart disease). Endorsed by the Society of Cardiovascular Anesthesiologists, Society for Cardiovascular Angiography and Interventions, and Society of Thoracic Surgeons. *J Am Coll Cardiol.* 2008;52:e1-142.
3. Roberts WC, Ko JM, Jones WH 3rd. Causes of pure aortic regurgitation in patients having isolated aortic valve replacement at a single US tertiary hospital (1993 to 2005). *Circulation.* 2006;114:422-429.

4. Griffin BP, Topol EJ. *Manual of Cardiovascular Medicine*. 3rd ed. Chapter 13. Aortic Valve Disease. Philadelphia, PA: Lippincott Williams & Wilkins; 2008:204-213.

5. Zoghbi WA, Enriquez-Sarano M, Foster E, et al. Recommendations for evaluation of the severity of native valvular regurgitation with two-dimensional and Doppler echocardiography. *J Am Soc Echocardiogr*. 2003;16:777-802.

6. Detaint D, Messika-Zeitoun D, Maalouf J, et al. Quantitative echocardiographic determinants of clinical outcome in asymptomatic patients with aortic regurgitation: a prospective study. *J Am Coll Cardiol Img*. 2008;1(1):1-11. doi:10.1016/j.jcmg.2007.10.008

7. Dujardin KS, Enriquez-Sarano M, Schaff HV, et al. Mortality and morbidity of aortic regurgitation in clinical practice: a long-term follow-up study. *Circulation*. 1999;99(14):1851-1857.

SECTION 6

Rheumatic Mitral Stenosis

Gina G. Mentzer, MD

CLINICAL CASE PRESENTATION

A 57-year-old woman presented with palpitations, transient memory loss, and vision changes. Over the past 8 months, she has noticed intermittent palpitations that were not triggered by exercise, caffeine, or medications. She used to be able to walk a mile to the grocery store, but she states that she gets tired and out of breath with even walking up one flight of stairs, so she has been driving rather than walking for the past 4 months. Her past medical history was significant for rheumatic fever when she was 3 years old, an appendectomy, and asthma.

On clinical exam, she demonstrated an irregular heart beat with an opening snap and a soft first heart sound (S_1) with a 2/6 diastolic murmur heard at the apex with the bell. There was also a 3/6 systolic murmur at the apex that radiated to the axilla. She had a slight right ventricular heave and a loud pulmonic closure sound at the 4th intercostal space consistent with elevated pulmonary pressures. The clinical suspicion for mitral stenosis (MS) was confirmed with echocardiography which demonstrated a rheumatic appearing MV with thickened leaflets and an elevated transmitral gradient (Figures 3-6-1 to 3-6-6).

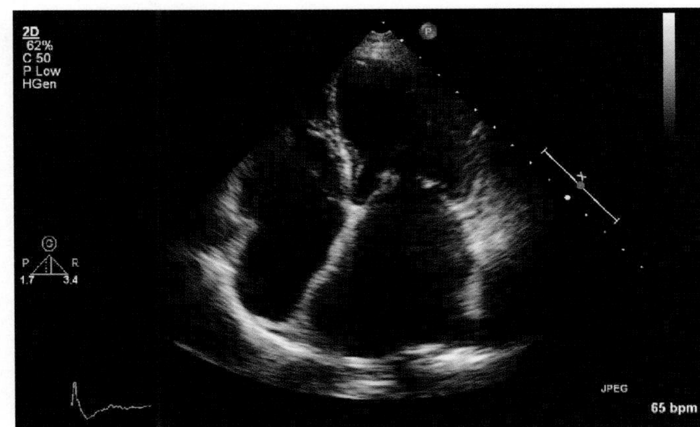

FIGURE 3-6-2 Two-dimensional transthoracic echocardiography apical 4 chamber view of severe MS. Note the severity of valve thickening and severely enlarged left atrium (LA) ► (see Video 3-6-2).

CLINICAL FEATURES

- New onset atrial fibrillation or embolic events are the most common presentations for MS.[1]

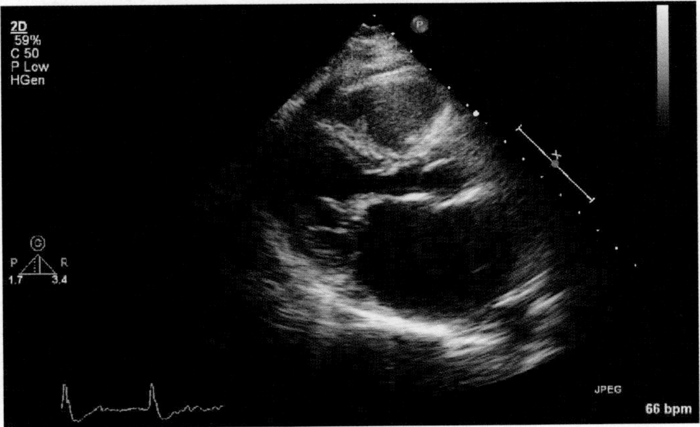

FIGURE 3-6-1 Two-dimensional transthoracic echocardiography parasternal long axis (PLAX) view of severe MS demonstrating thickened MV leaflets and LA enlargement ► (see Video 3-6-1).

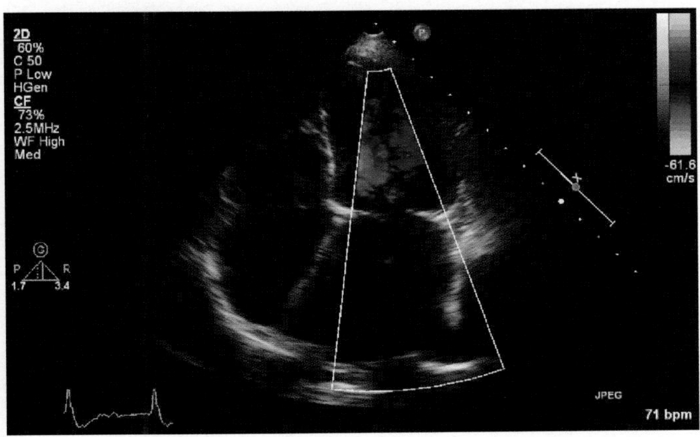

FIGURE 3-6-3 Two-dimensional transthoracic echocardiography with color Doppler in the apical 4-view. There is minimal MR ► (see Video 3-6-3).

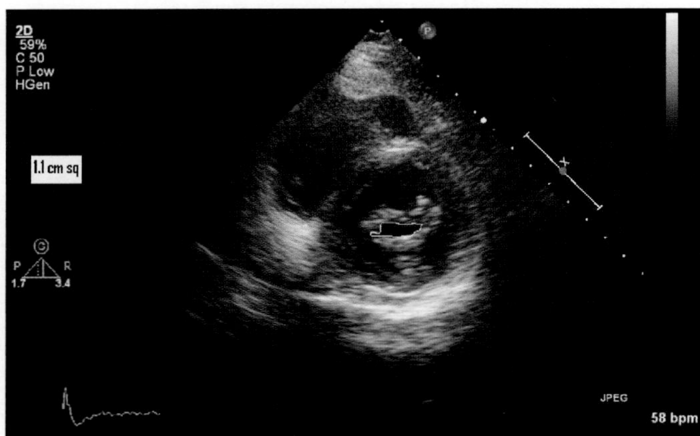

FIGURE 3-6-4 Planimetry of the MVA in the parasternal short axis (PSAX) window demonstrating severe MS. Valve area is 1.1 cm^2.

- Signs and symptoms of heart failure (HF) such as dyspnea, fatigue, or frank pulmonary edema can occur. Rare findings include hemoptysis, dysphagia, and hoarseness.
- Classic ausculatory findings include an accentuated first heart sound (S_1), opening snap (OS), low-pitched mid-diastolic rumble, and pre-systolic accentuation of the diastolic murmur primarily at the apex.[1,2]
- A shorter aortic valve (A2)-OS interval, soft S_1, loud pulmonary valve (P2) closure sound, right ventricular (RV) heave, and a longer duration of diastolic rumble indicates more severe MS.[3]

EPIDEMIOLOGY

- The primary cause of MS is rheumatic carditis (99%), and MS is the most frequent valvular complication of rheumatic fever (40% of those with rheumatic heart disease have isolated MS). The prevalence is 10% of left-sided valve diseases in Europe and is higher in developing countries.[2,4]
- The mean age of presentation is now in the fifth to sixth decade.
- In pure MS, a history of rheumatic fever is present in approximately 60% with a ratio of 2:1 women to men.[1]

PATHOPHYSIOLOGY AND ETIOLOGY

- Through an inflammatory, rheumatologic reaction to the *group A hemolytic streptococcus* species, a process of valvular fibrosis, commissural fusion, and calcification primarily affects the MV and causes LV inflow obstruction during diastole. This involves commissural and/or chordal fusion to create a funnel-shaped orifice that is decreased in size. Chordal thickening and shortening and progressive calcification cause further stenosis.
- It is a lifelong disease with a slow and stable course in the early years. If left untreated it can progressively accelerate into more fulminant disease in the later years. In developed countries, there can be a latent period of 20 to 40 years following illness with rheumatic fever until symptoms develop. These symptoms progress over 10 years leading to a more serious disabling clinical condition.[5]
- The survival rate is quite good for asymptomatic patients at 80% survival within 10 years and 50% if left untreated. In fact, 60% of patients may not develop symptoms and maintain a normal lifestyle. However, if severe symptoms present, the survival rate decreases to 0% to 15% at 10 years.[1]
- MS can progress more rapidly, presumably due to either a more severe rheumatic insult or repeated episodes of streptococcal infections, resulting in severe symptomatic MS in the late teens and early 20s.
- If MS is left untreated, mortality rates increase and can be due to a variety of confounding morbidities. Table 3-6-1 lists those morbidities with associated a percentage in MS patient mortality cases.[1,4]

ECHOCARDIOGRAPHY

- Transthoracic echocardiography (TTE) should be performed in patients for the diagnosis of MS, for the reevaluation of patients with known MS, and if new signs or symptoms develop. A thorough hemodynamic assessment including MV mean gradient MV area by

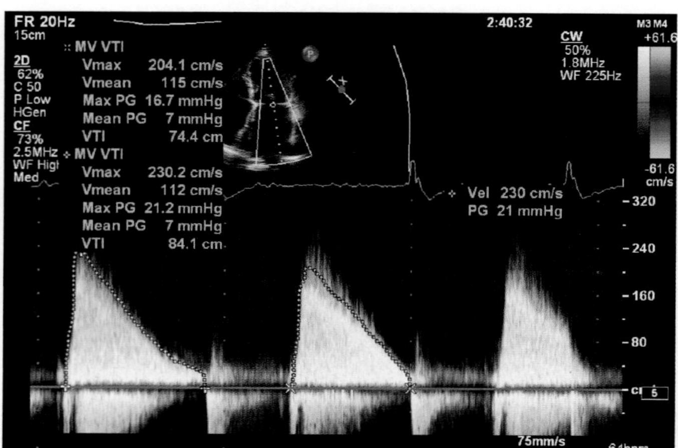

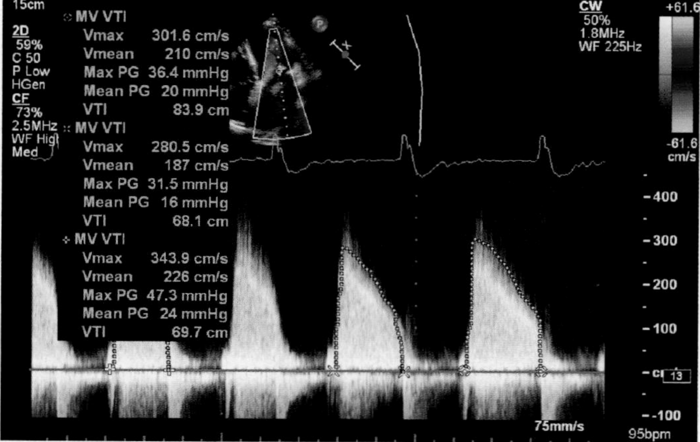

FIGURE 3-6-5 Continuous-wave Doppler (CWD) of the mitral inflow signal used to identify the maximal velocity (to determine the peak gradient as calculated by the modified Bernouli equation) as well as determine the mean transvalvular gradient by planimetry of the jet. Notice the significant influence of the heart rate on the gradients. With tachycardia (right panel) the peak and mean gradients are significantly higher.

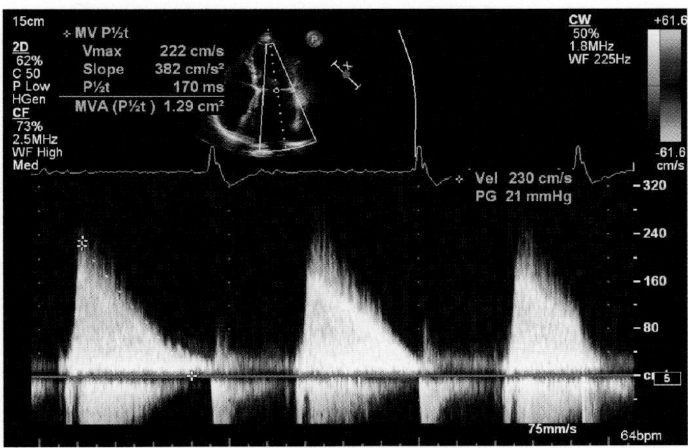

FIGURE 3-6-6 Pressure half-time (PHT) tracing used to determine mitral valve area. Valve area was determined to be approximately 1.3 cm^2.

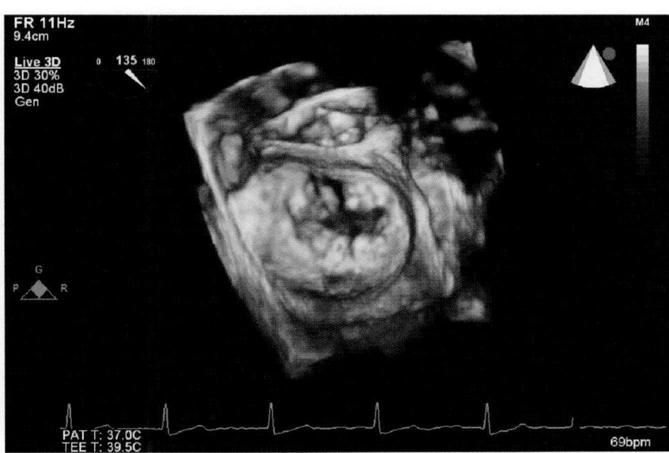

FIGURE 3-6-7 Three-dimensional transesophageal echocardiography of moderately-severe MS in the short-axis view ▶ (see Video 3-6-7).

planimetry, assessment of MV morphology, pulmonary artery systolic pressure (PASP), evaluation for concomitant valvular lesions, and left atrial size should be reported.[1,4]

- The reference measurement for MVA is determined by planimetry in the parasternal short-axis view, perpendicular to the mitral orifice at the tips of the leaflets (Figure 3-6-4).
- The diastolic mean pressure gradient is obtained using the simplified Bernoulli equation $\Delta P=4v^2$ and the transmitral velocity flow curve.[4]
- Continuous-wave Doppler (CWD) and pulse wave Doppler are used to evaluate the maximal velocities most commonly assessed in the apical windows (Figure 3-6-5). Color Doppler is used to identify the highest flow velocity zone to assist in finding the maximal velocity.[4]
- The mean gradient is helpful in the hemodynamic assessment, as the maximal gradient is influenced by left atrial compliance and LV diastolic function. Heart rate (HR), cardiac output (CO), MR and mitral valve area all affect the mean gradient and thus valve gradient alone is not the best assessment of severity.
- If the patient is in atrial fibrillation, a minimum of 5 cardiac cycles should be assessed with the least variation in R-R intervals.
- Pressure half time (PHT or $T_{½}$) is used to measure and calculate MVA (MVA=220/$T_{½}$). PHT is obtained by tracing the deceleration slope of the E-wave on the Doppler spectral display of the transmitral flow (Figure 3-6-6).

TABLE 3-6-1 Co-Morbid Conditions Associated with Increased Mortality in MS

Co-morbidity	%
Progressive pulmonary and systemic congestion	65%
Systemic embolism	25%
Pulmonary embolism	10%
Infections	3%

If MS is left untreated, mortality rates increase and can be due to a variety of confounding co-morbidities. This table lists those morbidities (%).[1,4]

- Stress echocardiography (exercise Doppler echocardiography) should be performed for the assessment of the hemodynamic response of the mean gradient and PASP in patients with MS when there is a discrepancy between resting Doppler echocardiographic findings and clinical findings, as well as patient signs and symptoms of dyspnea, fatigue, and exercise tolerance.[1,4]
- Valve anatomy should be directly assessed with either TTE or TEE. Commissural fusion is assessed in the parasternal short-axis view. At times, 3-D echocardiography can improve accuracy of this assessment (Figure 3-6-7). Leaflet thickening, mobility, and chordal shortening are assessed in the parasternal long-axis, apical 2 and 4 chamber views, which contribute to the decision for valvuloplasty or valve replacement.
- Among many scoring systems, the Wilkins and Cormier scores (used to assess MV anatomy, with the evaluation of leaflet thickness, calcification, mobility and subvalvular/chordal involvement) have been used most often to help predict the success as well as complications (especially the development of MR) of balloon valvuloplasty in patients being considered for this therapy. These scores have not been validated in large studies and have a limited predictive value of the results of balloon mitral commissurotomy; however, they have been found useful in the decision-making process.[1]
- Transesophageal echocardiography (TEE) in MS should be performed to evaluate for LA thrombus and assess the severity of MR in patients considered for percutaneous mitral balloon valvotomy, especially when TTE images are suboptimal.

OTHER DIAGNOSTIC TESTING AND PROCEDURES

- The electrocardiogram (ECG) may demonstrate left atrial enlargement (P-mitrale), atrial fibrillation, RV hypertrophy, and P-pulmonale.
- Computed tomography (CT) or magnetic resonance imaging (MRI) may be used to determine MVA by planimetry if the echocardiographic assessment is suboptimal and if the results will affect clinical management.

- Exercise testing is recommended in patients with MVA <1.5 cm^2 who claim to be asymptomatic or with doubtful symptoms. Parameters such as mean MV gradient and PASP are assessed during the testing.[4]
- Cardiac catheterization to diagnose MS is not indicated unless the clinical presentation does not correlate with the echocardiographic or noninvasive assessment. In appropriate patients, coronary angiography is warranted prior to MV replacement surgery.

DIFFERENTIAL DIAGNOSIS

- LA myxoma, ball valve thrombus, mucopolysaccharidosis, infective endocarditis, and severe annular calcification can cause rare cases of acquired MV obstruction.
- Congenital malformation is rare and causes leaflet thickening with restriction, but commissural fusion is rare in these patients.[4]
- Degenerative MS is due to annular calcification and more predominantly presents with a greater degree of MR. The leaflet bases are involved without the classical commissural fusion or leaflet tip involvement found in rheumatic MS.[4,6]

DIAGNOSIS

- The diagnosis is suspected based on history, physical examination, chest x-ray, and ECG.
- Echocardiography has the major role in confirmation of the diagnosis, evaluating valve anatomy and quantitation of severity of stenosis.
  - Normal MVA is 4.0 to 5.0 cm^2. MVA greater than 1.5 cm^2 and a mean gradient of less than 5 mm Hg typically does not produce symptoms at rest and requires no further work-up.
  - MS is generally classified as mild, moderate, or severe by echocardiography as demonstrated in Table 3-6-2.[1,4]
- Pulmonary vascular resistance is altered as the pulmonary venous pressure increases causing pulmonary artery hypertension and pathological changes of the vasculature. Despite measured mild MS and the absence of symptoms, PASP values greater than 50 mm Hg is an indication for further evaluation.
- The demonstration of an increase to ≥15 mm Hg in the transmitral gradient and ≥60 mm Hg in the PASP with exercise Doppler echocardiography are indications for percutaneous mitral valvotomy if the MV morphology is suitable.[1]

TABLE 3-6-2 Classification of the Severity of Mitral Stenosis[4]

	Mean gradient (mm Hg)	Mitral valve area (cm^2)	PHT (msec)	PASP (mmHg)
Mild	<5	1.6-2	<100	<30
Moderate	5-9	1.1-1.5	100-220	30-50
Severe	>10	<1	>220 msec	>50; exerc >60

MS is generally classified as mild, moderate, or severe by echocardiography as demonstrated in this table.[4]

MANAGEMENT [1,8]

Medical Therapy

- Anticoagulation is indicated in patients with MS and atrial fibrillation, prior embolic event even in sinus rhythm, or when an LA thrombus is present.[1]
- In those with a greater than mild degree of MS, avoidance of physical stresses is advised.
- β-blocker and calcium channel blockers (negative chronotropic agents) are recommended for those with exertional symptoms and tachycardia.
- With the presence of atrial fibrillation, anticoagulation and digoxin as well as a rate-control agent or antiarrhythmic medications should be used.

Imaging Surveillance

- Mild MS: a TTE should be performed every 3 to 5 years.
- Moderate MS: a TTE should be performed every 1 to 2 years.
- Severe MS: annual surveillance with a TTE is indicated.
- TTE should be performed at any time if symptoms of heart failure, palpitations, or fatigue develop or clinical deterioration occurs.

Percutaneous MV Commissurotomy and Valvotomy

- In patients with NYHA functional class II, II, and IV symptoms, percutaneous mitral balloon valvotomy is effective with moderate and severe MS. Intervention is not considered in patients with MS and MVA >1.5 cm^2 unless the patient is symptomatic with a large body size.[1]
- Valvuloplasty is contraindicated if an LA thrombus is present, if the degree of MR is mild-to-moderate or greater, and when the valve morphology is not amendable to the procedure.
- Mean MVA usually doubles with a 50% to 60% reduction in the transmitral gradient with greater than 90% remaining in the NYHA functional class I or II postvalvotomy.[1]
- The underlying MV morphology is the greatest factor in predicting outcomes after a valvotomy.
- Some evidence has suggested that a commissurotomy reduces the incidence of future embolic events, while other evidence states there is no decrease in the incidence of systemic emboli. Continued anticoagulation with warfarin is recommended.

Surgical Management

- In symptomatic patients with NYHA functional class III-IV with moderate or severe MS, surgical repair or replacement is indicated when percutaneous methods are unavailable or contraindicated.[1]
- MV repair is preferred (if feasible) over MV replacement when surgery is indicated.
- MV replacement is reasonable for patients with severe MS and severe pulmonary hypertension (PASP greater than 60 mm Hg) with NYHA functional class I-II symptoms who cannot undergo percutaneous MV valvuloplasty or MV repair.
- Symptomatic patients with moderate to severe MS and concomitant moderate to severe MR should receive a MV replacement.

PATIENT EDUCATION

- Even in asymptomatic patients, yearly surveillance with history, physical exam, chest x-ray and ECG should be performed.
- Symptoms of palpitations with the diagnosis of MS are an indication for ambulatory ECG monitoring to diagnose atrial fibrillation.
- Endocarditis prophylaxis in patients with MS is no longer indicated. For those who have prosthetic cardiac valves or material used for valve repair surgically, prophylactic antibiotics prior to dental procedures are indicated.[7]

FOLLOW-UP

Our 57-year-old female presented with NYHA functional class III symptoms. She was in atrial fibrillation and had an echocardiographic evaluation that demonstrated moderate-to-severe MS. The valve morphology was amendable to percutaneous balloon valvuloplasty (Figure 3-6-8). She tolerated the valvuloplasty (and subsequent cardioversion to sinus rhythm) well and has not had any further complications from systemic embolization or arrhythmias postprocedure. Her postprocedure echo demonstrated an improvement in valve mobility, lower gradients, and no significant MR (Figures 3-6-9 to 3-6-11). Her exercise capacity has greatly improved, and she no longer has symptoms of dyspnea and fatigue. She will be followed annually by clinical visits and TTE surveillance. Antibiotic prophylaxis prior to dental procedures is not indicated; however, she continued with secondary preventive therapy for rheumatic fever. She remains on warfarin for secondary prevention of stroke with MS and atrial fibrillation.

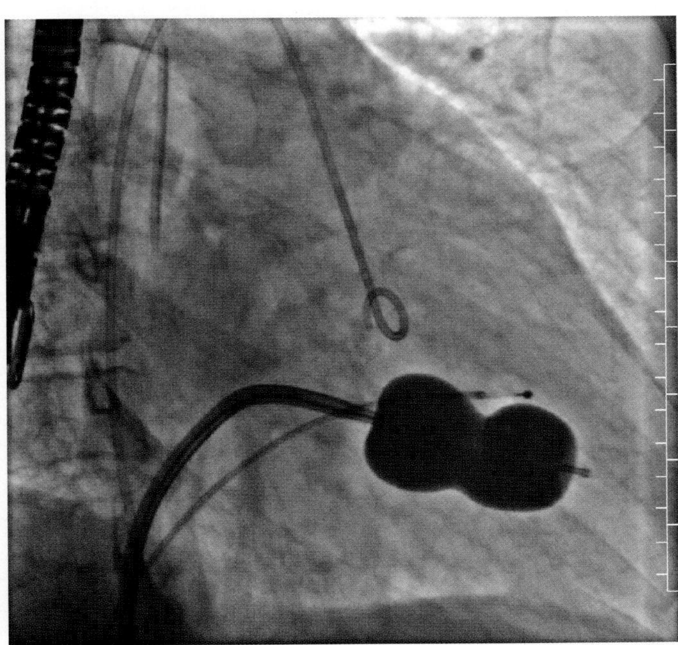

FIGURE 3-6-8 Case demonstration of mitral valve percutaneous balloon valvuloplasty by fluoroscopy. Note the "waist" of the balloon prior to full expansion. A TEE probe (used to monitor the patient during the procedure) is also seen ▶ (see Video 3-6-8).

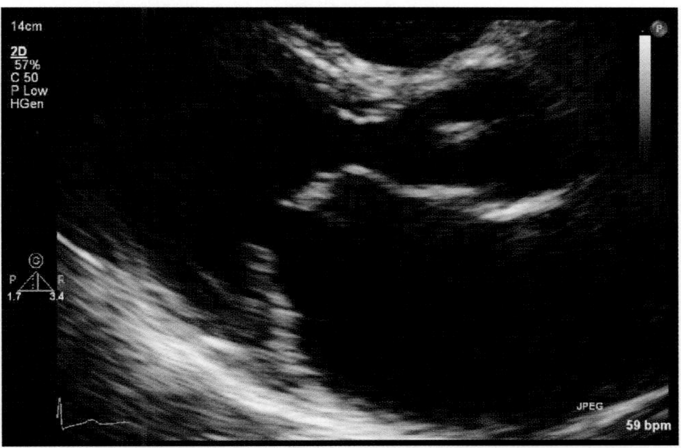

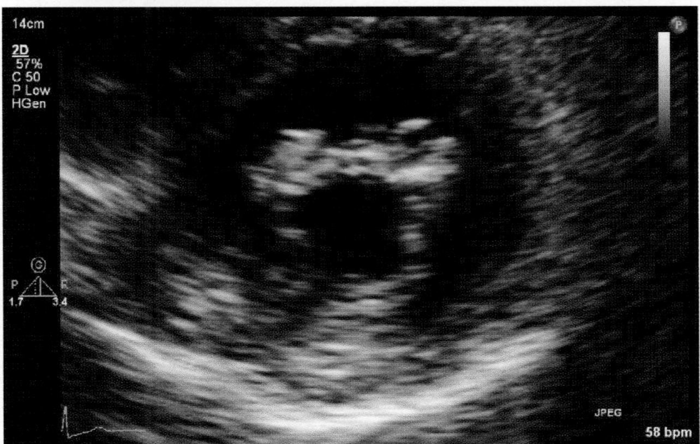

FIGURE 3-6-9 Two dimensional transthoracic echocardiography in PLAX view (top panel) and SAX view (bottom panel) postvalvuloplasty, demonstrating improved MV leaflet mobility ▶ (see Video 3-6-9).

VIDEO LEGENDS

1. Video 3-6-1: 2D transthoracic echocardiography parasternal long axis (PLAX) view of severe MS demonstrating thickened MV leaflets and LA enlargement
2. Video 3-6-2: 2D transthoracic echocardiography Apical 4 chamber view of severe MS. Note the severity of valve thickening and severely enlarged left atrium (LA)

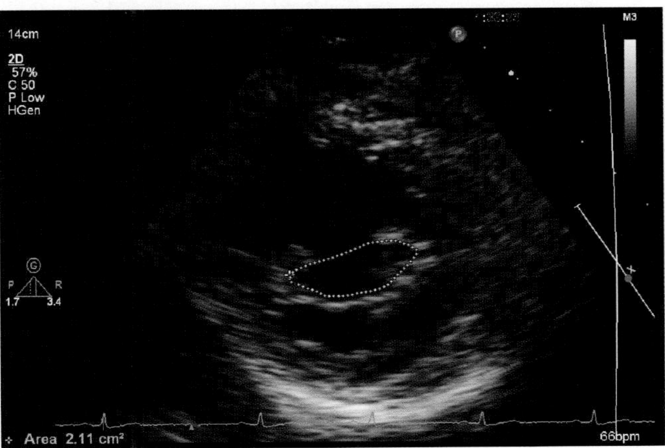

FIGURE 3-6-10 Planimetry of the MVA in the PSAX window demonstrating MS postvalvuloplasty. Valve area is 2.1 cm^2.

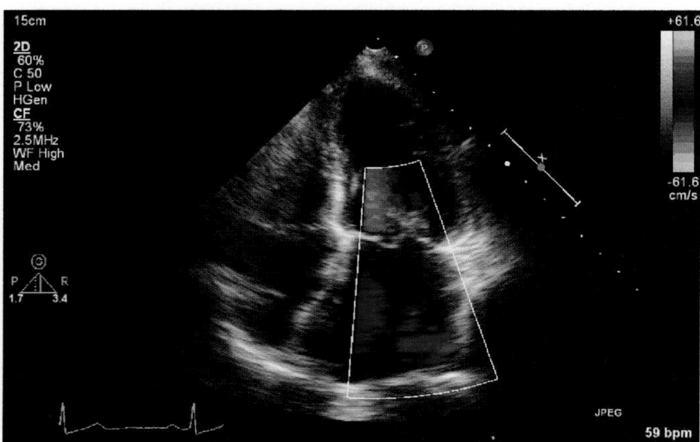

FIGURE 3-6-11 Two-dimensional transthoracic echocardiography postvalvuloplasty for MS in apical 4 chamber view. This demonstrates the desired outcome without significant MR postvalvuloplasty ▶ (see Video 3-6-11).

3. Video 3-6-3: 2D transthoracic echocardiography with color Doppler in the Apical 4 chamber view. There is minimal MR
4. Video 3-6-7: Three-dimensional transesophageal echocardiography of moderately-severe MS in the short-axis view
5. Video 3-6-8: Demonstration of mitral valve percutaneous balloon valvuloplasty by fluoroscopy. Note the "waist" of the balloon prior to full expansion. A TEE probe (used to monitor the patient during the procedure) is also seen
6. Video 3-6-9 L: 2D transthoracic echocardiography in PLAX view post-valvuloplasty demonstrating improved MV leaflet mobility
7. Video 3-6-9 R: 2D transthoracic echocardiography in SAX view post-valvuloplasty demonstrating improved MV leaflet mobility
8. Video 3-6-11: 2D transthoracic echocardiography post-valvuloplasty for MS in apical 4 chamber view. This demonstrates the desired outcome without significant MR post-valvuloplasty

REFERENCES

1. Bonow RO, Carabello BA, Chatterjee K, et al. 2008 focused update incorporated into the ACC/AHA 2006 guidelines for the management of patients with valvular heart disease: a report of the American College of Cardiology/American Heart Association Task Force on Practice Guidelines (Writing committee to develop guidelines for the management of patients with valvular heart disease). Endorsed by the Society of Cardiovascular Anesthesiologists, Society for Cardiovascular Angiography and Interventions, and Society of Thoracic Surgeons. *J Am Coll Cardiol*. 2008;52:e1-142.
2. Reynolds T. *The Echocardiographer's Pocket Reference*. 3rd ed. Phoenix, AZ: School of Cardiac Ultrasound-Arizona Heart Foundation; 2010:442.
3. Constant JM. *Bedside Cardiology*. 5th ed. Philadelphia, PA: Lippincott Williams and Wilkins; 1999:342.
4. Baumgartner H, Hung J, Bermejo J, et al. Echocardiographic assessment of valve stenosis: EAE/ASE recommendations for clinical practice. *Eur J Echocardiogr*. 2009;10(1):1-25.
5. Selzer A, Cohn KE. Natural history of mitral stenosis: a review. *Circulation*. 1972;45(4):878-890.
6. Libby P, Bonow RO, Mann DL, Zipes DP, Braunwald E, eds. *Braunwald's Heart Disease: A Textbook of Cardiovascular Medicine*. 8th ed. Philadelphia, PA: Saunders Elsevier; 2008; No.1-2.
7. Nishimura RA, Carabello BA, Faxon DP, et al. ACC/AHA 2008 guideline update on valvular heart disease: focused update on infective endocarditis: a report of the American College of Cardiology/American Heart Association Task Force on Practice Guidelines endorsed by the Society of Cardiovascular Anesthesiologists, Society for Cardiovascular Angiography and Interventions, and Society of Thoracic Surgeons. *J Am Coll Cardiol*. 2008;52(8):676-685.
8. Nishimura RA, Otto CM, Bonow RO, et al. 2014 AHA/ACC guideline for the management of patients with valvular heart disease:executive summary; a report of the American College of Cardiology/American Heart Association Task Force on Practice Guidelines. *J Am Coll Cardiol*. 2014; 63:2348-2388.

SECTION 7

Chronic Ischemic Mitral Regurgitation

Kavita Sharma, MD

CLINICAL CASE PRESENTATION

The patient is a 53-year-old man with a history of hypertension and hyperlipidemia. He has known coronary artery disease (high grade disease in the right coronary and circumflex arteries) and a prior myocardial infarction. He has not had ongoing medical follow-up. He has been having progressive dyspnea and lower extremity edema and presented to the emergency room with worsening symptoms including dyspnea at rest. On physical examination, his rhythm was irregular, with a normal S_1 and S_2. An S_3 gallop was present. There is displacement of the LV apical impulse. There is a holosystolic murmur heard throughout the precordium, loudest at the apex, radiating to the axilla. He has bilateral rales in his lung fields. There is 2+ pitting edema of the lower extremities. An ECG demonstrated sinus rhythm with premature atrial contractions and a prior inferior MI.

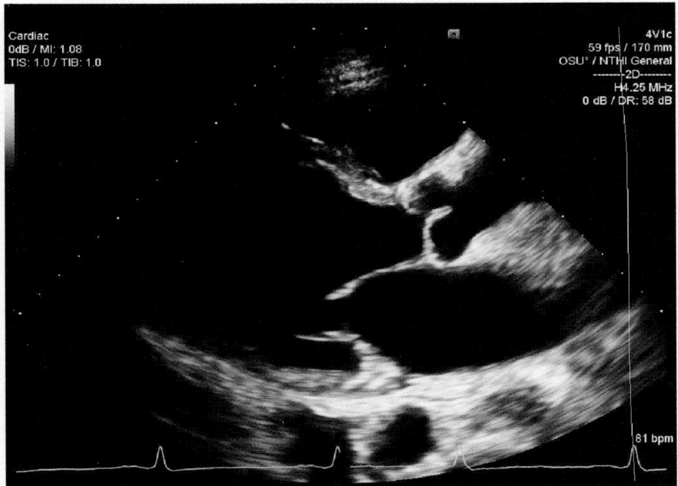

FIGURE 3-7-1 Parasternal long axis demonstrating a dilated LV with an inferolateral wall motion abnormality and tethering of the posterior MV leaflet ► (see Video 3-7-1).

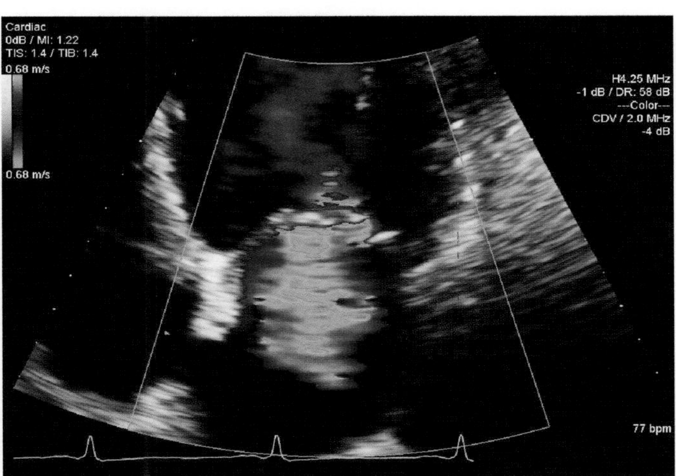

FIGURE 3-7-3 Apical 4 chamber view with color Doppler demonstrating severe MR ► (see Video 3-7-3).

Chest x-ray demonstrated evidence of pulmonary congestion. His echocardiogram demonstrated a dilated left ventricle with moderately severe segmental LV dysfunction. There were wall motion abnormalities involving the inferior and inferolateral walls. Color Doppler demonstrated severe mitral regurgitation (Figures 3-7-1 to 3-7-8). He was treated with IV diuretics with improvement of his symptoms. Cardiac catheterization demonstrated progression of his coronary artery disease. He was evaluated by cardiothoracic surgery and underwent successful mitral valve repair and coronary artery bypass grafting. Postoperatively, he has done well. Subsequent echocardiography demonstrated trivial mitral insufficiency, no significant MV gradient, and an improvement in his left ventricular ejection fraction.

PATHOPHYSIOLOGY AND ETIOLOGY

- Mitral regurgitation (MR) may occur from a disorder of the mitral valve, and causes include mitral valve prolapse, collagen vascular disease, certain drugs, rheumatic heart disease, endocarditis, and coronary artery disease.[1]
- MR due to ischemic heart disease may be due to ischemia/infarction of the papillary muscle, regional contractile dysfunction of the LV walls with disruption of the support of the papillary muscle, or, as in the current case, progressive LV dysfunction/remodeling with altered LV geometry.
- MR may occur from a dilated annulus secondary to a dilated left ventricle.
- MR may occur acutely (such as from endocarditis, ruptured papillary muscles or ruptured chordae tendineae), or may occur gradually.
- When MR occurs gradually, the left ventricle has time to adapt and develop compensatory hypertrophy. Cardiac output is maintained.[2] In addition, the left atrium will enlarge over time, and pulmonary congestion does not develop. Patients may remain asymptomatic for years.
- In time, however, the prolonged burden of volume may result in LV dysfunction.

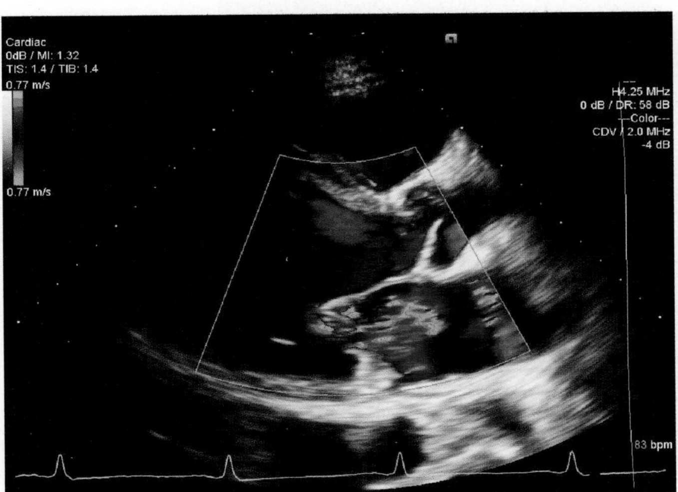

FIGURE 3-7-2 Parasternal long axis with color Doppler demonstrating severe MR. There is also mild AR ► (see Video 3-7-2).

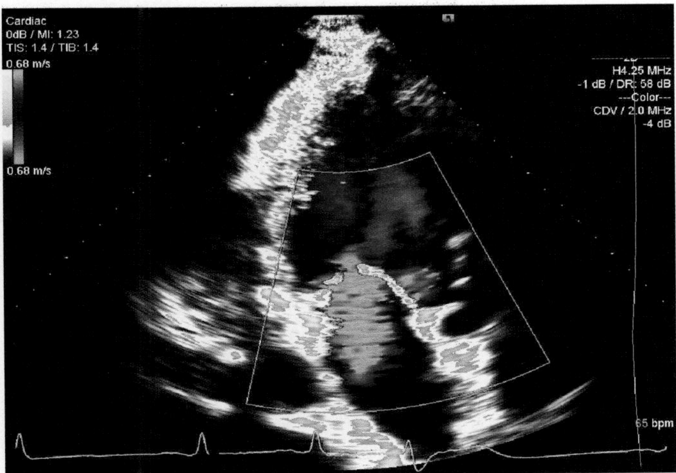

FIGURE 3-7-4 Apical 3 chamber view with color Doppler demonstrating the MR ► (see Video 3-7-4).

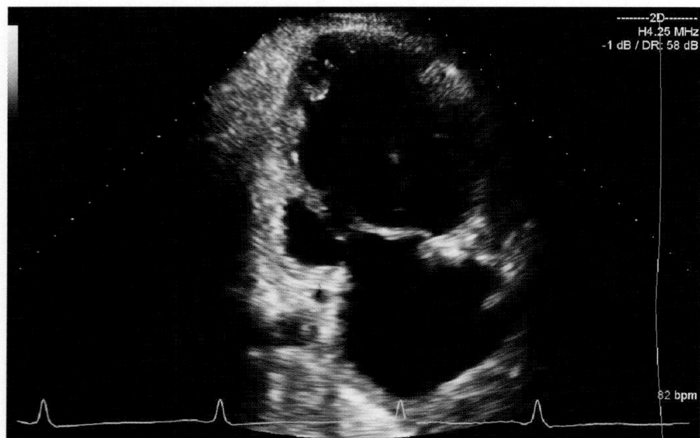

FIGURE 3-7-5 Apical 2 chamber view demonstrating the inferior wall motion abnormality ▶ (see Video 3-7-5).

NATURAL HISTORY AND CLINICAL FEATURES

- Patients with mild to moderate MR may remain asymptomatic for many years.[1]
- The progression of MR is variable and depends on the underlying lesion, LV function/geometry, and mitral annular size.[1]
- Patients with chronic severe MR have a high likelihood of developing symptoms or LV dysfunction over 6 to 10 years.[3]
- Patients at risk of death are those with ejection fractions <60% and those with NYHA functional class III-IV symptoms.[4]
- Patients with ischemic MR fare worse than those with non-ischemic MR. In ischemic MR, the MR results from papillary muscle displacement and tethering of the mitral leaflets.
- In ischemic MR, there is local remodeling of the LV (apical and posterior displacement of the papillary muscles), which results in abnormal valvular function.

EPIDEMIOLOGY

- A study at Duke University found that post-infarction mitral regurgitation occurred in 19% of 11,748 patients having significant coronary artery disease at cardiac catheterization.[5]

ECHOCARDIOGRAPHY (TABLE 3-7-1)

Echocardiography plays a vital role in the evaluation of MR. The valve structure, valve apparatus, and left ventricular function and wall motion are examined on 2-D echocardiography. Doppler echocardiography (spectral and color flow Doppler) provide information on the presence and severity of the mitral insufficiency. An integrative approach to quantitation of MR is supported in the guidelines.

- In ischemic MR, the regurgitant jet may result from LV annular dilation or from tethering of the posterior mitral leaflet because of regional LV dysfunction in patients with ischemic heart disease.[1]
- The size of the left ventricle and left atrium is obtained from 2-D echo. These are useful in determining whether the MR is acute or chronic, its severity, and whether surgery is indicated.[6] Normal LV end-diastolic volume is <82 ml/m2[7] and normal maximal LA volume is <36 ml/m2.[8]
- Left ventricular function and regional wall motion abnormalities are identified on 2-D echo.

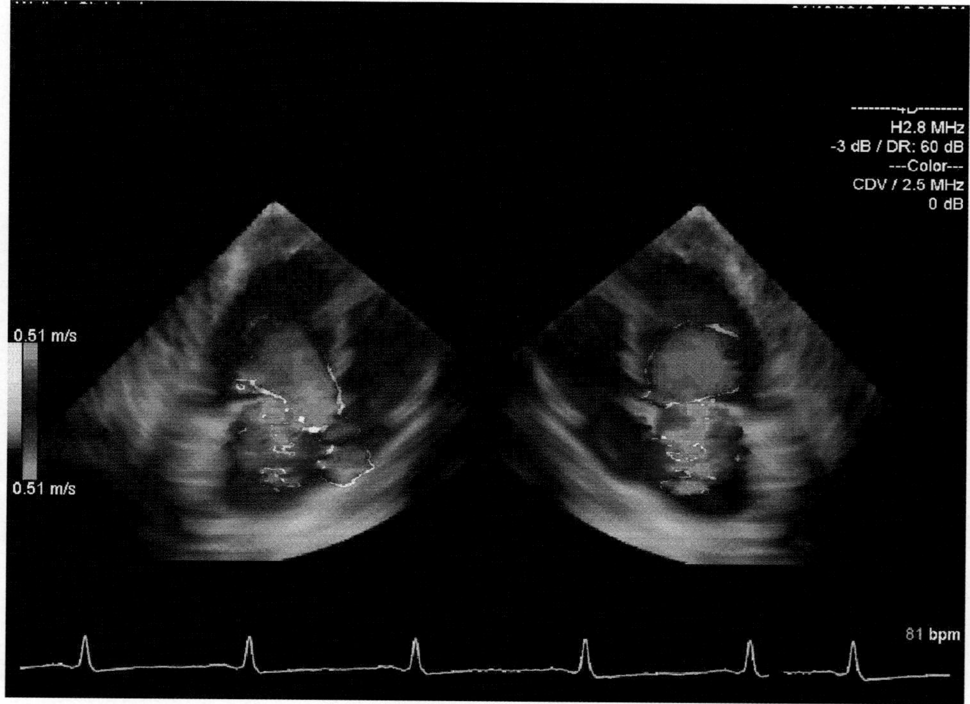

FIGURE 3-7-6 Three-dimensional echo with color Doppler demonstrating severe MR ▶ (see Video 3-7-6).

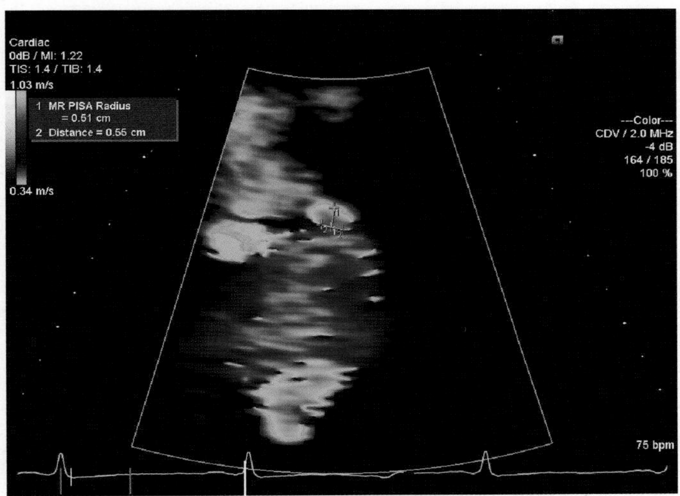

FIGURE 3-7-7 Color flow Doppler with the baseline shifted to measure the PISA radius.

- Color Doppler is used to obtain the regurgitant jet area, the vena contracta, and the proximal isovelocity surface area (PISA).
- Examination of the regurgitant area based on color Doppler assessment can be misleading in determining MR severity, as it depends on the preload and afterload of the patient,[9] and appears larger in central jets versus eccentric jets.[10]
- The vena contracta is the narrowest portion of the jet that occurs at or just downstream from the orifice.[11] A vena contracta <0.3 cm is associated with mild MR, and severe MR is associated with a vena contracta between 0.6 and 0.8 cm.[12]
- The PISA method for assessing MR is based on the assumption that as blood approaches a regurgitant orifice, its velocity increases, forming concentric, roughly hemispheric shells of increasing velocity and decreasing surface area.[13] With color Doppler, a hemispheric shape may be visualized at the Nyquist limit. The flow rate can then be calculated at the regugitant orifice, as the product of the surface area of the hemisphere and aliasing velocity. Using the peak velocity of the MR jet, the effective regurgitant orifice area (EROA) may be calculated. An EROA of ≥0.4 cm^2 is consistent with severe MR, 0.20 to 0.39 cm^2 is consistent with moderate MR, and <0.20 cm^2 is consistent with mild MR.[11]

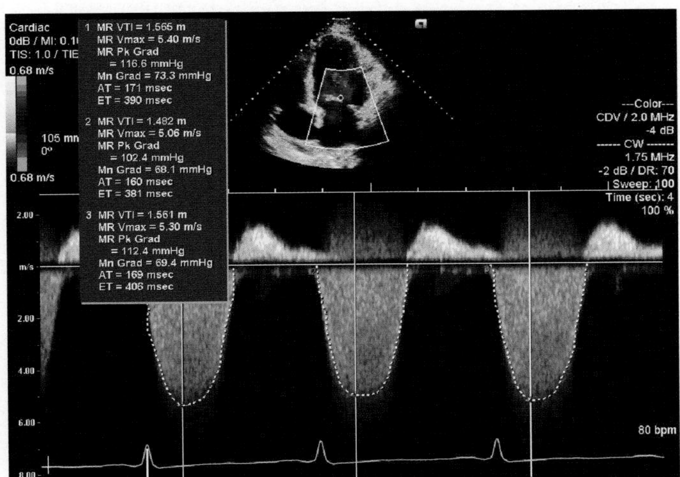

FIGURE 3-7-8 Continuous-wave Doppler of the mitral regurgitation jet.

- Useful information may be obtained from continuous-wave Doppler. A truncated, triangular jet contour with early peaking of the maximal velocity indicates elevated left atrial pressure or more severe MR.
- A dense MR envelope is consistent with severe MR.
- Pulmonary artery systolic pressure should also be estimated using the continuous-wave Doppler jet of tricuspid regurgitation, as pulmonary artery hypertension can indicate the presence of severe of MR.
- On pulsed wave Doppler, patients with severe MR often have a dominant early filling ("E" wave) on mitral inflow.[14]
- The stroke volume can be calculated at different valve sites via pulsed wave Doppler.[11] The cross-sectional area of a valve (or annulus) multipled by the time velocity integral (TVI) at the valve gives the stroke volume. It can be determined at both the regurgitant valve and another valve. The difference between the two is the regurgitant volume (RV). The RV divided by the stroke volume of the regurgitant valve gives the regurgitant fraction (RF). Severe MR is associated with a RV of >60 ml/beat and a RF of ≥50%.
- The pulmonary vein flow pattern has a characteristic pattern with severe MR. Normally the systolic component of pulmonary vein flow is higher than the diastolic component. In MR, there is a fall in the systolic velocity of pulmonary vein flow, and in severe MR, it becomes reversed.[11]
- TEE is useful in evaluating MR due to its improved resolution and the proximity of the mitral valve to the TEE probe.
- The complete evaluation of MR requires integration of these various components.

OTHER DIAGNOSTIC MODALITIES

- In cases where the severity of mitral regurgitation is unclear, left ventriculography is recommended.[1]
- When patients have severe MR and risk factors for coronary artery disease, cardiac catheterization is recommended prior to MV surgery.[1]
- When there is a discrepancy between physical exam and echocardiography regarding the severity of MR, left ventriculography, trans-esophageal echocardiography, or cardiac magnetic resonance is recommended.[1]

MANAGEMENT[1,16]

- The treatment of ischemic mitral regurgitation is a combination of medical and surgical treatment.
- There has been no proven benefit in the use of ACE inhibitors in the treatment of MR.
- Unless hypertension is present, ACE inhibitors are not indicated for MR.
- However, β-blockers and ACE inhibitors are recommended for the treatment of LV dysfunction.

TABLE 3-7-1 Selected Echocardiographic Parameters for the Evaluation of Mitral Regurgitation

Parameter	Advantages	Disadvantages
Left atrial and left ventricular size	Enlargement sensitive for chronic significant MR, important for outcomes. Normal size virtually excludes significant chronic MR.	Enlargement seen in other conditions. May be normal in acute significant MR.
Mitral valve leaflet/ support apparatus	Flail valve and ruptured papillary muscle specific for significant MR.	Other abnormalities do not imply significant MR.
Jet area-color flow	Simple, quick screen for mild or severe central MR. Evaluates spatial orientation of jet.	Subject to technical, hemodynamic variation. Significantly underestimates severity in wall-impinging jets.
Vena contracta width	Simple, quantitative, good at identifying mild or severe MR.	Not useful for multiple MR jets; intermediate values require confirmation. Small values, thus small error leads to large percentage error.
Proximal isovelocity surface area (PISA)	Quantitative. Presence of flow convergence at Nyquist limit of 50-60 cm/s alerts to significant MR. Provides both lesion severity (effective regurgitant orifice area and regurgitant fraction) and volume overload (regurgitant volume).	Less accurate in eccentric jets. Not valid in multiple jets. Provides peak flow and maximal effective regurgitant orifice area.
Flow quantitation-pulsed wave	Quantitative. Valid in multiple jets and eccentric jets. Provides both lesion severity (effective regurgitant orifice area and regurgitant fraction) and volume overload (regurgitant volume).	Measurement of flow at mitral valve annulus less reliable in calcific mitral valve and/ or annulus. Not valid with concomitant significant aortic regurgitation unless pulmonic site is used.
Jet profile–continuous-wave	Simple, readily available.	Qualitative, complementary data.
Peak mitral E velocity	Simple, readily available. A-wave dominance excludes severe MR.	Influenced by left atrial pressure, left ventricular relaxation, mitral valve area, and atrial fibrillation. Complementary data only, does not quantify MR severity.
Pulmonary vein flow	Simple, systolic flow reversal is specific for severe MR.	Influenced by left atrial pressure, atrial fibrillation. Not accurate if MR jet directed into the sampled vein.

MR = mitral regurgitation
Adapted with permission from Zoghbi WA, Enriquez-Sarano M, Foster E, Grayburn PA, Kraft CD, Levine RA, et al. Recommendations for evaluation of the severity of native valvular regurgitation with two-dimensional and Doppler echocardiography. *J Am Soc Echocardiogr.* 2003;16:777-802.[11]

- In general, MV repair is recommended over MV replacement when feasible
- MV surgery is recommended as a Class I indication in the ACC/ AHA Guidelines for the Management of Patients with Valvular Heart Disease in chronic severe MR when patients have NYHA functional class II, III, or IV symptoms (in the absence of severe LV dysfunction and/or end-systolic dimension >55 mm).[1,16]
- MV surgery is recommended as a Class I indication for asymptomatic patients with chronic severe MR and ejection fractions <60% (but greater than 30%) and/or end systolic dimension >40 mm.[1,16]
- In asymptomatic patients, other indications for surgery (when the likelihood of mitral valve repair is >95% and the expected mortality is <1%) include new onset atrial fibrillation, pulmonary hypertension and patients with an EF >60% with an LVESD <40 mm (Class IIa).[16]
- In patients with chronic ischemic MR, patients often benefit from MV annuloplasty at the time of CABG.
- The European Society of Cardiology guidelines recommend that patients with severe ischemic MR who are going to undergo coronary artery bypass grafting should undergo mitral valve surgery.[15]

FOLLOW-UP

- In asymptomatic patients with moderate to severe MR, annual or semiannual echocardiography is recommended to assess LV function (ejection fraction and end-systolic dimension).[1]

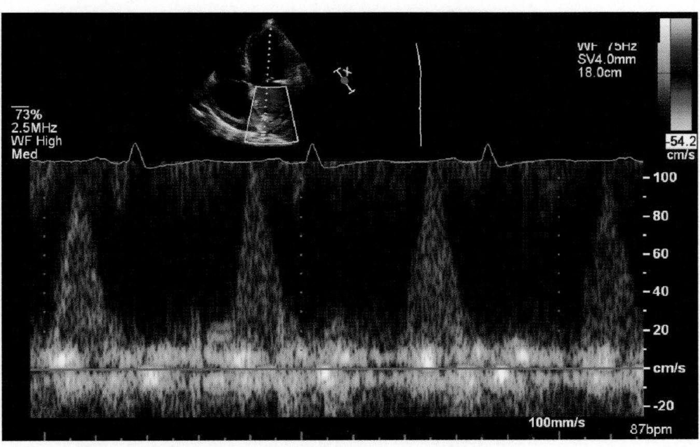

FIGURE 3-7-9 Pulsed wave Doppler of the pulmonary vein flow demonstrating diastolic predominance with blunted/reversed systolic flow.

- With a change in signs or symptoms in patients with MR, an echocardiogram is recommended.
- Exercise echocardiography is reasonable in asymptomatic patients with severe MR to assess exercise tolerance and the effects of exercise on pulmonary artery pressure and MR severity.
- Echocardiography is not indicated for routine follow-up evaluation of asymptomatic patients with mild MR and normal LV size and function.
- After mitral valve repair or replacement, patients should receive endocarditis prophylaxis, and those with atrial fibrillation should receive anticoagulation.
- During the first 3 months after mitral valve repair, it is reasonable for patients to receive oral anticoagulation. Long-term treatment with aspirin is reasonable after mitral valve repair or bioprosthetic valve replacement.
- After mechanical mitral valve replacement, long-term anticoagulation is required.
- Aspirin is recommended for all patients with prosthetic heart valves.
- Aspirin alone is recommended for patients with bioprosthetic heart valves and no risk factors.
- Aspirin combined with warfarin is recommended with patients with mechanical heart valves and high-risk patients with bioprostheses.
- A baseline echocardiogram is recommended after mitral valve repair or replacement.

SUMMARY

- Patients with ischemic mitral regurgitation have a poorer prognosis than those with nonischemic mitral regurgitation.
- Echocardiography is useful to evaluate the severity of mitral regurgitation, left ventricular function, and wall motion abnormalities.
- The treatment of ischemic mitral regurgitation includes medical therapy for heart failure and mitral valve surgery.

VIDEO LEGENDS

1. Video 3-7-1: Parasternal long axis demonstrating a dilated LV with an inferolateral wall motion abnormality and tethering of the posterior MV leaflet
2. Video 3-7-2: Parasternal long axis with color Doppler demonstrating severe MR. There is also mild AR
3. Video 3-7-3: Apical four chamber view with color Doppler demonstrating severe MR.
4. Video 3-7-4: Apical three-chamber with color Doppler demonstrating the MR
5. Video 3-7-5: Apical 2 chamber view demonstrating the inferior wall motion abnormality
6. Video 3-7-6: 3 D Echo with color Doppler demonstrating severe MR

REFERENCES

1. Bonow RO, Carabello BA, Chatterjee K, et al. 2008 focused update incorporated into the ACC/AHA 2006 guidelines for the management of patients with valvular heart disease: a report of the American College of Cardiology/American Heart Association Task Force on Practice Guidelines (Writing committee to develop guidelines for the management of patients with valvular heart disease). Endorsed by the Society of Cardiovascular Anesthesiologists, Society for Cardiovascular Angiography and Interventions, and Society of Thoracic Surgeons. *J Am Coll Cardiol*. 2008;52:e1-142.
2. Zile MR, Gaasch WH, Carroll JD, Levine HJ. Chronic mitral regurgitation: predictive value of preoperative echocardiographic indexes of left ventricular function and wall stress. *J Am Coll Cardiol*. 1984;3:235-242.
3. Rosenhek R, Rader F, Klaar U, et al. Outcome of watchful waiting in asymptomatic severe mitral regurgitation. *Circulation*. 2006;113:2238-2244.
4. Ling LH, Enriquez-Sarano M, Seward JB, et al. Clinical outcome of mitral regurgitation due to flail leaflet. *N Engl J Med*. 1996;335:1417-1423.
5. Hickey MS, Smith LR, Muhlbaier LH, et al. Current prognosis of ischemic mitral regurgitation. Implications for future management. *Circulation*. 1988;78:151-159.
6. Carabello BA, Crawford FA, Jr. Valvular heart disease. *N Engl J Med*. 1997;337:32-41.
7. Schiller NB, Shah PM, Crawford M, et al. Recommendations for quantitation of the left ventricle by two-dimensional echocardiography. American Society of Echocardiography Committee on Standards, Subcommittee on Quantitation of Two-Dimensional Echocardiograms. *J Am Soc Echocardiogr*. 1989;2:358-367.
8. Wang Y, Gutman JM, Heilbron D, Wahr D, Schiller NB. Atrial volume in a normal adult population by two-dimensional echocardiography. *Chest*. 1984;86:595-601.
9. Sahn DJ. Instrumentation and physical factors related to visualization of stenotic and regurgitant jets by Doppler color flow mapping. *J Am Coll Cardiol*. 1988;12:1354-1365.

10. Chen CG, Thomas JD, Anconina J, et al. Impact of impinging wall jet on color Doppler quantification of mitral regurgitation. *Circulation*. 1991;84:712-720.

11. Zoghbi WA, Enriquez-Sarano M, Foster E, et al. Recommendations for evaluation of the severity of native valvular regurgitation with two-dimensional and Doppler echocardiography. *J Am Soc Echocardiogr*. 2003;16:777-802.

12. Heinle SK, Hall SA, Brickner ME, Willett DL, Grayburn PA. Comparison of vena contracta width by multiplane transesophageal echocardiography with quantitative Doppler assessment of mitral regurgitation. *Am J Cardiol*. 1998;81:175-179.

13. Bargiggia GS, Tronconi L, Sahn DJ, et al. A new method for quantitation of mitral regurgitation based on color flow Doppler imaging of flow convergence proximal to regurgitant orifice. *Circulation*. 1991;84:1481-1489.

14. Thomas L, Foster E, Schiller NB. Peak mitral inflow velocity predicts mitral regurgitation severity. *J Am Coll Cardiol*. 1998;31:174-179.

15. Vahanian A, Baumgartner H, Bax J, et al. Guidelines on the management of valvular heart disease: The Task Force on the Management of Valvular Heart Disease of the European Society of Cardiology. *Eur Heart J*. 2007;28:230-268.

16. Nishimura RA, Otto CM, Bonow RO, et al. 2014 AHA/ACC guideline for the management of patients with valvular heart disease:executive summary; a report of the American College of Cardiology/American Heart Association Task Force on Practice Guidelines. *J Am Coll Cardiol*. 2014; 63:2348-2388.

SECTION 8

Mitral Regurgitation Secondary to Nonischemic Dilated Cardiomyopathy

Kavita Sharma, MD

CLINICAL CASE PRESENTATION

The patient is a 58-year-old man with a history of hypothyroidism who presents with progressive dyspnea, orthopnea, and edema. He is on thyroid supplementation. On examination, he has a soft S_1 and a normal S_2. He has an S_3 gallop. He has an apically displaced point of maximal impulse. There is a grade 3/6 holosystolic murmur, best heard at the apex and radiating to the axilla. His lungs have rales one-quarter of the way up bilaterally. He has 1+ pitting edema of both lower extremities. He was treated with intravenous diuretics with clinical improvement. An echocardiogram was obtained. This demonstrates a severely dilated left ventricle with severely reduced function, ejection fraction <20%. There is global left ventricular dysfunction with inferior and inferolateral wall akinesis. There is severe mitral regurgitation. There is mild aortic regurgitation and mild tricuspid regurgitation (Figures 3-8-1 to 3-8-4). Cardiac catheterization revealed no evidence of coronary artery disease. He underwent a myocardial biopsy, which demonstrated nonspecific fibrosis. He was treated with an ace-inhibitor, β-blocker and spironolactone, as well as furosemide. He has had improvement of his symptoms.

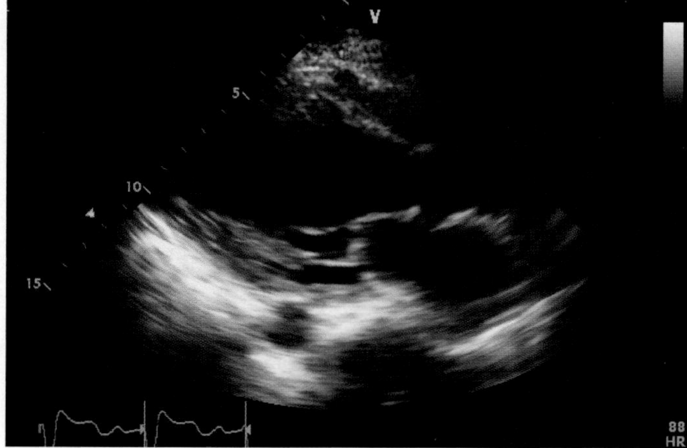

FIGURE 3-8-1 Parasternal long axis view demonstrating severe LV dysfunction and apical displacement of the mitral valve leaflets ▶ (see Video 3-8-1).

PATHOPHYSIOLOGY AND ETIOLOGY

- In dilated cardiomyopathy, the left ventricle or both ventricles show evidence of dilation and impaired function (left ventricular ejection fraction <40% or fractional shortening less than 25%).[1]
- The most common causes of dilated cardiomyopathy are idiopathic, myocarditis, and coronary artery disease.[2]
- Other causes are infiltrative disease, postpartum cardiomyopathy, stress-induced, infectious, toxic, genetic, tachycardia-induced, autoimmune, endocrine dysfunction, and nutritional deficiency.
- When primary and secondary causes of cardiomyopathy are ruled out, the diagnosis of idiopathic dilated cardiomyopathy is made.
- The mitral valve leaflets are structurally normal. Mitral insufficiency is due to abnormalities of the annulus (dilation) or

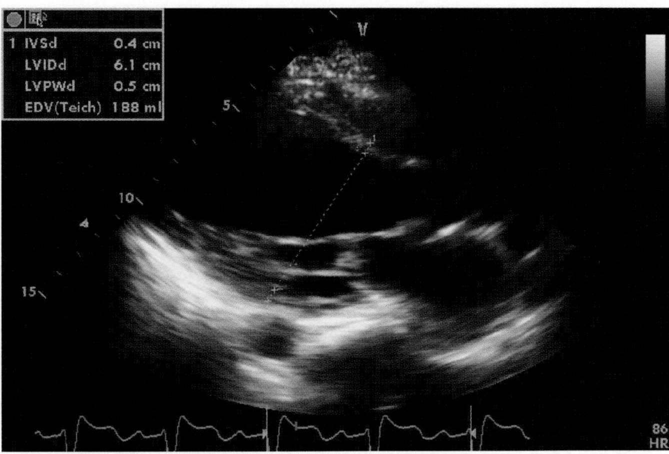

FIGURE 3-8-2 Parasternal long axis view demonstrating left ventricular dimensions.

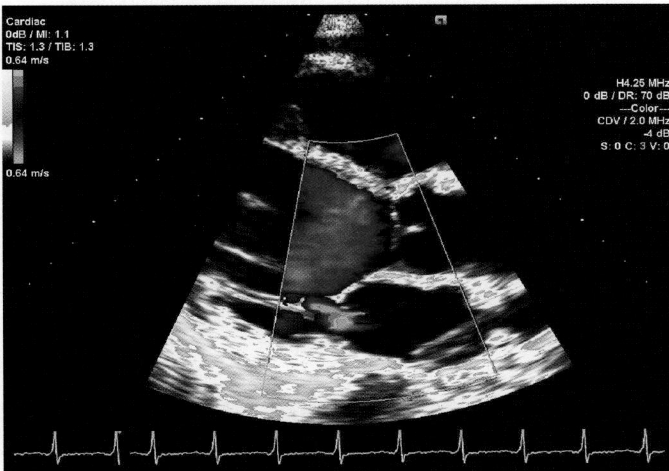

FIGURE 3-8-3 Parasternal long axis with color flow Doppler demonstrating mitral insufficiency ▶ (see Video 3-8-3).

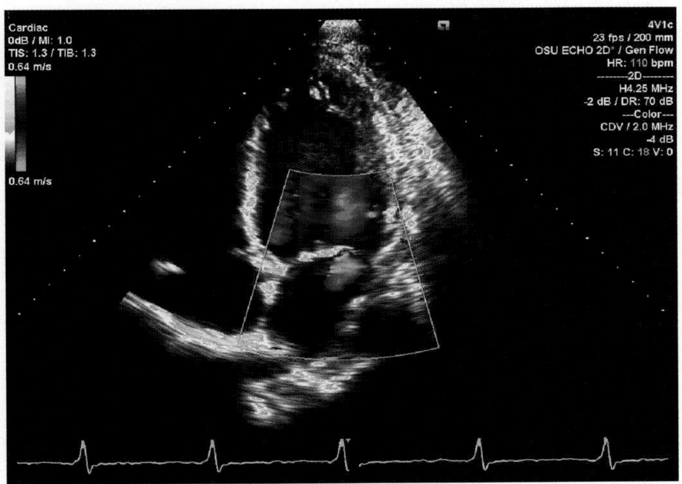

FIGURE 3-8-4 Apical 4 chamber with color flow Doppler demonstrating mitral insufficiency ▶ (see Video 3-8-4).

alterations in LV geometry (LV dilation and increased sphericity) and the papillary muscles which results in incomplete leaflet coaptation.[3]

EPIDEMIOLOGY

- The incidence of dilated cardiomyopathy has been estimated to be 5 to 8 cases per 100,000 population, with a prevalence of 36 per 100,000.[4]
- Among patients with nonischemic dilated cardiomyopathy, significant MR is common; approximately ⅓ of patients with nonischemic dilated cardiomyopathy have significant MR.[5]

ECHOCARDIOGRAPHY

Echocardiography plays a vital role in the evaluation of nonischemic MR. The valve structure, valve apparatus, and the left ventricular function and wall motion are examined on 2-dimensional echocardiography (2DE). Doppler echocardiography (spectral and color flow Doppler) provide information on the presence/severity of the mitral insufficiency. An integrative approach to quantitation of MR is supported in the guidelines (see Table3-7-1 in Section VII, Chronic Ischemic Mitral Regurgitation).

- The size of the left ventricle and left atrium is obtained from 2DE. These are useful in determining whether the MR is acute or chronic, its severity, and whether surgery is indicated.[6] Normal LV end-diastolic volume is <82 ml/m^2.[7] Normal maximal LA volume is <36 ml/m^2.[8]
- Left ventricular function and regional wall motion abnormalities are identified on 2DE.
- Color Doppler is used to obtain the regurgitant jet area, the vena contracta, and the proximal isovelocity surface area (PISA).
- Examination of the regurgitant area can be misleading in determining MR severity, as it depends on the preload and afterload of the patient,[9] and appears larger in central jets versus eccentric jets.[10]
- The vena contracta is the narrowest portion of the jet that occurs at or just downstream from the orifice.[11] A vena contracta <0.3 cm is associated with mild MR, and severe MR is associated with a vena contracta between 0.6 and 0.8 cm.[12]
- The PISA method (see Section VII: Chronic Ischemic Mitral Regurgitation) for assessing MR is based on the assumption that as blood approaches a regurgitant orifice, its velocity increases, forming concentric, roughly hemispheric shells of increasing velocity and decreasing surface area.[13] An EROA of ≥ 0.4 cm^2 is consistent with severe MR, 0.20 to 0.39 cm^2 consistent with moderate MR, and <0.20 cm^2 with mild MR.[11]
- Useful information may be obtained from continuous-wave Doppler. A truncated, triangular jet contour with early peaking of the maximal velocity indicates elevated left atrial pressure or more severe MR.
- A dense MR envelope is consistent with severe MR.
- Pulmonary artery systolic pressure should also be estimated using the continuous-wave Doppler jet of tricuspid regurgitation, as pulmonary artery hypertension can indicate the severity of MR.

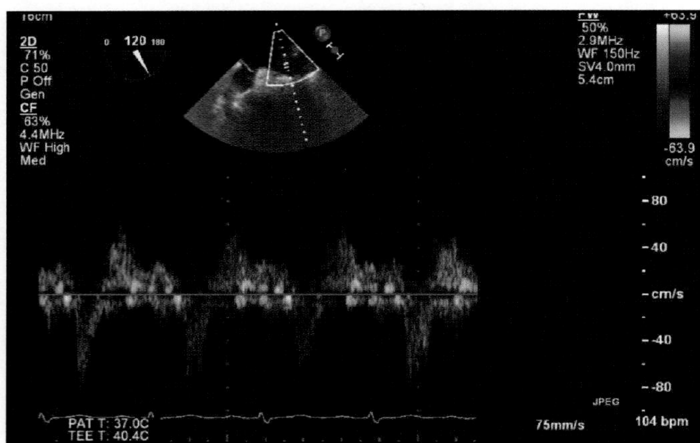

FIGURE 3-8-5 TEE image from a different patient. Doppler of the pulmonary vein is shown demonstrating systolic flow reversal of the pulmonary vein flow, an indicator of severe MR.

- On pulsed wave Doppler, patients with severe MR often have a dominant early filling on mitral inflow (increased E velocity).[14]
- The stroke volume can be calculated at different sites via pulsed Doppler.[11] It can be determined at both the regurgitant valve and another valve. The difference between the two is the regurgitant volume (RV). Severe MR is associated with a RV of >60 ml/beat and a RF of ≥50% (see Section VII: Chronic Ischemic Mitral Regurgitation).
- The pulmonary vein flow pattern has a characteristic pattern with severe MR (Figure 3-8-5). Normally, the systolic component of pulmonary vein flow is higher than the diastolic component. In MR, there is a fall in the systolic velocity of pulmonary vein flow, and in severe MR, it becomes reversed.[11]
- TEE is useful in evaluating MR due to its improved resolution and the proximity of the mitral valve to the TEE probe.
- The complete evaluation of MR requires integration of these various components.

OTHER DIAGNOSTIC MODALITIES

- In cases where the severity of mitral regurgitation is unclear, left ventriculography is recommended.[15]
- When there is a discrepancy between physical exam and echocardiography regarding the severity of MR, left ventriculography, transesophageal echocardiography or cardiac magnetic resonance is recommended.[15]

MANAGEMENT

- Medical therapies that reduce remodeling should restore the orientation of the papillary muscles.
- By reducing LV load, various intravenous and oral vasodilators (nitroprusside, angiotensin-converting enzyme inhibitors, hydralazine, and isosorbide dinitrate) along with loop diuretics may, in selected patients, reduce MR by as much as 1 to 2 echocardiographic grades[16] and substantially reduce vena contracta width.[17]
- Cardiac resynchronization therapy may reduce mitral regurgitation.
- MV surgery (MV repair is recommended over mitral valve replacement when possible) is a Class IIb indication in patients with severe secondary MR.[18]

FOLLOW-UP[18]

- In asymptomatic patients with moderate to severe MR, annual or bi-annual echocardiography is recommended to assess LV function (ejection fraction and end-systolic dimension).
- With a change in signs or symptoms in patients with MR, an echocardiogram is recommended.
- Exercise echocardiography is reasonable in asymptomatic patients with severe MR to assess exercise tolerance and the effects of exercise on pulmonary artery pressure and MR severity.
- Echocardiography is not indicated for routine follow-up evaluation of asymptomatic patients with mild MR and normal LV size and function.
- After mitral valve repair or replacement, patients should receive endocarditis prophylaxis and those with atrial fibrillation should receive anticoagulation.
- During the first 3 months after mitral valve replacement, it is reasonable for patients to receive oral anticoagulation. Long-term treatment with aspirin is reasonable after mitral valve repair or bioprosthetic valve replacement.
- After mechanical mitral valve replacement, long-term anticoagulation is required.
- A baseline echocardiogram is recommended after mitral valve repair or replacement.

SUMMARY

- Mitral regurgitation is common in patients with nonischemic dilated cardiomyopathy.
- Echocardiography is useful to evaluate the severity of mitral regurgitation, left ventricular function, and wall motion abnormalities.
- Medical therapy and surgical therapy may be useful in the management of nonischemic MR.

VIDEO LEGENDS

1. Video 3-8-1: Parasternal long axis view demonstrating severe LV dysfunction and apical displacement of the mitral valve leaflets
2. Video 3-8-3: Parasternal long axis with color flow Doppler demonstrating mitral insufficiency
3. Video 3-8-4: Apical four chamber with color flow Doppler demonstrating mitral insufficiency

REFERENCES

1. Richardson P, McKenna W, Bristow M, et al. Report of the 1995 World Health Organization/International Society and Federation of Cardiology Task Force on the definition and classification of cardiomyopathies. *Circulation*. 1996;93:841-842.
2. Kasper EK, Agema WR, Hutchins GM, Deckers JW, Hare JM, Baughman KL. The causes of dilated cardiomyopathy: a clinicopathologic review of 673 consecutive patients. *J Am Coll Cardiol*. 1994;23:586-590.

3. Levine RA, Schwammenthal E. Ischemic mitral regurgitation on the threshold of a solution: from paradoxes to unifying concepts. *Circulation*. 2005;112:745-758.
4. Dec GW, Fuster V. Idiopathic dilated cardiomyopathy. *N Engl J Med*. 1994;331:1564-1575.
5. Patel JB, Borgeson DD, Barnes ME, Rihal CS, Daly RC, Redfield MM. Mitral regurgitation in patients with advanced systolic heart failure. *J Card Fail*. 2004;10:285-291.
6. Carabello BA, Crawford FA Jr. Valvular heart disease. *N Engl J Med*. 1997;337:32-41.
7. Schiller NB, Shah PM, Crawford M, et al. Recommendations for quantitation of the left ventricle by two-dimensional echocardiography. American Society of Echocardiography Committee on Standards, Subcommittee on Quantitation of Two-Dimensional Echocardiograms. *J Am Soc Echocardiogr*. 1989;2:358-367.
8. Wang Y, Gutman JM, Heilbron D, Wahr D, Schiller NB. Atrial volume in a normal adult population by two-dimensional echocardiography. *Chest*. 1984;86:595-601.
9. Sahn DJ. Instrumentation and physical factors related to visualization of stenotic and regurgitant jets by Doppler color flow mapping. *J Am Coll Cardiol*. 1988;12:1354-1365.
10. Chen CG, Thomas JD, Anconina J, et al. Impact of impinging wall jet on color Doppler quantification of mitral regurgitation. *Circulation*. 1991;84:712-720.
11. Zoghbi WA, Enriquez-Sarano M, Foster E, et al. Recommendations for evaluation of the severity of native valvular regurgitation with two-dimensional and Doppler echocardiography. *J Am Soc Echocardiogr*. 2003;16:777-802.
12. Heinle SK, Hall SA, Brickner ME, Willett DL, Grayburn PA. Comparison of vena contracta width by multiplane transesophageal echocardiography with quantitative Doppler assessment of mitral regurgitation. *Am J Cardiol*. 1998;81:175-179.
13. Bargiggia GS, Tronconi L, Sahn DJ, et al. A new method for quantitation of mitral regurgitation based on color flow Doppler imaging of flow convergence proximal to regurgitant orifice. *Circulation*. 1991;84:1481-1489.
14. Thomas L, Foster E, Schiller NB. Peak mitral inflow velocity predicts mitral regurgitation severity. *J Am Coll Cardiol*. 1998;31:174-179.
15. Bonow RO, Carabello BA, Chatterjee K, et al. 2008 focused update incorporated into the ACC/AHA 2006 guidelines for the management of patients with valvular heart disease: a report of the American College of Cardiology/American Heart Association Task Force on Practice Guidelines (Writing committee to develop guidelines for the management of patients with valvular heart disease). Endorsed by the Society of Cardiovascular Anesthesiologists, Society for Cardiovascular Angiography and Interventions, and Society of Thoracic Surgeons. *J Am Coll Cardiol*. 2008;52:e1-142.
16. Hamilton MA, Stevenson LW, Child JS, Moriguchi JD, Walden J, Woo M. Sustained reduction in valvular regurgitation and atrial volumes with tailored vasodilator therapy in advanced congestive heart failure secondary to dilated (ischemic or idiopathic) cardiomyopathy. *Am J Cardiol*. 1991;67:259-263.
17. Kizilbash AM, Willett DL, Brickner ME, Heinle SK, Grayburn PA. Effects of afterload reduction on vena contracta width in mitral regurgitation. *J Am Coll Cardiol*. 1998;32:427-431.
18. Nishimura RA, Otto CM, Bonow RO, et al. 2014 AHA/ACC guideline for the management of patients with valvular heart disease: executive summary; a report of the American College of Cardiology/American Heart Association Task Force on Practice Guidelines. *J Am Coll Cardiol*. 2014;63:2348-2388.

SECTION 9

Mitral Valve Prolapse

Gina G. Mentzer, MD

CLINICAL CASE PRESENTATION

A 38-year-old woman presents to the outpatient clinic with chest palpitations, dizziness, and chest heaviness that has increased over the past 6 months. She has noticed that it has become harder for her to exercise on her bicycle, and she has decreased her activity due to shortness of breath and palpitations. She was concerned over the weekend when she felt anxious and then suddenly lost vision in her left eye for 3 minutes. On physical exam, she has a high-pitched mid-to-late systolic murmur heard best at the apex. In addition, there is a mid-systolic click heard at the apex, which occurs earlier in systole with Valsalva maneuver that is consistent with mitral valve prolapse (MVP). To confirm this diagnosis, an echocardiogram was performed, which demonstrated a thickened, anterior leaflet bowing into the left atrium (LA) during systole consistent with MVP as well as MR (Figures 3-9-1 to 3-9-5).

CLINICAL FEATURES

- Symptoms may be related to autonomic dysfunction. These can be quite bothersome and are associated with the term "MVP syndrome."
    - Autonomic dysfunction includes symptoms of anxiety, panic attacks, and arrhythmias with palpitations, exercise intolerance, atypical chest pain and presyncope.

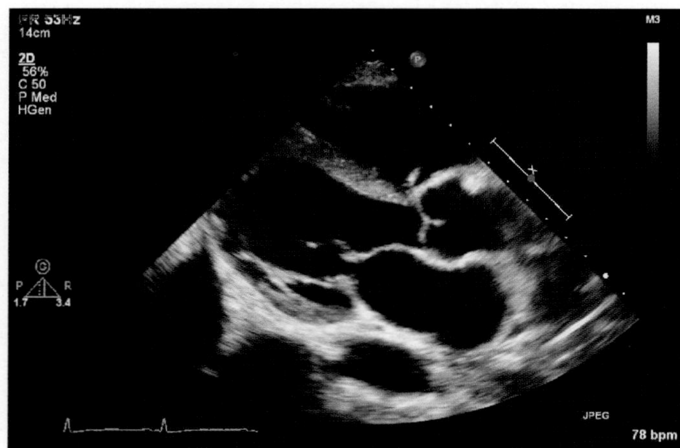
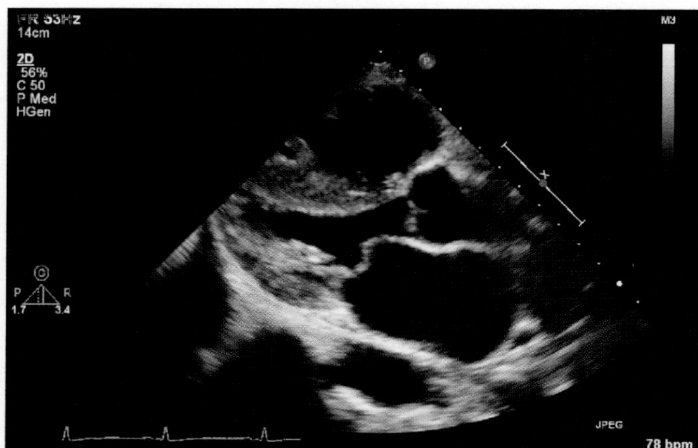

FIGURE 3-9-1 A 2-D transthoracic echocardiogram in the parasternal long axis (PLAX) view in diastole (top panel) and systole (bottom panel) with demonstration of leaflet thickening and anterior leaflet prolapse ► (see Video 3-9-1).

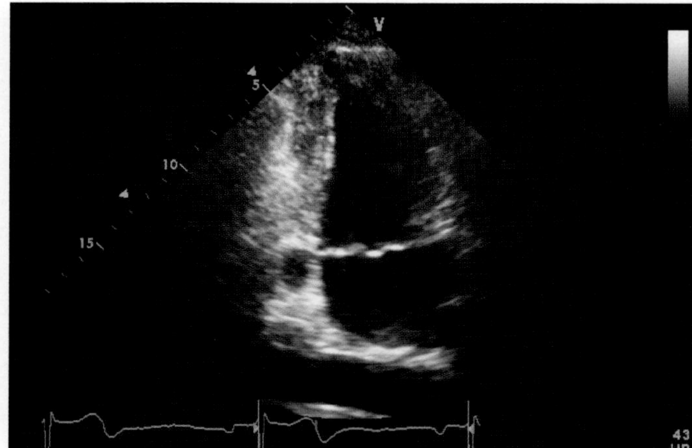
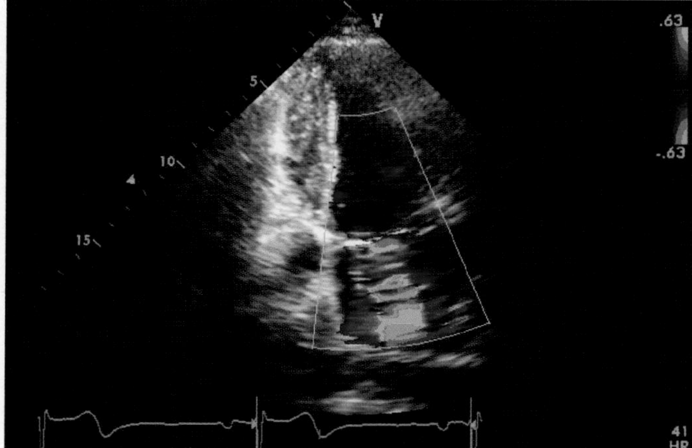

FIGURE 3-9-2 Apical 2 chamber view without (top panel) and with (bottom panel) color Doppler demonstrating MR ► (see Video 3-9-2).

- Symptoms directly attributed to the valvular pathology or its sequelae may include CHF (dyspnea especially with exertion, exercise intolerance, orthopnea, and paroxysmal nocturnal dyspnea) due to progression of MR with or without LV dysfunction, endocarditis, or neurological sequelae due to embolization from the valve.
- With severe MR, atrial fibrillation may occur due to LA enlargement.
- MVP is also associated with musculoskeletal disorders (eg, pectus excavatum) and connective tissue disorders (eg, Marfan Syndrome).[1,2]

EPIDEMIOLOGY

- MVP was first described by John Brereton Barlow in 1966 and may also be referred to as Barlow's Syndrome. It was termed MVP by J. Michael Criley.
- MVP is the most common cause of MR in developed countries and is found in 2% to 5% of the US population. The Framingham Heart Study found the prevalence to be 2.4% and some evidence demonstrating 2:1 women-to-men ratio.[3-5]
- Primary MVP is due to degenerative myxomatous changes of the valve in the absence of recognizable systemic connective tissue disorders. This is the most common form found with isolated MVP. In these cases, other valves can also be involved, including the tricuspid valve in 40% of cases and the aortic valve in 2% to 10% of cases with rare involvement of the pulmonary valve.[2]
    - Familial MVP is inherited in an autosomal dominant fashion with incomplete penetrance.

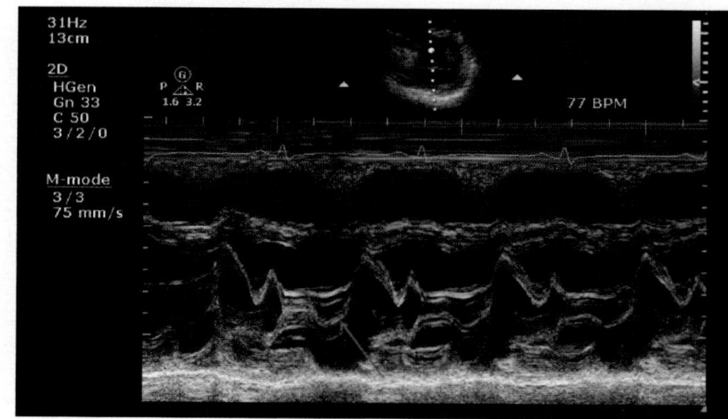

FIGURE 3-9-3 Demonstration of MVP by M-mode in the parasternal view.

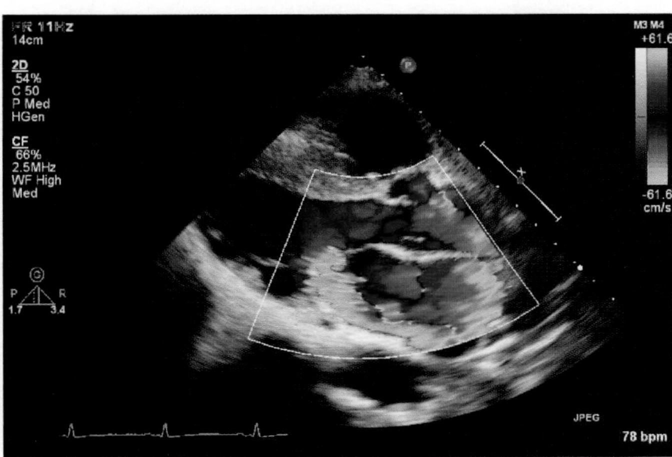

FIGURE 3-9-4 Two-dimensional transthoracic echocardiogram in the PLAX view with demonstration of severe MR by color Doppler due to anterior leaflet MVP ► (see Video 3-9-4).

- Secondary MVP is from myxomatous degeneration of the leaflets in association with an underlying connective tissue disorder. Only 1% to 2% of MVP patients have a connective tissue disorder, including Marfan syndrome, Ehlers-Danlos syndrome, adult polycystic kidney disease, osteogenesis imperfecta, pseudoxanthoma elasticium, and in association with some congenital heart diseases.[1,5]

PATHOPHYSIOLOGY AND ETIOLOGY

MVP is an organic heart disease associated with myxomatous thickening of the leaflets with the underlying etiology unknown. Anatomically, MVP is separated into 2 groups, including those with true organic heart disease with myxomatous thickening and those with a mild buckling of the MV without thickening or MR. MVP is typically a benign diagnosis, but in rare cases it can cause disabling symptoms from associated autonomic dysfunction or progression of disease with resultant severe MR and HF. Patients are also at risk for endocarditis and its sequelae.

ECHOCARDIOGRAPHY

- Echocardiography is utilized to evaluate the anatomy of the MV as well as assess for MR and left ventricular function. This assessment is a class I recommendation by the American College of Cardiology and American Heart Association as well as the American Society of Echocardiography.[2]
- In 2-D ecocardiography, the parasternal long axis (PLAX) has a higher sensitivity and specificity for diagnosis when one or more leaflets extend posterior to the plane of the mitral annulus into the LA, more classically in an asymmetric manner (see Figure 3-9-1).
- The apical 2 chamber is also an acceptable view; however, prolapse in this view is a less specific finding (Figure 3-9-2).
- In the apical 4 chamber view, due to the "saddle shape" of the MV annulus, prolapse of the valve into the LA may be seen. This tends to overdiagnose MVP (decreases specificity); therefore, this view should not be used to diagnose MVP.[2,6]
- In the PLAX, the M-mode beam is aligned directly across the area in the LA behind the MV annulus (Figure 3-9-3). Classically, asymmetric, posterior bowing of the leaflets into the LA by 3 mm (holosystolic excursion) or by 2 mm in late systole along with mid-anterior leaflet thickening of 5 mm confirms clinical suspicion.[2,6,7]
- Color Doppler and spectral Doppler are used to assess associated MR (Figure 3-9-4).
- Other valve pathology (eg, AV disease, TV prolapse) and an assessment of the aorta (especially in subjects with associated connective tissue diseases, including Marfan Syndrome) is warranted.

OTHER DIAGNOSTIC TESTING AND PROCEDURES

- With MVP, the EKG can demonstrate ST depression or T-wave inversion in the inferior leads, arrhythmias, or QT prolongation.[2,7,8]
- Event recorders and Holter monitors may demonstrate arrhythmias such as atrial fibrillation, premature atrial and ventricular beats, as well as sinus node dysfunction.
- Rarely is cardiac catheterization utilized to assess MVP, but it can be helpful to quantify MR, pulmonary hypertension, and right atrial pressures in advanced cases undergoing evaluation for surgery.
- An evaluation for associated aortopathies with computed tomography (CT) or magnetic resonance imaging (MRI) imaging of the aorta is recommended if adequate assessment cannot be made with echocardiography (see Chapter 7, Section IV: Marfan Syndrome and Chapter 7, Section V: Aortopathy in Bicuspid Aortic Valve Disease) (Figure 3-9-6).
- TEE may be used to better define the severity of the MR and to evaluate the valve for preoperative planning (Figures 3-9-7 to 3-9-9).

DIFFERENTIAL DIAGNOSIS

In the evaluation for MVP, a differential diagnosis is made to conduct a thorough evaluation and determine the diagnosis. Thickened leaflets can give the appearance of vegetations or masses suggestive of endocarditis. Furthermore, MVP is associated with higher rates of endocarditis; therefore, if indicated, clinical evaluation is recommended to evaluate. Other organic abnormalities, such as a dilated MV annulus from ischemic heart disease and chordae rupture, may mimic MVP.

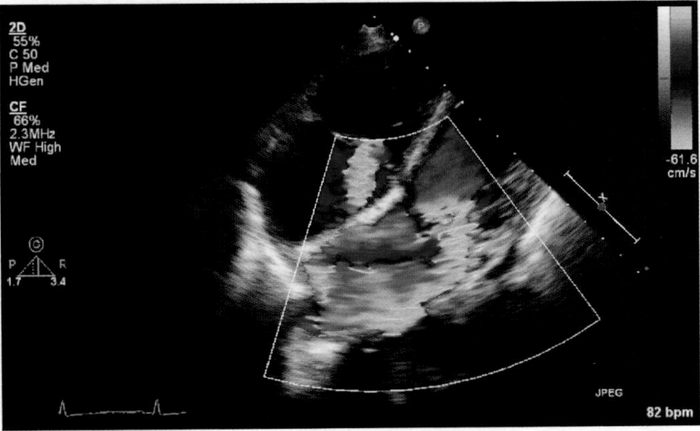

FIGURE 3-9-5 Subcostal 4 chamber view demonstrating an eccentric MR jet with color Doppler. TR is also noted ► (see Video 3-9-5).

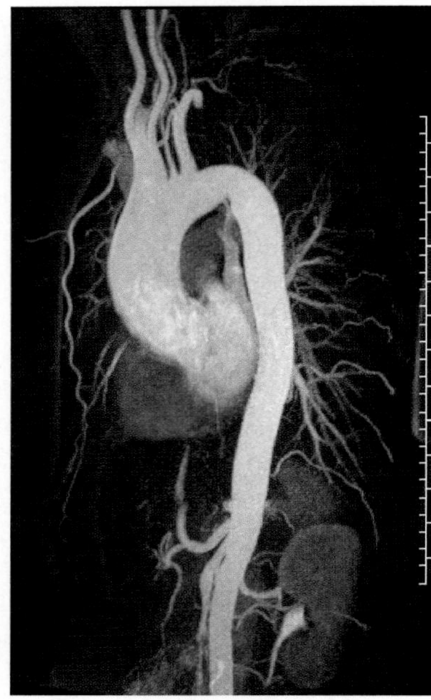

FIGURE 3-9-6 MRA with a time bolus of gadolinium contrast demonstrating a dilated ascending aorta in a patient with Marfan Syndrome.

DIAGNOSIS

MVP is classified as primary, secondary, or functional based upon the anatomic and/or physiologic defects found on echocardiography and clinical exam. As previously discussed, the valve must be thickened and demonstrate a buckling appearance that extends beyond the MV annulus into the LA.

MANAGEMENT

Medical Management

- Most patients with MVP are asymptomatic and the condition is benign. Reassurance is indicated as well as counseling on lifestyle improvements for a healthy diet and daily exercise.
- Antibiotic prophylaxis is not indicated, unless the patient is considered high risk, for example, by having a prior history of endocarditis.[9]

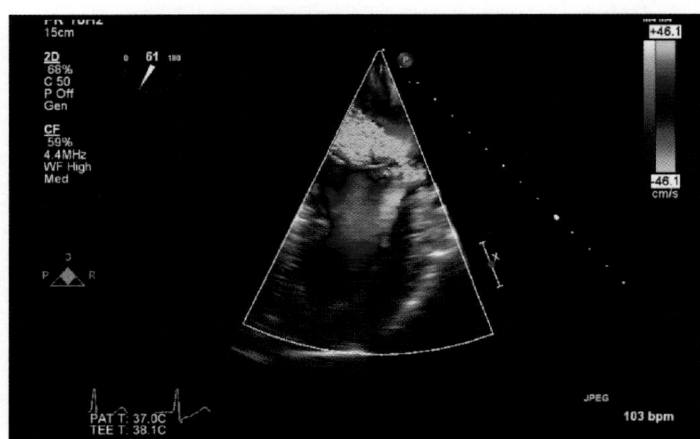

FIGURE 3-9-8 TEE image with color Doppler from the patient in Figure 3-9-7 demonstrating MR ► (see Video 3-9-8).

- Symptomatic patients, especially those with chest pain, anxiety, fatigue, and palpitations may respond to β-blocker therapy.
- Orthostatic symptoms improve with hydration, increased salt intake, and compression stockings.
- Aspirin or anticoagulants are not routinely recommended in patients with MVP, but are indicated in those with MVP who have had neurological events.[2,10]
- Wafarin is used in those who have had an embolic stroke while on aspirin and as determined by a cardiologist. Patients with associated atrial fibrillation also warrant anticoagulation. High-risk patients include those who are age older than 65, have MR, HTN, or a history of heart failure.[2]

Surgical Management[15]

- In certain cases, surgery is indicated. Symptomatic patients with severe MR warrant surgical MV repair or replacement. In the asymptomatic patient, findings that require further evaluation for surgery include moderate or severe MR along with an LV end systolic diameter greater than or equal to 40 mm, decreased EF less than 60% (but greater than 30%), atrial fibrillation, or pulmonary hypertension with a PA systolic pressure greater than 50 mm Hg at rest.

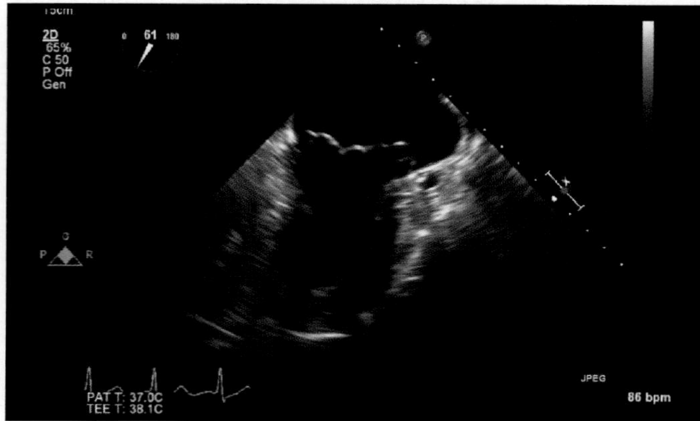

FIGURE 3-9-7 TEE image from a different patient demonstrating a myxomatous MV with prolapse of A1 ► (see Video 3-9-7).

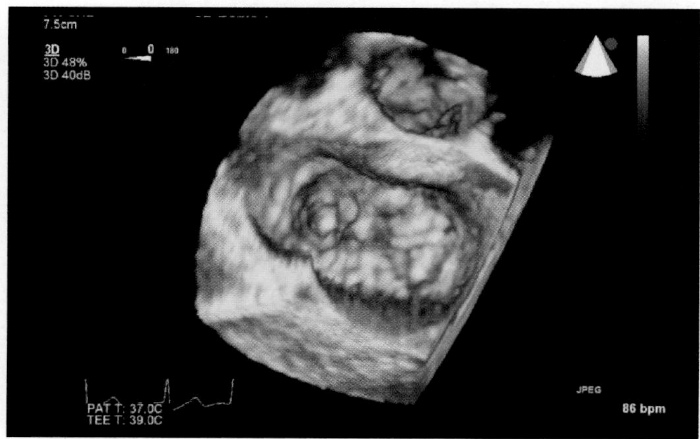

FIGURE 3-9-9 3-D TEE of a myxomatous MV with A1 prolapse ► (see Video 3-9-9).

- Spontaneous chordal rupture may result in severe MR due to the flail MV.[2,11] These patients may present with acute severe MR and surgical repair/replacement is warranted.
- If possible, MV repair is preferred over replacement as there are fewer complications and improved outcomes with repair versus replacement. There are certain anatomical features that direct the surgical therapy toward replacement, such as calcification, annular dilation, and papillary muscle function.[12,13]
- Surgical techniques such as Carpentier, quadrangular resection with annuloplasty, and sliding repair are used to repair the MV.[11,12]
- Preoperative and intraoperative TEE is utilized in this process for planning and in determination of surgical success.

Surveillance

- Clinical evaluation and echocardiography in patients with MVP should be performed to assess valvular progression, degree of MR, and LV function every 3 to 5 years. In addition, an exam is indicated at any point if the clinical condition changes.
- If high-risk characteristics are present, such as moderate to severe MR, increased LA or LV size, depressed LV function, or palpitations, an annual clinical exam is indicated.
- The recommended frequency of repeat echocardiography is based on the severity of the MR as well as LV dimensions and function

PATIENT EDUCATION

- Classic MVP is associated with higher risks of progressive mitral regurgitation, spontaneous chordal rupture, neurological events, and endocarditis. These occur only at a rate of 1 per 100 patient years.[7]
- Screening should be performed in those with a positive family history as well as those with underlying connective tissue disease. First-degree relatives of patients with MVP should be clinically evaluated and assessed with echocardiography.[7]
- Depending on the degree of MVP and related cardiac abnormalities, competitive sports may be restricted by a cardiologist. High-risk features include moderate LV dilation and dysfunction, arrhythmias, long-QT interval, and history of syncope.[2,14]
- Sudden cardiac death rarely occurs and occurs in less than 2% of known cases.[2]
- For the most part, patients with MVP alone can safely experience pregnancy.

FOLLOW-UP

The patient was diagnosed with symptomatic MVP complicated by neurological sequelae, but there was no evidence of a cerebral vascular accident on an MRI of the brain. Her LV size and function was preserved with mild-to-moderate MR. She has no evidence of an underlying connective tissue disorder, and her family history was unremarkable. She was started on aspirin, 81 mg daily, and a β-blocker with improved symptoms. She was given a 30-day event recorder for evaluation for arrhythmias, which proved negative, and will follow-up in the outpatient clinic for further evaluation.

VIDEO LEGENDS

1. Video 3-9-1: A 2-D transthoracic echocardiogram in the parasternal long axis (PLAX) view with demonstration of leaflet thickening and anterior leaflet prolapse.
2. Video 3-9-2: Apical 2 chamber view without (left) and with (right) color Doppler demonstrating MR in a "Zoom" mode
3. Video 3-9-4: 2-D transthoracic echocardiogram in the PLAX view with demonstration of severe MR by color Doppler due to anterior leaflet MVP
4. Video 3-9-5: Subcostal 4 chamber view demonstrating an eccentric MR jet with color Doppler. TR is also noted
5. Video 3-9-7: TEE image from a different patient demonstrating a myxomatous MV with prolapse of A1
6. Video 3-9-8: TEE image with color Doppler from the patient in Video 5 demonstrating MR
7. Video 3-9-9: 3 D TEE of a myxomatous MV with A1 prolapse

REFERENCES

1. Glesby MJ, Pyeritz RE. Association of mitral valve prolapse and systemic abnormalities of connective tissue. A phenotypic continuum. *JAMA*. 1989;262(4):523-528.
2. Bonow RO, Carabello BA, Chatterjee K, et al. 2008 focused update incorporated into the ACC/AHA 2006 guidelines for the management of patients with valvular heart disease: a report of the American College of Cardiology/American Heart Association Task Force on Practice Guidelines (Writing committee to develop guidelines for the management of patients with valvular heart disease). Endorsed by the Society of Cardiovascular Anesthesiologists, Society for Cardiovascular Angiography and Interventions, and Society of Thoracic Surgeons. *J Am Coll Cardiol*. 2008;52:e1-142.
3. Savage DD, Devereux RB, Garrison RJ, et al. Mitral valve prolapse in the general population. 2. Clinical features: the Framingham Study. *Am Heart J*. 1983;106(3):577-581.
4. Freed LA, Levy D, Levine RA, et al. Prevalence and clinical outcome of mitral-valve prolapse. *N Engl J Med*. 1999;341(1): 1-7.
5. Grau JB, Pirelli L, Yu PJ, Galloway AC, Ostrer H. The genetics of mitral valve prolapse. *Clin Genet*. 2007;72(4):288-295.
6. Levine RA, Stathogiannis E, Newell JB, Harrigan P, Weyman AE. Reconsideration of echocardiographic standards for mitral valve prolapse: lack of association between leaflet displacement isolated to the apical four chamber view and independent echocardiographic evidence of abnormality. *J Am Coll Cardiol*. 1988;11(5):1010-1019.
7. Libby P, Bonow RO, Mann DL, Zipes DP, Braunwald E, eds. *Braunwald's Heart Disease: A Textbook of Cardiovascular Medicine*. 8th ed. Philadelphia, PA: Saunders Elsevier; 2008; No. 1-2.
8. Bhutto ZR, Barron JT, Liebson PR, Uretz EF, Parrillo JE. Electrocardiographic abnormalities in mitral valve prolapse. *Am J Cardiol*. 1992;70(2):265-266.

9. Nishimura RA, Carabello BA, Faxon DP, et al. ACC/AHA 2008 guideline update on valvular heart disease: focused update on infective endocarditis: a report of the American College of Cardiology/American Heart Association Task Force on Practice Guidelines endorsed by the Society of Cardiovascular Anesthesiologists, Society for Cardiovascular Angiography and Interventions, and Society of Thoracic Surgeons. *J Am Coll Cardiol.* 2008;52(8):676-685.
10. Sacco RL, Adams R, Albers G, et al. Guidelines for prevention of stroke in patients with ischemic stroke or transient ischemic attack: a statement for healthcare professionals from the American Heart Association/American Stroke Association Council on Stroke: co-sponsored by the Council on Cardiovascular Radiology and Intervention: the American Academy of Neurology affirms the value of this guideline. *Circulation.* 2006;113(10):e409-449.
11. Gillinov AM, Blackstone EH, Nowicki ER, et al. Valve repair versus valve replacement for degenerative mitral valve disease. *J Thorac Cardiovasc Surg.* 2008;135(4):885-893,893.e1-2.
12. Braunberger E, Deloche A, Berrebi A, et al. Very long-term results (more than 20 years) of valve repair with carpentier's techniques in nonrheumatic mitral valve insufficiency. *Circulation.* 2001;104(12 Suppl 1):I8-11.
13. Cohn LH, Couper GS, Aranki SF, Rizzo RJ, Adams DH, Collins JJ Jr. The long-term results of mitral valve reconstruction for the "floppy" valve. *J Card Surg.* 1994;9(2 Suppl):278-281.
14. Mellwig KP, van Buuren F, Gohlke-Baerwolf C, Bjornstad HH. Recommendations for the management of individuals with acquired valvular heart diseases who are involved in leisure-time physical activities or competitive sports. *Eur J Cardiovasc Prev Rehabil.* 2008;15(1):95-103.
15. Nishimura RA, Otto CM, Bonow RO, et al. 2014 AHA/ACC guideline for the management of patients with valvular heart disease:executive summary; a report of the American College of Cardiology/American Heart Association Task Force on Practice Guidelines. *J Am Coll Cardiol.* 2014;63:2348-2388.

SECTION 10

Functional Tricuspid Valve Regurgitation

Kavita Sharma, MD

CLINICAL CASE PRESENTATION

A 78-year-old woman with a history of deep vein thrombosis and pulmonary embolism presented with progressive dyspnea, lower extremity edema, and ascites. Her physical examination demonstrated a right ventricular heave, a holosystolic left parasternal murmur that increased with inspiration, hepatomegaly, and lower extremity edema. An electrocardiogram demonstrated evidence of right ventricular hypertrophy. Her echocardiogram showed a severely dilated right ventricle (RV), with severely elevated RV systolic pressure and severe tricuspid regurgitation (TR) (Figures 3-10-1 to 3-10-5). She underwent right heart catheterization which demonstrated RV pressures of 51/23 mm Hg. Chronic pulmonary embolism was felt to be the etiology of her pulmonary hypertension and RV failure. She was seen by cardiothoracic surgery who felt that surgery for repair or replacement of the tricuspid valve was very high-risk due to her RV failure. The patient elected to return home with hospice care.

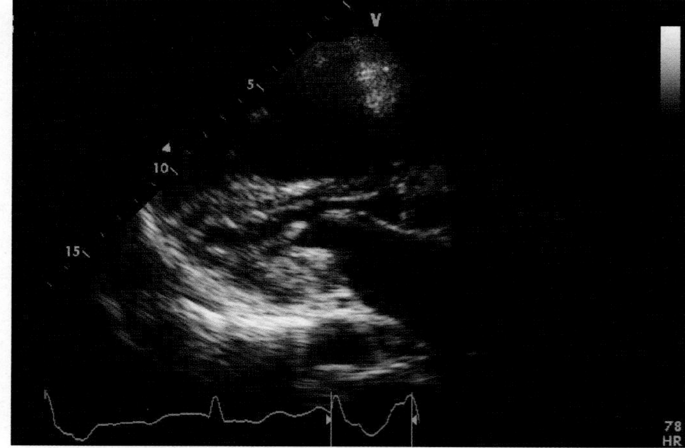

FIGURE 3-10-1 Parasternal long-axis demonstrating a relatively small LV with normal function. The RV is dilated and there is RV dysfunction ► (see Video 3-10-1).

PATHOPHYSIOLOGY AND ETIOLOGY

- The etiologies of tricuspid valve regurgitation can be separated into those involving a normal tricuspid valve (functional TR) and those with an abnormal tricuspid valve.[1]
- Causes of an abnormal tricuspid valve include Ebstein's anomaly, rheumatic valvulitis, infective endocarditis, carcinoid syndrome, rheumatoid arthritis, trauma, Marfan syndrome, and tricuspid valve prolapse.[2]
- When TR develops with a structurally normal tricuspid valve, the likely etiology is functional TR and is related to elevated.

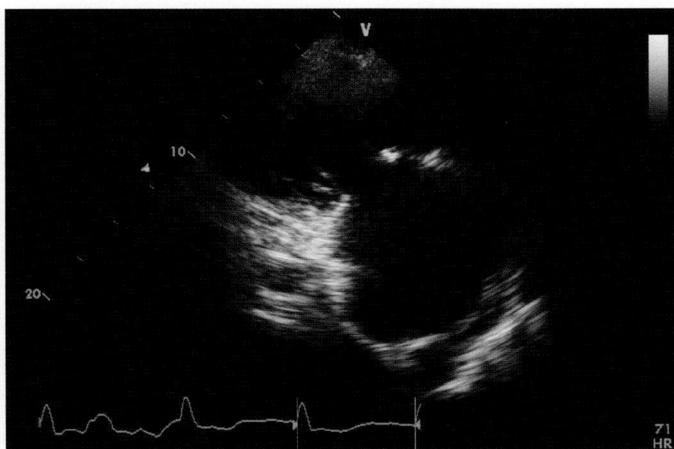

FIGURE 3-10-2 RV inflow demonstrating a dilated TV annulus and RV with inadequate tricuspid valve leaflet coaptation ▶ (see Video 3-10-2).

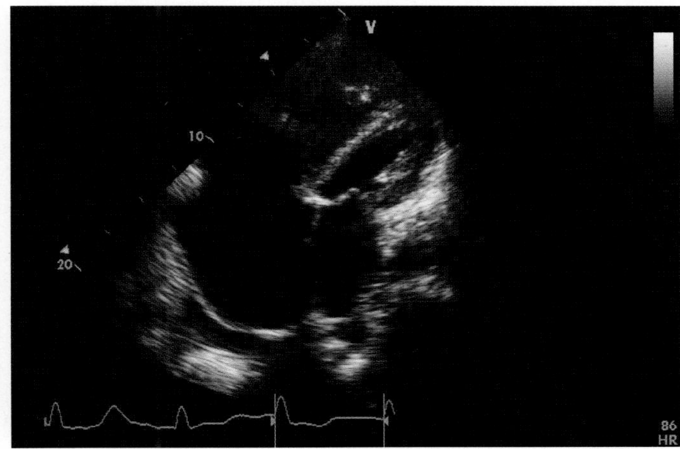

FIGURE 3-10-5 Apical 4 chamber demonstrating RV dilation, severe RV dysfunction, and TV annular dilation ▶ (see Video 3-10-5).

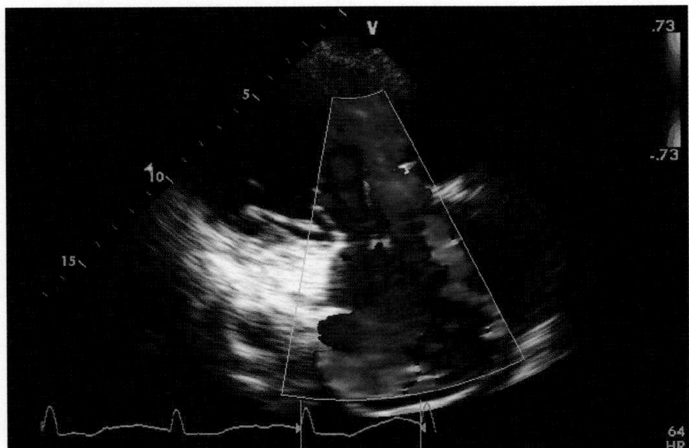

FIGURE 3-10-3 RV inflow view with color Doppler demonstrating severe tricuspid regurgitation ▶ (see Video 3-10-3).

RV pressure or RV dysfunction with resultant RV cavity enlargement and tricuspid annular dilation.[2,3]

- Pulmonary hypertension has many possible causes, including mitral valve stenosis, LV systolic and diastolic dysfunction, idiopathic (primary) pulmonary hypertension, pulmonary embolism, drug and toxin-induced, connective tissue disease-related, and chronic obstructive pulmonary disease.

EPIDEMIOLOGY

- On pathological analysis of cases of TR, 47% were due to functional TR.[1]

ECHOCARDIOGRAPHY

- The valve appearance and its functional status are evaluated with echocardiography, utilizing 2-D imaging, color flow Doppler, and spectral Doppler (continuous-wave and pulsed wave Doppler).
- The valve and its annulus are visualized using 2-D imaging. In cases of an abnormal tricuspid valve, the abnormal appearance is evident on 2-D imaging.

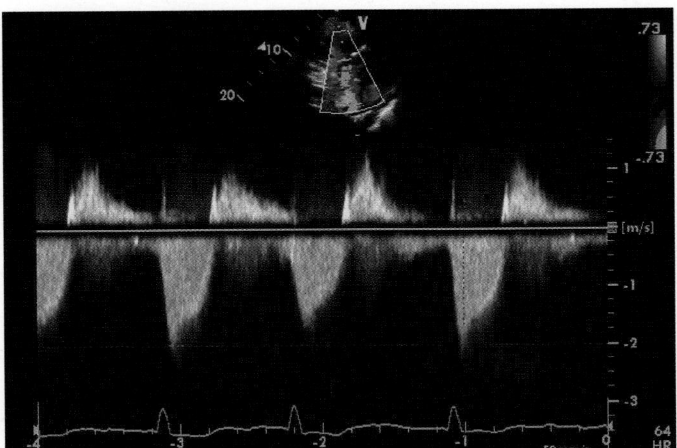

FIGURE 3-10-4 Continuous-wave Doppler showing severe TR. Note the triangular, early peaking nature of the regurgitant jet.

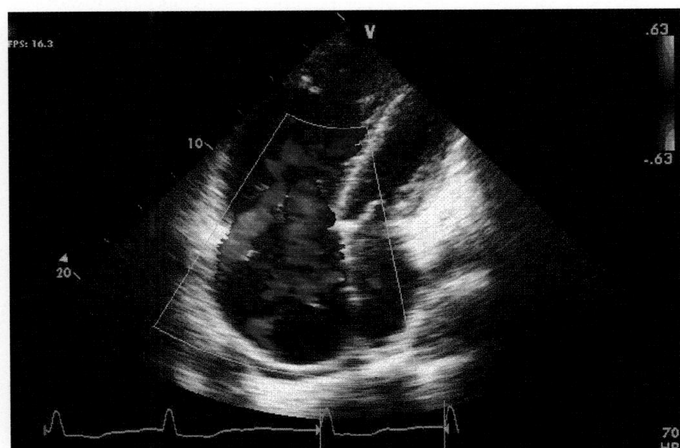

FIGURE 3-10-6 Apical 4 chamber view with color Doppler demonstrating severe TR ▶ (see Video 3-10-6).

- The size and appearance of the right ventricle (RV) and right atrium are also visually examined.
- Images of the RV are obtained in the parasternal RV inflow view, parasternal short axis, apical 4 chamber, and subcostal 4 chamber views.
- Color flow Doppler is useful to visualize the regurgitant jet.
- Generally, jets that extend deeper into the right atrium represent more severe tricuspid regurgitant jets.[3] Caution must taken, however, as clinically insignificant tricuspid regurgitant jets are often visualized in normal persons.[2]
- Color Doppler may be utilized to obtain the PISA value (see Section VII: Chronic Ischemic Mitral Regurgitation for details of the PISA method) to determine regurgitant severity.
- The vena contracta of the tricuspid regurgitant jet may be obtained to assess severity. A jet width >0.7 cm identifies severe triscuspid regurgitation with a sensitivity of 89% and a specificity of 93%.[4]
- On continuous-wave Doppler, the RV systolic pressure can be estimated by utilizing the tricuspid regurgitant jet velocity.
- RV systolic pressures greater than 55 mm Hg are likely to cause functional TR, whereas TR and a RV systolic pressure less than 40 mm Hg is associated with an abnormal tricuspid valve.[2]
- On continuous-wave Doppler, when severe TR is present, a dense spectral recording is seen, along with a triangular, early peaking velocity.[3]
- On pulsed Doppler, the severity of TR will affect the early diastolic triscuspid E velocity; values above 1.0 m/s are often seen in patients with severe triscuspid regurgitation, even without significant stenosis.
- Severe TR is associated with abnormal hepatic vein flow patterns; systolic flow reversal of the hepatic vein flow can be seen with severe TR.[3]

OTHER DIAGNOSTIC TESTING

- A right heart catheterization may be considered to invasively measure RV pressure, pulmonary artery pressures, and wedge pressure.
- Elevated pulmonary artery pressures may be related to pulmonary arterial hypertension versus pulmonary venous hypertension.
- During right heart catheterization, the transpulmonary gradient may be calculated, which can differentiate between the two entities.

MANAGEMENT

- Treatment of the underlying cause of the TR may improve the degree of insufficiency.
- Usually, functional tricuspid valve regurgitation is managed medically, unless the patient is undergoing surgery on another valve, at which time the tricuspid valve may be addressed as well (Class I for patients with severe TR, Class IIa for others with less than severe TR.[5,6]
- Some patients with symptomatic severe primary TR may benefit from surgery if they fail medical therapy (Class IIa).[6]
- Diuretic therapy can be used to relieve edema; however, aggressive therapy often leads to hypotension and/or pre-renal azotemia.
- In the case of mitral stenosis, with resultant elevated RV pressure, and subsequent functional TR, surgery on the mitral valve may result in improvement in the TR.[2]

FOLLOW-UP

- The patient's clinical status and the cause of the TR determine the appropriate follow-up.
- If the patient undergoes tricuspid valve repair or mitral valve surgery, baseline echocardiography is recommended, along with follow-up for endocarditis prophylaxis, anticoagulation, and follow-up echocardiography after a change in symptoms, as detailed elsewhere in this chapter.
- In patients who are being medically managed, periodic patient assessment and echocardiography is recommended to follow the valve regurgitation and right heart function.

SUMMARY

- Functional TR is due to elevated RV pressure with resultant tricuspid valve regurgitation or due to abnormalities (dilation) of the RV and/or the TV annulus. Its characteristics can be studied on echocardiography. Generally, patients with functional tricuspid valve regurgitation do not undergo surgery.

FIGURE LEGENDS

1. Video 3-10-1: Parasternal long-axis demonstrating a relatively small LV with normal function. The RV is dilated and there is RV dysfunction
2. Video 3-10-2: RV inflow demonstrating a dilated TV annulus and RV with inadequate tricuspid valve leaflet coaptation
3. Video 3-10-3: RV inflow view with color Doppler demonstrating severe tricuspid regurgitation
4. Video 3-10-5: Apical four-chamber demonstrating RV dilation, severe RV dysfunction and TV annular dilation
5. Video 3-10-6: Apical 4 chamber view with color Doppler demonstrating severe TR

REFERENCES

1. Waller BF. Etiology of pure tricuspid regurgitation. *Cardiovasc Clin*. 1987;17:53-95.
2. Bonow RO, Carabello BA, Chatterjee K, et al. 2008 focused update incorporated into the ACC/AHA 2006 guidelines for the management of patients with valvular heart disease: a report of the American College of Cardiology/American Heart Association Task Force on Practice Guidelines (Writing committee to develop guidelines for the management of patients with valvular heart disease). Endorsed by the Society of Cardiovascular Anesthesiologists, Society for Cardiovascular Angiography and Interventions, and Society of Thoracic Surgeons. *J Am Coll Cardiol*. 2008;52:e1-142.

3. Zoghbi WA, Enriquez-Sarano M, Foster E. Recommendations for evaluation of the severity of native valvular regurgitation with two-dimensional and Doppler echocardiography. *J Am Soc Echocardiogr*. 2003;16:777-802.
4. Tribouilloy CM, Enriquez-Sarano M, Bailey KR, Tajik AJ, Seward JB. Quantification of tricuspid regurgitation by measuring the width of the vena contracta with Doppler color flow imaging: a clinical study. *J Am Coll Cardiol*. 2000;36:472-478.
5. Pellegrini A, Colombo T, Donatelli F, et al. Evaluation and treatment of secondary tricuspid insufficiency. *Eur J Cardiothorac Surg*. 1992;6:288-296.
6. Nishimura RA, Otto CM, Bonow RO, et al. 2014 AHA/ACC guideline for the management of patients with valvular heart disease: executive summary; a report of the American College of Cardiology/American Heart Association Task Force on Practice Guidelines. *J Am Coll Cardiol*. 2014;63:2348-2388.

SECTION 11

Severe Tricuspid Valve Insufficiency Following Valve Resection For Endocarditis

David A. Orsinelli, MD, FACC, FASE

CLINICAL CASE PRESENTATION

A 34-year-old woman presented for inpatient drug rehabilitation. She complained of mild dyspnea on exertion and intermittent lower extremity edema. She had a history of intravenous drug abuse (IVDA) and had undergone tricuspid valve (TV) resection at another institution 10 years prior to her presentation for staphylococcal endocarditis. She has had minimal medical follow-up.

Physical examination was remarkable for markedly elevated jugular venous pressure with neck vein distention well above the angle of the jaw at 45°. She had a marked left parasternal lift, a grade II-III/VI holosystolic murmur along the left sternal border which increased with inspiration, and RV S_3 gallop. Her lungs were clear. Abdominal examination revealed an enlarged, pulsatile liver. She had 1+ lower extremity edema.

A transthoracic echocardiogram revealed a dilated, hypokinetic RV, severe TV insufficiency, absence of significant TV leaflet tissue and echocardiographic features of RV volume overload (Figures 3-11-1 to 3-11-9).

She was treated with low dose oral diuretics, as well as sodium and fluid restriction. Her edema improved; however, she remained mildy dyspneic with activity.

She was referred to a cardiac surgeon who felt that she was not a candidate for tricuspid valve replacement due to her ongoing drug use as well her surgical risk in view of her right ventricular failure. She was lost to follow-up.

CLINICAL FEATURES AND NATURAL HISTORY

- Severe tricuspid insufficiency may be asymptomatic.
- With the development of right ventricular dysfunction, symptoms may occur.

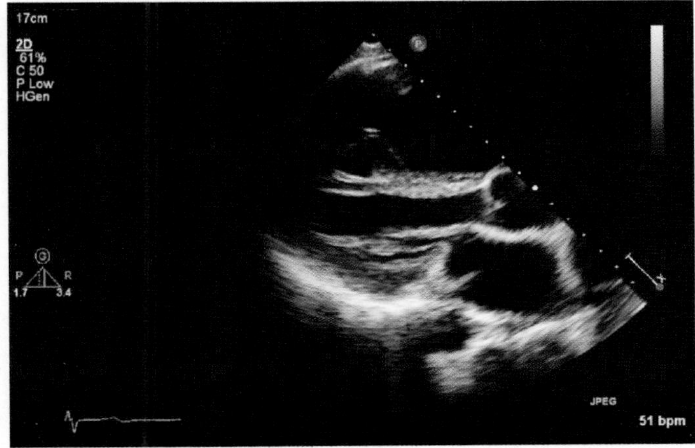

FIGURE 3-11-1 Parasternal long axis demonstrating a relatively small LV, RV enlargement, and hypokinesis as well as abnormal septal motion due to RV volume overload ▶ (see Video 3-11-1).

- Patients may present with evidence of right heart failure (edema, fatigue, dyspnea).
- Tricuspid valve resection was performed in the late 1970s and early 1980s as a treatment for TV endocarditis (which most often occurs in patients who inject drugs). The rationale was that TV replacement carried a high risk of prosthetic valve endocarditis in this patient population and that due to the low pressures in the RV, absence of a functional TV would be well tolerated.[1,2]
    - Acutely, most patients tolerate the TR. Unfortunately, many patients over time develop significant right heart failure.

EPIDEMIOLOGY

- Infectious endocarditis can involve any of the cardiac valves, prosthetic valves, as well as the endocardial surfaces of the cardiac

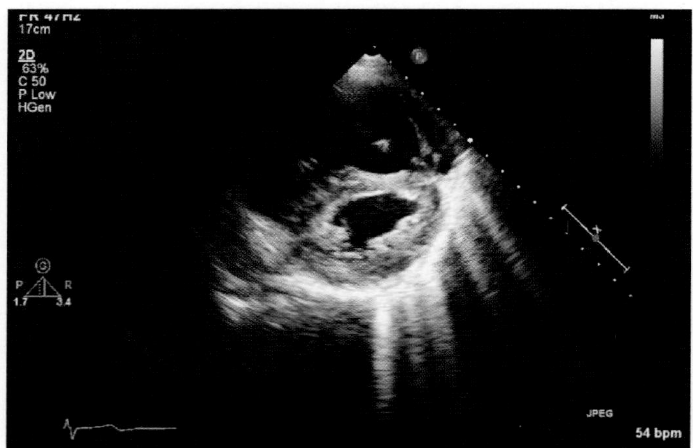

FIGURE 3-11-2 Parasternal short axis demonstrating a relatively small LV, RV enlargement, and hypokinesis as well as abnormal septal motion due to RV volume overload ► (see Video 3-11-2).

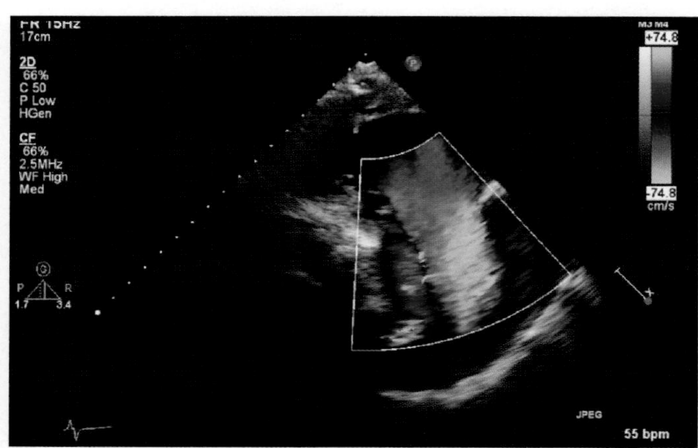

FIGURE 3-11-5 RV inflow view with color Doppler demonstrating severe TR with "to and fro" flow across the TV. Note the lack of turbulent flow ►(see Video 3-11-5).

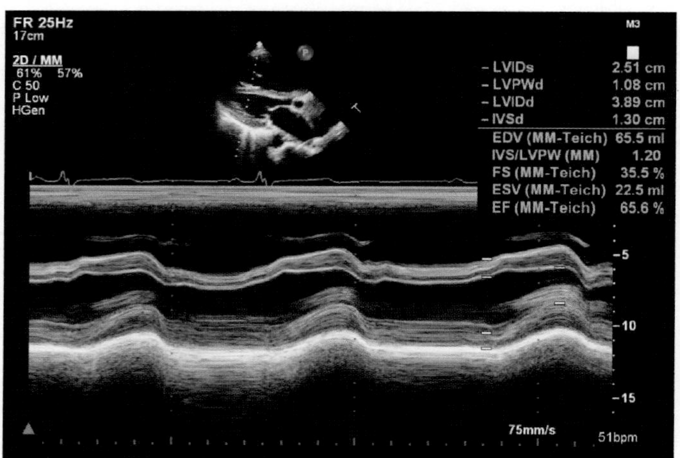

FIGURE 3-11-3 M-mode echocardiogram demonstrating diastolic flattening of the septum consistent with RV volume overload.

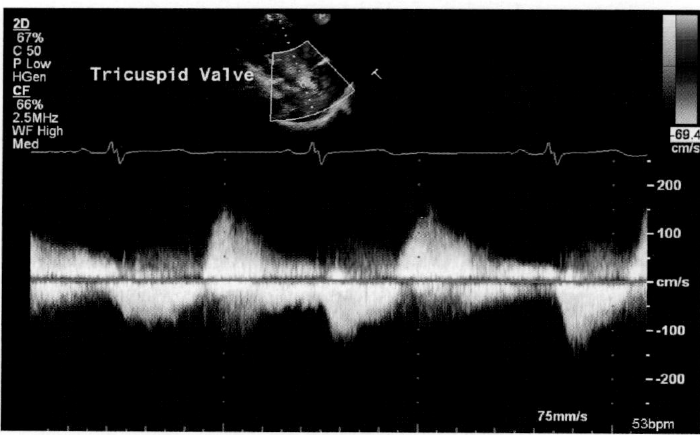

FIGURE 3-11-6 Continuous-wave Doppler from the RV inflow view demonstrating "to and fro" flow across the TV. Note the lack of a gradient in systole (peak velocity 1.4 m/sec) as there is no valve tissue to create a gradient between the RV and the RA.

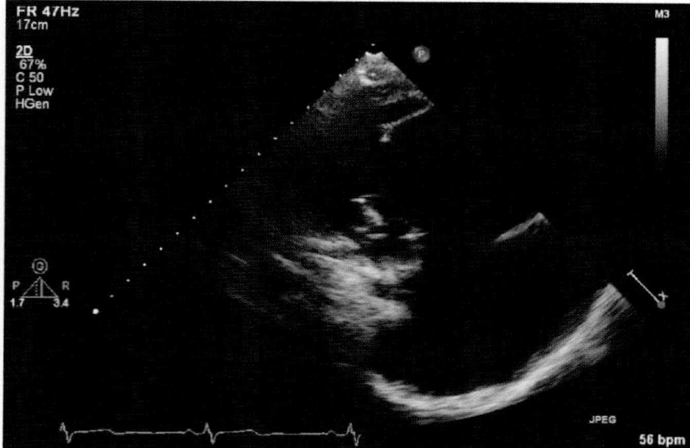

FIGURE 3-11-4 RV inflow view demonstrating RA and RV enlargement. Note the dilated TV annulus and minimal TV leaflet tissue ► (see Video 3-11-4).

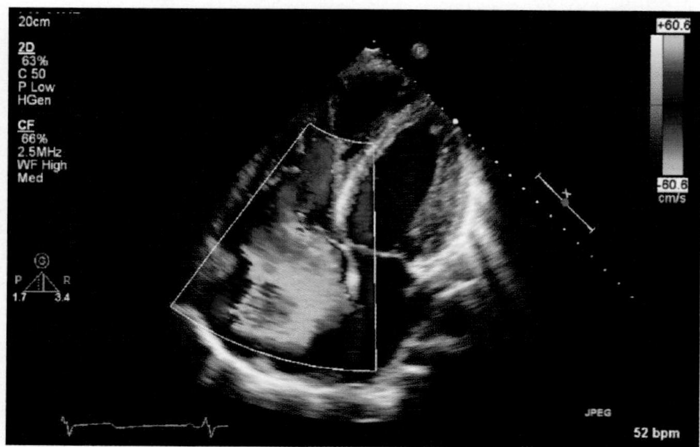

FIGURE 3-11-7 Apical 4 chamber view demonstrating a dilated, hypokinetic RV which is heavily trabeculated. Color Doppler demonstrates severe TR ► (see Videos 3-11-7).

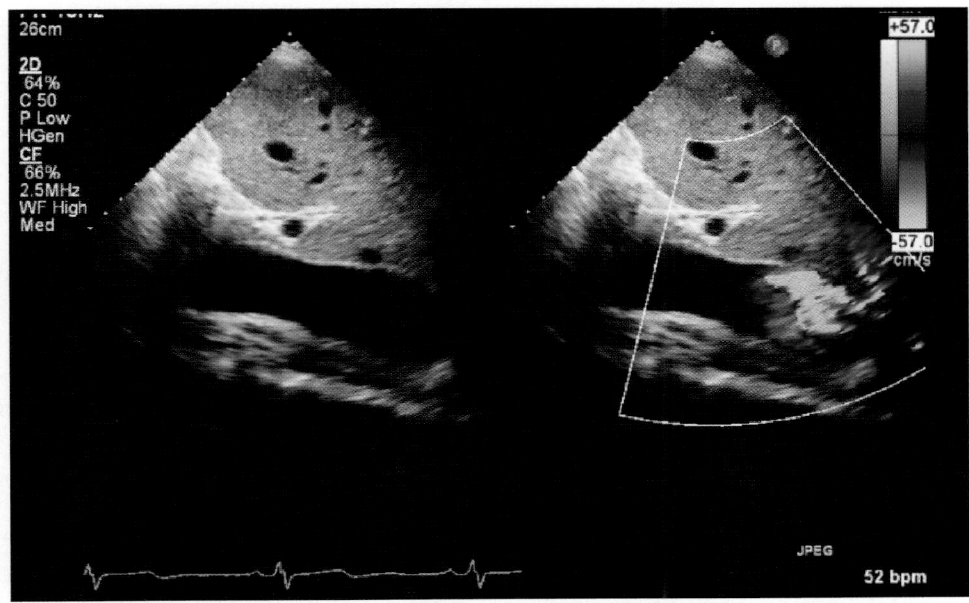

FIGURE 3-11-8 Subcostal view demonstrating a dilated, pulsatile IVC. Color Doppler demonstrates retrograde flow in systole into the IVC and hepatic vein ► (see Video 3-11-8).

chambers, most often the RA, as well as implanted cardiac devices such as pacemakers and ICD leads (see Section XIV: Native and Prosthetic Valve Endocarditis).

- TV endocarditis is most often seen in patients with a history of IVDA.
- Involvement of the TV is also seen in patients with implanted cardiac devices and indwelling central venous catheters.
- Severe TR can be due to abnormalities of the valve itself, the supporting chordae and the RV (see Section X: Functional Tricuspid Valve Regurgitation).

PATHOPHYSIOLOGY[1,3]

- Acutely, tricuspid valvectomy is usually well tolerated unless there is pre-existing right ventricular dysfunction or pulmonary hypertension.

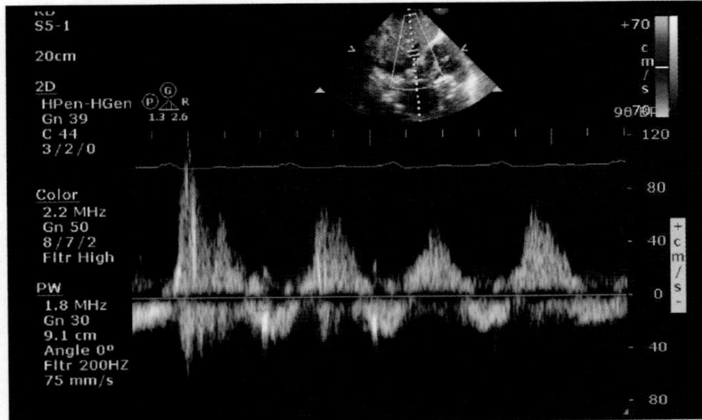

FIGURE 3-11-9 Pulsed wave Doppler demonstrating systolic flow reversal in the hepatic vein.

- Severe TV insufficiency results in RV volume overload.
- Over time, the RV dilates and systolic function is impaired. Further RV and TV annular dilation results in increasingly severe TR.
- Clinically, patients develop evidence of right heart failure with impaired exercise capacity, dyspnea, and edema.
- Liver dysfunction, including cirrhosis, can develop.

ECHOCARDIOGRAPHIC FINDINGS[4]

- Two-dimensional imaging reveals minimal or absent TV tissue.
- The RA and RV are dilated.
- Abnormal septal motion due to RV volume overload is present.
- The LV may be abnormally small (due to poor LV filling from low right sided stroke volume).
- The IVC is dilated and may demonstrate pulsatility.
- Color Doppler demonstrates regurgitant flow from the RV to the RA. The flow is often not turbulent due to lack of significant obstruction between the 2 chambers.
- Spectral Doppler reveals a dense TR signal that is often triangular rather than parabolic.
- PW Doppler of the IVC and HV demonstrates systolic flow reversal.

OTHER DIAGNOSTIC TESTING

- The ECG may demonstrate evidence of RA enlargement or RV enlargement.
- Atrial dysrhythmias may occur.
- CXR demonstrates an enlarged cardiac silhouette with evidence of RA and RV enlargement. The lung fields are typically clear.

- Cardiac MRI may be used to better assess the RV.
- Cardiac catheterization may be considered to assess right sided pressures and evaluate the patient for pulmonary hypertension and assess pulmonary vascular resistance.
  - Coronary angiography may be warranted if the patient is being evaluated for TV surgery.

DIFFERENTIAL DIAGNOSIS

- The differential diagnosis of severe TR includes any cause of right heart failure or edema.
  - Tricuspid stenosis
  - Pulmonary hypertension
  - Severe lung disease (COPD, interstitial lung disease)
  - Liver failure/cirrhosis
  - Renal failure
  - Nephrotic syndrome
- The etiology of severe TR includes functional TR (see Section 10: Functional Tricuspid Valve Regurgitation), congenital abnormalities such as Ebstein anomaly, myxomatous TV disease, ruptured TV chordae due to trauma, complications of cardiac biopsy with damage to the TV chordae from the bioptome, and pacemaker lead entrapment of the TV.

DIAGNOSIS

- The diagnosis of severe TR is made based on the history, physical examination, and echocardiography.

MANAGEMENT

- When patients present acutely with TV endocarditis and have indications for surgery (persistent sepsis, recurrent embolic events, heart block, severe TR), current guidelines recommend TV repair if feasible. If TV replacement is needed, most surgeons prefer a bioprosthetic valve.[2]
  - While some groups have favored TV resection, this procedure is rarely performed for TV endocarditis at the present time due to the long-term complications.
  - It may be considered as a planned 2 stage procedure with valvectomy followed by TV replacement if the patient abstains from drug use and there is no pulmonary hypertension or severe RV failure.
- In patients who have undergone TV resection and have significant TR:
  - Diuretic therapy and sodium restriction.
  - The role of TV replacement is controversial.
    - Patients are at risk of prosthetic valve endocarditis, especially if they continue to abuse drugs.
  - Since RV dysfunction can develop, careful follow-up is needed.

FOLLOW-UP AND PATIENT EDUCATION

- Patients should be monitored for the development of RV dysfunction with serial examinations and echocardiography.
- Complete abstinence from substance abuse (IVDA) is imperative.
- Endocarditis prophylaxis is warranted for patients with prior TV endocarditis and those with TV replacement or repair.

VIDEO LEGENDS

1. Video 3-11-1: Parasternal long axis demonstrating a relatively small LV, RV enlargement and hypokinesis as well as abnormal septal motion due to RV volume overload.
2. Video 3-11-2: Parasternal short axis demonstrating a relatively small LV, RV enlargement and hypokinesis as well as abnormal septal motion due to RV volume overload.
3. Video 3-11-4: RV inflow view demonstrating RA and RV enlargement. Note the dilated TV annulus and minimal TV leaflet tissue.
4. Video 3-11-5: RV inflow view with color Doppler demonstrating severe TR with "to and fro" flow across the TV. Note the lack of turbulent flow
5. Video 3-11-7 A: Apical 4 chamber view demonstrating a dilated, hypokinetic RV which is heavily trabeculated.
6. Video 3-11-7 B: Apical 4 chamber view. Color Doppler demonstrates severe TR.
7. Video 3-11-8: Subcostal view demonstrating a dilated, pulsatile IVC. Color Doppler demonstrates retrograde flow in systole into the IVC and hepatic vein.

REFERENCES

1. Arbulu A, Holmes RJ, Asfaw I. Tricuspid valvectomy without replacement. Twenty years' experience. *J Thorac Cardiovasc Surg*. 1990;49:845-857.
2. Byrne JG, Rezai K, Sanchez JA, et al. Surgical management of endocarditis: The Society of Thoracic Surgeons clinical practice guideline. *Ann Thorac Surg*. 2011;91:2012-2019.
3. Bonow RO, Carabello BA, Chatterjee K, et al. 2008 focused update incorporated into the ACC/AHA 2006 guidelines for the management of patients with valvular heart disease: a report of the American College of Cardiology/American Heart Association Task Force on Practice Guidelines (Writing committee to develop guidelines for the management of patients with valvular heart disease). Endorsed by the Society of Cardiovascular Anesthesiologists, Society for Cardiovascular Angiography and Interventions, and Society of Thoracic Surgeons. *J Am Coll Cardiol*. 2008;52:e1-142.
4. Rudski LG, Lai WW, Afilalo J, et al. Guidelines for the echocardiographic assessment of the right heart in adults: a report for the American Society of Echocardiography. *J Am Soc Echocardiogr*. 2010;23:685-713.

SECTION 12

Pulmonary Valve Stenosis

Kavita Sharma, MD

CLINICAL CASE PRESENTATION

A 20-year-old white female presents for routine care. She reports no problems as a child. She has no symptoms and is on no medications. On physical examination, she has a normal S_1 and S_2, with no S_3 or S_4 gallops. A pulmonary ejection click is noted. She has a systolic ejection murmur, with maximal intensity at the left upper sternal border. She has a prominent right ventricular impulse with a parasternal lift. An echocardiogram is performed to evaluate the murmur and her right ventricle. On the echocardiogram, she has normal left ventricular size and function, mild right ventricular dilation with normal function, a thickened pulmonic valve with moderate to severe stenosis (peak gradient 68 mm Hg) and mild to moderate pulmonary regurgitation (Figures 3-12-1 to 3-12-4). A referral for balloon valvotomy was placed; however, she was lost to follow-up and thus far has not had the recommended procedure.

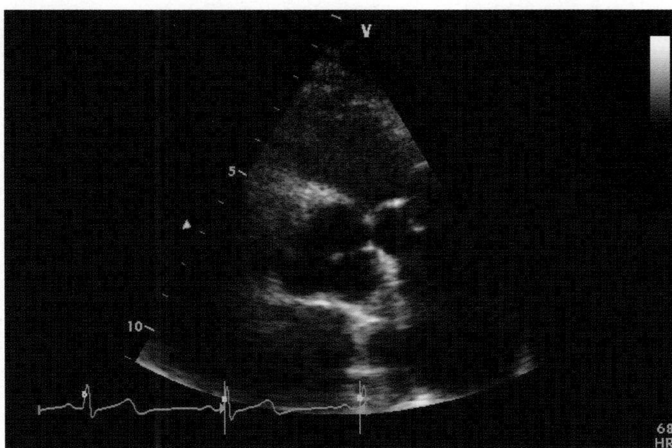

FIGURE 3-12-2 Parasternal short axis demonstrating the thickened pulmonary valve with doming in systole. The main pulmonary artery is dilated ▶ (see Video 3-12-2).

PATHOPHYSIOLOGY AND ETIOLOGY

- Virtually all cases of pulmonary stenosis (PS) are congenital.
  - Most commonly, a dome-shaped pulmonary valve with a narrow central opening is present. Less frequently, the pulmonary valve is dysplastic.[1] PS may occur as part of a congenital syndrome, such as Tetralogy of Fallot.
  - Less commonly than congenital causes, acquired PS can occur. Causes include rheumatic disease and carcinoid disease.[2]
- Stenosis above or below the pulmonary valve may occur as well.
  - Subvalvular stenosis (in the right ventricular outflow tract) is often seen in patients with Tetralogy of Fallot.
  - It may be caused by a ventricular septal defect with right ventricular outflow tract obstruction. Any cause of right ventricular hypertrophy may cause stenosis below the pulmonary valve.
  - Additionally, stenosis may occur in the pulmonary artery; this may occur in the main pulmonary artery, at the bifurcation, or more distally in the branches.[2]

EPIDEMIOLOGY

- In the general population, PS is rare. However, in the population of patients with congenital heart disease, PS is relatively common. It occurs in approximately 10% of children with congenital heart disease.[3]

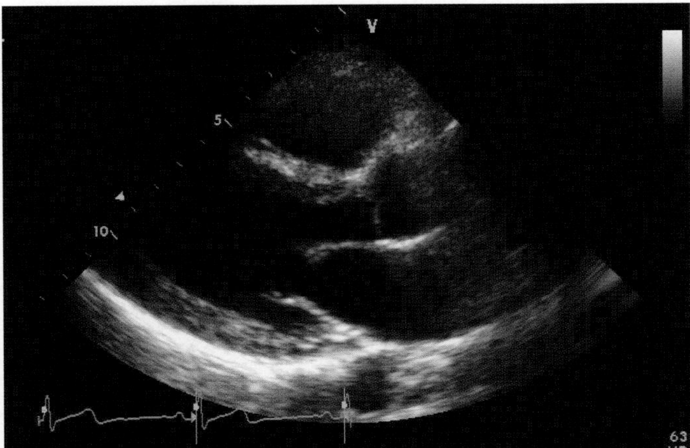

FIGURE 3-12-1 Parasternal long axis demonstrating RV hypertrophy, mild RV enlargement, and normal LV size and function ▶ (see Video 3-12-1).

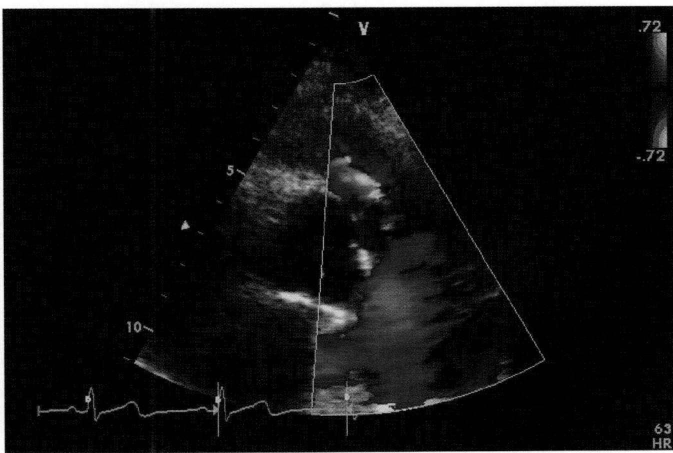

FIGURE 3-12-3 Parasternal short axis with color Doppler across the pulmonary valve demonstrating turbulent flow in systole and mild pulmonary insufficiency ▶ (see Video 3-12-3).

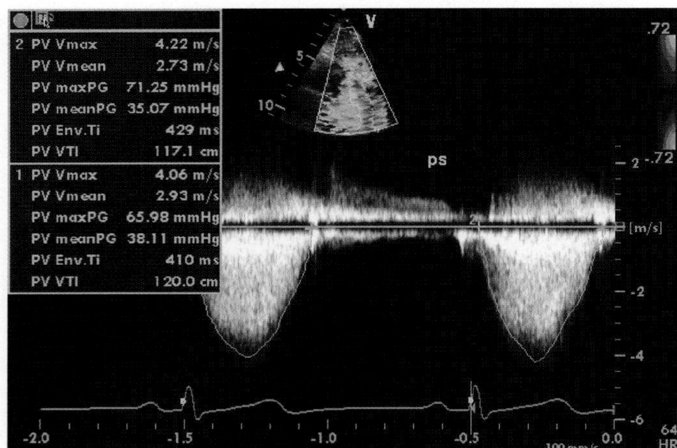

FIGURE 3-12-4 Continuous-wave Doppler of the gradient across the pulmonary valve demonstrating a markedly elevated peak and mean gradient.

ECHOCARDIOGRAPHY

The pulmonary valve is assessed using 2-D echocardiography, color flow Doppler, continuous-wave Doppler, and pulsed Doppler.

- Using 2-D imaging, the morphology of the pulmonary valve is evaluated, looking for doming or dysplasia.
- Right ventricular hypertrophy is assessed using 2-D imaging. A thickness of >5 mm of the right ventricle is considered abnormal.[4]
- The severity of PS is defined by the velocity and systolic gradient across the valve, using continuous-wave Doppler. The systolic pressure gradient is estimated from the transpulmonary velocity using the modified Bernoulli equation.

$$\Delta P = 4V^2$$

- Severe stenosis is defined as a peak velocity >4m/s or peak gradient >64 mm Hg. Moderate stenosis is a peak velocity of 3 to 4 m/s or peak gradient 36 to 64 mm Hg. Mild stenosis is a peak velocity <3m/s or peak gradient <36 mm Hg.[5]
- Pulsed wave Doppler may be used to evaluate serial stenotic lesions.
- Color flow Doppler and spectral Doppler are employed to assess concomitant PR.

OTHER DIAGNOSTIC TESTING AND PROCEDURES

- In patients with moderate or severe pulmonic stenosis, cardiac catheterization is indicated for further evaluation of the transpulmonary gradient if balloon dilation is being considered.[6]

MANAGEMENT

- Patients with mild pulmonic stenosis are managed medically, as the disease rarely progresses.[7]
- Balloon valvotomy is recommended for symptomatic patients with a mean transpulmonary gradient of >30 mm Hg or asymptomatic patients with a mean gradient >40 mm Hg, based on the ACC/AHA 2008 guidelines for the management of adults with congenital heart disease.[5]
- Balloon valvotomy is the procedure of choice due to its high success rate and low complication rate.[8]

FOLLOW-UP

- For asymptomatic patients with peak Doppler gradient <30 mm Hg, follow-up physical examination, Doppler echocardiography, and electrocardiogram are recommended at 5-year intervals.[5]
- For asymptomatic patients with a peak instantaneous Doppler gradient >30 mm Hg, follow-up Doppler echocardiography is recommended every 2 to 3 years.
- After valvotomy, periodic echocardiography of the pulmonic valve is recommended, for assessment of pulmonic valve stenosis, regurgitation, and right heart function.

SUMMARY

- PS commonly occurs as a congenital lesion. Echocardiography is useful to demonstrate valve morphology and severity of stenosis. In select patients, balloon valvotomy is recommended due to a high success rate and low complication rate.

VIDEO LEGENDS

1. Video 3-12-1: Parasternal long axis demonstrating RV hypertrophy, mild RV enlargement and normal LV size and function
2. Video 3-12-2: Parasternal short axis demonstrating the thickened pulmonary valve with doming in systole. The main pulmonary artery is dilated
3. Video 3-12-3: Parasternal short axis with color Doppler across the pulmonary valve demonstrating turbulent flow in systole and mild pulmonary insufficiency

REFERENCES

1. Koretzky ED, Moller JH, Korns ME, Schwartz CJ, Edwards JE. Congenital pulmonary stenosis resulting from dysplasia of valve. *Circulation*. 1969;40:43-53.
2. Baumgartner H, Hung J, Bermejo J, et al. Echocardiographic assessment of valve stenosis: EAE/ASE recommendations for clinical practice. *Eur J Echocardiogr*. 2009;10:1-25.
3. Rocchini AP, Emmanouilides EG. In Emmanouilides GC, Riemenschneider TA, Allen HD, Gutgesell HP, eds. *Moss and Adams Heart Disease in Infants, Children and Adolescents*. Baltimore, MD: Williams & Wilkins; 1995.
4. Lang RM, Bierig M, Devereux RB, et al. Recommendations for chamber quantification. *Eur J Echocardiogr*. 2006;7:79-108.
5. Warnes CA, Williams RG, Bashore TM, et al. ACC/AHA 2008 guidelines for the management of adults with congenital heart disease: executive summary: a report of the American College of Cardiology/American Heart Association Task Force on practice guidelines (Writing committee to develop guidelines for the management of adults with congenital heart disease). *Circulation*. 2008;118:2395-2451.
6. Bonow RO, Carabello BA, Chatterjee K, et al. 2008 focused update incorporated into the ACC/AHA 2006 guidelines for the management of patients with valvular heart disease: a report of the American College of Cardiology/American Heart Association Task Force on Practice Guidelines (Writing committee to develop

guidelines for the management of patients with valvular heart disease). Endorsed by the Society of Cardiovascular Anesthesiologists, Society for Cardiovascular Angiography and Interventions, and Society of Thoracic Surgeons. *J Am Coll Cardiol*. 2008;52:e1-142.

7. Nadas AS. Report from the joint study on the natural history of congenital heart defects. I. General introduction. *Circulation*. 1977;56:I3-4.

8. Stanger P, Cassidy SC, Girod DA, Kan JS, Lababidi Z, Shapiro SR. Balloon pulmonary valvuloplasty: results of the Valvuloplasty and Angioplasty of Congenital Anomalies Registry. *Am J Cardiol*. 1990;65:775-783.

SECTION 13

Prosthetic Mitral Valve Dysfunction

Kavita Sharma, MD

CLINICAL CASE PRESENTATION

The patient is a 48-year-old woman with a history of rheumatic heart disease who underwent prosthetic mitral valve replacement with a bi-leaflet mechanical valve and coronary artery bypass grafting 2 years ago. She was lost to follow-up and has had little medical care. She has not been regularly taking her warfarin or other cardiac medications. She presents with progressive shortness of breath and chest pain. On exam, the mechanical valve sounds are dull in nature. A diastolic murmur is appreciated in the mitral position. She underwent a transthoracic echocardiogram (TTE), which demonstrated an elevated mean gradient across the prosthetic mitral valve of 7 mm Hg (Figures 3-13-1 to 3-13-2). The time velocity integral of the prosthetic mitral valve (TVI PrMV) and the time velocity integral of the left ventricular outflow tract (TVI LVOT) are obtained. The TVI PrMV/TVI LVOT ratio is approximately 3.0. The left atrium is shadowed by the prosthetic mitral valve. The patient underwent fluoroscopy of the mitral valve which demonstrated immobile mitral valve leaflets. She underwent a transesophageal echocardiogram (TEE) which demonstrated a large thrombus obstructing the mechanical mitral valve and confirmation of an elevated mean gradient (13 mm Hg) (Figures 3-13-3 to 3-13-5). She underwent emergent mitral valve replacement surgery and did well post-operatively (Figure 3-13-6).

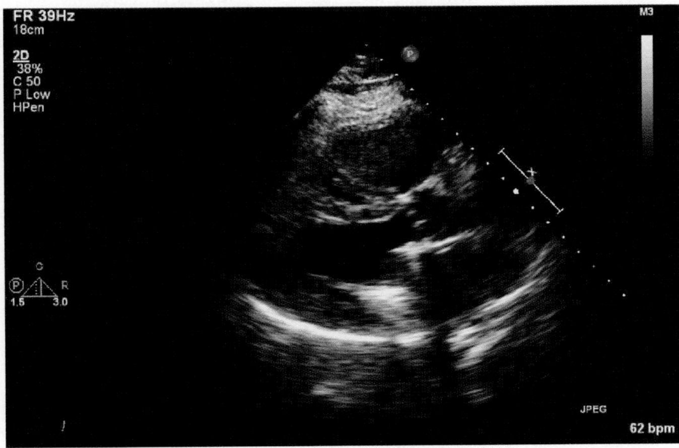

FIGURE 3-13-1 Parasternal long axis TTE demonstrated preserved LVEF but no obvious mass on the prosthetic mitral valve ▶ (see Video 3-13-1).

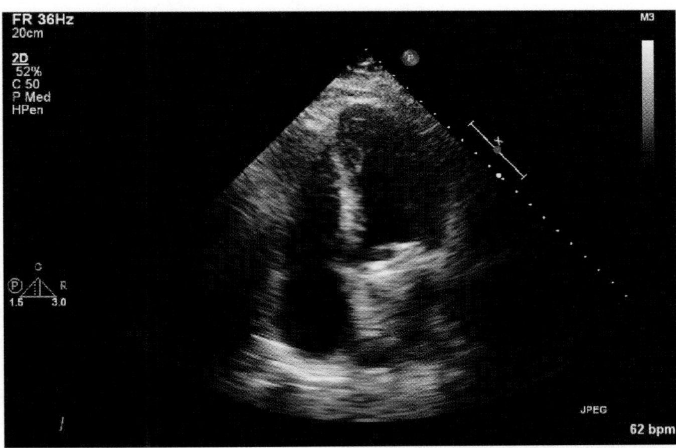

FIGURE 3-13-2 Apical 4 chamber TTE again demonstrated preserved LVEF but no obvious mass on the prosthetic mitral valve. Leaflet mobility is not well assessed ▶ (see Video 3-13-2).

EPIDEMIOLOGY

- Approximately 4000 mitral valve replacement surgeries are performed annually for isolated mitral valve disease.[1]
- An additional 2800 mitral valve replacements are performed in combination with coronary artery bypass grafting annually.[1]
- The incidence of thromboembolic complications of mechanical prosthetic valves ranges from 0.03% to 4.3% patient-years, depending on the prosthesis used, the location of the valve, and the quality of anticoagulation.[2,3]

PATHOPHYSIOLOGY AND ETIOLOGY

- Prosthetic valves are divided into 2 broad types: mechanical valves and bioprosthetic valves.

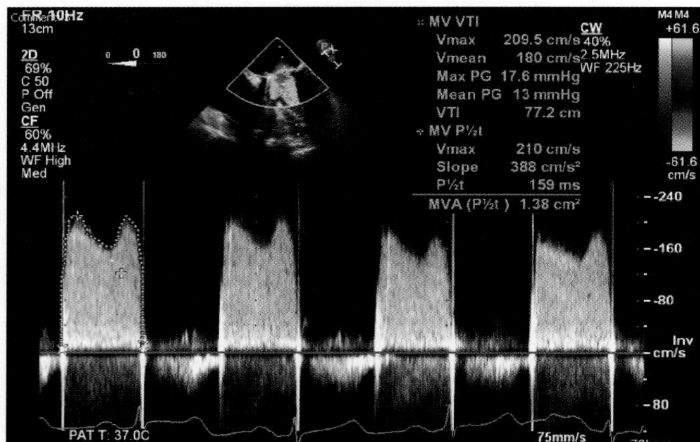

FIGURE 3-13-3 Continuous-wave Doppler from the TEE demonstrating an elevated prosthetic mitral valve gradient (mean gradient 13 mm Hg).

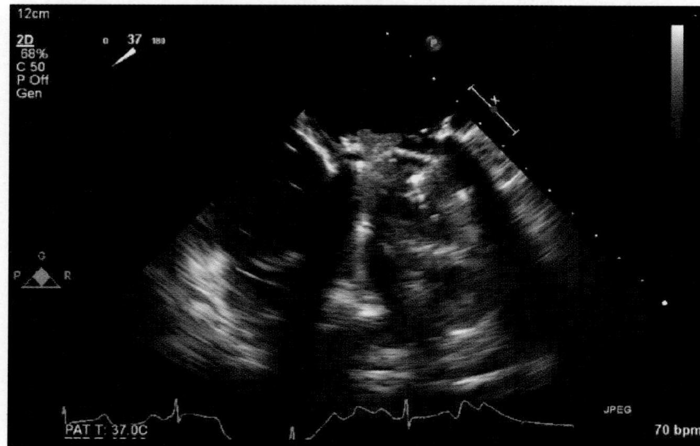

FIGURE 3-13-4 TEE 4 chamber view demonstrating thrombus (still frame).

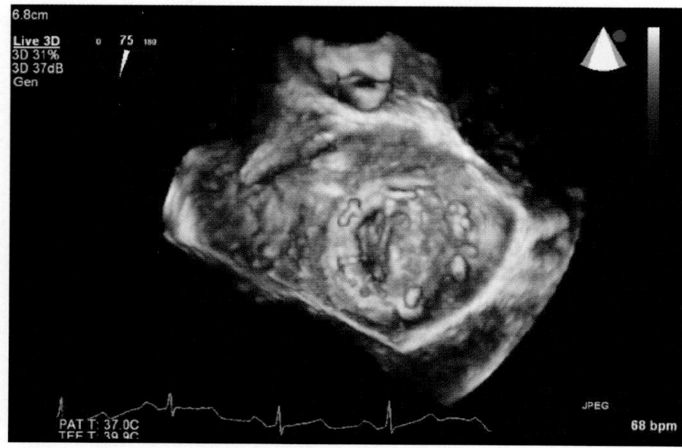

FIGURE 3-13-5 TEE 3-dimensional image of the prosthetic mitral valve (still frame).

- The major complications of prosthetic valves are patient-prosthesis mismatch, geometric mismatch, dehiscence, primary failure, thrombosis and thromboembolism, pannus formation, pseudoaneurysm formation, endocarditis, and hemolysis.
- Mechanical valves may develop thrombi, most often related to inadequate anticoagulation.[4]
- Pannus formation may occur on both bioprosthetic and mechanical valves.
- Bioprosthetic valves may degenerate over time, with resultant stenosis or regurgitation.[4]
- Patients with prosthetic mitral valves are at risk for developing endocarditis and abscesses.
- Thrombosis is much more common with mechanical prosthetic valves than bioprosthetic valves.[4]

ECHOCARDIOGRAPHY

- All patients who have undergone valve replacement surgery should have a baseline study performed postoperatively and follow-up studies as detailed in Section I: Asymptomatic Severe Aortic Stenosis.
- A major consideration in the evaluation of prosthetic valves is the effect of shadowing by the valve.[5]
- On TTE, a prosthetic mitral valve often obscures the appearance of mitral regurgitation (MR) and of the left atrium. On TEE, the left ventricle is often obscured by the prosthetic mitral valve. Therefore, both TTE and TEE imaging is often required when prosthetic mitral valve dysfunction is suspected.[5]
- On 2-D imaging, the valve should be examined for leaflet excursion. The valve should be examined for thrombus, pannus, or vegetation. The valve should be examined for abnormal rocking motion.
- The size of the left ventricle, right ventricle, and left atrium should be established.
- One should look for transvalvular mitral regurgitation with color Doppler, as well as paravalvular leaks.
- Mild thickening is often the first sign of bioprosthetic valve failure.[6]
- On continuous-wave and pulse Doppler, the following parameters should be obtained: peak early mitral velocity, estimated mean pressure gradient, and pressure half-time.
- The heart rate of the cardiac cycle used for Doppler measurements is very important for mitral prosthetic valves because the mean gradient is influenced by the diastolic filling period.[5]
- The relationship between velocity and pressure gradient is defined by $\Delta P = 4V^2$ (the Bernoulli equation).
- In normal bioprosthetic mitral valves, the peak early mitral velocity should range from 1.0 to 2.7 m/s.[7]
- In mechanical mitral valves, a peak velocity <1.9 m/s is likely to be normal.[8]
- Elevated velocities suggest valve stenosis or regurgitation.[8]
- The mean gradient across a prosthetic mitral valve is usually <5 to 6 mm Hg.[9]

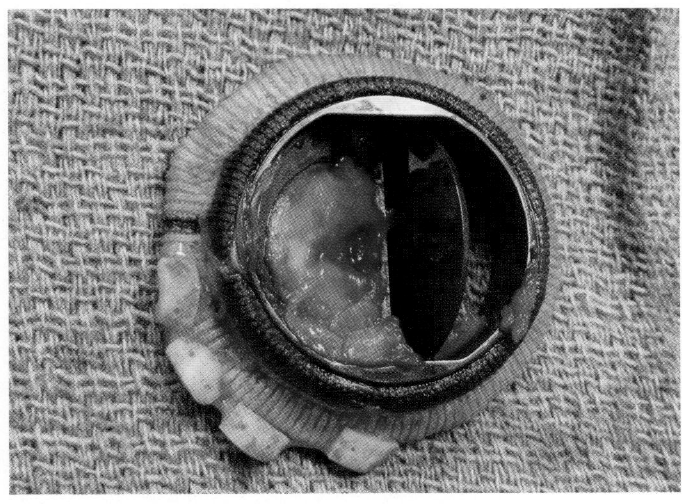

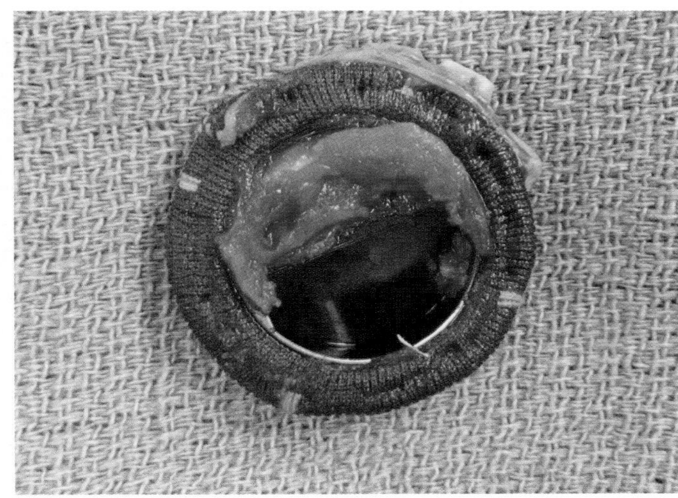

FIGURE 3-13-6 Explanted valve demonstrating a large thrombus as seen from the LV (L) and LA (R) aspects. One leaflet was encased in thrombus.

- High mean velocities may be due to hyperdynamic states, tachycardia, patient-prosthesis mismatch, valvular regurgitation, or stenosis.[4]
- A pressure half time >130 ms is rare in a normally functioning prosthetic mitral valve.[8]
- Calculation of the effective orifice area (EOA) using the pressure half-time method is not valid in prosthetic valves.[10]
- Calculation of the EOA by the continuity equation is preferable in prosthetic mitral valves.[10]
- The EOA is equal to the stroke volume across the mitral valve/velocity time integral (TVI). The stroke volume is calculated at the LV outflow tract.
- The ratio of the TVIs of the mitral prosthesis to the LV outflow tract (TVI PrMV/TVI LVOT) is useful. Elevated mitral velocities may occur in stenosis, regurgitation or high output states. However, the TVI PrMV/TVI LVOT is elevated only in stenosis or regurgitation.[4]
- In mechanical mitral valves, a TVI PrMV/TVI LVOT <2.2 is most often normal.[8]
- It is vital to compare any abnormal hemodynamic findings on the echo to the baseline characteristics on the initial postoperative echo or any prior echocardiographic studies.[4]
- In evaluating for prosthetic valve dysfunction, all of the above information should be assessed comprehensively.
- TEE can be very useful in evaluation of prosthetic mitral valve dysfunction as the mitral valve is well visualized on TEE (Figures 3-13-7, 3-13-8).
- On TEE, paravalvular leaks on color Doppler typically pass outside the surgical ring in an eccentric jet.[4]
- The vena contracta is useful in the assessment of prosthetic mitral valve regurgitation; a vena contract ≥6 mm is defined as large prosthetic mitral valve regurgitation.[11]

OTHER DIAGNOSTIC MODALITIES

- Fluoroscopy is indicated as a Class IIa indication in the 2014 ACC/AHA Valvular Heart Disease Guidelines to assess suspected valve thrombosis by evaluating valve motion.[14]

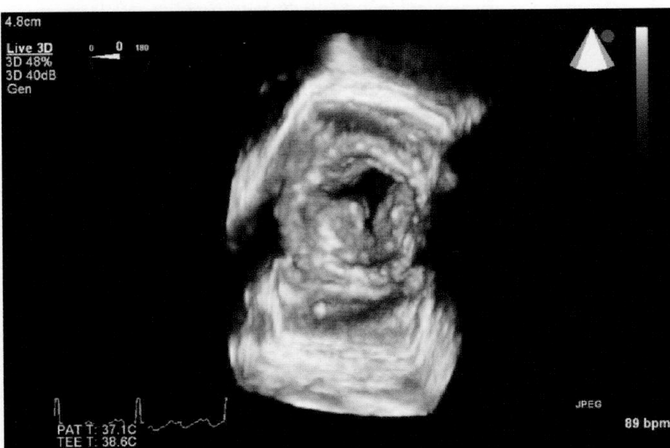

FIGURE 3-13-7 TEE (live 3-D) view of a thickened, calcified stenotic bioprosthetic MV from a different patient who presented with CHF ► (see Video 3-13-7). All 3 leaflets are thickened, and two of the leaflets have limited mobility. Doppler demonstrated an elevated gradient.

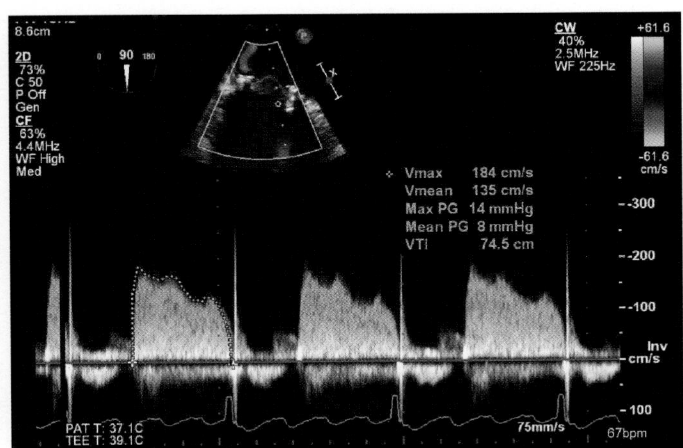

FIGURE 3-13-8 Continuous-wave Doppler from the patient in Figure 3-13-7 demonstrating a mean gradient of 8 mm Hg consistent with moderate stenosis

- Multidetector computed tomography (MDCT) has been shown to be of value in visualizing prosthetic valves and possible causes of dysfunction.[12]

MANAGEMENT

- All patients with mechanical prosthetic valves should be anticoagulated with warfarin. The target INR varies depending on valve type, position, and concomitant risks for thromboembolism, such as LV dysfunction and atrial fibrillation.[14]
- There are higher INR goals for mitral mechanical prostheses and those patients with risk factors such as atrial fibrillation, prior thromboembolism, or hypercoaguable state.[14]
- In addition, patients with mechanical prosthetic valves should be on an aspirin, 81 mg.[14]
- Patients with bioprosthetic valves should be on low dose aspirin. Warfarin is indicated in patients with additional thrombo-embolic risk factors, especially atrial fibrillation, and should be considered in the first 3 months after valve surgery.[14]
- Emergency surgery is recommended (Class I) for patients with a thrombosed left-sided prostheses and NYHA functional class III-IV symptoms or patients with a large clot burden (> 0.8 cm^2), in whom surgery is a Class IIa indication.[14]
- Fibrinolytic therapy is recommended as a Class IIa indication for patients with left-sided prosthetic valve thrombosis with a small thrombus burden (<0.8 cm^2) and recent onset NYHA class I to II symtoms, as well as patients with thrombosed right-sided valves.[14]
- Fibrinolytic therapy for a thrombosed left-sided valve is associated with a high risk.[13]

FOLLOW-UP

- A baseline echocardiogram is recommended after valve replacement.[14]
- After valve replacement, asymptomatic patients need to be seen only at 1-year intervals, at which time a complete history and thorough physical examination should be performed.
- Follow-up echocardiography is recommended thereafter if there is a change in the patient's clinical condition. In patients with suspected LV dysfunction, prosthetic valve dysfunction, or dysfunction of other heart valves, echocardiography is recommended.
- Once regurgitation is detected, close follow-up with 2-D and Doppler echocardiography every 3 to 6 months is indicated.

SUMMARY

- The major complications of prosthetic valves are patient-prosthesis mismatch, geometric mismatch, dehiscence, primary failure, thrombosis and thromboembolism, pannus formation, pseudoaneurysm formation, endocarditis, and hemolysis.
- Echocardiography provides vital information in the assessment of prosthetic valves, in the form of both transthoracic echocardiography and transesophageal echocardiography.
- In thrombosed prosthetic valves, emergent surgery or fibrinolytic therapy may be considered, depending on the location of the valve, size of the thrombus and patient symptoms.

VIDEO LEGENDS

1. Video 3-13-1: Parasternal long axis TTE demonstrated preserved LVEF but no obvious mass on the prosthetic mitral valve.
2. Video 3-13-2: Apical four chamber TTE again demonstrates preserved LVEF but no obvious mass on the prosthetic mitral valve. Leaflet mobility is not well assessed
3. Video 3-13-7: TEE (live 3-D) view of a thickened, calcified stenotic bioprosthetic MV from a different patient who presented with CHF. All 3 leaflets are thickened and two of the leaflets have limited mobility. Doppler demonstrated an elevated gradient.

REFERENCES

1. Bonow RO, Carabello BA, Chatterjee K, et al. 2008 focused update incorporated into the ACC/AHA 2006 guidelines for the management of patients with valvular heart disease: a report of the American College of Cardiology/American Heart Association Task Force on Practice Guidelines (Writing committee to develop guidelines for the management of patients with valvular heart disease). Endorsed by the Society of Cardiovascular Anesthesiologists, Society for Cardiovascular Angiography and Interventions, and Society of Thoracic Surgeons. *J Am Coll Cardiol*. 2008;52:e1-142.
2. Horstkotte D, Burckhardt D. Prosthetic valve thrombosis. *J Heart Valve Dis*. 1995;4:141-153.
3. Stein PD, Alpert JS, Bussey HI, Dalen JE, Turpie AG. Antithrombotic therapy in patients with mechanical and biological prosthetic heart valves. *Chest*. 2001;119:220S-227S.
4. Zoghbi WA, Chambers JB, Dumesnil JG, et al. Recommendations for evaluation of prosthetic valves with echocardiography and doppler ultrasound: a report from the American Society of Echocardiography's Guidelines and Standards Committee and the Task Force on Prosthetic Valves, developed in conjunction with the American College of Cardiology Cardiovascular Imaging Committee, Cardiac Imaging Committee of the American Heart Association, the European Association of Echocardiography, a registered branch of the European Society of Cardiology, the Japanese Society of Echocardiography and the Canadian Society of Echocardiography, endorsed by the American College of Cardiology Foundation, American Heart Association, European Association of Echocardiography, a registered branch of the European Society of Cardiology, the Japanese Society of Echocardiography, and Canadian Society of Echocardiography. *J Am Soc Echocardiogr*. 2009;22:975-1014; quiz 1082-1014.
5. Sprecher DL, Adamick R, Adams D, Kisslo J. In vitro color flow, pulsed and continuous-wave Doppler ultrasound masking of flow by prosthetic valves. *J Am Coll Cardiol*. 1987;9:1306-1310.
6. Alam M, Goldstein S, Lakier JB. Echocardiographic changes in the thickness of porcine valves with time. *Chest*. 1981;79:663-668.

7. Goetze S, Brechtken J, Agler DA, Thomas JD, Sabik JF 3rd, Jaber WA. In vivo short-term Doppler hemodynamic profiles of 189 Carpentier-Edwards Perimount pericardial bioprosthetic valves in the mitral position. *J Am Soc Echocardiogr*. 2004;17:981-987.
8. Fernandes V, Olmos L, Nagueh SF, Quinones MA, Zoghbi WA. Peak early diastolic velocity rather than pressure half-time is the best index of mechanical prosthetic mitral valve function. *Am J Cardiol*. 2002;89:704-710.
9. Bitar JN, Lechin ME, Salazar G, Zoghbi WA. Doppler echocardiographic assessment with the continuity equation of St. Jude Medical mechanical prostheses in the mitral valve position. *Am J Cardiol*. 1995;76:287-293.
10. Dumesnil JG, Honos GN, Lemieux M, Beauchemin J. Validation and applications of mitral prosthetic valvular areas calculated by Doppler echocardiography. *Am J Cardiol*. 1990;65:1443-1448.
11. Vitarelli A, Conde Y, Cimino E, et al. Assessment of severity of mechanical prosthetic mitral regurgitation by transoesophageal echocardiography. *Heart*. 2004;90:539-544.
12. Habets J, Symersky P, van Herwerden LA, et al. Prosthetic heart valve assessment with multidetector-row CT: imaging characteristics of 91 valves in 83 patients. *Eur Radiol*. 2011;21:1390-1396.
13. Birdi I, Angelini GD, Bryan AJ. Thrombolytic therapy for left sided prosthetic heart valve thrombosis. *J Heart Valve Dis*. 1995;4:154-159.
14. Nishimura RA, Otto CM, Bonow RO, et al. 2014 AHA/ACC guideline for the management of patients with valvular heart disease:executive summary; a report of the American College of Cardiology/American Heart Association Task Force on Practice Guidelines. *J Am Coll Cardiol*. 2014;63:2348-2388.

SECTION 14

Native and Prosthetic Valve Endocarditis

Gbemiga Sofowora, MBChB, FACC, Nkechinyere N. Ijioma, MBBS, and David A. Orsinelli, MD, FACC, FASE

Native and prosthetic valve endocarditis share many epidemiologic and pathologic features. We will present 2 representative cases of endocarditis to highlight the role of echocardiography in the evaluation and management of such patients.

CLINICAL CASE PRESENTATION 1

NATIVE VALVE ENDOCARDITIS

The patient is a 29-year-old man with a history of chronic intravenous drug abuse (IVDA) who presented to an outside hospital with a 1 week history of malaise, dyspnea, and chest pain that was worse lying flat and improved sitting up. He had no significant past medical history, but had not seen a physician for several years. He was transferred to our institution with a presumed diagnosis of pericarditis. On arrival, he appeared chronically ill and was in moderate respiratory distress. He was pale and diaphoretic. Physical examination revealed a blood pressure of 140/50 mm Hg, a pulse of 100 beats/min, and a temperature of 101.4° F (38.5° C). He had rales approximately ½ way up bilaterally. His neck veins were elevated. Cardiac examination revealed a prominent two component friction rub, a soft systolic murmur at the base of the heart with a grade 3/6 blowing diastolic murmur heard along the left sternal boarder. There was a grade 3/6 holosystolic murmur at the apex which radiated to the axilla and was also appreciated posteriorly in the left chest. An S_3 gallop was appreciated. He had hepatomegaly, scleral icterus, and 1+ pedal edema. Laboratory data included a microcytic anemia (Hgb 6.8), leukocytosis, elevated transaminases, and bilirubin. Chest x-ray revealed pulmonary edema. Blood cultures were obtained (which subsequently grew *Staph aureus*) and he was started immediately on broad spectrum antibiotics. A stat transthoracic echocardiogram (Figures 3-14-1 to 3-14-9) was obtained which revealed a moderate to large pericardial effusion, vegetations on the aortic valve

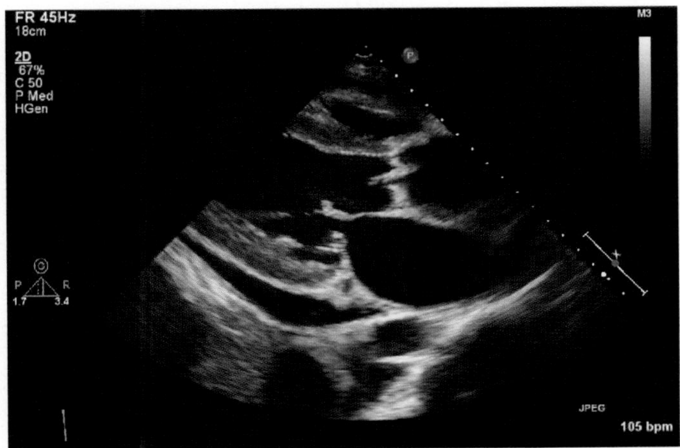

FIGURE 3-14-1 Parasternal long axis demonstrating vegetations on the aortic valve and thickening of the mitral valve. There is also evidence of a pericardial effusion and a left pleural effusion ▶ (see Video 3-14-1).

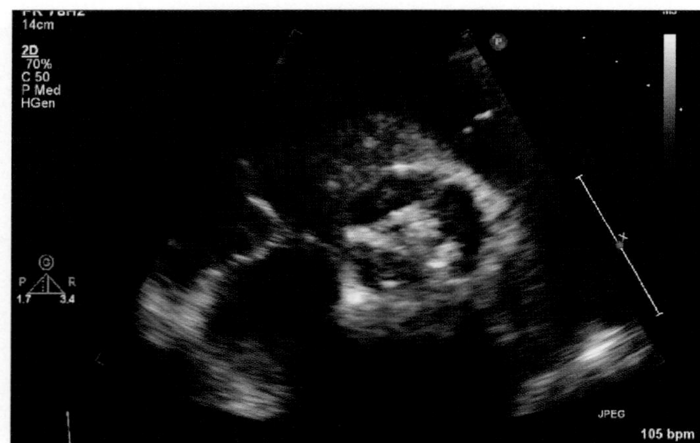

FIGURE 3-14-2 Parasternal short axis demonstrating vegetations on the aortic valve. There is also periaortic "fullness" which correlated with the root abscess identified at the time of surgery ▶ (see Video 3-14-2).

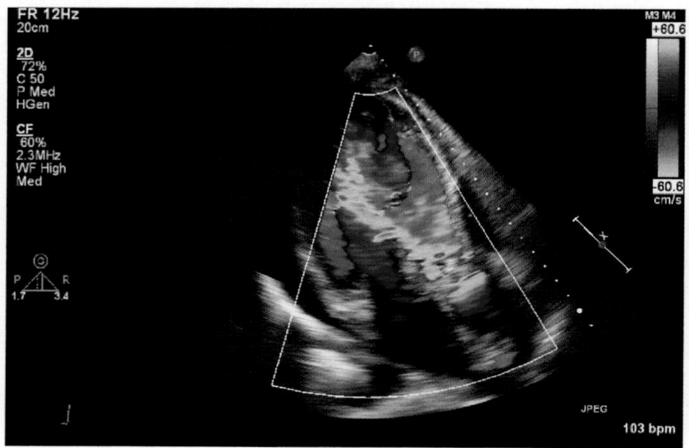

FIGURE 3-14-3 Apical 3 chamber view with color Doppler demonstrating severe AR ▶ (see Video 3-14-3).

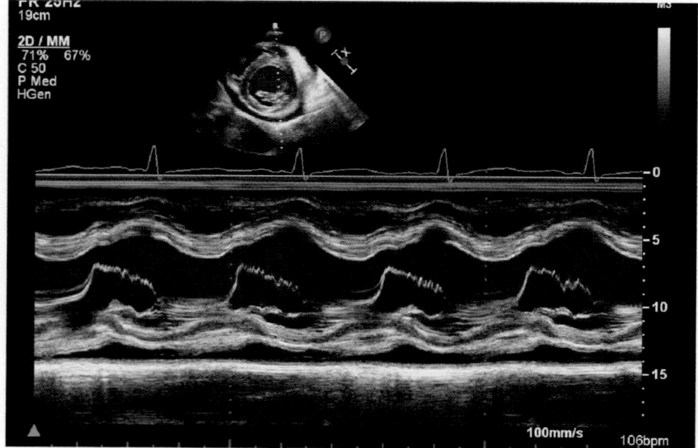

FIGURE 3-14-4 M-mode of the MV demonstrating diastolic fluttering of the anterior leaflet as a result of the severe AR jet impacting the anterior MV leaflet.

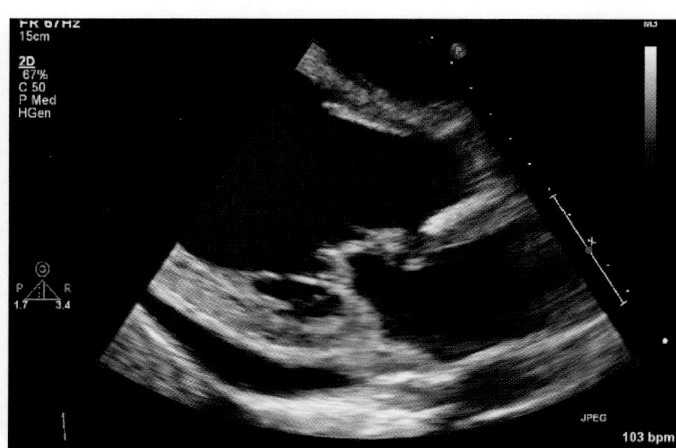

FIGURE 3-14-5 Parasternal long axis demonstrating the thickened mitral valve with evidence of a perforation of the anterior mitral valve leaflet ▶ (see Video 3-14-5).

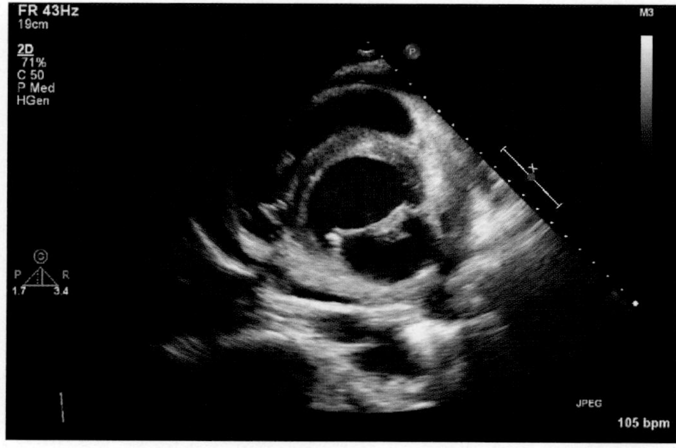

FIGURE 3-14-6 Parasternal short axis view of the MV anterior leaflet perforation ▶ (see Video 3-14-6).

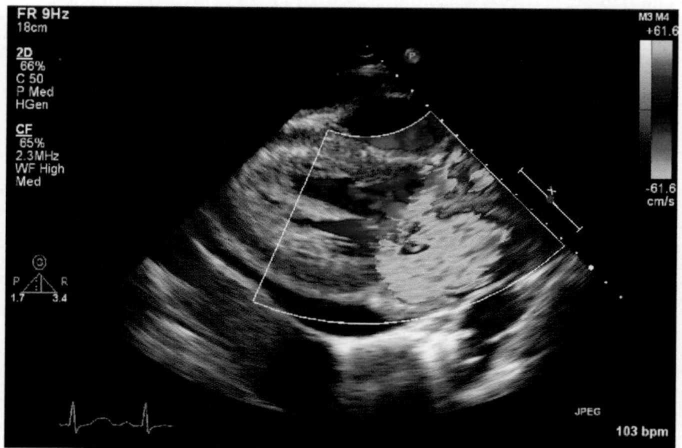

FIGURE 3-14-7 Parasternal long axis view of the MV with color Doppler demonstrating severe MR ▶ (see Video 3-14-7).

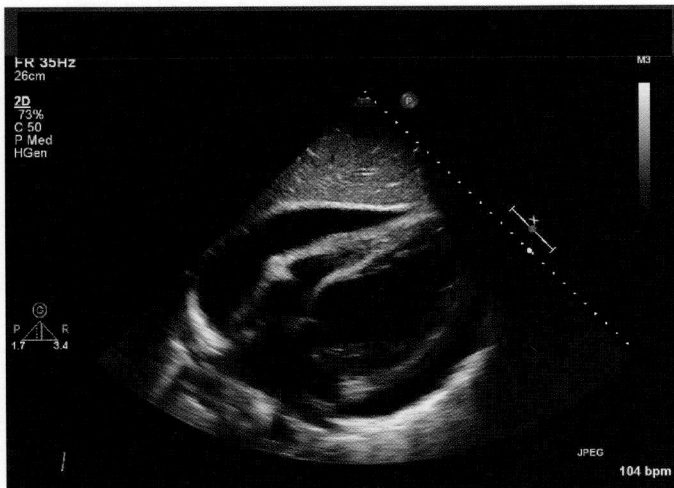

FIGURE 3-14-8 Subcostal view demonstrating the moderate to large pericardial effusion.

(which was bicuspid) with severe AR, a perforation of the anterior MV leaflet with severe MR, and mild global LV dysfunction. Urgent consultation with cardiac surgery was obtained, and he was taken emergently to the operating room where intraoperative TEE confirmed the above findings (Figures 3-14-10 and 3-14-11). There was hemorrhagic pericardial effusion with evidence of pericardial inflammation. Large vegetations were found on the bicuspid AV, as well as an aortic root abscess. There was a perforation of the anterior MV leaflet with vegetations at the site of the perforation. He underwent debridement of the root abscess. The aortic and mitral valves were replaced using bioprosthetic valves. He developed complete heart block postoperatively and required permanent pacemaker placement. He was discharged to a skilled nursing facility for rehabilitation and to complete a 6-week course of antibiotics. He unfortunately left the facility against medical advice and was lost to follow-up.

CLINICAL CASE PRESENTATION 2

PROSTHETIC VALVE ENDOCARDITIS

The patient is a 30-year-old woman who underwent tricuspid valve replacement 1 year prior to presentation for tricuspid insufficiency. She had a history of IVDA and was found to have endocarditis with severe TR at that time. She was lost to follow-up, but reported taking her medications. She presented to the hospital with fevers, chills, and malaise, as well as intermittent chest discomfort. She denied current IVDA; however, needle marks were noted on her arms. She was febrile with a temperature of 102.2° F (39° C) and tachycardic but normotensive. She appeared chronically ill. Her lung exam was remarkable for scattered rhonchi. Auscultation of the heart revealed a holosystolic murmur located over the tricuspid region which was louder with inspiration. A mitral insufficiency murmur was also appreciated. She had no abdominal findings and no edema. Laboratory studies were remarkable for a leukocytosis. A transthoracic echo was of suboptimal quality. Blood cultures grew Methicillin resistant *Staphylococcus aureus*. She was placed on IV vancomycin. A subsequent TEE revealed vegetations on her prosthetic tricuspid valve as well as her mitral valve (Figures 3-14-12 to 3-14-14). She improved clinically with resolution of her fevers. Three days later however, a watchful nurse noted that the patient had new onset slurred speech which resolved spontaneously. A head CT revealed no intraparenchymal bleed or mass. After several more days of IV antibiotics, during which time her neurologic status remained stable and her blood cultures became negative, she was taken to the operating room. The previously placed prosthetic TV was explanted and replaced with a bioprosthetic valve. She also underwent bioprosthetic MV replacement. She was discharged to a rehabilitation facility to complete a course of IV antibiotics. After completing her course of IV antibiotics, she was discharged home and has done well. At follow-up, she has remained compliant with medical therapy and has thus far abstained from IVDA.

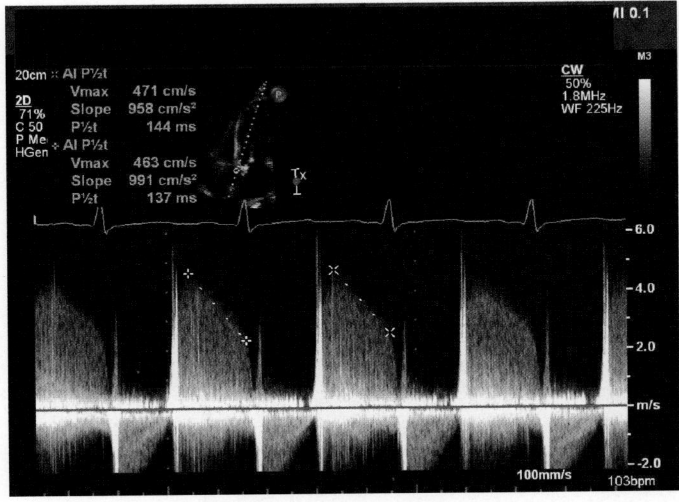

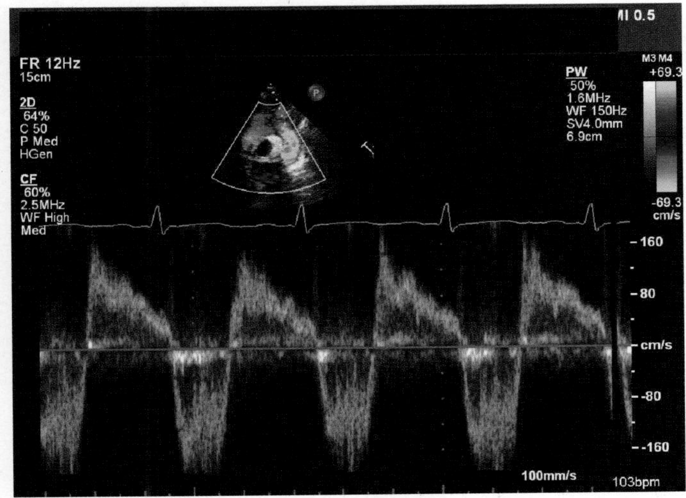

FIGURE 3-14-9 Continuous-wave Doppler (L) of the AR consistent with severe AR. Pulsed wave Doppler of the flow in the descending aorta (R) demonstrating holodiastolic flow reversal.

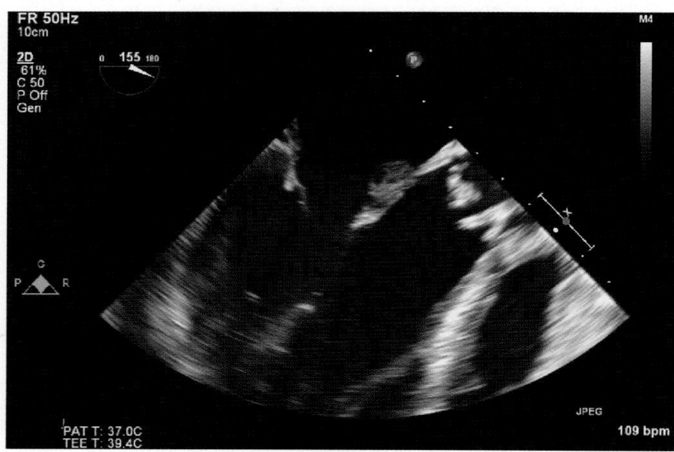

FIGURE 3-14-10 Intraoperative TEE demonstrating vegetations on the AV and MV with the MV perforation ► (see Video 3-14-10).

CLINICAL FEATURES AND NATURAL HISTORY OF ENDOCARDITIS

- Constitutional symptoms:
  - malaise
  - anorexia
  - fatigue
  - night sweats
  - myalgias
  - fevers and chills
- Symptoms that may be related to cardiac complications or embolic events:
  - cough
  - dyspnea
  - chest pain
  - abdominal or back pain
  - stroke, seizures[1-3]
- Infective endocarditis may be acute or subacute.
  - Acute infective endocarditis: abrupt and rapidly progressive. Symptoms are related to embolic events or cardiac complications. High-grade fever is a common feature.
  - Subacute infective endocarditis: subtle, non-specific symptoms. Cardiac murmurs are a common feature.
- May involve native or prosthetic valves. Native valve endocarditis (NVE) and prosthetic valve endocarditis (PVE) features:
  - Native valve endocarditis: The mitral valve is most common valve affected, followed by the aortic valve, and, less commonly, the right-sided valves.
  - Prosthetic valve endocarditis (PVE): Occurs in up to 15% to 34% of cases.[4] Is classified as early when valve infection occurs within 2 months of valve surgery, and late when valve infection occurs after 2 months of valve surgery.[5] Mechanical prosthetic valves are at higher risk for early PVE,[6] while bioprosthetic valves are at higher risk for late PVE.[7] Overall, the risk for PVE is similar for both mechanical and bioprosthetic valves.
- Endocarditis in users of IV drugs:
  - The right-sided valves are most commonly affected (predominantly the TV). Initial presentation may be symptoms of pneumonia/empyema or septic pulmonary emboli (pleuritic chest pain, hemoptysis).
  - When left-sided valves are affected, the clinical presentation is similar to non-IV drug use endocarditis.
  - *Staphylococcus aureus* is the most common organism.
- Culture negative infective endocarditis: negative blood cultures, usually due to prior antibiotic use or infection with fastidious organisms (*Bartonella*, *Coxiella burnetti*, *Chlamydia psittaci*).

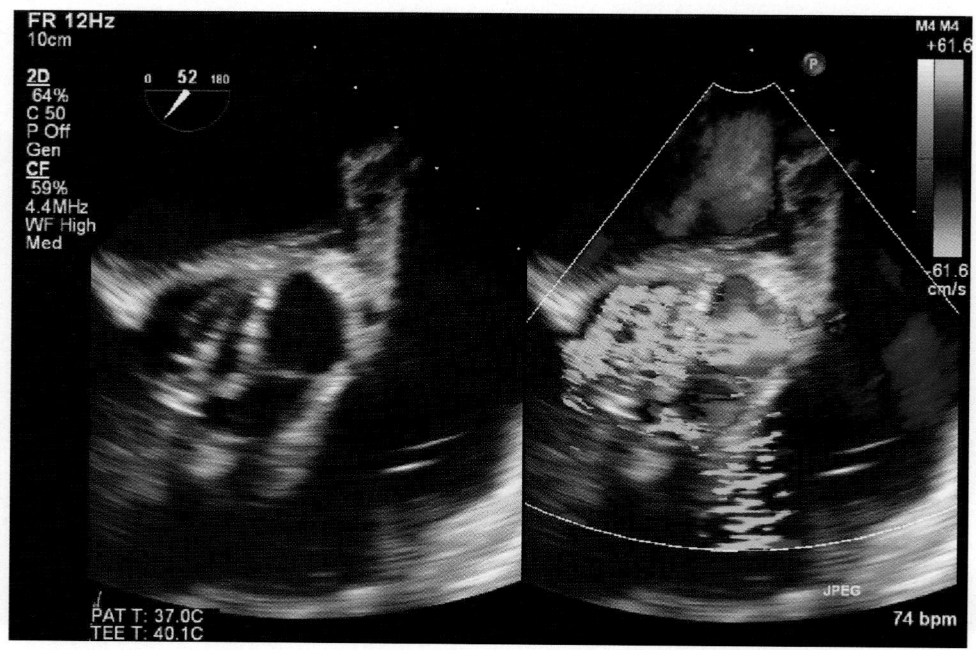

FIGURE 3-14-11 Intraoperative TEE demonstrating the bicuspid AV (L) with severe AR seen with Color Doppler imaging (R) ► (see Video 3-14-11).

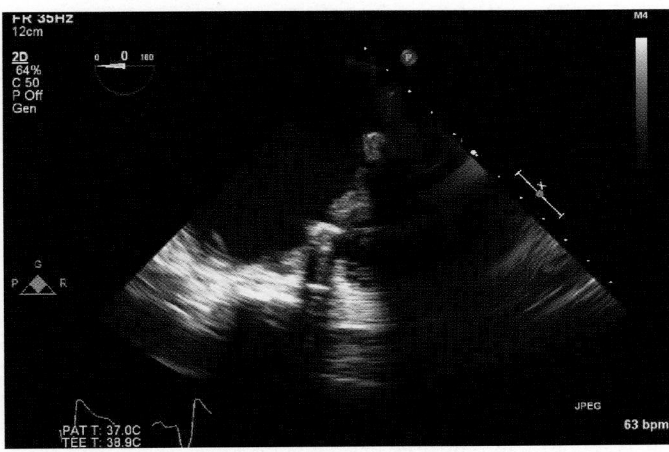

FIGURE 3-14-12 TEE demonstrating a large vegetation on the prosthetic TV in the patient presented ► (see Video 3-14-12).

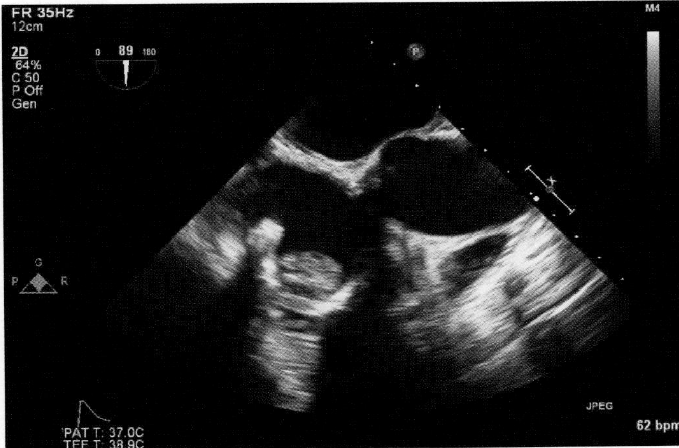

FIGURE 3-14-13 Modified bi-caval TEE image of the prosthetic TV with large vegetations ► (see Video 3-14-13). Doppler imaging (not shown) demonstrated significant TR as well as a 6 mm Hg gradient across the valve.

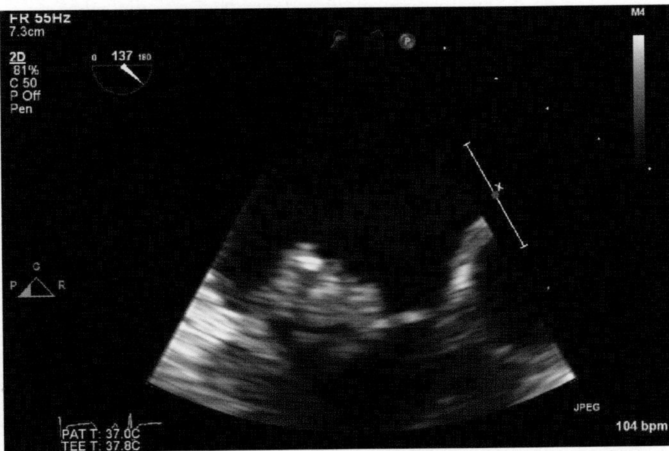

FIGURE 3-14-14 Zoomed view of the MV in this patient demonstrating multiple vegetations ► (see Video 3-14-14). Color Doppler demonstrated severe MR (not shown).

- Pacemaker/Implanted Electrical Cardiac Device infective endocarditis: Fever is a common presentation. Other clinical features depend on site of pacemaker affected (leads/generator) and source of infection (bacteremia, pocket infection).
- Healthcare associated infective endocarditis: This is infective endocarditis which develops in a patient after >48 hours of hospitalization or associated with a health-care facility procedure performed in the preceding 4 weeks (eg, placement of hemodialysis catheters or shunts).
- Complications:
  - Embolic events occur in up to 20% to 50% of patients. The central nervous system is the most common site of embolization, followed by the spleen, kidneys, and lung.
  - Congestive heart failure is the most common complication. It is usually caused by valvular dysfunction and has the greatest effect on mortality.
  - Cardiac abscesses may involve the aortic root and are common with aortic valvular lesions and PVE. Aortic valve abscesses can lead to heart block. They may spread down the mitral aortic intervalvular fibrosa (MAIVF).
  - Pseudoaneurysms and fistulae: Pseudoaneurysms may affect the coronary sinuses. These may then rupture to form fistulae. The mitral aortic intervalvular fibrosa may rupture leading to a communication between the ascending aorta and left atrium.

EPIDEMIOLOGY

- The incidence of infective endocarditis is one admission per 1000 admissions.
- The pattern of infective endocarditis in the western world has shifted over the past few decades. In the past, the predominant underlying valvular pathology was rheumatic valvular heart disease. More recently, the predisposing conditions relate to the presence of prosthetic material in the heart, such as prosthetic valves or intracardiac devices. This has coincided with the relative increase in invasive cardiac procedures, including placement of prosthetic valves and pacemakers and the eradication of rheumatic heart disease.
- In one series,[8] 34% of cases involved prosthetic valves, 33% were nosocomial.
- The 6-month mortality rate was 22%.
- Male preponderance was noted.
- Incidence increases with age.

PATHOPHYSIOLOGY

- The initial lesion in infective endocarditis is a defect in the endothelial lining. This is most commonly caused by a high velocity blood jet or turbulent blood flow. Endothelial damage attracts fibrin and platelets which clump together to form a sterile thrombus. The sterile thrombus can become secondarily seeded by microorganisms leading to vegetation. These microorganisms proliferate and stimulate inflammation of the valvular endothelium. Further deposition of fibrin and platelets stimulated by bacterial proliferation and inflammatory activation leads to vegetation maturation.

- These micro-organisms enter the body through:
  - Use of intravascular catheters
  - Previous surgery
  - Urinary or GI tract procedures
  - Dental procedures
  - IV drug use
- Typical organisms that cause infective endocarditis include *Streptococcus viridians*, *Streptococcus bovis*, *Enterococcus*, *Staphylococcus aureus*, and the HACEK organisms.
- Other organisms include coagulase negative *staphylococcus* and gram negative *bacilli*.
- The valves affected in order of frequency in native valve endocarditis are:
  - Mitral
  - Aortic
  - Tricuspid valve
- The most frequent predisposing cardiac conditions for native valve endocarditis are[8]:
  - Degenerative valvular disease: 55%
  - Immune suppression: 13%
  - Prior endocarditis:12%
  - Mitral valve prolapse: 9%
  - Bicuspid aortic valve: 5%

PHYSICAL EXAMINATION

- Vitals signs: Fever is the most common clinical feature. Tachycardia is not uncommon.
- Eye: Roth spots.
- Cardiac findings: Increased jugular venous pulse, new cardiac murmur (valvular destruction), or a change in a prior murmur, S_3 gallop (reflecting development of congestive heart failure), pericardial rub.
- Neurologic findings: signs of embolic stroke with neurologic deficits (paresis, paralysis).
- Pulmonary findings include pneumonia from embolic pulmonary infection, rales (due to congestive heart failure), pleural rub.
- Abdominal findings: enlarged spleen.
- Skin findings include: petechiae, splinter hemorrhages, Janeway lesions (flat, nontender, blanching red spots on palms and soles), Osler nodes (subcutaneous nodes).

LABORATORY EVALUATION

- Positive blood cultures, increased erythrocyte sedimentation rate, elevated C-reactive protein, leukocytosis (acute endocarditis), normocytic normochromic anemia (subacute endocarditis), decreased complement levels in subacute endocarditis (C3, C4, CH50), positive Rheumatoid factor (subacute endocarditis).

CHEST X-RAY

- Lung infiltrates with central cavitation occur with septic emboli (right sided endocarditis).
- Evidence of CHF

ELECTROCARDIOGRAM

- Conduction abnormalities such as varying degrees of AV block due to abscess formation near the atrioventricular node or right-bundle branch block.
- Myocardial infarction due to coronary artery emboli.

ECHOCARDIOGRAPHY

- The defining characteristic of endocarditis is a vegetation. The echocardiographic features of a vegetation include:
  - Amorphous. A discrete well-defined mass is evidence against a vegetation.
  - An independently mobile mass.
  - Presence of valvular destruction usually resulting in regurgitation.
  - Location on the upstream portion of the valve. This is the atrial side for the mitral and tricuspid valves and the ventricular side of the aortic and pulmonic valves.
- Echocardiography may also detect complications of endocarditis such as:
  - Abscesses
  - Sinuses/fistulae
  - Valve perforation and resultant regurgitation
  - Flail leaflets
  - Pericardial effusion
- May be needed to assess the hemodynamic effects of endocarditis such as heart failure or tamponade.
- Detect underlying predisposing factors like classical mitral valve prolapse and congenital heart disease.
- Transthoracic echocardiography (TTE) has a lower sensitivity compared to transesophageal echocardiography (46%-63% versus 93%-100%) for native valves.[6,9] Both have similar specificity (95% versus 96%, respectively).[6] Advanced harmonic imaging and digital processing may increase the sensitivity of TTE to 82% for NVE.[10]
- When the pretest probability is low, TTE is an appropriate initial test, while trans-esophageal echocardiography (TEE) is an appropriate initial test for patients with higher pretest probability.[11]
- Algorithms exist for use of echocardiography for diagnosis of IE and are based on the pretest probability (IE risk factors, clinical exam, microorganism involved, and bacteremia).[12,13]
- The appropriate use criteria indicate that the use of TTE is appropriate for initial evaluation of suspected IE (native/prosthetic valve) with bacteremia and new murmur, and for reevaluation of IE.[14]
- The appropriate use criteria indicate that the use of TEE is appropriate in patients with an intracardiac device and persistent fever, or for evaluation where the pretest probability is high.[14] TEE is an appropriate modality to evaluate for periannular extension.
- TEE is, however, not superior to TTE for right-sided valvular lesions.[15]
- In the case of a prosthetic valve, dehiscence, or evidence of obstruction in the right clinical scenario: TEE has higher sensitivity and specificity than TTE for detecting valvular and perivalvular lesions in PVE.[11] However, the sensitivity of TEE for PVE is lower than for NVE. In PVE, abscesses are more common than valvular vegetations.[4]

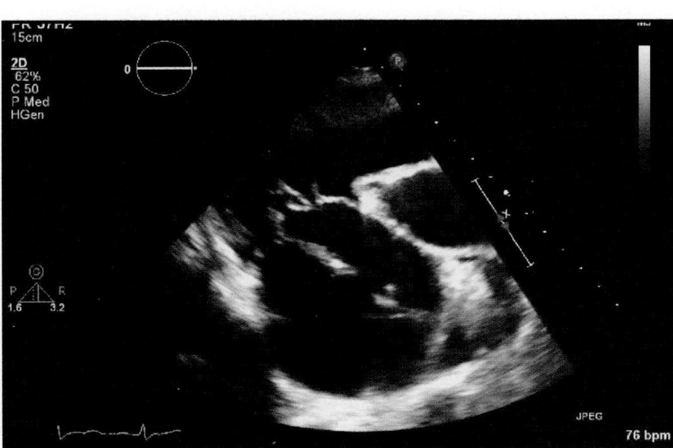

FIGURE 3-14-15 TTE image of a patient with a vegetation on the TV in the setting of pacemaker infection. There is also a small vegetation on one of the device wires ► (see Video 3-14-15). Infectious complications of implanted cardiac electrical devices is becoming a more frequent cause of endocarditis.

- TEE is more sensitive than TTE (80% versus <30%, respectively, for lead vegetations) for diagnosis of device-related (pacemaker/ICD) IE.[16]
- Figures 3-14-15 to 3-14-20 demonstrate additional echocardiographic images of endocarditis and its complications.

DIAGNOSIS

The Modified Duke criteria are used to confirm the diagnosis, based on the presence of major and minor criteria.

- Major criteria include blood culture data and imaging (echocardiographic) data.
  - The presence of blood cultures positive for typical organisms causative for infective endocarditis.
  - The presence of persistently positive blood cultures such as:
    - *Staph aureus*
    - *Streptococcus* species
    - *Enterococcus faecalis*
    - The HACEK organisms:
    - *Hemophilus* sp.
    - *Actinobacillus* sp.
    - *Cardiobacterium* sp.
    - *Eikenella* sp.
    - *Kingella* sp.
  - Any positive blood culture for *Coxiella burnetii*.
  - Positive IgG antibodies with titers of >1:800.
  - Endocardial involvement which requires demonstration of a vegetation, abscess, fistula, or prosthetic valve dehiscence with echocardiography.
- Minor criteria include:
  - Presence of predisposing conditions, eg IV drug abuse or preexisting valvular pathology
  - Fever >100.4° F (38° C)
  - Vascular phenomena:
    - Arterial emboli
    - Conjunctival hemorrhage
    - Mycotic aneurysms
    - Janeway lesions
  - Immunological phenomena
    - Osler's nodes
    - Roth's spots
    - Positive rheumatoid factor
    - Glomerulonephritis
  - Microbiological criteria which do not meet any of the major criteria

DIAGNOSTIC CRITERIA REQUIREMENTS

- Definite endocarditis is diagnosed when both major criteria, one major and 3 minor, or 5 minor criteria are present.
- Possible endocarditis is diagnosed with the presence of one major and one minor, or 3 minor criteria.
- The diagnosis of endocarditis is rejected is when you have:
  - Probable alternate diagnosis
  - Resolution of symptoms with ≤4 days of antibiotic therapy
  - Absence of histological or bacteriological confirmation at autopsy

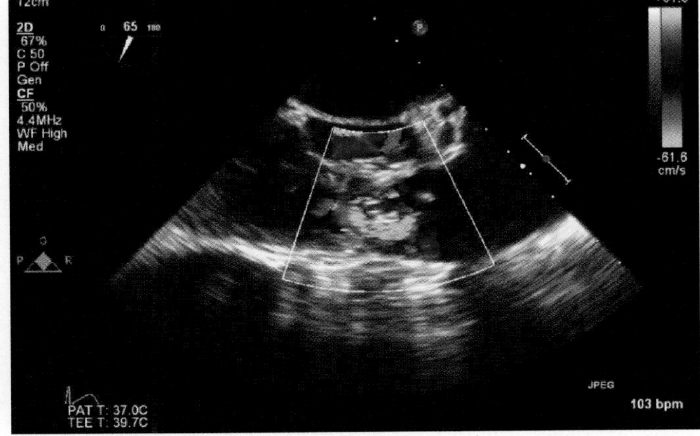

FIGURE 3-14-16 TEE images of a patient with isolated pulmonary valve endocarditis, which is quite rare, especially in the absence of a congenitally abnormal valve, as was the situation in this patient who presented with respiratory failure due to septic pulmonary emboli. The left panel demonstrates vegetations on the valve in a short axis view. The right panel demonstrates pulmonary insufficiency detected with color Doppler imaging ► (see Video 3-14-16).

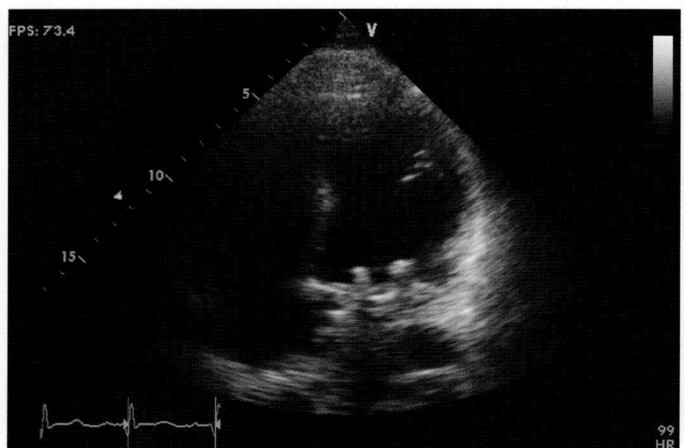

FIGURE 3-14-17 Apical 4 chamber demonstrating "rocking" of a prosthetic MV, a sign of valve dehiscence ▶ (see Video 3-14-17).

FIGURE 3-14-18 TEE image of aortic root abscess due to *staph aureus* in a patient with a mechanical aortic valve.

DIFFERENTIAL DIAGNOSIS OF MASSES DETECTED WITH ECHOCARDIOGRAPHY

- Echocardiography is critical in the assessment of patients with suspected endocarditis. Intracardiac masses on valves (native and prosthetic), the endocardial surface of the cardiac chambers, and associated implanted devices/catheters are not infrequently detected and may represent several different pathologies.
- The differential diagnosis of a mass seen on echocardiography that may be confused with a vegetation/abscess include:
  - Thrombus: Sometimes this can only be distinguished from a vegetation by the clinical scenario.
  - Papillary fibroelastoma: This is usually found on the aortic or mitral valve. This benign tumor may be differentiated from vegetation by its location on the downstream portion of the valve and often causes little or no regurgitation.
  - Lambl's excrescences: Usually found of the downstream portion of the aortic valve at the leaflet coaptation point.
  - Mitral annular calcification: May be difficult to distinguish from an abscess of the mitral valve. The clinical scenario and clinical predisposing factors, ie, age, presence of hypertension, and renal failure may suggest mitral annular calcification over a mitral valve abscess.
  - Recent aortic valve prostheses implanted by the inclusion technique may be indistinguishable from an aortic root abscess.
  - Primary cardiac lymphoma may be difficult to distinguish from an aortic root abscess.

MANAGEMENT

- Medical: Three sets of aerobic and anaerobic blood cultures should be drawn within 24 hours.
  - Broad spectrum IV antibiotics appropriate for the underlying cause should be started.
    - The common causative organisms are identical for native valve endocarditis and late prosthetic valve endocarditis. These include: Methicillin sensitive *staphylococcus aureus*, *Streptococcus* sp., and *Enterococcus* sp.
    - The causative organisms for early prosthetic valve endocarditis are: Methicillin resistant *staphylococcus aureus*, Coagulase negative *staphylococcus aureus*, and gram negative pathogens.

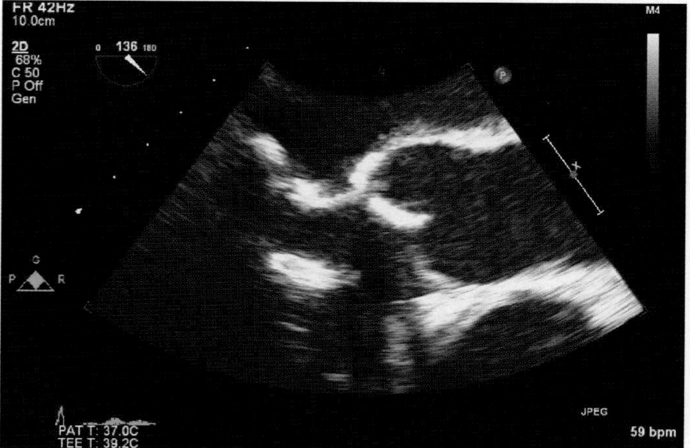

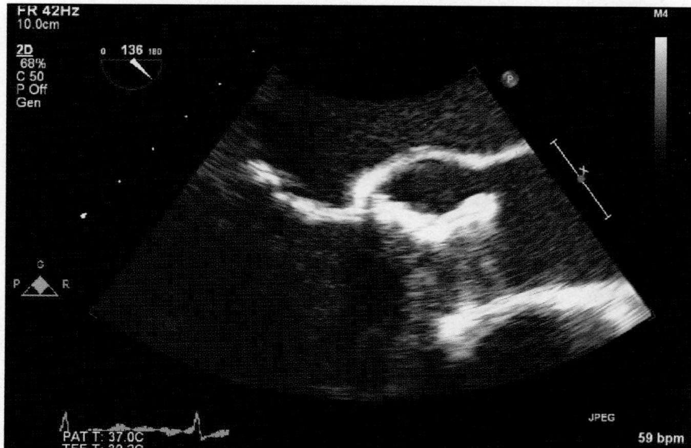

FIGURE 3-14-19 TEE image of a large mitral valve vegetation caused by *staph aureus* which crosses the AV in systole. The left panel demonstrates the mass during diastole. In the right panel, the vegetation is seen across the AV ▶ (see Video 3-14-19).

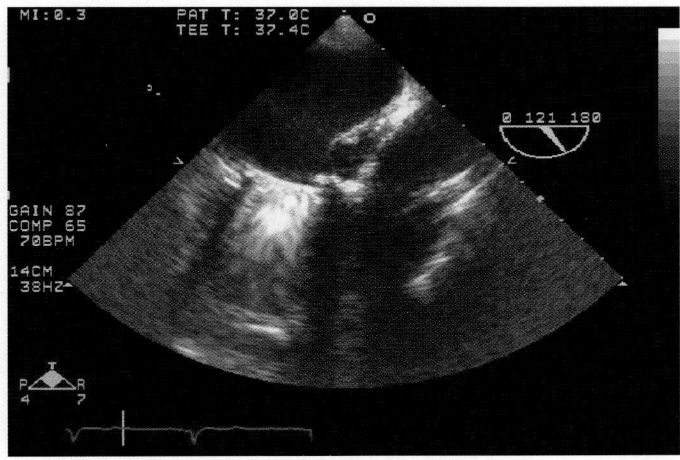

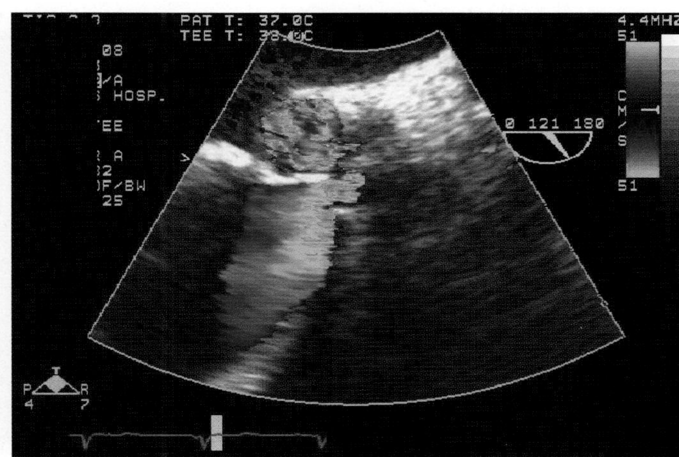

FIGURE 3-14-20 TEE images of a patient with mitral and aortic prosthetic valves with an abscess. Color Doppler (right panel) demonstrates flow in to the abscess cavity ▶ (see Videos 3-14-20).

- These antibiotics can then be narrowed down once the causative organism has been identified.
- Duration of therapy is at least 6 weeks.

- Surgical: The indications for surgery include:
  - Congestive heart failure
  - Failure of medical management, ie, persistent systemic emboli or sepsis despite appropriate antibiotics
  - Severe acute mitral regurgitation and aortic regurgitation
  - Spread of infection with abscesses, fistulae, periannular extension, septic embolization, new onset atrioventricular block
  - Prosthetic valve endocarditis
  - Fungal endocarditis or other highly resistant microorganisms
  - Hemodynamic instability secondary to valvular damage

FOLLOW-UP

- All patients must be educated on the importance of good oral hygiene, the use of prophylactic antibiotics prior to dental procedures, and the signs and symptoms of endocarditis.
- Patients with native valve endocarditis (treated medically) who have residual valve dysfunction should be evaluated clinically and by serial echocardiography (frequency determined by the severity of the residual valvular pathology) for evidence of progressive valve dysfunction and the development of CHF.
- Patients who undergo valve replacement should be monitored clinically and with serial echocardiography.

VIDEO LEGENDS

1. Video 3-14-1: Parasternal long axis demonstrating vegetations on the aortic valve and thickening of the mitral valve. There is also evidence of a pericardial effusion and a left pleural effusion.
2. Video 3-14-2: Parasternal short axis demonstrating vegetations on the aortic valve. There is also peri-aortic "fullness" which correlated with the root abscess identified at the time of surgery.
3. Video 3-14-3: Apical 3 chamber view with color Doppler demonstrating severe AR
4. Video 3-14-5: Parasternal long axis demonstrating the thickened mitral valve with evidence of a perforation of the anterior mitral valve leaflet
5. Video 3-14-6: Parasternal short axis view of the MV anterior leaflet perforation
6. Video 3-14-7: Parasternal long axis view of the MV with color Doppler demonstrating severe MR
7. Video 3-14-10: Intraoperative TEE demonstrating vegetations on the AV and MV with the MV perforation
8. Video 3-14-11: Intraoperative TEE demonstrating the bicuspid AV (L) with severe AR seen with Color Doppler imaging (R)
9. Video 3-14-12: TEE demonstrating a large vegetation on the prosthetic TV in the patient presented
10. Video 3-14-13: Modified bi-caval TEE image of the prosthetic TV with large vegetations
11. Video 3-14-14: Zoomed view of the MV in this patient demonstrating multiple vegetations. Color Doppler demonstrated severe MR
12. Video 3-14-15: TTE image of a patient with a vegetation on the TV in the setting of pacemaker infection. There is also a small vegetation on one of the device wires
13. Video 3-14-16 L: TEE images of a patient with isolated pulmonary valve endocarditis. The video demonstrates vegetations on the valve in a short axis view.
14. Video 3-14-16 R: TEE images of a patient with isolated pulmonary valve endocarditis. The video demonstrates pulmonary insufficiency detected with color Doppler imaging
15. Video 3-14-16 A: TEE images of PV endocarditis in a long axis view demonstrating multiple vegetations
16. Video 3-14-16 B: TEE image of PV endocarditis in a horizontal plane demonstrating the vegetations in the main PA
17. Video 3-14-17: Apical four chamber demonstrating "rocking" of a prosthetic MV, a sign of valve dehiscence
18. Video 3-14-19: TEE image of a large mitral valve vegetation caused by staph aureus which crosses the AV in systole.

19. Video 3-14-20 L: TEE images of a patient with mitral and aortic prosthetic valves with an abscess
20. Video 3-14-20 R: TEE images of a patient with mitral and aortic prosthetic valves with an abscess. Color Doppler demonstrates flow into the abscess cavity

REFERENCES

1. Anderson DJ, Goldstein LB, Wilkinson WE, et al. Stroke location, characterization, severity, and outcome in mitral vs aortic valve endocarditis. *Neurology*. 2003;61(10):1341-1346.
2. Heiro M, Nikoskelainen J, Engblom E, Kotilainen E, Marttila R, Kotilainen P. Neurologic manifestations of infective endocarditis: a 17-year experience in a teaching hospital in Finland. *Archives of Internal Medicine*. 2000;160(18):2781-2787.
3. Murdoch DR, Corey GR, Hoen B, et al. Clinical presentation, etiology, and outcome of infective endocarditis in the 21st century: the International Collaboration on Endocarditis-Prospective Cohort Study. *Archives of Internal Medicine*. 2009;169(5):463-473.
4. Wang A, Athan E, Pappas PA, et al. Contemporary clinical profile and outcome of prosthetic valve endocarditis. *JAMA*. 2007;297(12):1354-1361.
5. Moreillon P, Que YA. Infective endocarditis. *Lancet*. 2004;363(9403):139-149.
6. Bashore TM, Cabell C, Fowler V Jr. Update on infective endocarditis. *Current Problems in Cardiology*. 2006;31(4):274-352.
7. Piper C, Korfer R, Horstkotte D. Prosthetic valve endocarditis. *Heart*. 2001;85(5):590-593.
8. Hill EE, Herijgers P, Claus P, Vanderschueren S, Herregods MC, Peetermans WE. Infective endocarditis: changing epidemiology and predictors of 6-month mortality: a prospective cohort study. *European Heart Journal*. 2007;28(2):196-203.
9. Hill EE, Herijgers P, Claus P, Vanderschueren S, Peetermans WE, Herregods MC. Abscess in infective endocarditis: the value of transesophageal echocardiography and outcome: a 5-year study. *American Heart Journal*. 2007;154(5):923-928.
10. Casella F, Rana B, Casazza G, et al. The potential impact of contemporary transthoracic echocardiography on the management of patients with native valve endocarditis: a comparison with transesophageal echocardiography. *Echocardiography*. 2009;26(8):900-906.
11. Baddour LM, Wilson WR, Bayer AS, et al. Infective endocarditis: diagnosis, antimicrobial therapy, and management of complications: a statement for healthcare professionals from the Committee on Rheumatic Fever, Endocarditis, and Kawasaki Disease, Council on Cardiovascular Disease in the Young, and the Councils on Clinical Cardiology, Stroke, and Cardiovascular Surgery and Anesthesia, American Heart Association: endorsed by the Infectious Diseases Society of America. *Circulation*. 2005;111(23):e394-434.
12. Kuruppu JC, Corretti M, Mackowiak P, Roghmann MC. Overuse of transthoracic echocardiography in the diagnosis of native valve endocarditis. *Archives of Internal Medicine*. 2002;162(15):1715-1720.
13. Greaves K, Mou D, Patel A, Celermajer DS. Clinical criteria and the appropriate use of transthoracic echocardiography for the exclusion of infective endocarditis. *Heart*. 2003;89(3):273-275.
14. Douglas PS, Garcia MJ, Haines DE, et al. ACCF/ASE/AHA/ASNC/HFSA/HRS/SCAI/SCCM/SCCT/SCMR 2011 appropriate use criteria for echocardiography: a report of the American College of Cardiology Foundation Appropriate Use Criteria Task Force, American Society of Echocardiography, American Heart Association, American Society of Nuclear Cardiology, Heart Failure Society of America, Heart Rhythm Society, Society of Cardiovascular Angiography and Interventions, Society of Critical Care Medicine, Society of Cardiovascular Computed Tomography, and Society of Cardiovascular Magnetic Resonance. *J Am Coll Cardiol*. 2011;57(9):1126-1166. doi: 10.1016/j.jacc.2010.11.002.
15. San Roman JA, Vilacosta I, Lopez J, et al. Role of transthoracic and transesophageal echocardiography in right-sided endocarditis: one echocardiographic modality does not fit all. *J Am Soc Echocardiogr*. 2012;25(8):807-814.
16. Baddour LM, Bettmann MA, Bolger AF, et al. Nonvalvular cardiovascular device-related infections. *Circulation*. 2003;108(16):2015-2031.

4 ECHOCARDIOGRAPHIC ASSESSMENT OF THE PATIENT WITH KNOWN OR SUSPECTED CONGESTIVE HEART FAILURE

Gerard P. Aurigemma, MD, FAHA, FASE, FACC

INTRODUCTION

Echocardiography is the principal imaging method employed to assess patients with known or suspected congestive heart failure. The appropriate use criteria for echocardiography highlight the important and appropriate role of echocardiography in the evaluation of these patients, as do the guidelines for the use of imaging in heart failure.[1,2] The recently published guidelines for the management of patients with CHF as well as the guidelines for the use of imaging in CHF both emphasize the central role that echocardiography plays in the initial evaluation and ongoing management of these patients.[2,3] "Although a complete history and physical examination are important first steps, the most useful diagnostic test in the evaluation of patients with or at risk for HF (eg, postacute MI) is a comprehensive 2-dimensional echocardiogram; coupled with Doppler flow studies, the transthoracic echocardiogram can identify abnormalities of myocardium, heart valves, and pericardium."[3]

In this chapter, Dr. Aurigemma and his colleagues will provide insight into the role of echocardiography in the clinical management of these patients, including the evaluation of the patient presenting with dyspnea, CHF due to systolic and diastolic dysfunction, and the critical role that echocardiography plays in the decision-making process for device therapy (ICD and CRT). In addition, we will visit the important role of echocardiography in the evaluation and management of patients with left ventricular assist devices (LVAD) and the cardiac transplant patient.

SECTION 1

Echocardiography in the Evaluation of the Dyspneic Patient

Gerard P. Aurigemma, MD, FAHA, FASE, FACC

CLINICAL CASE PRESENTATION

A 71-year-old woman, who was brought by her family to the emergency room, was admitted to the cardiology service for the evaluation of progressive dyspnea. She is visiting her family from a foreign country. Her major complaint is dyspnea on exertion and episodes of chest pain. The chest pain is nonexertional. The dyspnea began approximately 6 months ago and was thought to be due to deconditioning. However, it has progressed to the point where she can barely walk 50 feet without becoming severely short of breath. The emergency department has diagnosed congestive heart failure, and you are asked to direct further evaluation.

She denies paroxysmal nocturnal dyspnea or orthopnea and is able to lie flat in bed. There is mild peripheral edema. She has occasional spasms of coughing; the cough is not productive. She has lost 8 pounds since the shortness of breath was first noted. The medical history is significant only for hypertension for which she has been prescribed lisinopril and hydrochlorothiazide. She takes these medications faithfully. She is a lifelong nonsmoker and does not drink alcohol.

Examination revealed a frail, elderly woman in no respiratory distress. She becomes dyspneic, however, in moving from her chair to the bed for examination. Vital signs: her blood pressure is 155/70 mm Hg, her heart rate is 92 beats/min and regular, her room air pulse oximetry is 94%, and she is afebrile.

Pertinent exam findings include normal jugular venous pressure, a prominent innominate artery pulsation in the right supraclavicular region, scattered rhonchi, and coarse rales heard throughout the lung fields. The S_1 is normal, as is the S_2. The P_2 is accentuated. There are no murmurs, and there is mild peripheral edema.

Laboratory data is significant for a slightly elevated Troponin I of 0.09 mg/dL and a BNP of 176.

The chest x-ray (Figure 4-1-1) is interpreted as showing prominent interstitial markings, consistent with pulmonary edema. There is also engorgement of the pulmonary vasculature.

Her ECG (Figure 4-1-2) shows biatrial enlargement and precordial T-wave inversions, consistent with anterior wall ischemia.

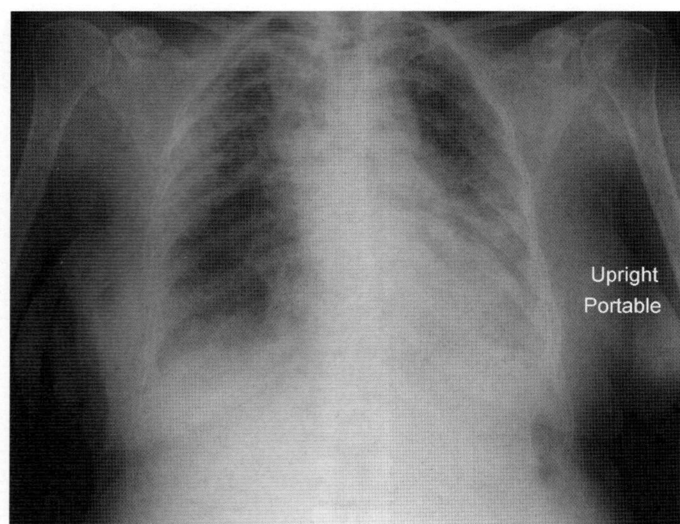

FIGURE 4-1-1 Chest x-ray, which was interpreted as showing diffuse interstitial markings, consistent with pulmonary edema and cardiomegaly, with prominent pulmonary artery and venous silhouette.

ECHOCARDIOGRAPHIC EVALUATION

The patient underwent comprehensive echocardiography (Figures 4-1-3 to 4-1-7).

- The findings include normal LV ejection fraction, RV hypertrophy, and pulmonary hypertension, with an RV-RA gradient of 59 mm Hg. The IVC was not well visualized, so the peak pulmonary artery systolic pressure cannot be more precisely assessed, but it is certainly elevated.
- Doppler examination yields clues concerning LA and LV diastolic pressures: the transmitral pattern is A dominant, consistent with abnormal relaxation. The pulmonary venous inflow (Figure 4-1-4) shows clear-cut S dominance. The tissue Doppler early (e') velocity is 5 cm/s, yielding an E/e' ratio of 10, which suggests that LA pressure is not elevated.[4]

The clinical and echocardiographic examinations of this patient were consistent with the notion of a noncardiac cause of dyspnea.

- This is based on the findings of LA pressure which is not elevated, based on the transmitral inflow pattern of low E/A ratio; the pulmonary venous inflow pattern, which is S dominant; and the E/e' which is not elevated.[4]

DIAGNOSIS

Based on the cardiologist's clinical evaluation and the results of the echocardiogram, the dyspnea was felt most likely due to the pulmonary disease, and pulmonary hypertension was felt not to be passive, ie, due to elevated LA pressure[5]. Electrocardiographic findings were deemed to be consistent with idiopathic pulmonary hypertension. These include right atrial enlargement and precordial T-wave inversions, thought to represent an RV strain pattern.

HOSPITAL COURSE

The patient was evaluated by the pulmonary medicine service. She underwent CT scanning of the chest (Figure 4-1-8). This study demonstrated diffuse interstitial fibrosis, and eventually the diagnosis of idiopathic pulmonary fibrosis was made. She was subsequently discharged with follow-up with the pulmonary medicine team.

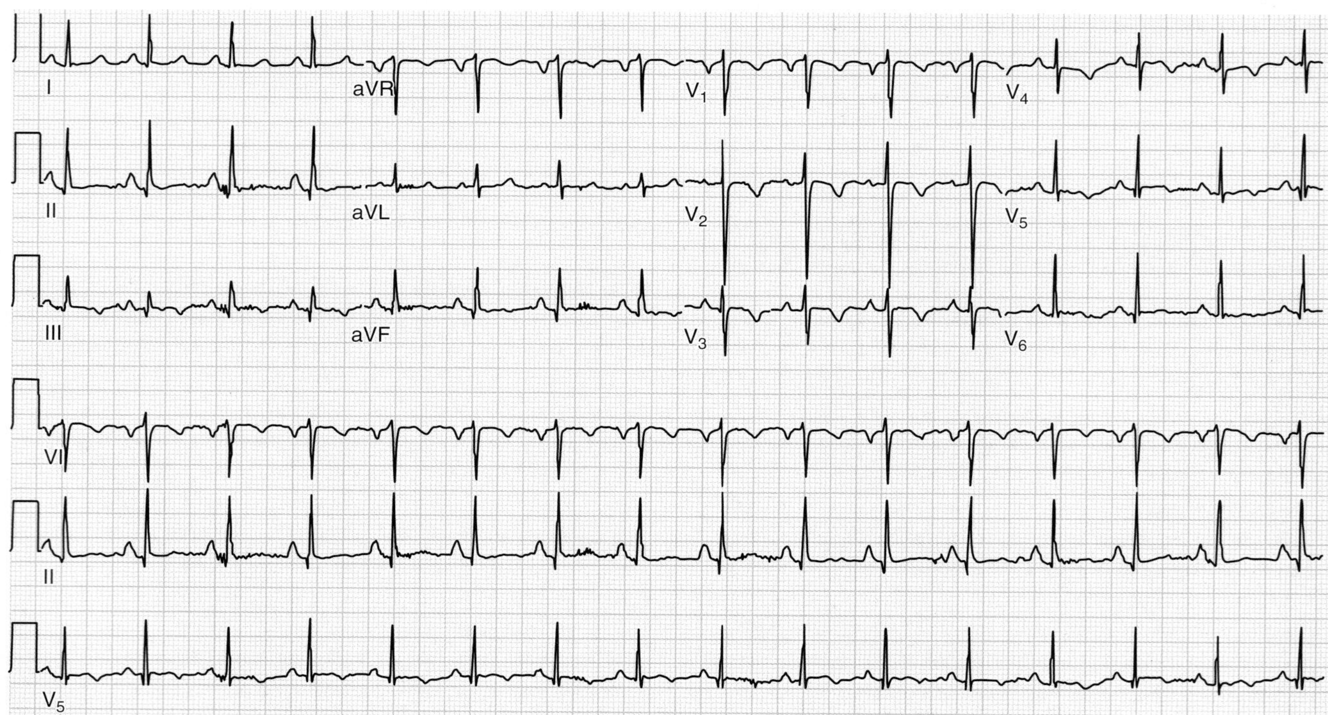

FIGURE 4-1-2 ECG obtained on admission, showing sinus rhythm, right atrial enlargement, and precordial T-wave inversions, consistent with anterior ischemia. Left atrial abnormality is also present.

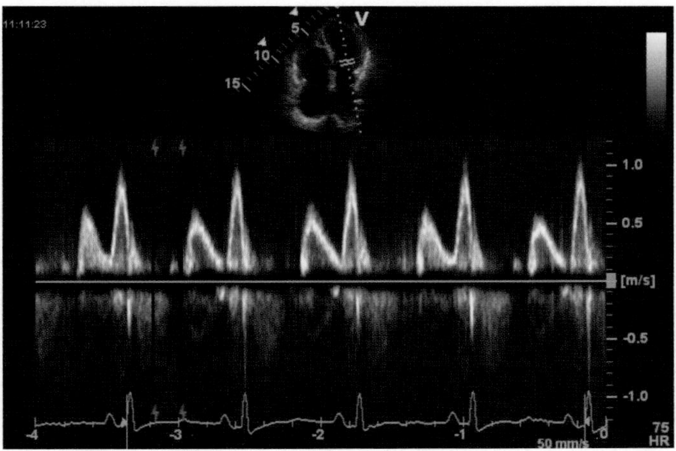

FIGURE 4-1-3 Transmitral inflow profile, showing low E/A ratio and low absolute E velocity.

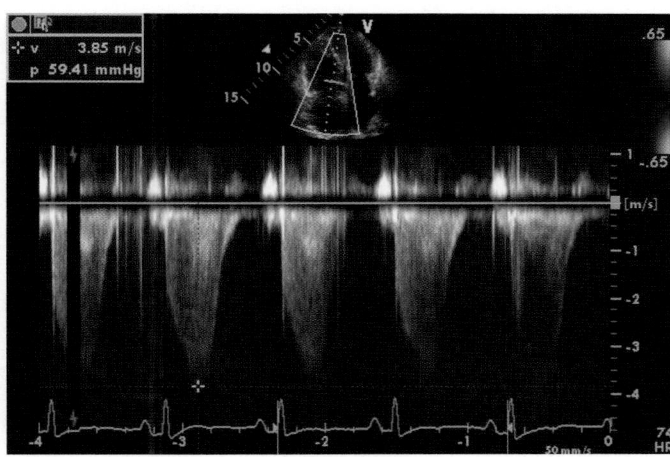

FIGURE 4-1-6 TR profile showing peak RV to RA gradient of 59 mm Hg, consistent with elevated RV systolic pressure.

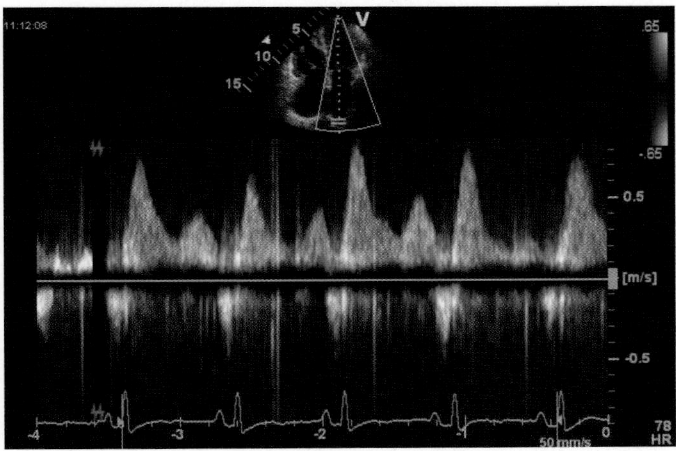

FIGURE 4-1-4 Pulmonary venous inflow pattern obtained with the sample volume in the right upper pulmonary vein; this was interpreted as showing low left atrial pressure.

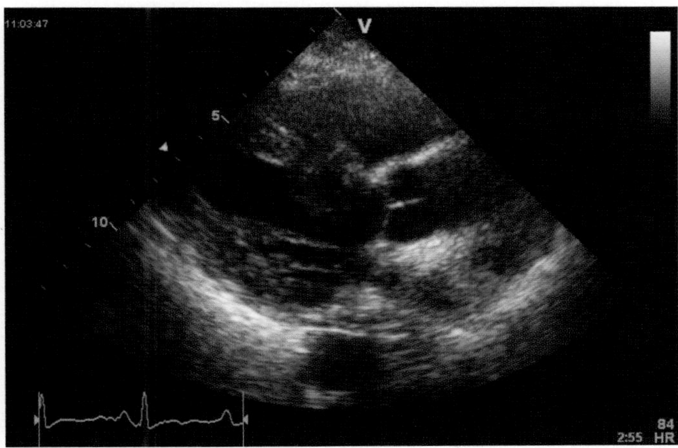

FIGURE 4-1-7 Parasternal long axis demonstrating normal LV size and EF. The RV outflow tract appears dilated and hypertrophied ► (see Video 4-1-7 A-D)

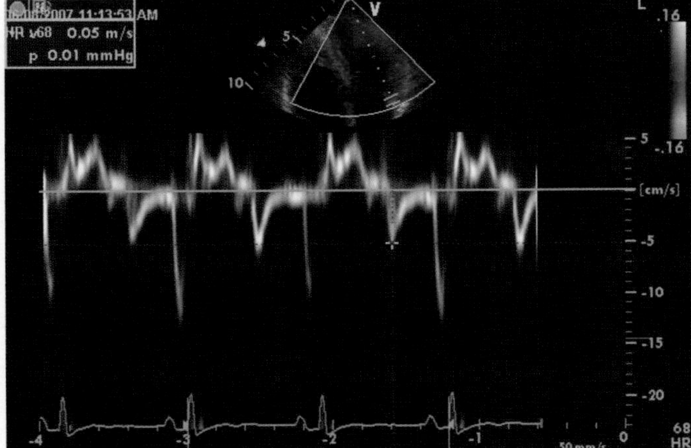

FIGURE 4-1-5 Tissue Doppler spectral profile obtained with the sample volume in the lateral annulus. While this velocity is low at 5 cm/s, the E/e' ratio is 50 cm/s ÷ 5 cm/s = 10, which is not consistent with elevated LA pressure.

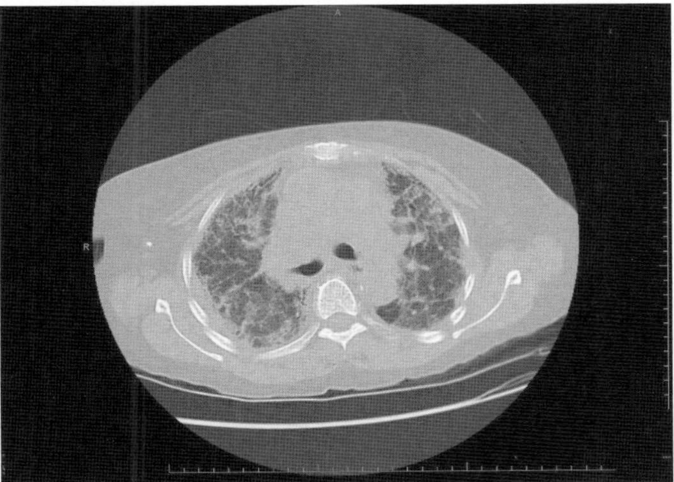

FIGURE 4-1-8 CT scan of chest obtained on third hospital day; this was interpreted as showing evidence of diffuse interstitial fibrosis, consistent with the diagnosis of idiopathic pulmonary fibrosis.

DYSPNEA

- Dyspnea was the presenting symptom for this patient. Whether it occurs either at rest or with exertion, dyspnea is a cardinal symptom of heart disease.
- It can be difficult, at the bedside, to distinguish among the various etiologies of dyspnea, which, in addition to heart and lung disease, include deconditioning, anemia, or anxiety/hyperventilation.
- Dyspnea accompanying obvious signs of left heart disease strongly suggests a cardiac etiology, but these signs were not present in this patient.
- As was shown in this case, echocardiography is an essential component of the initial evaluation of the patient with dyspnea. It may help to elucidate the origin of dyspnea by documenting or ruling out the common cardiac causes of pulmonary congestion: left-sided valvular disease, depressed systolic function, diastolic dysfunction, and cardiomyopathy.
- For this reason, echocardiography is an important initial diagnostic test when the history, physical examination, and routine laboratory tests suggest or cannot eliminate cardiac disease.

ADDITIONAL DIAGNOSTIC TESTS IN THE EVALUATION OF DYSPNEA

Depending on the initial history and physician examination findings, as well as baseline laboratory studies (cbc, chemistries), further diagnostic tests may be warranted:

- Chest x-ray (to assess for pneumonia, underlying lung disease)
- Pulmonary function studies
- 6-minute walk test
- Cardio-pulmonary exercise test (to differentiate pulmonary from cardiac etiologies)
- Cardiac stress test (to assess for myocardial ischemia)
- Chest CT
- CT pulmonary angiogram or ventilation-perfusion scan to rule out pulmonary emboli

ECHOCARDIOGRAPHY IN THE EVALUATION OF THE DYSPNEIC PATIENT

Echocardiography is clearly indicated in the evaluation of the dyspneic patient when there is a clinical suspicion for a cardiac contribution to the patient's symptoms.[1,2,3,6]

- The 2011 Appropriate Use Guidelines for echocardiography lists: "Symptoms or conditions potentially related to suspected cardiac etiology including but not limited to chest pain, shortness of breath, palpitations, TIA, stroke, or peripheral embolic event" and "Prior testing that is concerning for heart disease or structural abnormality including but not limited to chest X-ray, baseline scout images for stress echocardiogram, ECG, or cardiac biomarkers" as appropriate indications for echocardiography, with a score of 9 (the highest possible) for each.[1]
- One of the principal findings in this patient was that systolic function was normal. In fact, of all the indications for echocardiography, the evaluation of ventricular systolic function is the most common. Krumholz, et al,[7] has shown that evaluation of LV systolic function was the primary indication for TTE in 26% of inpatients studied, a frequency at least twice that of the next most common indication.
- A comprehensive echocardiographic examination includes assessment of LV size and function, as well as information concerning diastolic function[4,6] filling pressures, and an estimate of pulmonary artery systolic pressure.[8]
- In this instance, as we have seen, resting diastolic function was consistent with grade I diastolic dysfunction. Such diastolic dysfunction is usually not associated with elevated filling pressures at rest.[4,9] Furthermore, while many if not most patients with pulmonary hypertension in clinical practice have elevated left-sided filling pressures as the etiology,[10] this was most likely not the case in this patient.
- Other cardiac etiologies that might account for dyspnea include valvular heart disease, especially mitral valve stenosis and/or regurgitation, aortic valve disease, tricuspid regurgitation, and pericardial disease. The echocardiogram in this patient quickly ruled out these etiologies.

VIDEO LEGENDS

1. Video 4-1-7 A: Parasternal long axis demonstrating normal LV size and EF
2. Video 4-1-7 B: Apical 4-chamber view demonstrating a dilated, hypertrophied and hypokinetic RV. The LV is normal.
3. Video 4-1-7 C: Apical long axis demonstrating normal LV size and EF
4. Video 4-1-7 D: Subcostal view again demonstrating a normal LV. RV hypertrophy is noted.

REFERENCES

1. Douglas PS, Garcia MJ, Haines DE, et al. ACCF/ASE/AHA/ASNC/HFSA/HRS/SCAI/SCCM/SCCT/SCMR 2011 appropriate use criteria for echocardiography: a report of the American College of Cardiology Foundation Appropriate Use Criteria Task Force, American Society of Echocardiography, American Heart Association, American Society of Nuclear Cardiology, Heart Failure Society of America, Heart Rhythm Society, Society for Cardiovascular Angiography and Interventions, Society of Critical Care Medicine, Society of Cardiovascular Computed Tomography, and Society for Cardiovascular Magnetic Resonance. *J Am Coll Cardiol*. 2011;57(9):1126-1166. doi:10.1016/j.jacc.2010.11.002.
2. Patel MR, White RD, Abbara S, et al. 2013 ACCF/ACR/ASE/ASNC/SCCT/SCMR appropriate utilization of cardiovascular imaging in heart failure: a joint report of the American College of Radiology Appropriateness Criteria Committee and the American College of Cardiology Foundation Appropriate Use Criteria Task Force. *J Am Coll Cardiol*. 2013;61:2207–2231. doi:10.1016/j.jacc.2013.02.005. This document is available on the World Wide Web sites of the American College of Cardiology (http://www.cardiosource.org) and the American College of Radiology (http://www.acr.org).

3. Yancy CW, Jessup M, Bozkurt B, et al. 2013 ACCF/AHA guideline for the management of heart failure: a report of the American College of Cardiology Foundation/American Heart Association Task Force on Practice Guidelines. *J Am Coll Cardiol*. 2013;62:e147–239. This document is available on the World Wide Web sites of the American College of Cardiology (www.cardiosource.org) and the American Heart Association (my.americanheart.org).
4. Nagueh SF, Appleton CP, Gillebert TC, et al. Recommendations for the evaluation of left ventricular diastolic function by echocardiography. *Eur J Echocardiogr*. 2009;10(2):165-193.
5. Bouchard JL, Aurigemma GP, Hill JC, Ennis CA, Tighe DA. Usefulness of the pulmonary arterial systolic pressure to predict pulmonary arterial wedge pressure in patients with normal left ventricular systolic function. *Am J Cardiol*. 2008;101(11):1673-1676.
6. Douglas PS, Hendel RC, Cummings JE, et al. ACCF/ACR/AHA/ASE/ASNC/HRS/NASCI/RSNA/SAIP/SCAI/SCCT/SCMR 2008 Health Policy Statement on Structured Reporting in Cardiovascular Imaging. Endorsed by the Society of Nuclear Medicine [added]. *Circulation*. 2009;119(1): 187-200.
7. Krumholz HM, Douglas PS, Goldman L, Waksmonski C, Clinical utility of transthoracic two-dimensional and Doppler echocardiography. *J Am Coll Cardiol*. 1994;24(1):125-131.
8. Lang RM, Bierig M, Devereux RB, et al. Recommendations for chamber quantification: a report from the American Society of Echocardiography's Guidelines and Standards Committee and the Chamber Quantification Writing Group, developed in conjunction with the European Association of Echocardiography, a branch of the European Society of Cardiology. *J Am Soc Echocardiogr*. 2005;18(12):1440-1463.
9. Aurigemma GP, Gaasch WH. Clinical practice. Diastolic heart failure. *N Engl J Med*. 2004;351(11):1097-1105.
10. Lam CS, Lyass A, Kraigher-Krainer E., et al. Cardiac dysfunction and noncardiac dysfunction as precursors of heart failure with reduced and preserved ejection fraction in the community. *Circulation*. 2011;124(1):24-30.

SECTION 2

Alcoholic Cardiomyopathy

Rebecca Baumann, MD, and Gerard P. Aurigemma, MD, FAHA, FASE, FACC

CLINICAL CASE PRESENTATION

A 48-year-old man with paroxysmal atrial fibrillation (not on anticoagulation), hypertension, hyperlipidemia, Type 2 diabetes mellitus, COPD, longstanding heavy tobacco and alcohol use, and dialysis-dependent end-stage renal disease presented to the emergency department with chest pressure, palpitations, shortness of breath and a nonproductive cough of 1 day's duration. The symptoms began after carrying a bicycle upstairs. He had had similar but much less intense dyspnea and coughing in the past. He denied any change in the chest discomfort with inspiration or position, lightheadedness, swelling, fevers, chills, sweating, or nausea. That day he had opted to forgo his dialysis as it was his daughter's birthday. His last dialysis session had been 3 days prior to presentation. On further review of his social history, the patient volunteered that for the past 6 to 9 months he had been drinking heavily, consuming up to 1 quart of vodka per day.

An initial ECG showed atrial fibrillation with an average ventricular rate of 143 bpm and a left bundle branch block (Figure 4-2-1). After the administration of intravenous diltiazem, his heart rate and blood pressure stabilized. His breathing was not labored or rapid, but he did require 2 L/min of oxygen. His exam was remarkable for bibasilar crackles and an S_3 gallop. A chest x-ray demonstrated mild cardiomegaly, pulmonary vascular congestion, and pulmonary edema. His troponin I peaked at 0.17 ng/mL and BNP was 4537 pg/mL. Electrolytes were within normal limits. CBC was significant for a mild leukocytosis. A repeat ECG confirmed that normal sinus rhythm had been restored (Figure 4-2-2).Over the next 24 hours his respiratory status worsened, and he was eventually transferred to the ICU for BiPAP and emergent dialysis.

A transthoracic echocardiogram at the time of dialysis revealed LV dilatation with LVEF of 30%, global hypokinesis, increased wall thickness, restrictive diastolic physiology, a moderately dilated left atrium and mild pulmonary hypertension. Doppler analysis was consistent with elevated mean left atrial pressure (Figures 4-2-3 to 4-2-7).

The patient had undergone cardiac catheterization 4 months prior to this admission (performed as a follow-up of an equivocal nuclear stress test results, which had been ordered as part of an evaluation for kidney transplant). The coronary arteriogram demonstrated minor luminal irregularities.

On review of his previous ECGs it was noted that the LBBB had been present 2 months prior but that his QRS complexes were normal 1 year ago (Figure 4-2-8).

Given his echocardiographic findings and social history in addition to his lack of significant coronary artery disease, he was presumptively diagnosed with an alcoholic cardiomyopathy. His decompensation was attributed to a combination of volume overload due to missed dialysis, exercise, and tachycardia due to paroxysmal atrial fibrillation with poor rate control, as well as the malefic effects on LV filling of the left bundle branch block.

With medical management of his heart failure, initiation of amiodarone to maintain sinus rhythm, and more aggressive ultrafiltration, the patient's clinical status soon improved dramatically, with

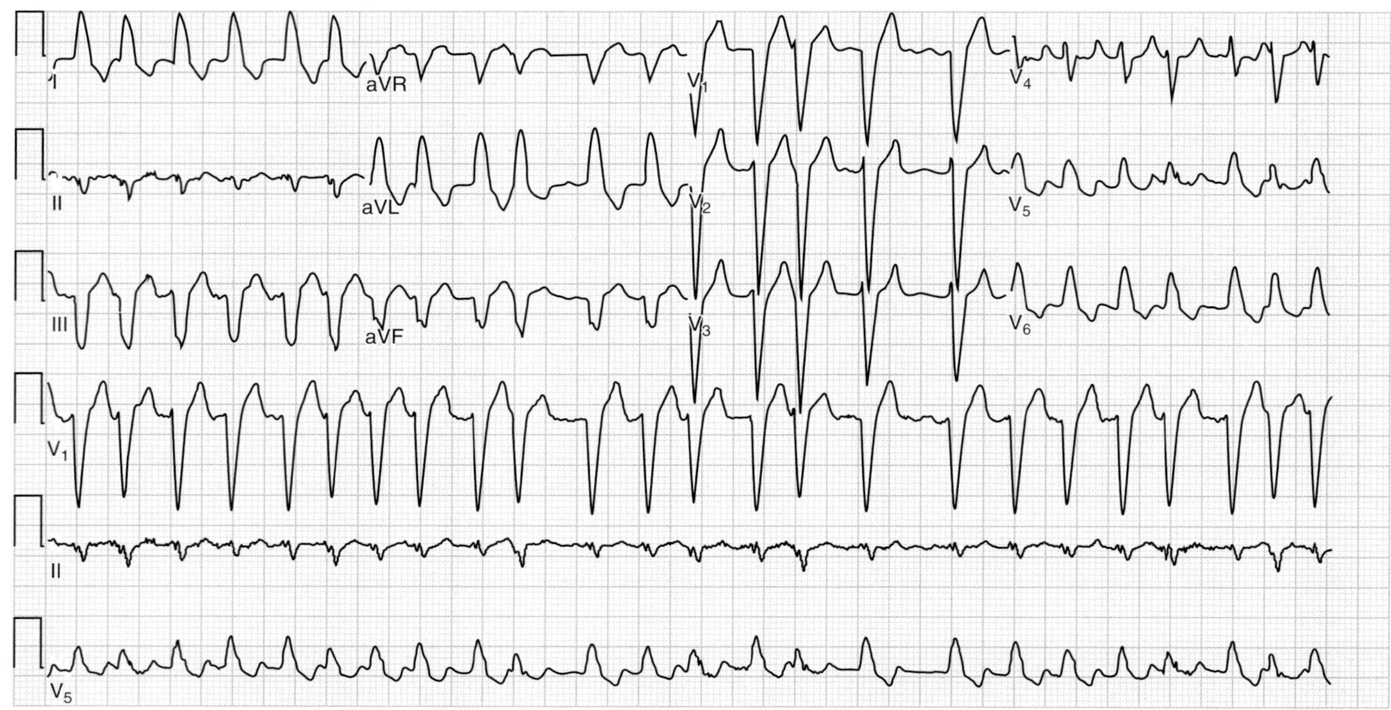

FIGURE 4-2-1 Admission ECG demonstrating rapid atrial fibrillation and left bundle branch block

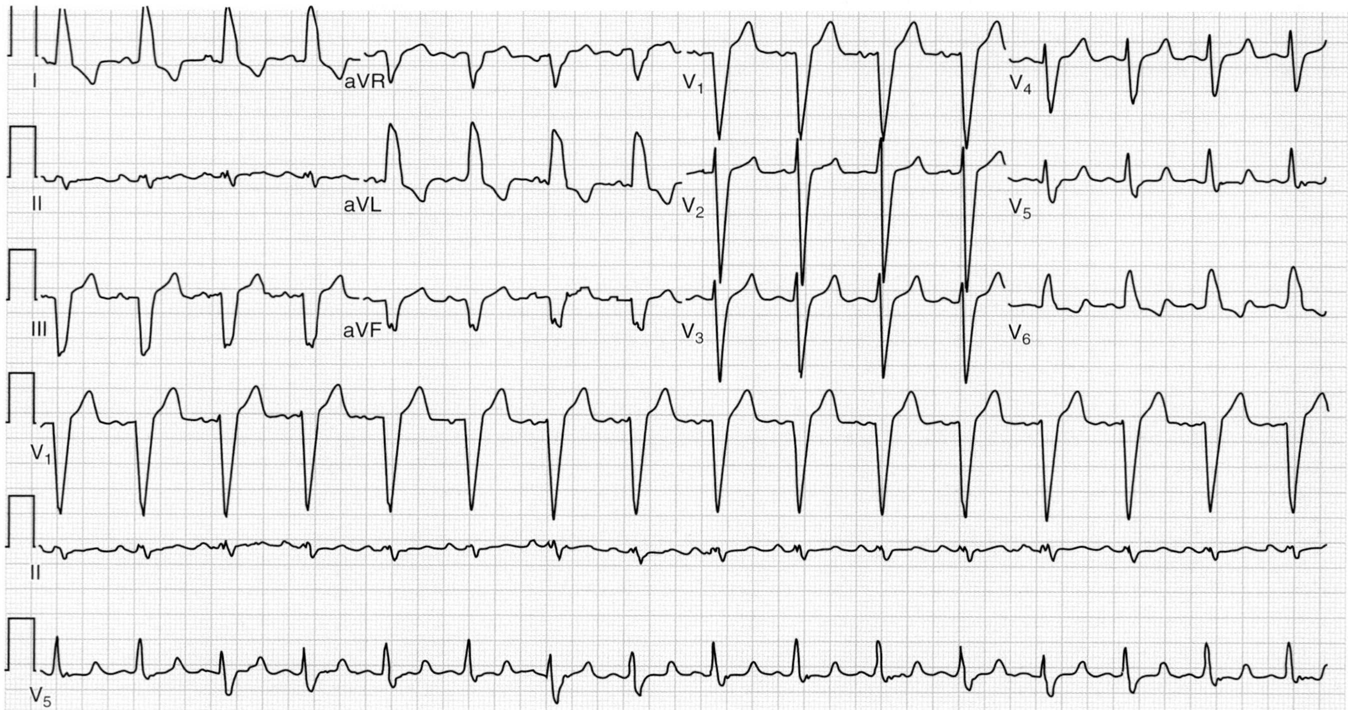

FIGURE 4-2-2 Repeat ECG demonstrates restoration of normal sinus rhythm; however, left bundle branch block persists.

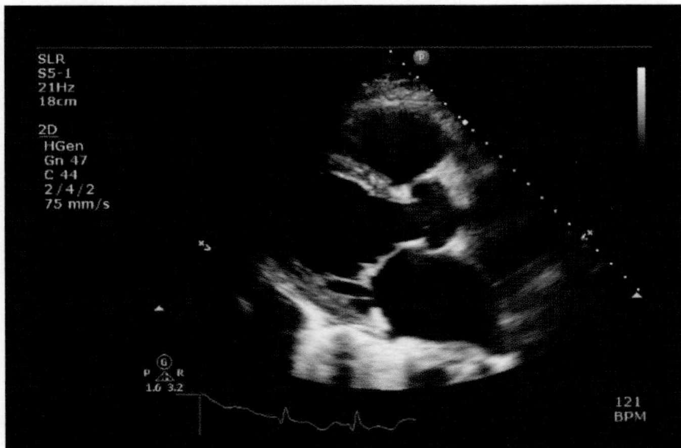

FIGURE 4-2-3 Parasternal long axis view demonstrating a dilated, hypokinetic LV ► (see Video 4-2-3 A-D).

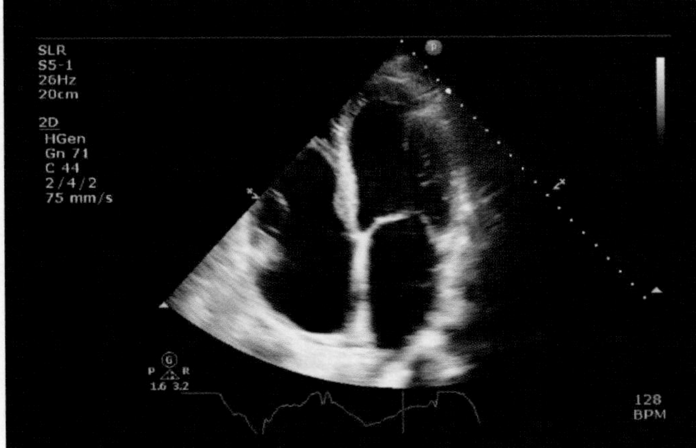

FIGURE 4-2-4 Apical 4 chamber view demonstrating 4 chamber enlargement. There is significant LV and RV hypokinesis.

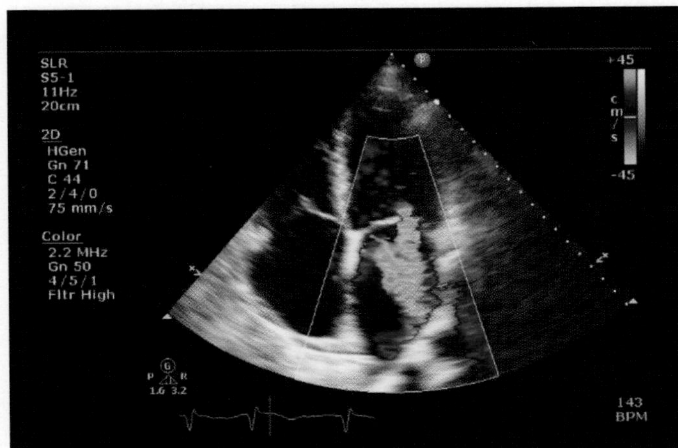

FIGURE 4-2-5 Apical 4 chamber view with color Doppler demonstrating significant MR.

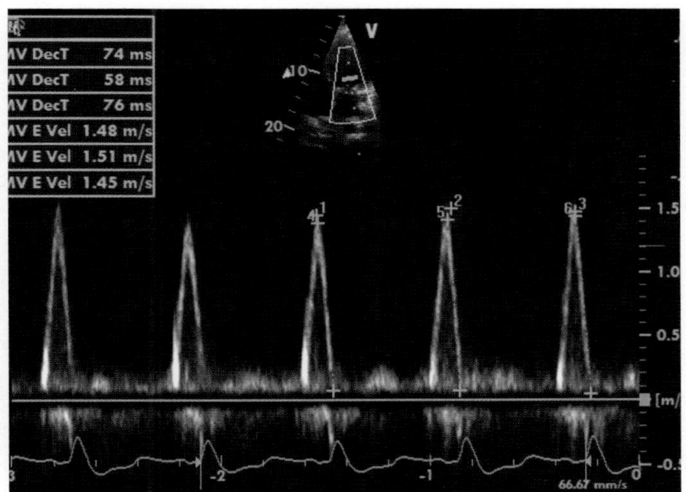

FIGURE 4-2-6 Pulsed Doppler at level of the mitral valve after normal sinus rhythm has been restored; this filling pattern is "restrictive" with high E velocity, rapid deceleration time, and absent A wave. The lack of an A wave despite restoration of normal sinus rhythm is consistent with either an atrial myopathy or atrial stunning.

resolution of his dyspnea and chest pain syndrome. The patient has abstained from alcohol use. A follow-up echocardiogram, performed 6 months later, demonstrated normal LV function and reduction in the severity of mitral regurgitation (Figures 4-2-9 and 4-2-10).

EPIDEMIOLOGY

Alcoholic cardiomyopathy (ACM) is the most common cause of non-ischemic dilated cardiomyopathy in the western world, comprising 21% to 36% of all cases.[1]

- Both systolic and diastolic LV dysfunction as well as systolic RV dysfunction can occur.
- It is believed that diastolic impairment may be an early harbinger of ACM as this is seen in 30% to 40% of alcoholics with normal systolic function and in two-thirds of those with systolic dysfunction.[2,3]

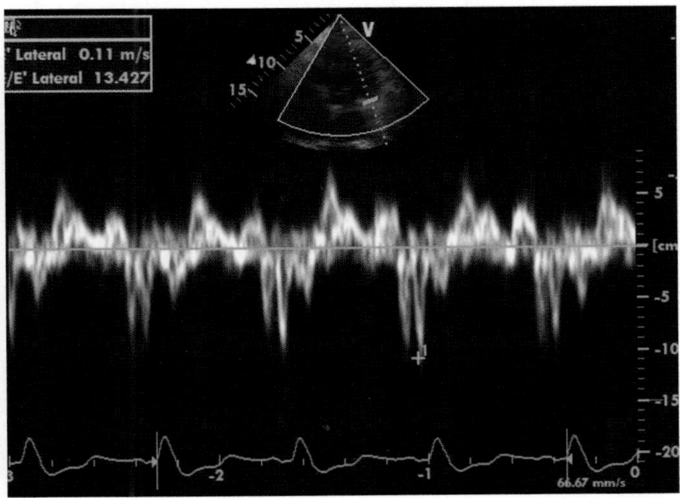

FIGURE 4-2-7 Tissue Doppler obtained at the lateral mitral annulus. The E/e' ratio is consistent with elevated mean LA pressure.

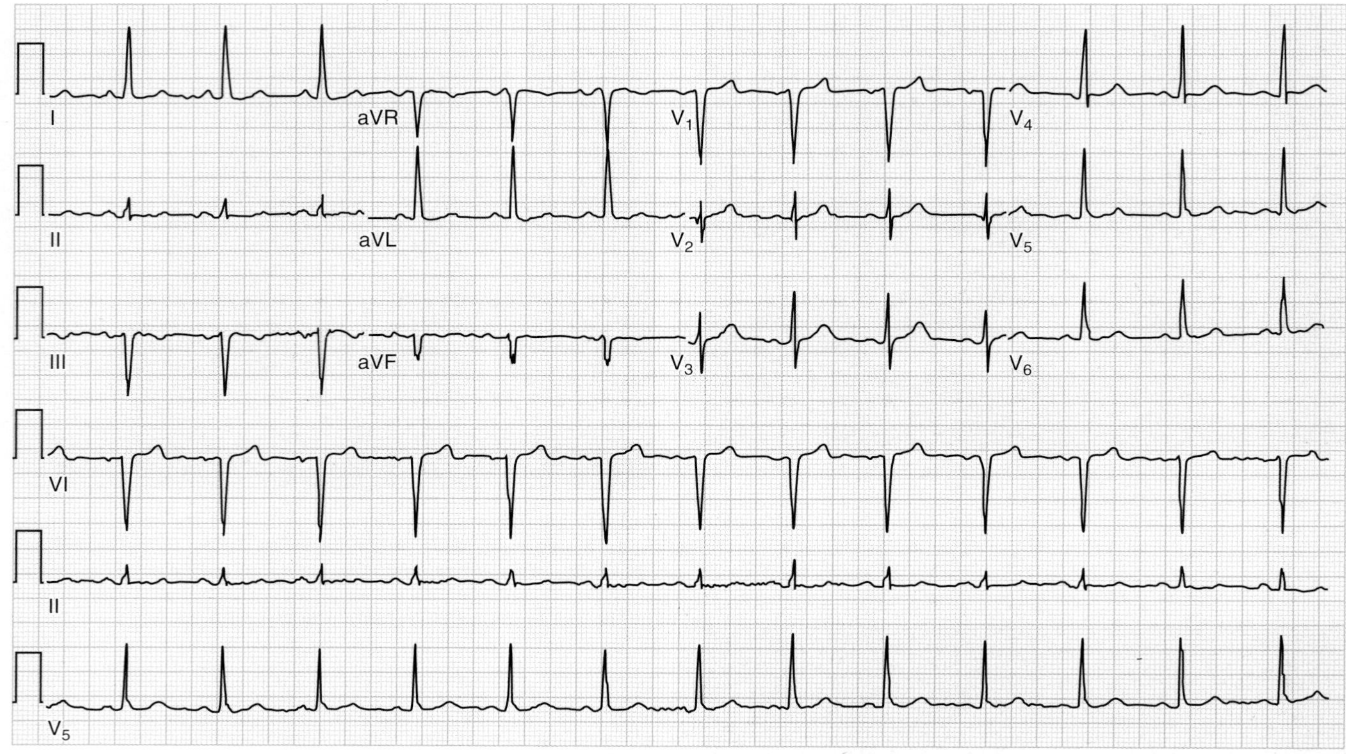

FIGURE 4-2-8 ECG performed approximately 1 year prior to admission demonstrating normal sinus rhythm and narrow QRS complex.

- An EF ≤50% has been reported in approximately 13% of heavy drinkers (lifetime alcohol consumption of 9 kg/kg body weight),[3] while another study claims the incidence of cardiomyopathy in chronic alcoholics is as high as 50%.[4]
- Men comprise the majority of ACM cases at roughly 86%[5] despite the increased sensitivity to toxic effects of alcohol in women.[6]
- In ACM patients, the 4-year mortality without alcohol abstinence is estimated at 50%.[5]

ETIOLOGY AND PATHOPHYSIOLOGY

Cardiotoxicity varies with both the amount of alcohol ingested and the duration of drinking above this threshold.[7] There is wide variation among studies as to what constitutes a "drink" and "mild," "moderate," and "heavy" drinking.

- In the US the common definition of a standard alcoholic drink is 14 g of alcohol (12 oz beer, 5 oz wine, 1.5 oz or "shot" of 80-proof distilled spirits or liquor).[2] It is thought that in order to develop

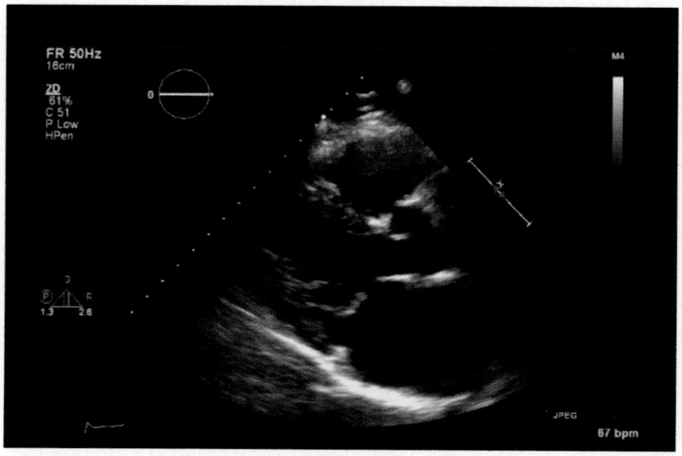

FIGURE 4-2-9 Parasternal long axis follow-up echo demonstrating improvement in LV dimensions and EF. The atria remain dilated ▶ (see Videos 4-2-9 A-D).

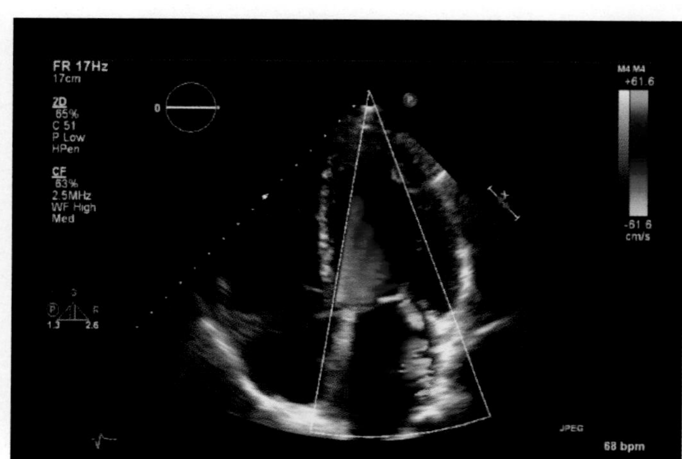

FIGURE 4-2-10 Apical 4 chamber view with color Doppler demonstrating an improvement in the MR.

ACM, men must consume on average 80 g of ethanol per day for a period of 5 to 15 years.[1,7] Women require less to achieve the same cardiotoxic effects.[6] The increased sensitivity to alcohol seen in women is possibly due to slower gastric metabolism and accelerated hepatic metabolism, leading to a net increase in the level of toxic metabolites.

There are many putative mechanisms leading from excessive alcohol consumption to ACM, but it is also fair to say that the mechanism is not fully understood.

- Nutritional deficiencies are no longer thought to play a major role.
- Proposed mechanisms of direct injury include oxidative stress with buildup of reactive oxygen species (ROS). These ROS cause myocyte hypertrophy and apoptosis, which lead to remodeling.[8]
- Changes in the myofibrillary architecture and decreased myocardial contractility occur as well.[4]
    - On electron microscopic studies of animals with induced ACM histologic findings include dilated sarcoplasmic reticula, swollen mitochondria with fragmented cristae and glycogen-filled vacuoles, myofibrillar degeneration and fibrosis, and collagen accumulation in the extracellular matrix.
- It is also believed that increases in norepinephrine levels and derangements in the renin-angiotensin-aldosterone system contribute.
- Finally, structural changes may reflect other cardiovascular effects of alcohol including hypertension, hyperlipidemia, and arrhythmias.
- Several genetic mechanisms which may predispose to ACM have also been proposed, prompted by the observation that only a minority of chronic alcohol abusers will go on to develop this condition.
    - It is well established that a certain genotype of the angiotensin converting enzyme (ACE-*DD*) is associated with heart failure in patients with both ischemic and dilated cardiomyopathy. One study showed the prevalence of this allele in alcohol abusers with symptomatic dilated cardiomyopathy to be 57% versus only 7% in abusers with normal systolic function. The odds ratio for development of ACM in alcoholics with the *DD* allele was 16.4 compared to those with the *I* allele.[9,10]
    - Other genetic polymorphisms implicated in development of ACM are involved in the metabolism of ethanol. Defective variants of acetaldehyde dehydrogenase and alcohol dehydrogenase (ADH) lead to accumulation of the highly cardiotoxic metabolite, acetaldehyde,[8] which concentrates in the heart and is far more reactive than ethanol. Increased levels of acetaldehyde due to overexpression of ADH have been demonstrated in alcoholics.[4] The acetaldehyde was also shown to hinder the coupling of myocyte excitation and contraction by inhibiting release of intracellular calcium from the sarcoplasmic reticulum.
- Illegally produced alcohol often contains additives such as lead and cobalt, which themselves are cardiotoxic.
- Heavy alcohol consumption is also frequently accompanied by electrolyte imbalances (hypokalemia, hypomagnesemia, hypophosphatemia), which further contribute to myocyte dysfunction, arrhythmias and structural alterations.

DIAGNOSIS

Clinical Features

Obtaining a careful clinical history is imperative. Of singular importance is the presence of long-standing heavy alcohol consumption. Frequently, patients will downplay this, and repeated, pointed, yet nonjudgmental questioning may be necessary to elicit this history.[1]

Patients with ACM will exhibit typical signs and symptoms of both systolic and/or diastolic heart failure. As mentioned, a significant number will have impaired LV function long before symptoms become apparent.[5]

- Dyspnea with exertion (and eventually at rest), dry cough, orthopnea, PND, chest heaviness, and fatigue all signal the transition to decompensation.
- Palpitations may occur and are usually due to supraventricular tachyarhythmias.
- Physical exam may reveal an S_3 or S_4 gallop, a systolic apical murmur of mitral regurgitation (due to papillary muscle dysfunction), crackles, and decreased pulse pressure from elevated diastolic pressure secondary to peripheral vasoconstriction.
- In advanced stages, signs and symptoms of RV dysfunction may also become evident including elevated JVP, peripheral edema, and ascites.

ECHOCARDIOGRAPHY

One definition of alcoholic cardiomyopathy is LV dilatation, increased LV mass, normal or decreased wall thickness in the setting of 5 to 10 years of heavy drinking, and absence of ischemia or other causes.[5,7]

- As in all forms of non-ischemic cardiomyopathy, systolic dysfunction is a hallmark. Diastolic impairment, however, often precedes this and even more frequently accompanies systolic dysfunction.[3]
- Early in the course of ACM, an increase in the relative wall thickness is found, with 4 chamber dilatation with associated valvular regurgitation eventually supervening.
- An elevated LV mass index, atrial contraction (A wave), and deceleration time with a reduced E wave and E/A ratio.[3]
- The fate of the RV in ACM has not been widely researched; however, one study showed a U-shaped dose-response curve with both LV and RV size where RV dilatation occurred only with very heavy drinking (>180 g/d) and paralleled the increase in LV size.[11]

OTHER LABORATORY STUDIES

All patients with a suspected cardiomyopathy should undergo a basic evaluation including a CXR, ECG and a basic metabolic panel. Nonspecific findings in ACM may include elevated BNP, ESR, and CRP, as well as low potassium, magnesium, sodium, and phosphorous.

- Laboratory studies suggestive of alcohol abuse may help to support the diagnosis:
    - Typical hematologic and chemical abnormalities found in alcohol abuse include abnormal levels of B12, folic acid, thiamine and zinc, as well as elevated MCV, MCH, transaminases, γ-glutamyltranspeptidase, PT/INR, and a low platelet count.

- Endomyocardial biopsy:
  - Usually not necessary as the echocardiographic findings along with the clinical history generally suffice to make the diagnosis of ACM.
  - Biopsy may be useful to distinguish certain types of myocarditis-induced or infiltrative cardiomyopathies. Once fibrosis has set in, the utility of this study declines significantly.

DIFFERENTIAL DIAGNOSIS

The differential diagnosis of a dilated cardiomyopathy includes:

- Tachycardia-mediated cardiomyopathy
- Stress-induced cardiomyopathy
- Idiopathic dilated cardiomyopathy
- Chronic volume overload due to inadequate dialysis
- Chemotherapy-related cardiomyopathy

MANAGEMENT

Conventional medical therapy for heart failure is warranted. This includes β-blockers, ACE-inhibitors/ARBs, diuretics, digoxin, fluid and sodium restriction. Nutritional deficiencies (thiamine, B12, and folate deficiencies) and electrolyte abnormalities, often seen in chronic alcoholism, should also be corrected.

Essential for the treatment of ACM is abstinence from or significant reduction in alcohol consumption. It has been well demonstrated that this can lead to partial or even full recovery of LV function.[7]

- After 1 year of abstinence, LVEF has been shown to improve by 13% with similar results in patients who reduced their consumption to 20 to 60 g/d.[12] Seventy-five percent of those who continued to drink >80 g/d (even if they had significantly cut down from their previous consumption) passed away within 4 years of follow-up.

PATIENT EDUCATION AND FOLLOW-UP

Patients must be educated on the adverse effects of alcohol on the heart. Referral to an alcohol treatment program is appropriate. The importance of compliance with an ongoing medical regimen for chronic CHF must be emphasized. Regular follow-up with a cardiologist is warranted. As noted above, the LVEF may improve with cessation of alcohol use and/or the institution of medical therapy, which may allow for a tailoring of medical therapy. A repeat echocardiogram after 3 to 6 months of therapy is thus warranted to reassess LVEF and guide the need for other therapies such as CRT and/or ICD placement (see other sections in this chapter).

VIDEO LEGENDS

1. Video 4-2-3 A : Parasternal long axis demonstrating a dilated, hypokinetic LV
2. Video 4-2-3 B: Parasternal short axis view demonstrating severe global LV dysfunction
3. Video 4-2-3 C: Apical 4 chamber view demonstrating 4 chamber enlargement. There is significant LV and RV hypokinesis.
4. Video 4-2-3 D: Apical 4 chamber view with color Doppler demonstrating significant MR
5. Video 4-2-9 A: Parasternal long axis follow-up echo demonstrating improvement in LV dimensions and EF
6. Video 4-2-9 B: Parasternal short axis view follow up echo demonstrating improved global LV function
7. Video 4-2-9 C: Apical 4 chamber view from the follow up echo demonstrating improvement in the LV function. The atria remain dilated.
8. Video 4-2-9 D: Apical four chamber view with color Doppler demonstrating an improvement in the MR.

REFERENCES

1. Skotzko CE. Alcohol use and congestive heart failure: incidence, importance, and approaches to improved history taking, *Heart Fail Rev*. 2009;14:51-55.
2. Kloner RA. To drink or not to drink? That is the question. *Circulation*. 2007;116(11):1306-1317.
3. Fernandez-Sola J. Diastolic function impairment in alcoholics. *Alcohol Clin Exp Res*. 2000;12(24):1830-1835.
4. Duan J. Overexpression of alcohol dehydrogenase exacerbates ethanol-induced contractile defect in cardiac myocytes. *Am J Physiol Heart Circ Physiol*. 2002;282(4):H1216-H1222.
5. Laonigro I. Alcohol abuse and heart failure, *Eur J Heart Fail*. 2009;11(5):453-462.
6. Urbano-Màrquez A. The greater risk of alcoholic cardiomyopathy and myopathy in women compared with men. *JAMA*. 1995;274:149-154.
7. Djousse L. Alcohol consumption and heart failure: a systematic review. *Curr Atheroscler Rep*. 2008;10(2):117-120.
8. Lucas DL. Alcohol and the cardiovascular system: research challenges and opportunities. *J Am Coll Cardiol*. 2005;45(12):1916-1924.
9. Fernandez-Sola J. Angiotensin-converting enzyme gene polymorphism is associated with vulnerability to alcoholic cardiomyopathy. *Ann Intern Med*. 2002;137:321-326.
10. Pilati M. The role of angiotensin-converting enzyme polymorphism in congestive heart failure. *CHF*. 2004;10:87-95.
11. Kajander OA. Dose dependent but non-linear effects of alcohol on the left and right ventricle. *Heart*. 2001;86:417-423.
12. Nicolàs JM. The effect of controlled drinking in alcoholic cardiomyopathy. *Ann Intern Med*. 2002;136:192-200.

SECTION 3

Tachycardia-Mediated Cardiomyopathy

Gaurav R Parikh, MD, MRCP (UK) and Gerard P. Aurigemma, MD, FAHA, FASE, FACC

CLINICAL CASE PRESENTATION

A 65-year-old woman with a history of mitral valve prolapse, treated breast cancer, hypothyroidism, and hyperlipidemia presented to her physician with symptoms of dyspnea. She was initially treated with antibiotics for a presumptive diagnosis of pneumonia. However, she continued to have symptoms of significant dyspnea and was referred for further workup. Upon presentation to the echo lab, she was noted to be tachycardic, and an ECG confirmed her to be in atrial fibrillation with rapid ventricular rate of 150 bpm (Figure 4-3-1). A chest radiograph (Figure 4-3-2) showed cardiomegaly, bilateral pleural effusions, and vascular congestion. An echocardiogram revealed a dilated, spherical left ventricle with severely reduced LV ejection fraction and severe mitral regurgitation (Figures 4-3-3 and 4-3-4). Right and left heart cardiac catheterization was performed, which demonstrated no obstructive coronary disease. Tracings from that procedure are seen in Figure 4-3-5 A and B; pulmonary hypertension was noted, and there was a sizeable 'v' wave noted in the pulmonary capillary wedge tracing.

The patient underwent successful cardioversion back to normal sinus rhythm, and a heart failure medical regimen was initiated. Echocardiography performed approximately 4 weeks later demonstrated improved systolic function, but also persistent chamber dilation (Figure 4-3-6). In addition, there was persistent severe mitral regurgitation. A subsequent echocardiogram performed 4 months later demonstrated normalization of LV size but there was persistent severe mitral regurgitation (Figure 4-3-7). Accordingly, she subsequently underwent mitral valve repair with annuloplasty and a modified biatrial Cox procedure and left atrial appendage resection. Upon follow-up, she was remarkably better without any symptoms or signs of heart failure, and her echocardiogram showed eventual normalization of LV cavity dimensions and normal LV ejection fraction.

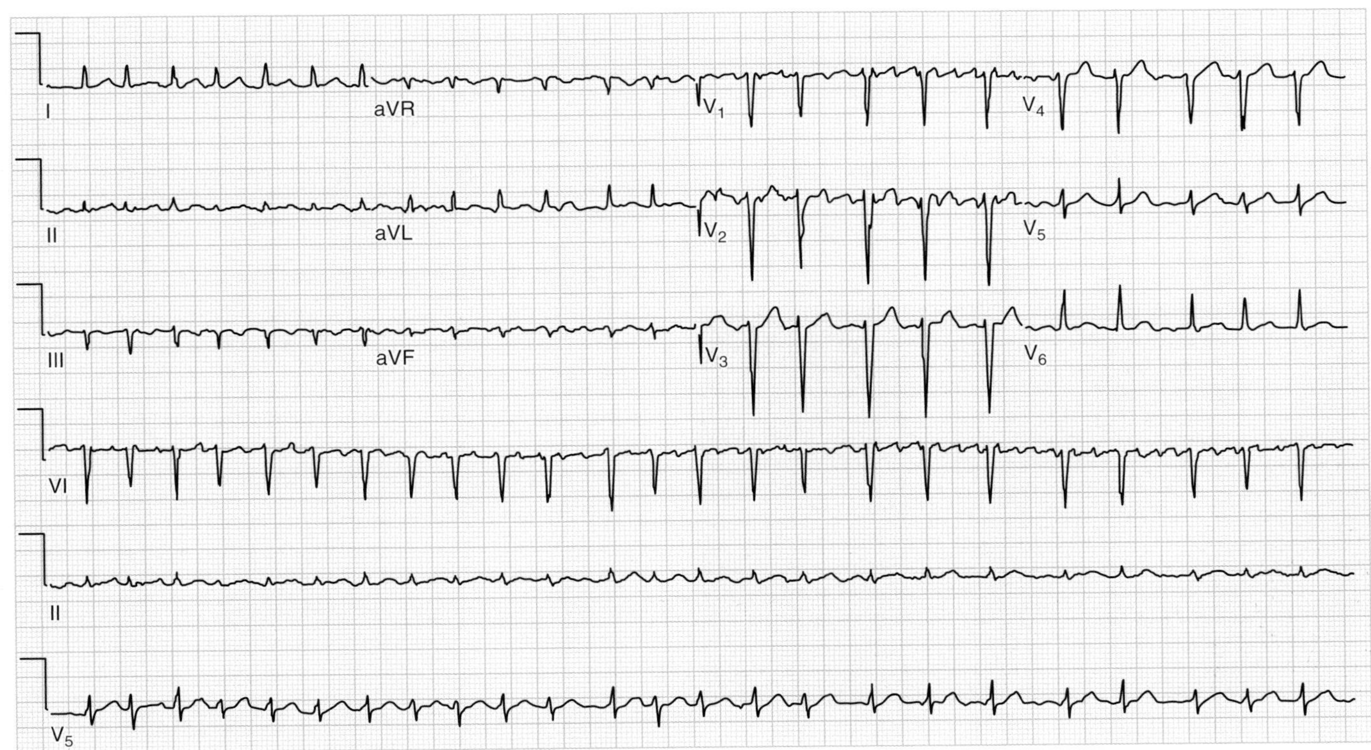

FIGURE 4-3-1 ECG showing atrial fibrillation with rapid ventricular response.

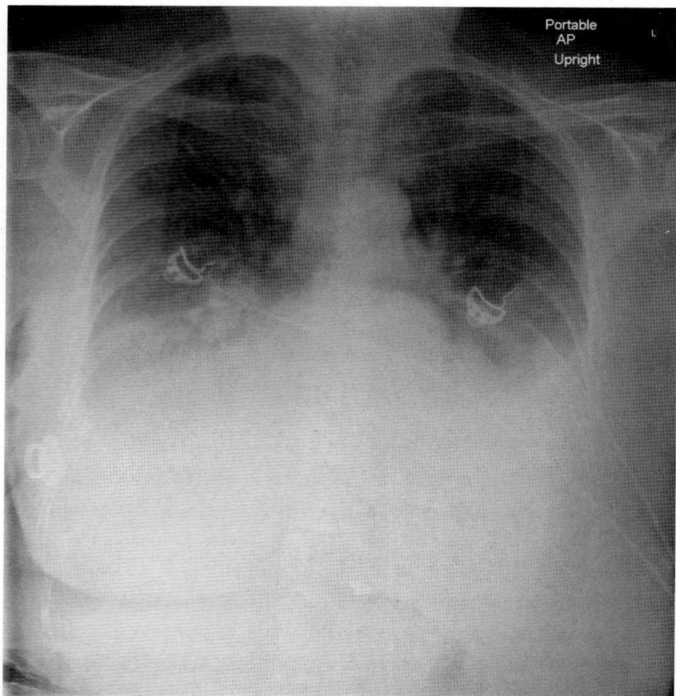

FIGURE 4-3-2 CXR showing bilateral pleural effusions and pulmonary vascular congestion.

CLINICAL FEATURES

- The clinical presentation of tachycardia-mediated cardiomyopathy can be extremely variable.
- Patients may present with palpitations related to the uncontrolled heart rate and irregularity of the underlying arrhythmia.
- Alternatively, they may present with signs and symptoms of congestive heart failure: fatigue, shortness of breath, paroxysmal nocturnal dyspnea, orthopnea, and pedal edema.
- Accordingly, the physical examination, apart from the rapid heart rate, can be variable. If heart failure is the presentation, there will be elevated JVP, S_3 gallop, mitral regurgitation murmur, and pedal edema. Lung examination may show the presence of pleural effusion and basilar rales.

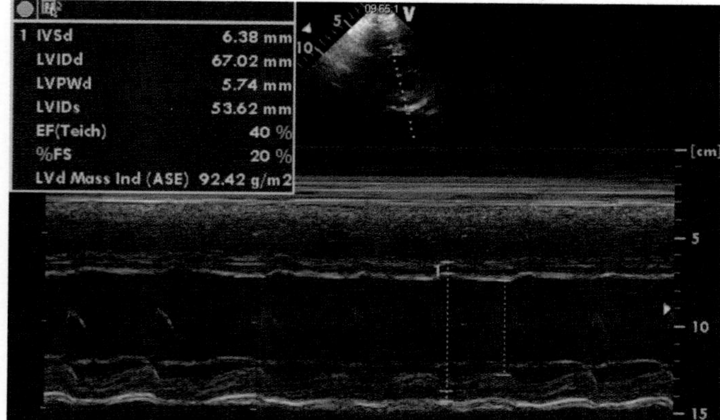

FIGURE 4-3-3 M-mode taken from the initial echocardiogram; M-mode cursor is directed through the LV showing the dilated LV cavity. There is marked LV dilation; diastolic dimension is 6.7 cm.

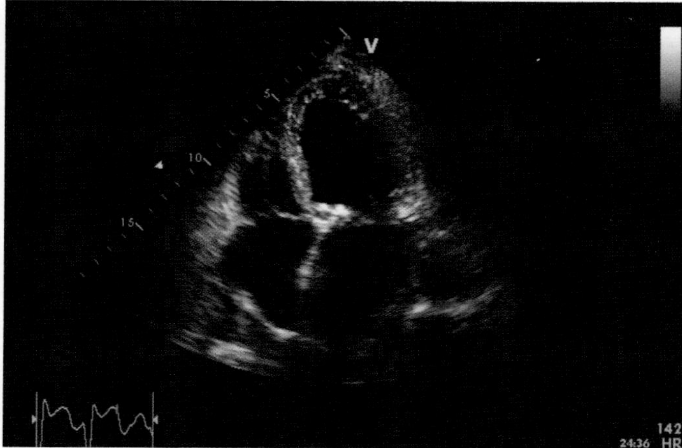

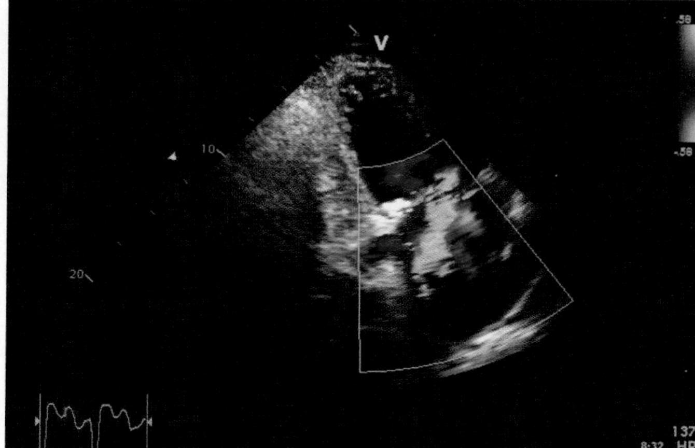

FIGURE 4-3-4 Apical 4 chamber view (top panel) and 2 chamber view with color Doppler (bottom panel). The echo shows LV dilation, tachycardia, and marked diminution of global systolic function. Note also, biatrial enlargement, severe mitral annular calcification, and myxomatous degeneration of the mitral valve. Apical 2 chamber view with color flow Doppler mapping demonstrates a broad area of flow turbulence in the left atrium in systole, indicative of severe mitral regurgitation. There is a large area of flow convergence in the left ventricle. Note also rapid heart rate and severe systolic dysfunction ▶ (see Videos 4-3-4 A and B).

BACKGROUND AND EPIDEMIOLOGY

Cardiomyopathy is a group of disorders caused by abnormal myocardial structure and function in absence of ischemic heart disease, hypertension, or valvular disease.

- Phenotypic classification is based on the anatomy and physiology. Categories include dilated, hypertrophic, restrictive, arrhythmogenic right ventricular and unclassified.[1]
- It has been known for some time that chronic rapid heart rates can cause a dilated type of cardiomyopathy that is highly reversible upon control of the tachycardia. While the exact incidence of tachycardia-mediated cardiomyopathy is not known, it is being increasingly recognized as an important cause of dilated cardiomyopathy.[1,2]

PATHOPHYSIOLOGY AND ETIOLOGY

- Dilated cardiomyopathy has been described in chronic and incessant tachycardia from atrial fibrillation, atrial flutter, atrial tachycardia,

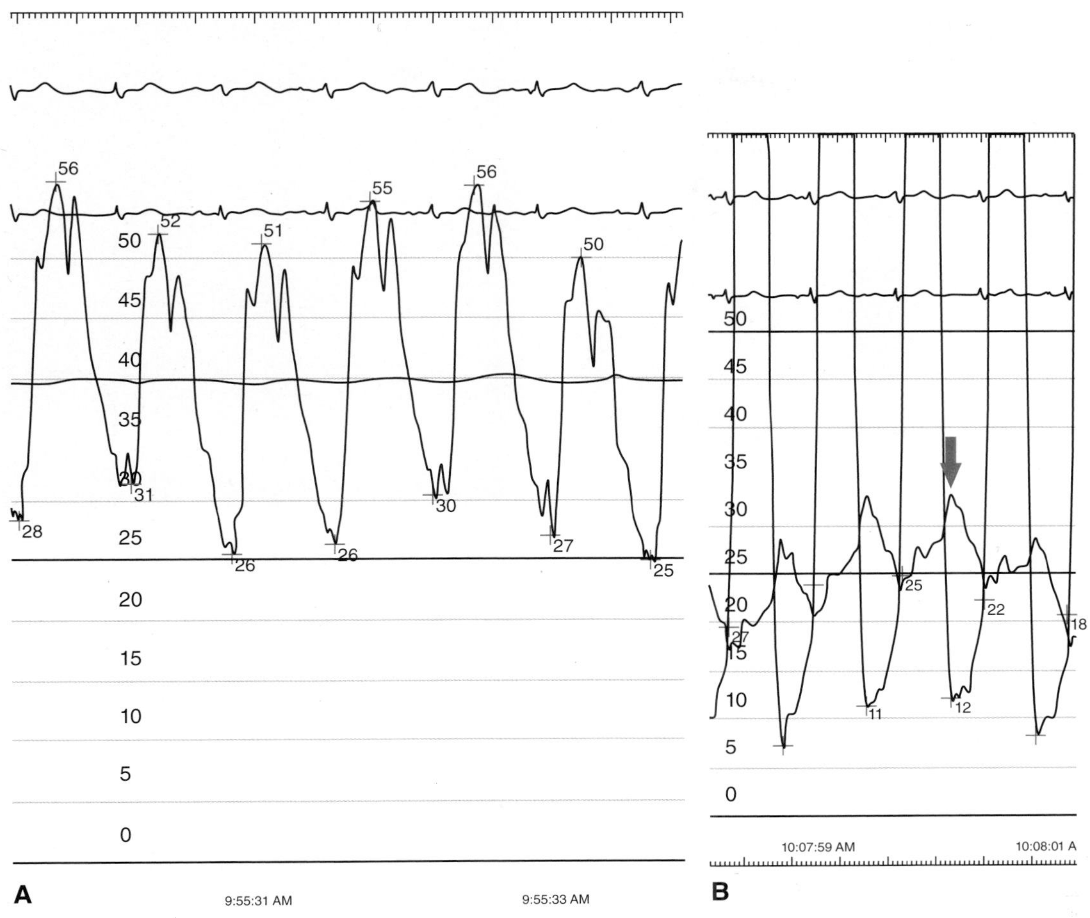

FIGURE 4-3-5 A Pulmonary artery pressure tracing documenting significant pulmonary hypertension, with peak systolic pressure in the 50 to 56 mm Hg range, and pulmonary artery diastolic pressure averaging 28 to 30 mm Hg. **B** Composite of pulmonary capillary wedge and left ventricular pressure tracings. (The PCW tracing is phase delayed, so the peak 'v' wave does not coincide with diastole.) Note the high mean pulmonary PCW pressures with elevated v waves to as much as 30 mm Hg.

accessory pathway mediated tachycardia, and AV nodal reentry tachycardia as well as with incessant ventricular tachycardia.[2-4]

- Animal models that were originally developed to investigate heart failure have helped immensely to understand tachycardia-mediated cardiomyopathy.

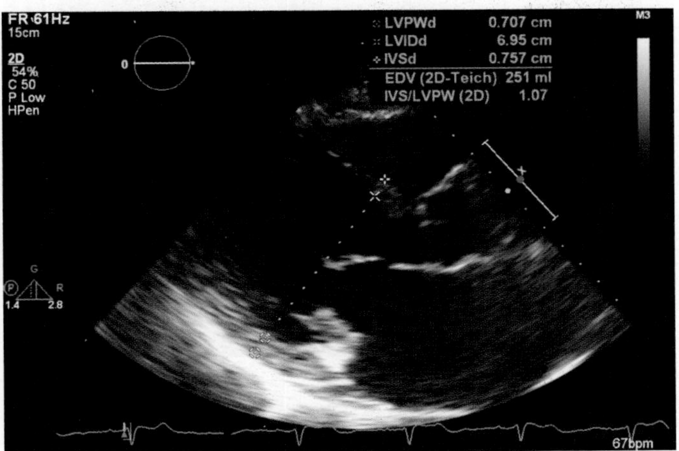

FIGURE 4-3-6 Parasternal long axis view 4 weeks postcardioversion showing persistently dilated LV cavity (LVIDD 6.9 cm).

  - In experimental animal models, rapid pacing produces hemodynamic changes such as a fall in blood pressure and a drop in cardiac output as early as 24 hours with continued deterioration in ventricular function for up to 3 to 5 weeks, leading to marked biventricular dilatation and end-stage heart failure.
  - The LV assumes a more spherical shape with thinning of the LV walls. There is apical and lateral displacement of the papillary muscles leading to tenting and tethering of mitral leaflets causing secondary mitral regurgitation.[2]
- Several mechanisms have been described to account for contractile dysfunction and structural changes:
  - Myocardial energy depletion and impaired utilization, abnormal calcium handling, myocardial ischemia, and myocyte and extracellular matrix remodeling have all been described.
  - At the cellular level, there is disruption of extracellular matrix architecture and myocyte basement membrane-sarcolemmal interface. There are morphologic changes in myocyte itself with myocyte loss and increase in volume of the remaining myocytes.[2]
- There is intense neurohumoral activation with marked elevation of atrial natriuretic peptide, epinephrine, norepinephrine, renin activity, and aldosterone levels.[2]

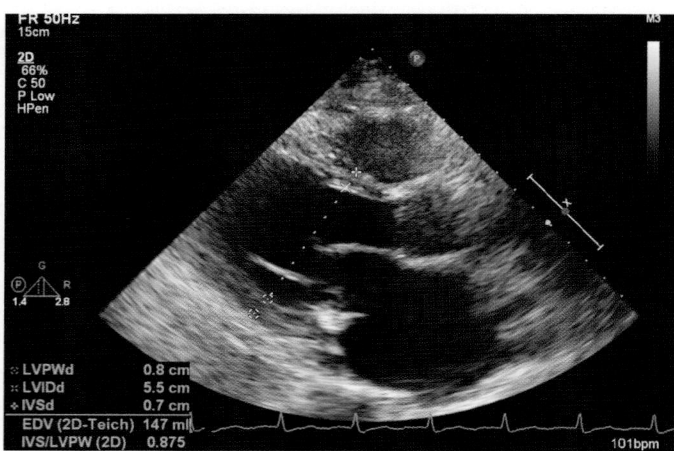

FIGURE 4-3-7 An echocardiogram performed 4 months post cardioversion demonstrated marked improvement in LV dilatation (LVIDD 5.5 cm). The accompanying 2 videos demonstrate improved LVEF but persistent significant MR ▶ (see Videos 4-3-7 A and B).

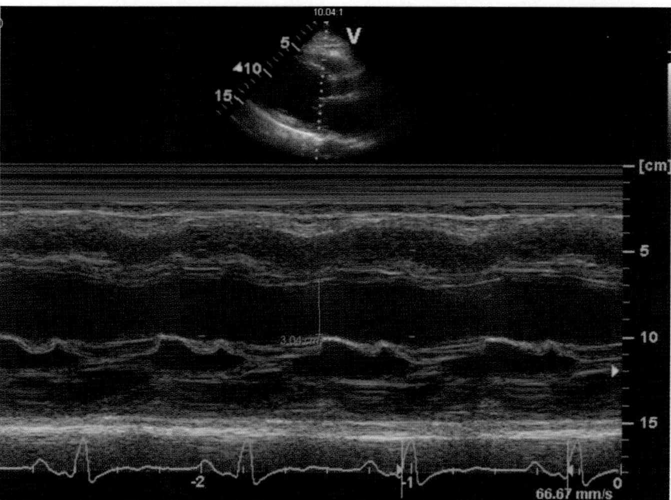

FIGURE 4-3-8 M-mode at the level of mitral leaflet tips in a patient with dilated cardiomyopathy with severely reduced systolic function showing increased EPSS = 3cm.

ECHOCARDIOGRAPHY

Patients with signs and symptoms of heart failure should be evaluated with an echocardiogram. There are several features of a dilated cardiomyopathy that can be assessed.[5]

- 2-D and M-mode echocardiography will show marked biventricular dilatation. The left ventricle assumes spherical geometry with sphericity index <1.5:1.
- Thinning of the ventricular walls is noted.
- There can be enlargement of the right ventricle and both the atria.
- There is markedly increased end-systolic and end-diastolic LV volumes and markedly reduced systolic function.
- Geometric changes in the shape of the LV as well as geometric changes resulting in apical and lateral displacement of the papillary muscles are seen. This may lead to apical tenting of the mitral apparatus causing functional mitral regurgitation.
- The LV apex should be examined carefully in cases with severely reduced systolic function to look for apical thrombus.
- M-mode echocardiography at the level of mitral leaflet tips will show increased E-point to septal separation (EPSS) distance indicating dilated LV cavity and reduced LV systolic function (Figure 4-3-8).
- Reduced mitral leaflet opening and premature tapering and closure of aortic cups are noted on M-mode consistent with reduced stroke volume.
- A "B-bump" (Figure 4-3-9) may be noted at the level of mitral tips indicating elevated LV filling pressures.
- Doppler echocardiography will help assess the LV filling pressure by looking at the mitral inflow pattern.
  - A steep mitral E wave deceleration slope of <130 ms and a ratio of E/e' >20 is associated with elevated left atrial pressures and elevated left ventricular filling pressures.
  - An E/e' <10 is associated with normal left atrial pressure.
- The presence and severity of mitral and tricuspid regurgitation add prognostic value, with a general rule of thumb being worse prognosis with worsening mitral and tricuspid regurgitation.[6]

OTHER DIAGNOSTIC TESTING AND PROCEDURES

A clinical evaluation should always begin with a careful history concerning the onset and type of symptoms.

- An ECG will give crucial information regarding the heart rate and rhythm.
- Holter monitoring or telemetry are used to diagnose any and all arrhythmias and to better understand the heart rate variability.
- Chest radiograph will show evidence of cardiomegaly. It may show right-sided pleural effusion and/or pulmonary vascular congestion.
- Radionuclide imaging may be of value in ruling out myocardial ischemia as well as assessing ventricular volumes and ejection fraction in cases where echocardiogram is suboptimal.

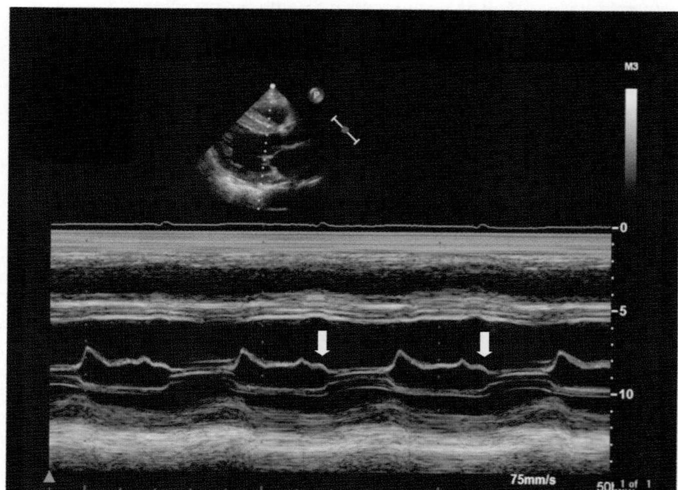

FIGURE 4-3-9 M-mode at the level of mitral leaflet tips in a patient with dilated cardiomyopathy with severely reduced systolic function. Broad arrows indicate an interruption in the smooth closure motion of the anterior leaflet of the mitral valve in late diastole, indicating a "B-bump" or "A-C" shoulder. This finding denotes an elevation in post-atrial systole ventricular diastolic pressure.

- Cardiac MRI can not only accurately assesses ventricular function, but it can also be immensely helpful in distinguishing inflammatory from infiltrative cardiomyopathies, as well as identify patients who have evidence of replacement fibrosis and are at high risk of sudden cardiac death due to electrical instability.[7]
- Cardiac catheterization, in this era, is generally reserved for assessing the presence and extent of coronary artery disease and to document filling pressures, as was done in this case.

DIFFERENTIAL DIAGNOSIS

The main differential diagnosis of tachycardia-mediated cardiomyopathy is a dilated cardiomyopathy from other causes: idiopathic, post-viral, HIV-related, familial, drugs, alcohol, and chemotherapy. Echocardiographically, these may exhibit a very similar phenotype, and the differentiation is provided by the history and other clinical features.

DIAGNOSIS

The diagnosis is usually made by careful history, physical examination, an ECG showing tachycardia with the echocardiographic features outlined above. Cardiac catheterization is useful to rule out underlying coronary disease.[8]

MANAGEMENT

The main emphasis of management of tachycardia-mediated cardiomyopathy is to terminate the arrhythmia and either establish sinus rhythm or control the ventricular response, either with medications or an AV nodal ablation/pacemaker. A secondary emphasis is on treating the heart failure with a medical regimen of diuretics, angiotensin converting enzyme inhibitor or angiotensin receptor antagonist, β-blockers, and an aldosterone antagonist.[8]

FOLLOW-UP

The patient should be followed up closely with a cardiologist/primary care physician. It should be reemphasized that tachycardia-mediated cardiomyopathy is highly reversible once the underlying arrhythmia is treated. The majority of cases will normalize their left ventricular size and systolic function.

VIDEO LEGENDS

1. Video 4-3-4 A: Apical 4 chamber view taken from the initial echocardiogram of this patient. The echo shows LV dilation, tachycardia, and marked diminution of global systolic function. Note, also, biatrial enlargement, severe mitral annular calcification and myxomatous degeneration of the mitral valve.
2. Video 4-3-4 B: Apical 2 chamber view taken from the initial study of this patient, with color flow Doppler mapping demonstrating a broad area of flow turbulence in the left atrium in systole, indicative of severe mitral regurgitation. There is a large area of flow convergence in the left ventricle. Note also the rapid heart rate and severe systolic dysfunction.
3. Video 4-3-7 A: Apical 4 chamber view taken from the 4 month post-cardioversion echocardiogram of this patient. There is a marked improvement in systolic function in association with a slower heart rate and the restoration of sinus rhythm.
4. Video 4-3-7 B: Composite of the apical 2 chamber view taken from the 4 month post-cardioversion study of this patient. Systolic function has improved, but there is still significant mitral regurgitation.

REFERENCES

1. Maron BJ, Towbin JA, Thiene G, et al. Contemporary definitions and classification of the cardiomyopathies: an American Heart Association Scientific Statement from the Council on Clinical Cardiology, Heart Failure and Transplantation Committee; Quality of Care and Outcomes Research and Functional Genomics and Translational Biology Interdisciplinary Working Groups; and Council on Epidemiology and Prevention. *Circulation*. 2006;113:1807.
2. Shinbane JS, Wood MA, Jensen DN, et al. Tachycardia-induced cardiomyopathy: a review of animal models and clinical studies. *J Am Coll Cardiol*. 1997;29:709.
3. Kasper EK, Agema WR, Hutchins GM, et al. The causes of dilated cardiomyopathy: a clinicopathologic review of 673 consecutive patients. *J Am Coll Cardiol*. 1994;23:586.
4. Redfield MM, Kay GN, Jenkins LS, et al. Tachycardia-related cardiomyopathy: a common cause of ventricular dysfunction in patients with atrial fibrillation referred for an atrioventricular ablation. *Mayo Clinic Proc*. 2000;75:790.
5. Armstrong WF, Ryan T. *Feigenbaum's Echocardiography* 7th ed. Philadelphia, PA: Lippincott Williams & Wilkins; 2009.
6. Koelling TM, Aaronson KD, Cody RJ, Bach DS, Armstrong WF. Prognostic significance of mitral regurgitation and tricuspid regurgitation in patients with left ventricular systolic dysfunction. *Am Heart J*. 2002;144:524-529.
7. Nazarian S, Bluemke DA, Lardo AC, et al. Magnetic resonance assessment of the substrate for inducible ventricular tachycardia in nonischemic cardiomyopathy. *Circulation*. 2005;112:2821.
8. Jessup M, Abraham WT, Casey DE, et al. 2009 focused update: ACCF/AHA Guidelines for the Diagnosis and Management of Heart Failure in Adults: a report of the American College of Cardiology Foundation/American Heart Association Task Force on Practice Guidelines: developed in collaboration with the International Society for Heart and Lung Transplantation. *Circulation*. 2009;119:1977.

SECTION 4

Heart Failure With Preserved Ejection Fraction

Jarrod Ferrara, MD, and Gerard P. Aurigemma, MD, FAHA, FASE, FACC

CLINICAL CASE PRESENTATION

A 65-year-old woman with a history of hypertension, Type 2 diabetes mellitus, paroxysmal atrial fibrillation, and obesity presented to the hospital with a chief complaint of shortness of breath. She reported dyspnea on exertion and orthopnea for several days prior to admission. She denied any chest pain or pressure, lower extremity edema, productive cough, or fever. There had been no recent medication changes. She had not weighed herself recently and was therefore not able to relate a recent change in weight.

She was found to be markedly hypertensive with a BP of 204/46 mm Hg. Her exam was notable for jugular venous distention, bibasilar crackles on lung exam, a systolic ejection murmur with radiation to the carotids, and no significant lower extremity edema. Her chest x-ray (Figure 4-4-1) showed pulmonary vascular congestion. Chest CT angiography showed no evidence of pulmonary embolism but did reveal bilateral pleural effusions and scattered patchy ground-glass opacities consistent with interstitial edema and a likely diagnosis of heart failure. The ECG showed sinus rhythm with a first degree AV block and nonspecific ST-T-wave abnormalities (Figure 4-4-2). Her BNP level was greater than 800.

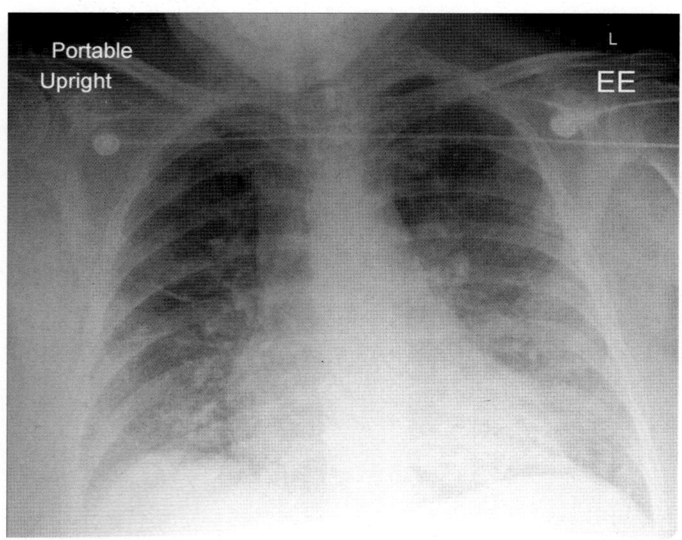

FIGURE 4-4-1 Admission chest x-ray. This study demonstrates a normal size cardiac silhouette, diffuse interstitial markings, and upper lobe redistribution. This x-ray was read as being consistent with acute pulmonary edema.

An echocardiogram was performed the following day, after diuresis and clinical improvement (Figure 4-4-3). It demonstrated normal LV size, with a normal to hyperdynamic ejection fraction. Left ventricular wall thickness was mildly increased at 12 mm, and LV mass index was 115 g/M^2; the ratio of wall thickness to cavity radius (relative wall thickness) was elevated at 0.50. These findings are consistent with concentric LV remodeling, commonly found in patients with hypertensive heart disease. LV diastolic function (Figure 4-4-4 A-C) was interpreted as follows: the E/A ratio was normal, but the pulmonary venous flow showed marked dominance of the diastolic wave. The tissue Doppler e' velocity at the lateral annulus was 5 cm/s, yielding an E/e' ratio of 25. These data are consistent with the diagnosis of elevated mean LA pressure. Pulmonary artery systolic pressure (data not shown) was estimated at 70 mm Hg. Left atrial volume index was 40 cc/M^2, consistent with mild LA dilation. There was mild mitral regurgitation and mild aortic stenosis.

She was treated for an acute heart failure exacerbation with intravenous diuresis and aggressive blood pressure control. On the second day after admission, she underwent cardiac catheterization. Coronary angiography showed no obstructive coronary artery disease. Right heart catheterization and hemodynamic assessment revealed severe systemic hypertension, an elevated pulmonary capillary wedge pressure, with a normal cardiac output. These findings supported the diagnosis of heart failure with preserved ejection fraction.

EPIDEMIOLOGY

Until the widespread use of echocardiography, congestive heart failure was considered to be synonymous with reduced left ventricular ejection fraction (LVEF), usually below 40%.

- Over the past two and a half decades, this paradigm has changed, and it is now recognized that the syndrome of congestive heart failure severe enough to require hospitalization is, at least half of the time, associated with an LVEF exceeding 50%.
- Patients with this syndrome of heart failure with a preserved LVEF (HFpEF) tend to be older, female, and obese. They are more likely to have a history of hypertension and atrial fibrillation, and they are less likely to have a history of coronary artery disease or significant valvular disease.[1,2] These same patient characteristics have been observed in multiple investigations, including in the three largest randomized trials to date that examined interventions in HFpEF.[4,5]

Some, but not all, clinical investigations into HFpEF have used an LVEF cutoff of 50% to define HFpEF.

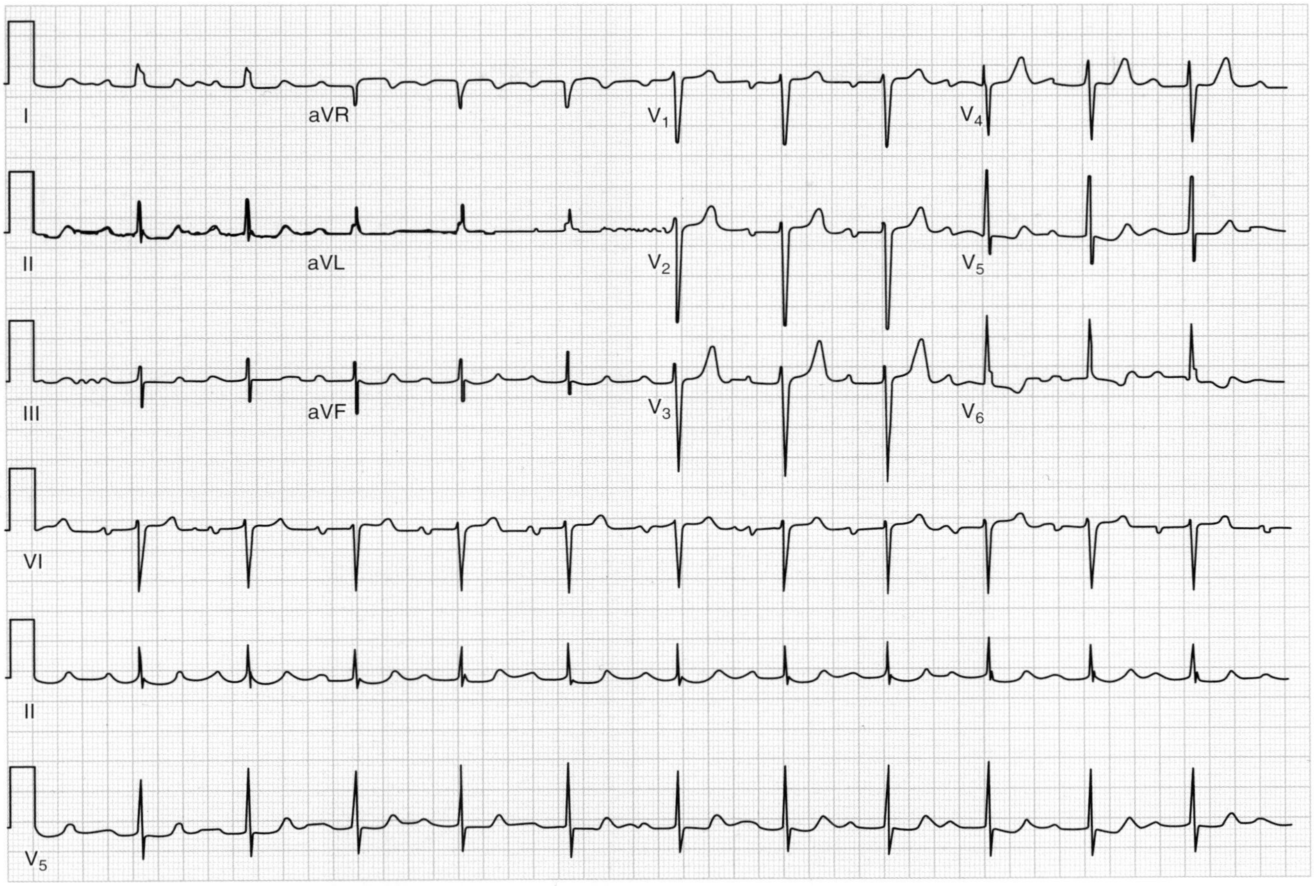

FIGURE 4-4-2 Admission 12 lead ECG. This study shows normal sinus rhythm, first-degree AV block, and evidence of left atrial abnormality. There is lateral ST-segment depression, consistent either with lateral wall myocardial ischemia or repolarization changes from left ventricular hypertrophy.

- The studies have also differed in their primary as well as their secondary endpoints, which has likely contributed to some degree in the differences in outcome that have been observed among the different studies of HFpEF.
- Earlier studies that examined outcomes in HFpEF found these patients to have a similar prognosis to those with HFREF.[1,2]

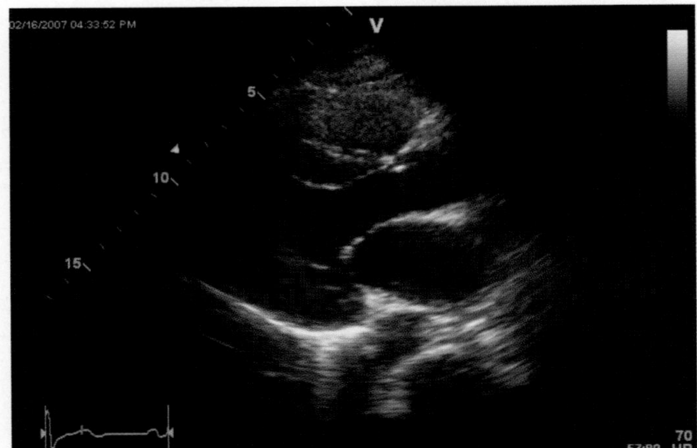

FIGURE 4-4-3 Parasternal long axis view of our patient. Left ventricular wall thickness was mildly increased, LV mass index was 115 g/M^2. The relative wall thickness was 0.50. The accompanying 4 videos demonstrate normal to hyperdynamic LV function ▶ (see Videos 4-4-3 A-D).

However, subsequent studies have suggested that a preserved EF confers a somewhat more favorable outcome.[4]

A report from the Framingham Study investigators identified risk factors associated with the development of HFpEF. Risk factors include:

- increased systolic blood pressure
- atrial fibrillation
- female gender

Not surprisingly, a history of prior myocardial infarction or left bundle-branch block QRS morphology was associated with HF with a reduced EF (HFrEF). The long-term prognosis was equally poor in both types of HF, and among men and women in the study cohort.[5]

While there has been variation in the literature regarding the prognosis for patients with HFpEF, it seems clear that they are representative of a distinct clinical syndrome, with a worse prognosis as compared to patients with hypertension or other disease states that raise cardiovascular risk.[4]

- In patients with clinical heart failure, the stage of diastolic dysfunction is a stronger predictor of mortality than the LVEF.[6] It is interesting that the progression of LV diastolic dysfunction has been found to be a strong predictor of all-cause mortality. Many studies and databases have found that a substantial number of these patients

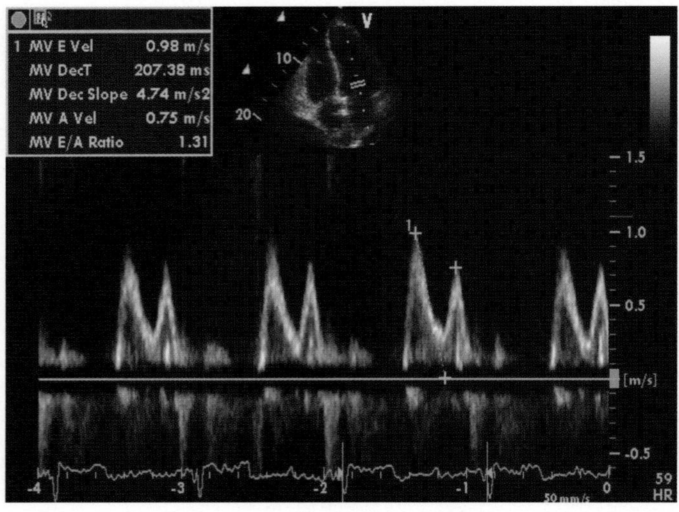

A

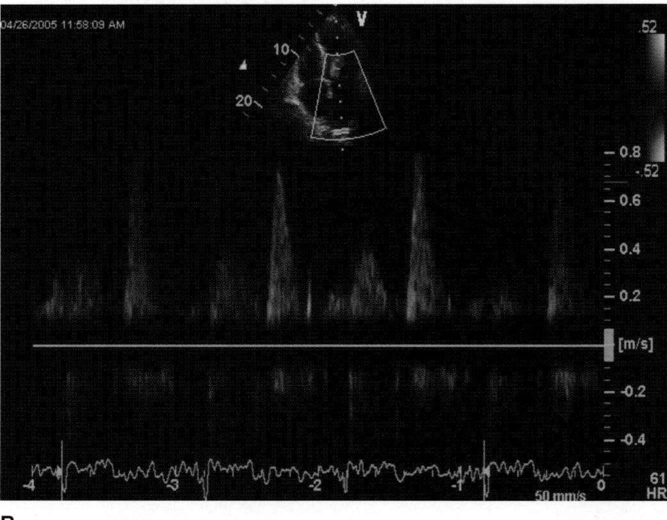

B

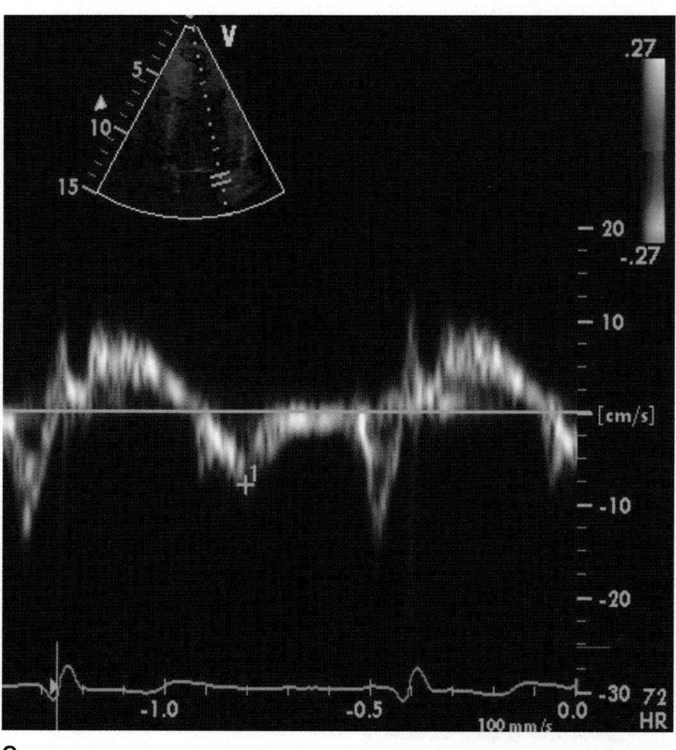

C

FIGURE 4-4-4 A Transmitral inflow pattern obtained on the inpatient echocardiogram. This spectral Doppler profile, obtained with the sample volume located at the leaflet tips, shows normal E wave velocity, E/A ratio, and E wave deceleration time. B Pulmonary venous inflow pattern obtained with the sample volume located in the ostium of the right upper pulmonary vein. This profile shows marked dominance of the diastolic (D) wave. This tracing is consistent with elevation in the left atrial pressure. C Tissue Doppler profile with the sample volume placed in the lateral annulus. In absolute terms the e wave velocity (e') is low, and the E/e' ratio is approximately 25. This is consistent with elevation in the left atrial pressure. This finding supports what was shown with the pulmonary venous tracing and the clinical diagnosis of heart failure.

die from noncardiovascular causes.[4-7] The presence of diastolic dysfunction with a preserved EF, therefore, likely represents a marker of increased risk more generally, above and beyond risk of cardiovascular complications.[7]

ETIOLOGY AND PATHOPHYSIOLOGY

Many studies have examined the pathophysiological basis that underlies HFpEF.

- As has been the case with regard to other aspects of this clinical syndrome, controversy persists as to the predominant mechanism of cardiac dysfunction that leads to HF.[6]
- Recently, attention has been focused on the role of the cardiac interstitium. Zile and colleagues have shown a panel of plasma biomarkers related to extracellular matrix (ECM) fibrillar collagen synthesis and degradation are more predictive of HFpEF than the use of N-terminal pro-B-type natriuretic peptide or clinical variables.[8]

- Other studies have identified other biomarkers reflective of myocardial fibrosis that are elevated in patients with HFpEF as well as in those with HFREF.
- Inflammation has been found to contribute to ECM remodeling and correlates with diastolic dysfunction.[8,9]
- Hypertension and the development of LV hypertrophy have been recognized as a major risk factor for HFpEF, although many patients with LVH and similar LV mass and left atrial volume do not have HF. Newer techniques to estimate left atrial strain and left atrial stiffness have been shown to be useful in differentiating patients with HFpEF from those with LVH without HF.[6]
- Investigators have looked at the pathophysiology in HFpEF patients under physical stress. Chronotropic incompetence, abnormal heart rate recovery, exercise-induced elevations in pulmonary capillary wedge pressure, and LV end-diastolic pressure, as well as pulmonary artery pressure, have been shown to be potentially useful measures of HFpEF.[6]

Whatever the predominant mechanism(s), the hallmark of diastolic dysfunction is the inability of the LV to fill at normal pressures.

- A study by Kumar, et al,[10] elegantly examined how diastolic dysfunction may progress to acute decompensated HF and the development of pulmonary edema, particularly in the presence of severe systemic hypertension, as in the case of our patient described above.
- In chronic congestive HF (CHF), the left atrial pressure can be elevated without clinical signs or symptoms of HF due to the adaptive response of the pulmonary lymphatic vessels.
- Acute pulmonary edema results when there is a sudden increase in left atrial and, consequently, pulmonary capillary pressure that overwhelms the adaptive capacity of the pulmonary lymphatics. An acute rise in systemic blood pressure (BP) is a common trigger.

With an acute rise in BP, as with other forms of physiologic stress, there is an increase in venous return to the right side of the heart.

- With normal right ventricular (RV) function, there is an acute increase in RV stroke volume into the pulmonary vasculature. In the setting of LV diastolic dysfunction, the increased volume results in an increase in left atrial pressure. This in turn leads to pulmonary vascular congestion, which promotes neurohumoral activation and elevated levels of catecholamines and activation of the renin-angiotensin system, further increasing systemic BP and venous return.
- Patient distress due to dyspnea and hypoxia also drives activation of these responses. This leads to a downward spiral ending in pulmonary edema and decompensated HF.
- Other factors that may also contribute include slowing of LV relaxation and increased LV stiffness due to increased myocardial turgor, and possibly ischemia resulting from compression of the coronary microvasculature from increased diastolic pressures.

DIAGNOSIS

Clinical Features

The clinical features that characterize an acute exacerbation of diastolic HF are essentially the same as those that accompany acute CHF from any cause. The patient reports dyspnea and is usually tachypneic and tachycardic. The patient may report cough and recent progressive weight gain, though this may not be present in the case of diastolic HF resulting from an acute rise in BP. On physical exam, bilateral rales, an S_3 gallop, and elevated jugular venous pressure and peripheral edema may be present.

Echocardiography

Echocardiography is the most important diagnostic test in the patient with suspected heart failure (see Section I, Echocardiography in the Evaluation of the Dyspneic Patient). This is due in part because of the limitations inherent in the clinical assessment of heart failure patients (in differentiating systolic from diastolic CHF), and in part because of the wealth of diagnostic information a comprehensive echo can provide.[11-14]

- The echocardiographic evaluation can rapidly rule out other important diagnoses that may be present in patients with HFpEF, such as severe left sided valvular heart disease or constrictive pericarditis.
- Doppler echocardiography has been used for the past 2 decades, to assess diastolic function and to estimate filling pressures (Figure 4-4-5). A detailed description of how Doppler patterns are used for this purpose can be found elsewhere.[11-14] Some points bear emphasis.
  - The standard transmitral velocity patterns give insight into left ventricular diastolic function and prognosis,[11] but are extremely sensitive to loading conditions, eg, left atrial pressure. For that reason, the standard transmitral flow data must be augmented by pulmonary vein flow data and tissue Doppler imaging (TDI).
  - TDI permits the direct measurement of the velocity of change in myocardial length, which is related to the integrity of left ventricular relaxation. A virtue of this technique is that it tends to be less sensitive to preload than the transmitral flow velocity Doppler approach and, accordingly, permits more accurate estimation of the filling pressures.

DIFFERENTIAL DIAGNOSIS

The differential diagnosis in a patient presenting with acute pulmonary edema includes acute (decompensation) of systolic CHF, acute myocardial ischemia, acute valvular dysfunction such as acute aortic or mitral regurgitation, and atrial fibrillation in the presence of mitral stenosis. In all patients with HFpEF, it is also important to investigate for potentially reversible causes, such as constrictive pericarditis, mitral stenosis, and primary mitral regurgitation.

FOLLOW-UP

Our patient was discharged after a 5-day hospitalization. Oral diuretics and an aggressive regimen to treat her BP was instituted. She was instructed on the importance of good BP control and sodium restriction and was advised to seek medical attention early if she develops recurrent symptoms. Early intervention in the outpatient setting may decrease the need for readmission. She was scheduled to follow up with her primary care physician and a cardiologist.

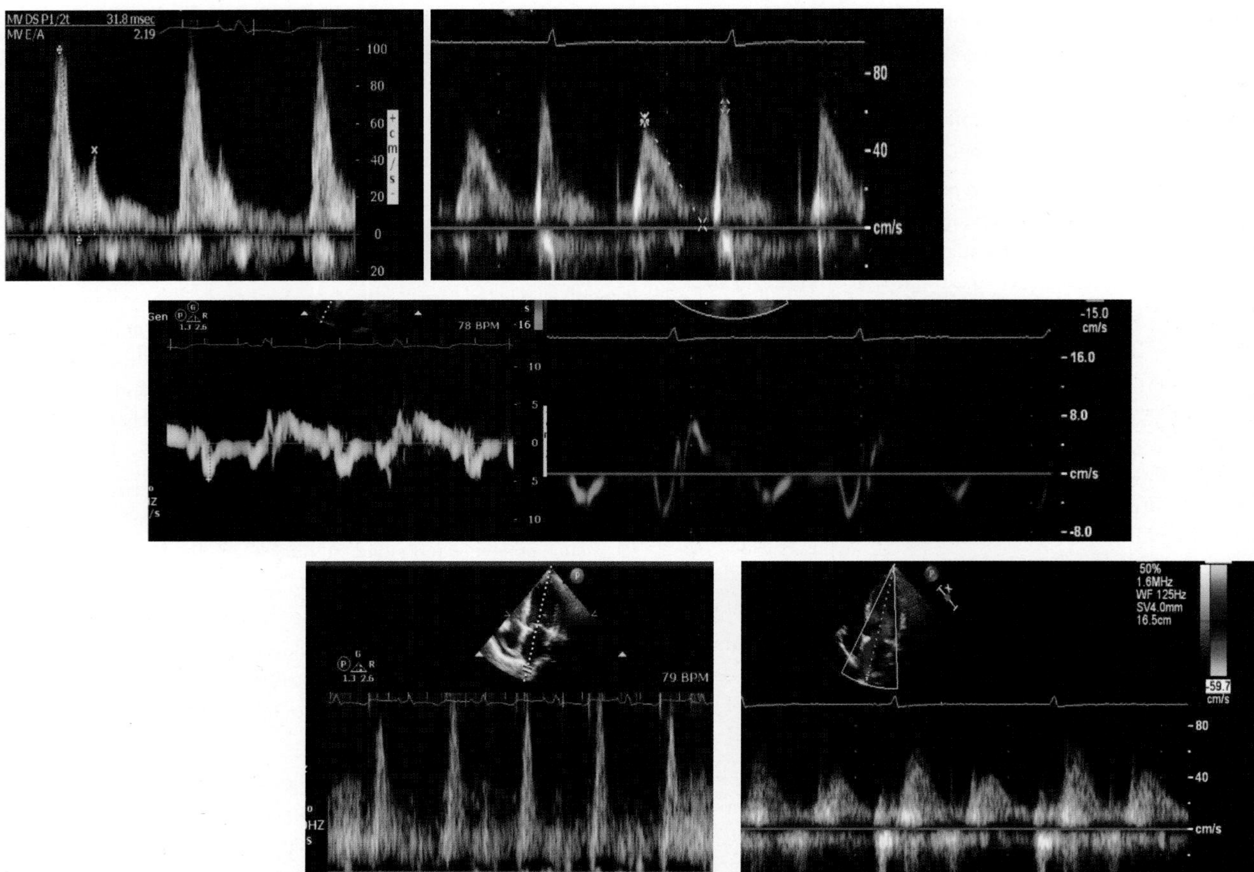

FIGURE 4-4-5 Transmitral inflow patterns (upper two panels), tissue Doppler profiles (middle two panels), and pulmonary venous inflow patterns (lower two panels) before (left panel in each pair) and after (right panel in each pair) treatment for heart failure. These parameters can be employed to assess diastolic function and filling pressures. Note that the restrictive pattern (tall E wave, rapid deceleration time, high E/e′ ratio, "D dominant" pulmonary venous pattern) changes after treatment. The E/A ratio is reduced, the pulmonary venous pattern becomes "S dominant", and the E/e′ ratio decreases. However, the absolute value of the e′ velocity does not change with treatment. This reflects the relative preload insensitivity of the tissue Doppler velocity. It is this property which allows the E/e′ ratio to be used to follow the effects of treatment for CHF. If the e′ velocity changed with treatment, the E/e′ ratio would be less useful as a gauge of left atrial pressure.

VIDEO LEGENDS

1. Video 4-4-3 A: Parasternal long axis demonstrating a normal EF
2. Video 4-4-3 B: Parasternal short axis demonstrating a normal EF. The relative wall thickness is increased
3. Video 4-4-3 C: Apical 4 chamber view demonstrating a normal to hyperdynamic LVEF. Note the LA enlargement.
4. Video 4-4-3 D: Apical 2 chamber view demonstrating a normal to hyperdynamic LVEF.

REFERENCES

1. Owan TE, Hodge DO, Herges RM, et al. Trends in prevalence and outcome of heart failure with preserved ejection fraction. *N Engl J Med*. 2006;355:251-259.
2. Bhatia RS, Tu JV, Lee DS, et al. Outcome of heart failure with preserved ejection fraction in a population-based study. *N Engl J Med*. 2006;355:260-269.
3. Redfield M M, Jacobsen S J, Burnett JC Jr, Mahoney DW, Bailey KR, Rodeheffer RJ. Burden of systolic and diastolic ventricular dysfunction in the community: appreciating the scope of the heart failure epidemic. *JAMA*. 2003;289(2):194-202.
4. Yancy CW, Lopatin M, Stevenson LW, DeMarco T, Fonarow GC. Clinical presentation, management, and in-hospital outcomes of patients admitted with acute decompensated heart failure with preserved systolic function: a report from the Acute Decompensated Heart Failure National Registry (ADHERE) Database. *J Am Coll Cardiol*. 2006;47:76-84.
5. Campbell RT, Jhund PS, Castagno D, Hawkins NM, Petrie MC, McMurray JJ. What have we learned about patients with heart failure and preserved ejection fraction from DIG-PEF, CHARM-Preserved, and I-PRESERVE? *J Am Coll Cardiol*. 2012;60:2349-2356.
6. Udelson JE. Heart failure with preserved ejection fraction. *Circulation*. 2011;124:e540-e543.
7. Kitzman DW, Little WC. Left ventricle diastolic dysfunction and prognosis. *Circulation*. 2012;125:743-745.
8. Zile, MR, Baicu CF, Gaasch WH, et al. Diastolic heart failure—abnormalities in active relaxation and passive stiffness of the left ventricle. *N Engl J Med*. 2004;350(19):1953-1959.

9. Barasch E, Gottdiener JS, Aurigemma GP, et al. The relationship between serum markers of collagen turnover and cardiovascular outcome in the elderly: the Cardiovascular Health Study. *Circ Heart Fail*. 2011;4(6):733-739.
10. Kumar R, Gandhi SK, Little WC. Acute heart failure with preserved systolic function. *Crit Care Med*. 2008;36(1 Suppl):S52-6.
11. Nagueh SF, Appleton CP, Gillebert TC, et al. Recommendations for the evaluation of left ventricular diastolic function by echocardiography. *Eur J Echocardiogr* 2009;10:165-193.
12. Aurigemma GP, Gaasch WH. Clinical practice. Diastolic heart failure. *N Engl J Med*. 2004;351(11):1097-1105.
13. Little WC, Oh JK. Echocardiographic evaluation of diastolic function can be used to guide clinical care. *Circulation*. 2009;120(9):802-809.
14. Oh JK, Hatle L, Tajik AJ, Little WC. Diastolic heart failure can be diagnosed by comprehensive two-dimensional and Doppler echocardiography. *J Am Coll Cardiol*. 2006;47(3):500-506.

SECTION 5

Echocardiography in Congestive Heart Failure: Utility in Patient Selection for Device Therapy

Brigid M. Carlson, MD, and Gerard. P. Aurigemma, MD, FAHA, FASE, FACC

CLINICAL CASE PRESENTATION

A 50-year-old man with a history of severe hypertension and significant alcohol consumption is hospitalized for shortness of breath. He has a long-standing history of hypertension which began in his late twenties. The hypertension is considered to be resistant in that he has been prescribed more than 3 drugs without success. The medications include a thiazide diuretic, β-blocker, and ACE inhibitor. He also consumes approximately 2 to 3 cans of beer per day and has untreated sleep apnea. He smokes 1 to 2 packs of cigarettes per day. There is no history of chest discomfort, syncope, or pre-syncope. The family history is positive for coronary artery disease in both parents.

Physical examination reveals a disheveled, middle-aged, man in mild respiratory distress. His blood pressure is 240/116 mm Hg, his heart rate 78 beats/min, and his respirations 20 breaths/min. He has increased jugular venous pressure to the angle of the jaw sitting upright. The exam is otherwise remarkable for diffuse rales, normal first and second heart sounds, and a summation gallop. He has a grade 2/6 holosystolic apical murmur radiating to the apex. There is 2+ non-pitting edema of both lower extremities. The electrocardiogram (Figure 4-5-1) shows sinus rhythm, left ventricular hypertrophy with nonspecific ST-wave changes, and borderline LV hypertrophy. The admission chest x-ray (Figure 4-5-2) shows cardiomegaly but no significant parenchymal lung disease or significant pulmonary edema. Laboratory examination is remarkable for normal glomerular filtration rate. BNP is 825 ng/L

The patient was admitted to the hospital, and an echocardiogram was performed, which demonstrated a thick walled LV with globally reduced EF, estimated to be in the 25% to 30% range, both visually and by biplane method of disks. Eccentric hypertrophy is evident (Figure 4-5-3). Figure 4-5-4 shows the transmitral filling pattern. The transmitral E wave is 100 cm/s. There is a rapid deceleration time (120 ms). These findings of a tall E wave, elevated E/A ratio, and rapid deceleration time constitute a restrictive filling pattern. Figure 4-5-5 shows the right upper pulmonary vein spectral Doppler pattern. There is a diastolic (D) dominant pattern, indicative of an elevated mean left atrial pressure. Tissue Doppler, obtained with the sample volume in the left lateral annulus, shows a peak diastolic velocity (e') of 5.4 cm/s (Figure 4-5-6). The E/e' ratio is approximately 25, consistent with elevated filling pressures. These Doppler findings are concordant in indicating elevated filling pressures and support both the clinical and x-ray findings.

In order to investigate the reason for heart failure, he undergoes left and right heart catheterization. His ejection fraction by ventriculography is judged to be 25%, and there are areas of hypokinesis and akinesis. There is no obstructive coronary artery disease. His left ventricular end-diastolic pressure is 22 mm Hg, and the pulmonary capillary wedge pressure is 18 mm Hg.

In view of the profoundly reduced systolic function found on this echocardiogram, as well as evidence of elevated filling pressures, he is treated for acute left- and right-sided heart failure with intravenous and then oral furosemide. He is also treated with amlodipine, lisinopril, and metoprolol succinate.

In the course of his hospital stay, it becomes clear he has been noncompliant with his medical regimen, and he confesses that he takes his medications sporadically, if at all. Consideration is given for implantation of an automatic implantable cardioverter defibrillator (AICD) because of the finding of nonischemic cardiomyopathy. The patient states he will do anything in his power to avoid "cardiac surgery." It is suggested to him that aggressive treatment of his hypertension and cessation of alcohol intake will conceivably help him avert an AICD.

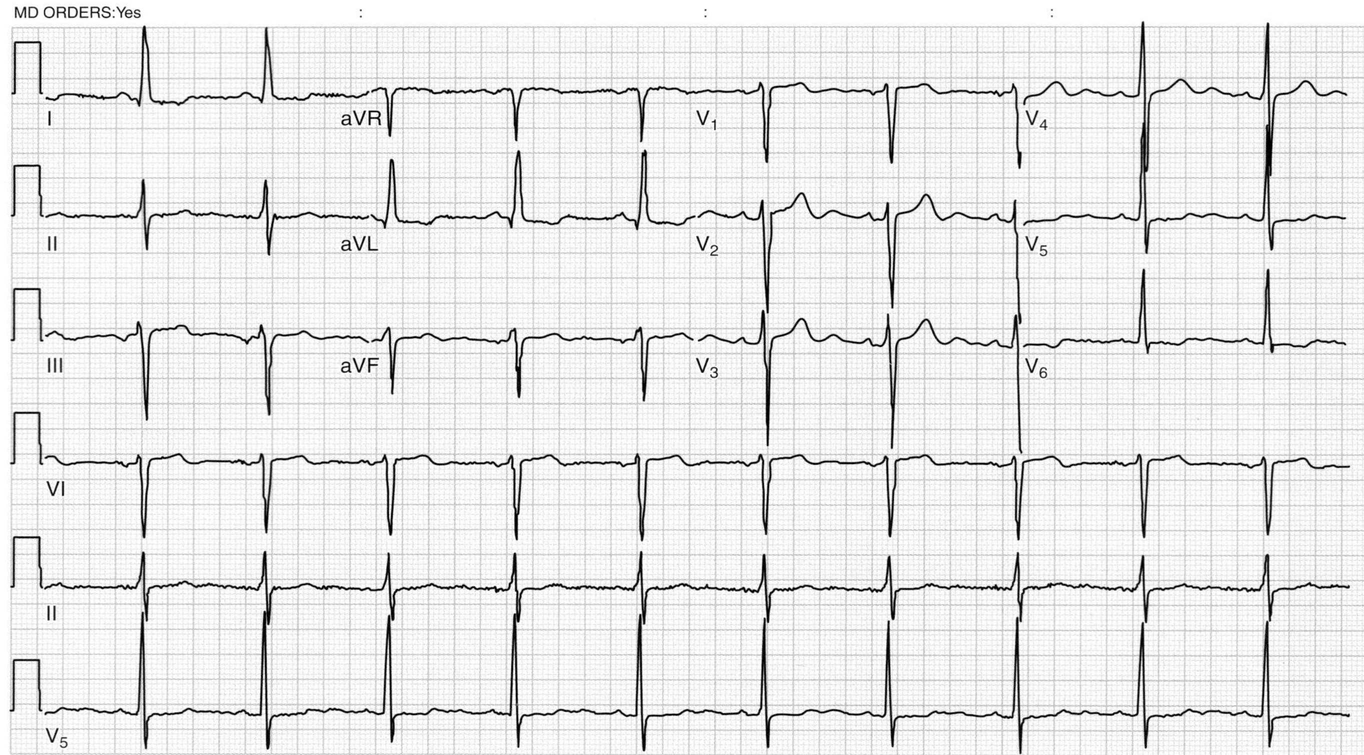

FIGURE 4-5-1 The ECG from our patient demonstrates sinus rhythm, left ventricular hypertrophy with nonspecific ST-wave changes, and borderline LV hypertrophy.

He promises that he will be more faithful with his medical regimen and follow-up visits with the doctor.

FOLLOW-UP

He is compliant with follow-up visits. Six months after the index hospitalization, he undergoes a repeat echo to reassess his LVEF to determine if he is a candidate for an AICD. Figure 4-5-7 and the accompanying videos demonstrate the apical 4 and apical 2 chamber view from that study. There is now evidence of low-normal systolic function, with an ejection fraction, estimated by biplane method of disks, at 55%. Figures 4-5-8 to 4-5-10 show the results of Doppler interrogation of diastolic function. Doppler examination no longer shows a restrictive filling pattern. The tissue Doppler e' is now 7 cm/s; the pulmonary venous flow pattern is now consistent with normal left atrial pressure. The E/e' ratio is now approximately 11.

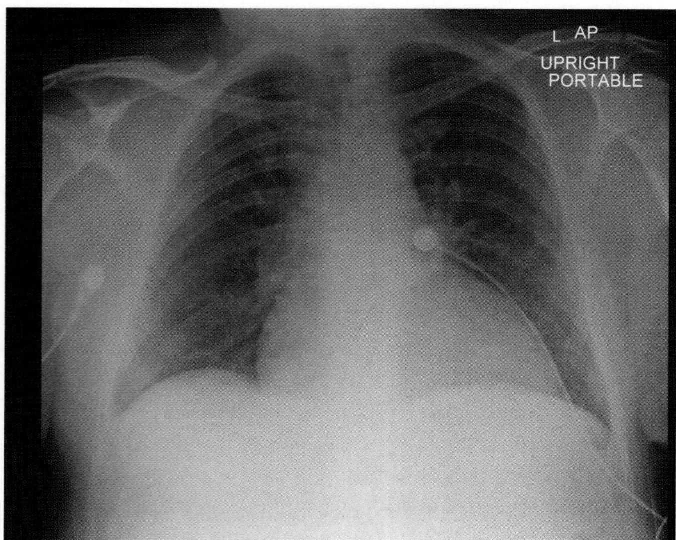

FIGURE 4-5-2 The admission chest x-ray shows cardiomegaly but no significant parenchymal lung disease or significant pulmonary edema.

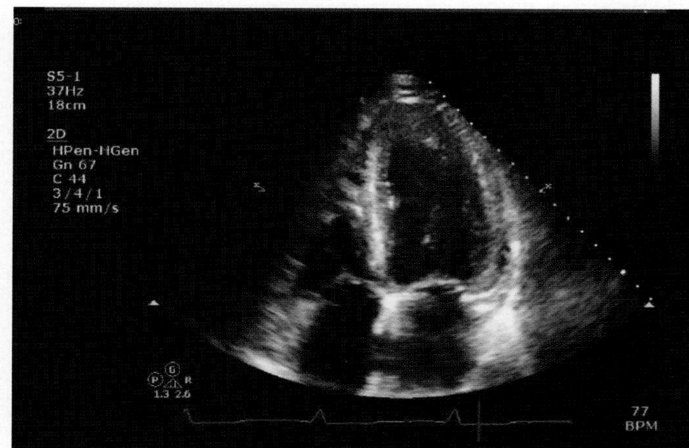

FIGURE 4-5-3 The apical 4 chamber view demonstrates global LV dysfunction ▶ (see Videos 4-5-3 A and B).

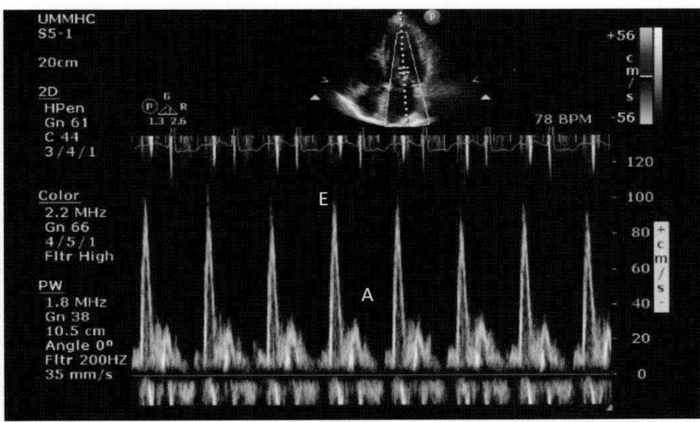

FIGURE 4-5-4 Transmitral Doppler flow pattern demonstrates an increased E/A ratio and short deceleration time (see text for details).

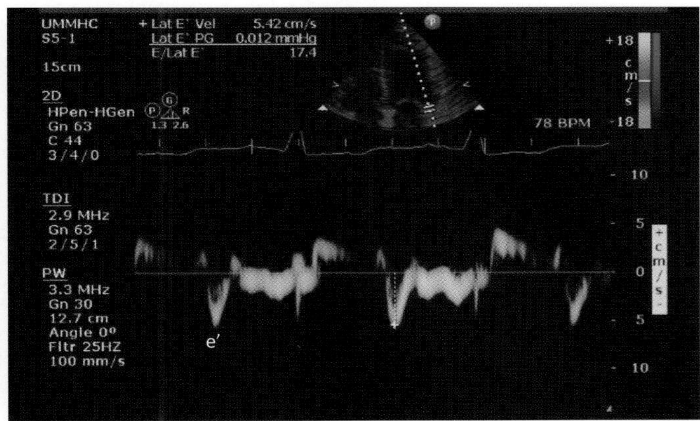

FIGURE 4-5-6 Tissue Doppler, obtained with the sample volume in the left lateral annulus, shows a peak diastolic velocity (e′) of 5.4 cm/s (see text for details).

DIAGNOSIS, MANAGEMENT/DECISION MAKING AND THE ROLE OF ECHOCARDIOGRAPHY

The epidemiology, etiology and pathophysiology, Diagnostic evaluation and the role of echocardiography, laboratory evaluation and patient management in a patient with new onset systolic dysfunction are addressed in other sections of this chapter as well as in Chapter 5 and will not be reviewed here.

This case highlights many issues which a clinician will encounter in practice. These issues include the importance of patient education (eg, medication compliance), a comprehensive initial evaluation (including a detailed social history), and the importance of follow-up.

Two major points are made concerning the role of comprehensive echocardiography in this situation:

- The first is that certain types of left ventricular dysfunction are reversible. Certain conditions that feature reversible dysfunction and are reasonably common include stress cardiomyopathy and tachycardia-mediated cardiomyopathy, as discussed elsewhere in this chapter and in Chapter 5.[1] Our patient most likely had left ventricular systolic and diastolic dysfunction due to a combination of poorly treated hypertension and the toxic effects of alcohol (see Section II, Alcoholic Cardiomyopathy).
- It is difficult to tell on the initial echocardiogram whether systolic dysfunction is reversible.[1] In hypertensive cardiomyopathy, the finding of a thick-walled ventricle with global systolic dysfunction is suggestive of unrelieved pressure overload.
- Predicting recovery of systolic function is more challenging when there is a picture of eccentric hypertrophy and/or of wall motion abnormality, as was the case here.

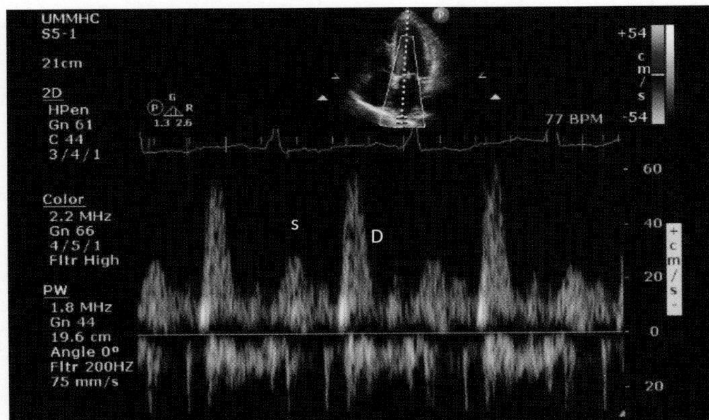

FIGURE 4-5-5 Pulmonary vein Doppler signal demonstrates systolic blunting with diastolic predominance (see text for details).

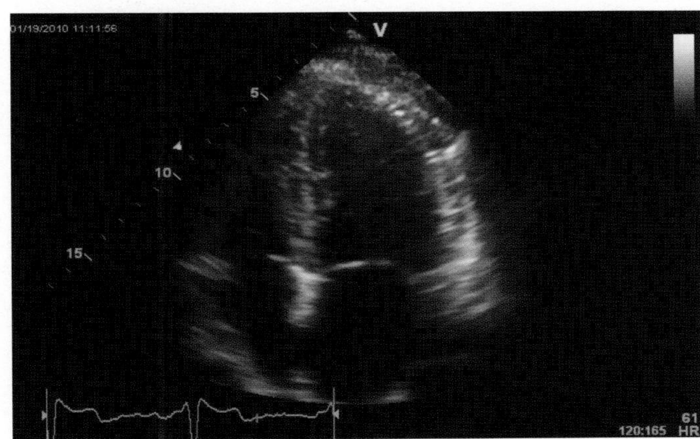

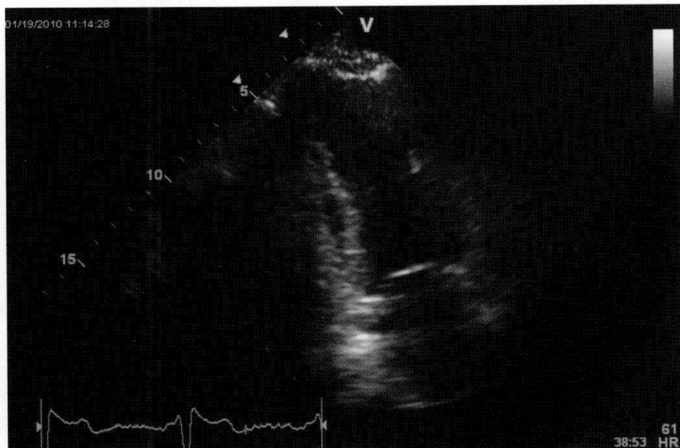

FIGURE 4-5-7 Apical 4 chamber view (top panel) and 2 chamber view (bottom panel) from the follow-up echo demonstrating improvement in LV EF (see Videos 4-5-7 A and B).

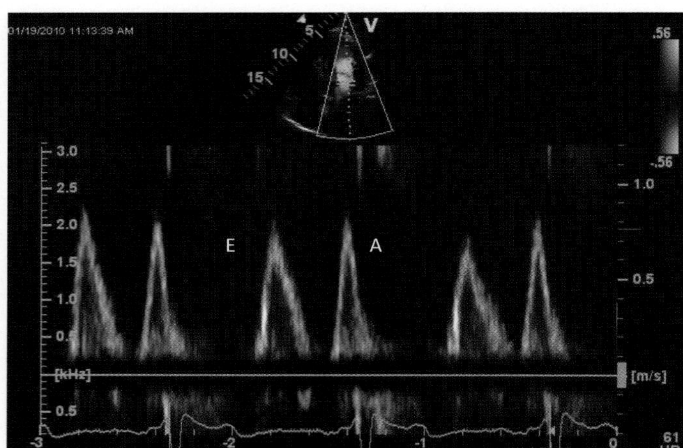

FIGURE 4-5-8 Transmitral Doppler flow pattern from the follow-up echo demonstrating a much lower E/A ratio and more normal deceleration time indicative of improved hemodynamics (see text for details).

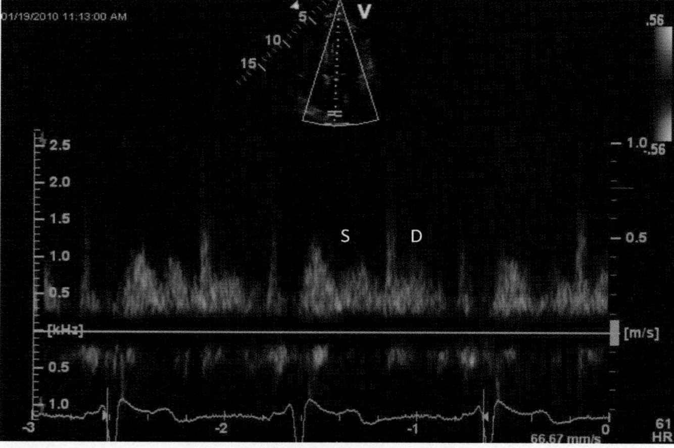

FIGURE 4-5-9 Pulmonary vein Doppler signal from the follow-up echo demonstrates a normal and diastolic flow pattern (see text for details).

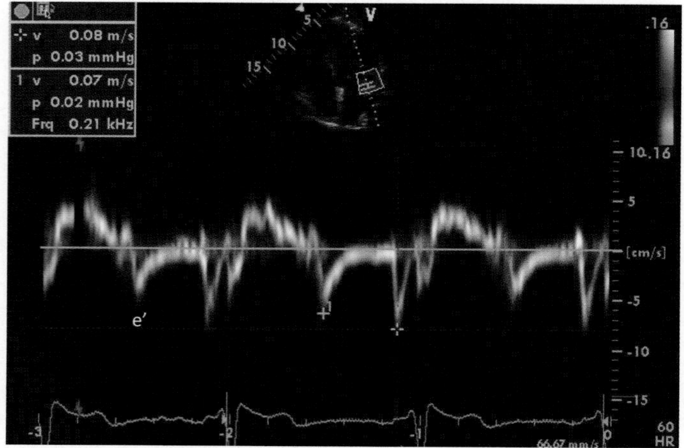

FIGURE 4-5-10 Tissue Doppler, obtained from the follow-up echo, shows a peak diastolic velocity (e') of 7 cm/s (see text for details).

- The diastolic function changes are quite illustrative in this case. The findings on the initial study supported the diagnosis of severe diastolic dysfunction with elevated filling pressure.[2] This was confirmed by the invasive study.
- With treatment of hypertension and cessation of alcohol intake, however, the patient improved clinically, and the Doppler findings mirrored this clinical improvement. The transmitral flow pattern changed from "restrictive" to normal; the E/e' ratio, used as an index of left atrial pressure, changed dramatically. These findings are mirrored by the pulmonary venous flow, which also supports a shift from elevated left atrial pressure to normal left atrial pressure.
- The absolute value for the tissue Doppler e' did not change significantly. This is because in abnormal hearts, the e' velocity is relatively preload insensitive.[2] The E/e' ratio is preload sensitive, and this is the key to its utility in following filling pressures in patients undergoing medical treatment for heart failure.
- The second management point related to echocardiography is that the selection of patients for AICD therapy usually depends on the two-dimensional echocardiogram.
- In most recent heart failure guidelines, AICD is recommended for patients with an LVEF (based in large part on an echocardiographic assessment) of less than or equal to 35% and mild to moderate symptoms of HF "in whom survival with good functional capacity is otherwise anticipated to extend beyond 1 year."[3]
- This recommendation is supported by two clinical trials which enrolled patients with cardiomyopathy: SCD-HeFT and DEFINITE.[4,5] Both ischemic and nonischemic etiologies of heart failure were included in SCD-HeFT (EF ≤30%), while DEFINITE enrolled only patients with nonischemic cardiomyopathy (EF <36%). Implantation of an AICD was associated with a 23% reduction in overall death in SCD-HeFT and a significant reduction in death from cardiac arrhythmia in DEFINITE, but only a borderline reduction in all cause mortality in that study.[5]
- Unfortunately, there is study to study variability in EF by echo, caused by both clinical factors and the inherent variability of the technique.[6,7] In these regards, echocardiography is no different than any other diagnostic test. When this has been studied in "real world" clinical practice, the variability in EF, in patients where no important clinical change had occurred, averaged 6%.[7]
- For these reasons, the ESC guidelines recommend that AICD implantation "should be considered only after a sufficient period of optimization of medical therapy (at least 3 months) and only if the EF remains persistently low."[8] This case illustrates the wisdom in this recommendation.

FOLLOW-UP

At one year following the initial hospitalization, the patient continues to feel well; his blood pressure is well-controlled, and he is compliant with his medical regimen. He has cut down on his drinking. His echocardiogram is now completely normal, with a normal EF and normal Doppler flow patterns, other than a low but improved e' velocity. There is no further discussion concerning an AICD. He continues to follow up with his primary care physician who continues to stress the importance of medication compliance and avoidance of alcohol.

VIDEO LEGENDS

1. Video 4-5-3 A: Apical four chamber view from the initial echo demonstrating globally reduced LVEF
2. Video 4-5-3 B: Apical two chamber view from the initial echo demonstrating globally reduced LVEF
3. Video 4-5-7 A: Apical four chamber view from the follow up echo demonstrating improved global LVEF
4. Video 4-5-7 B: Apical two chamber view from the follow up echo demonstrating improved global LVEF

REFERENCES

1. Aurigemma GP, Tighe DA. Echocardiography and reversible left ventricular dysfunction. *Am J Med*. 2006;119(1):18-21.
2. Nagueh SF, Appleton CP, Gillebert TC, et al. Recommendations for the evaluation of left ventricular diastolic function by echocardiography. *J Am Soc Echocardiogr*. 2009;22(2):107-133.
3. Hunt SA, Abraham WT, Chin MH, et al. 2009 Focused update incorporated into the ACC/AHA 2005 Guidelines for the Diagnosis and Management of Heart Failure in Adults: a report of the American College of Cardiology Foundation/American Heart Association Task Force on Practice Guidelines: developed in collaboration with the International Society for Heart and Lung Transplantation. *J Am Coll Cardiol*. 2009;53(15):e1-e90.
4. Bardy GH, Lee KL, Mark DB, et al. Amiodarone or an implantable cardioverter-defibrillator for congestive heart failure. *N Engl J Med*. 2005;352:225-237.
5. Kadish A, Dyer A, Daubert J, et al. Prophylactic defibrillator implantation in patients with nonischemic dilated cardiomyopathy. *N Engl J Med*. 2004;350:2151-2158. doi: 10.1056/NEJMoa033088.
6. Hare, JL, Brown JK, Marwick TH. Performance of conventional echocardiographic parameters and myocardial measurements in the sequential evaluation of left ventricular function. *Am J Cardiol*. 2008;101(5):706-711.
7. Joffe SW, Ferrara J, Chalian A, Tighe DA, Aurigemma GP, Goldberg RJ. Are ejection fraction measurements by echocardiography and left ventriculography equivalent? *Am Heart J*. 2009;158(3):496-502.
8. McMurray JJ, Adamopoulos S, Anker SD, et al. ESC guidelines for the diagnosis and treatment of acute and chronic heart failure 2012: The Task Force for the Diagnosis and Treatment of Acute and Chronic Heart Failure. *Eur J Heart Fail*. 2012;14(8):803-69. doi: 10.1093/eurjhf/hfs105.

SECTION 6

Ventricular Dyssynchrony and Cardiac Resynchronization Therapy

Anthony Garcia, MD, and Gerard P. Aurigemma, MD, FAHA, FASE, FACC

CLINICAL CASE PRESENTATION

An 88-year-old woman was admitted to the hospital for the third time in one month for an episode of rapid onset pulmonary edema. She has a longstanding history of hypertension, but no history of myocardial infarction or heart failure, until recently. Two months prior to this admission, she was hospitalized in another city, while on vacation with her children, for syncope. At that time, she underwent permanent pacemaker implantation and was discharged after an uneventful hospital stay. Six weeks prior to admission she was moved by her daughter and son to an assisted living facility. She was subsequently hospitalized at our institution for "pneumonia," treated with antibiotics, and discharged. However, she subsequently had three episodes of pulmonary edema, each associated with a rapid onset of symptoms of breathlessness, all of which were treated successfully with diuresis. At the time of the fourth admission, a cardiac work up was initiated.

At the time of examination, the patient had improved considerably after the administration of intravenous furosemide and nitrates. Vital signs were notable for a blood pressure of 168/70 mg Hg, pulse 80 beats/min and regular, and O_2 saturation on 2 L of oxygen by nasal cannula was 96%. There were rales throughout all lung fields, a paradoxically split S_2, a systolic ejection murmur, and a holosystolic murmur at the apex. There was no increase in jugular venous pressure, nor was there peripheral edema. The admission ECG showed evidence of a dual chamber pacemaker, and the chest x-ray was notable for signs of pulmonary edema (Figures 4-6-1 and 4-6-2). She underwent echocardiography (Figures 4-6-3 and 4-6-4) and dipyridamole nuclear stress imaging (Figure 4-6-5).

The constellation of findings of severe LV dysfunction in the absence of severe coronary artery disease by perfusion imaging, and the clinical circumstances of recurrent pulmonary edema following closely upon the insertion of a dual chamber pacemaker, led to speculation that cardiac dyssynchrony was partially responsible for the patient's signs and symptoms. The echocardiogram was consistent

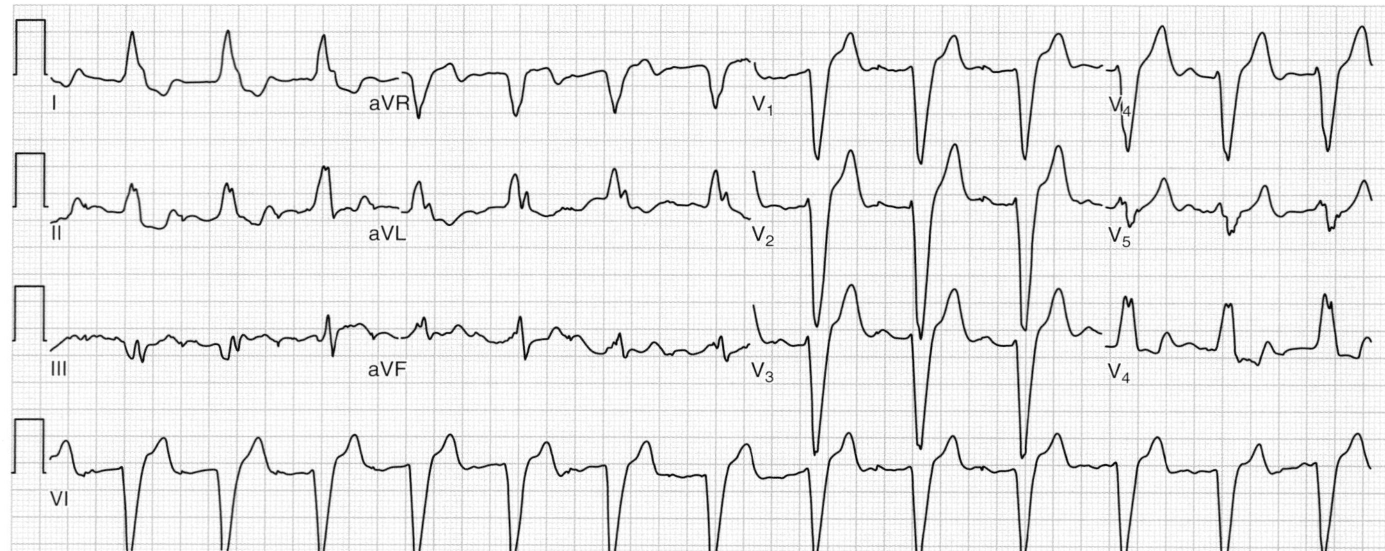

FIGURE 4-6-1 Twelve lead ECG at the time of the current admission showing evidence of dual chamber pacing and left bundle branch block morphology.

with this hypothesis. After a period of optimal medical therapy, she eventually underwent cardiac resynchronization therapy with a biventricular pacemaker. Over the ensuing 18 months, she has only had one episode of recurrent heart failure, and her echocardiogram. demonstrates a remarkable improvement in systolic function (Figures 4-6-6 and 4-6-7).

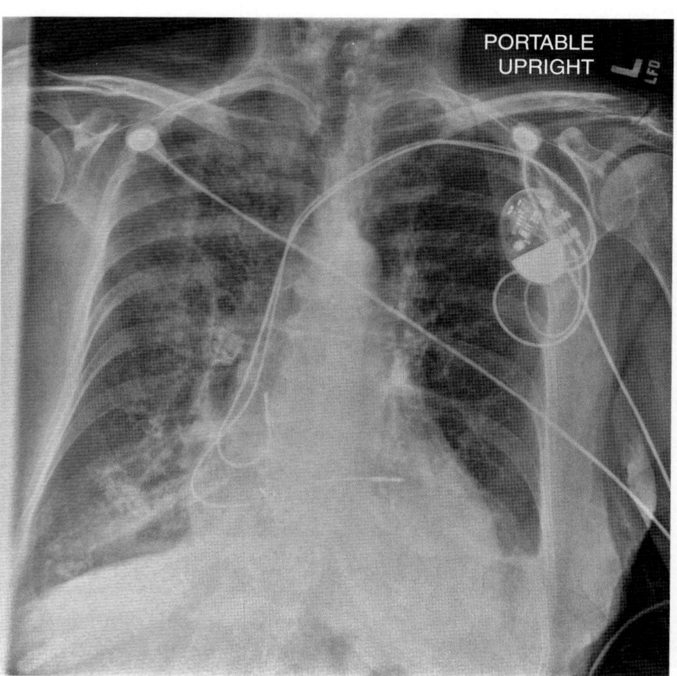

FIGURE 4-6-2 Admission chest radiograph showing evidence of pulmonary vascular congestion, as well as evidence of right atrial and right ventricular pacemaker leads. The cardiac silhouette is minimally enlarged.

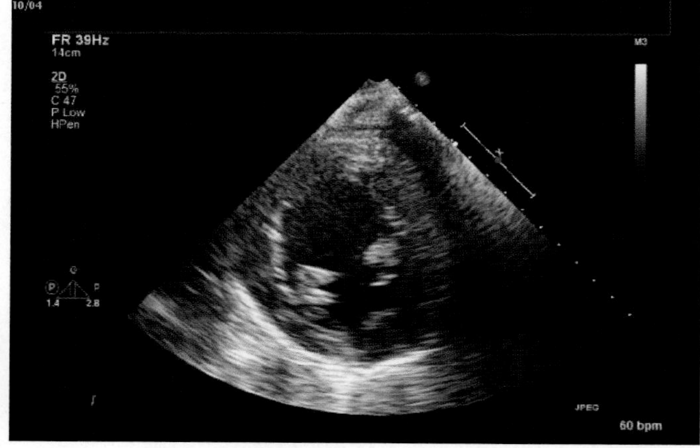

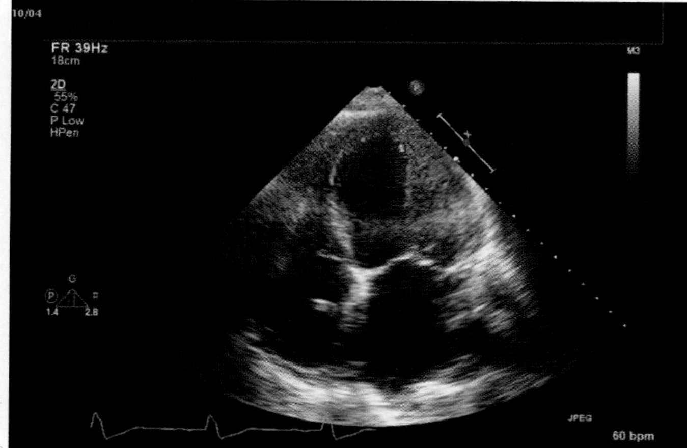

FIGURE 4-6-3 Parasternal short axis (upper panel) and apical four chamber (lower panel) views ▶ (see Videos 4-6-3 L and R) demonstrating LV dysfunction and marked dyssynchrony. Pacemaker wires are seen in the right heart.

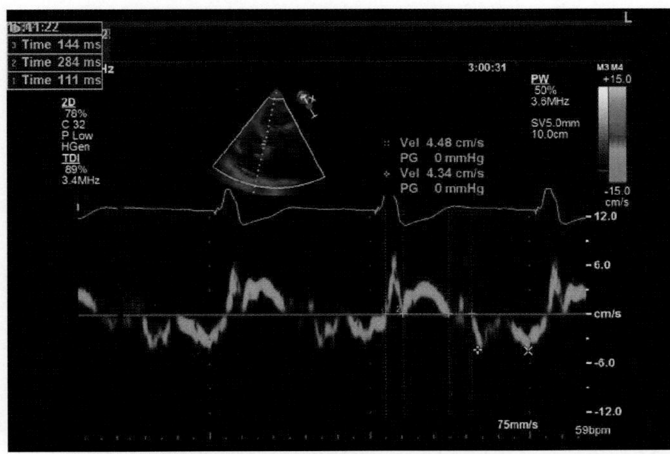

FIGURE 4-6-4 From the patient's echocardiogram, obtained prior to cardiac resynchronization therapy, a tissue Doppler tracing from the septal mitral annulus is shown. Based on the measured intervals of isovolumic relaxation time (IVRT), isovolumic contraction time (IVCT), and left ventricular ejection time (LVET), the Tei index [(IVRT + IVCT)/LVET] is calculated to be 0.90. A higher Tei index, as in this case, has been shown to be a marker of dyssynchrony.

PHYSIOLOGY

To transfer the energy of myocardial contraction to the ejection of blood requires coordinated electrical activation of the ventricles. Conduction system disease can lead to a perturbation in this finely tuned pump mechanism.[1]

- A large proportion of heart failure patients who undergo cardiac imaging show signs of dyssynchrony.
- Pacing the heart from multiple locations, termed cardiac resynchronization therapy (CRT), is designed to re-establish more efficient ventricular activation.
- In the majority of patients with advanced systolic dysfunction, CRT improves symptoms, decreases hospitalizations, and increases survival.[2]
- However, up to 30% of heart failure patients derive little, if any, clinical benefit,[3] underscoring the need for better strategies to identify CRT responders.

PATHOPHYSIOLOGY

Conduction through an intact His-Purkinje system allows the ventricle to efficiently translate myocardial contraction into mechanical work in a "synchronous" fashion.

- Conduction delays caused by left bundle branch block (LBBB), either spontaneous or caused by right ventricular pacing, can lead to dyssynchronous contraction. This mechanical dyssynchrony, in turn, leads to a decrease in stroke work, stroke volume, and rate of rise of left ventricular pressure.
- In a series of elegant electromechanical timing studies, Prinzen and coworkers have shown that in patients with LBBB, the interventricular septum begins depolarization more than 100 ms before the basal lateral wall, with the result that the septum contracts before the aortic valve opens. Instead of contributing to the ejection of blood, the work of septal contraction leads to elevations in regional preload along the lateral wall. The significant delay in regional activation subverts the accumulated Starling forces along the lateral wall, as they act after left ventricular ejection nears completion.[1]
- Dyssynchrony also impairs ventricular diastolic function. Delayed depolarization of certain wall segments prolongs isovolumic contraction. Likewise, segmental delays in repolarization lead to prolonged isovolumic relaxation. Longer isovolumic times reduce the time for diastolic filling. The result is a decrease in preload as the ventricle enters its next systolic cycle.[1]
- Measures of mechanical and electrical dyssynchrony do not correlate well with one another. While no imaging parameter for mechanical dyssynchrony has emerged as predictive of CRT response, clinical trials show that heart failure patients with QRS durations >150 ms and LBBB stand to benefit the most from CRT.[4]

ECHOCARDIOGRAPHY

As has been explored elsewhere in this chapter, echocardiography plays a critical role in the evaluation and management of the patient with CHF. In patients with conduction disturbances (wide QRS), echocardiography may play a role in the assessment of dyssynchrony.

- Patients with dyssynchrony due to LBBB display numerous echocardiographic abnormalities. Although not specific, increased LV end-diastolic volume, increased LV end-systolic volume, and slightly diminished left ventricular ejection fraction (LVEF) are all associated with LBBB.[5,6]
- The loss of synchronous repolarization also leads to Doppler patterns characteristic of diastolic dysfunction, including decreases in E velocity, E/A ratio, and deceleration time.[5,7]
- Furthermore, total isovolumic time (T-IVT), measured from Doppler signals at the mitral leaflet tips, is typically prolonged, evidence of inefficient LV contraction and relaxation.
- In addition, the Tei index, typically used as a global marker of systolic and diastolic function, turns out to be abnormally high in patients with isolated LBBB.[8]
- Approximately 30% of all patients who meet clinical criteria for biventricular pacing do not achieve any of the endpoints used in CRT trials: improvement in functional status by at least one NYHA class, decrease in hospitalizations, or decrease in mortality.[3]
- Predicting who may benefit from CRT remains an area of active research, and a variety of echocardiographic features have been explored in an effort to improve patient selection for CRT.
    - In the presence of dyssynchrony, the time from the start of the QRS complex to peak strain (radial or longitudinal) varies substantially by LV region.[4,9] Thus, strain imaging may emerge as a tool for predicting response to CRT.[4]
    - Earlier research using an index of time to peak tissue velocity did not consistently correlate with severity of dyssynchrony.[7,8]
    - On the other hand, longer T-IVTs during native conduction at peak pharmacologic stress were associated with larger gains in peak oxygen consumption with CRT.[10]
    - Although numerous echocardiographic parameters are associated with mechanical dyssynchrony, no single measurement can, as of yet, accurately predict which patients will derive clinical benefit from CRT.[4] Thus, at the present time patient selection for CRT

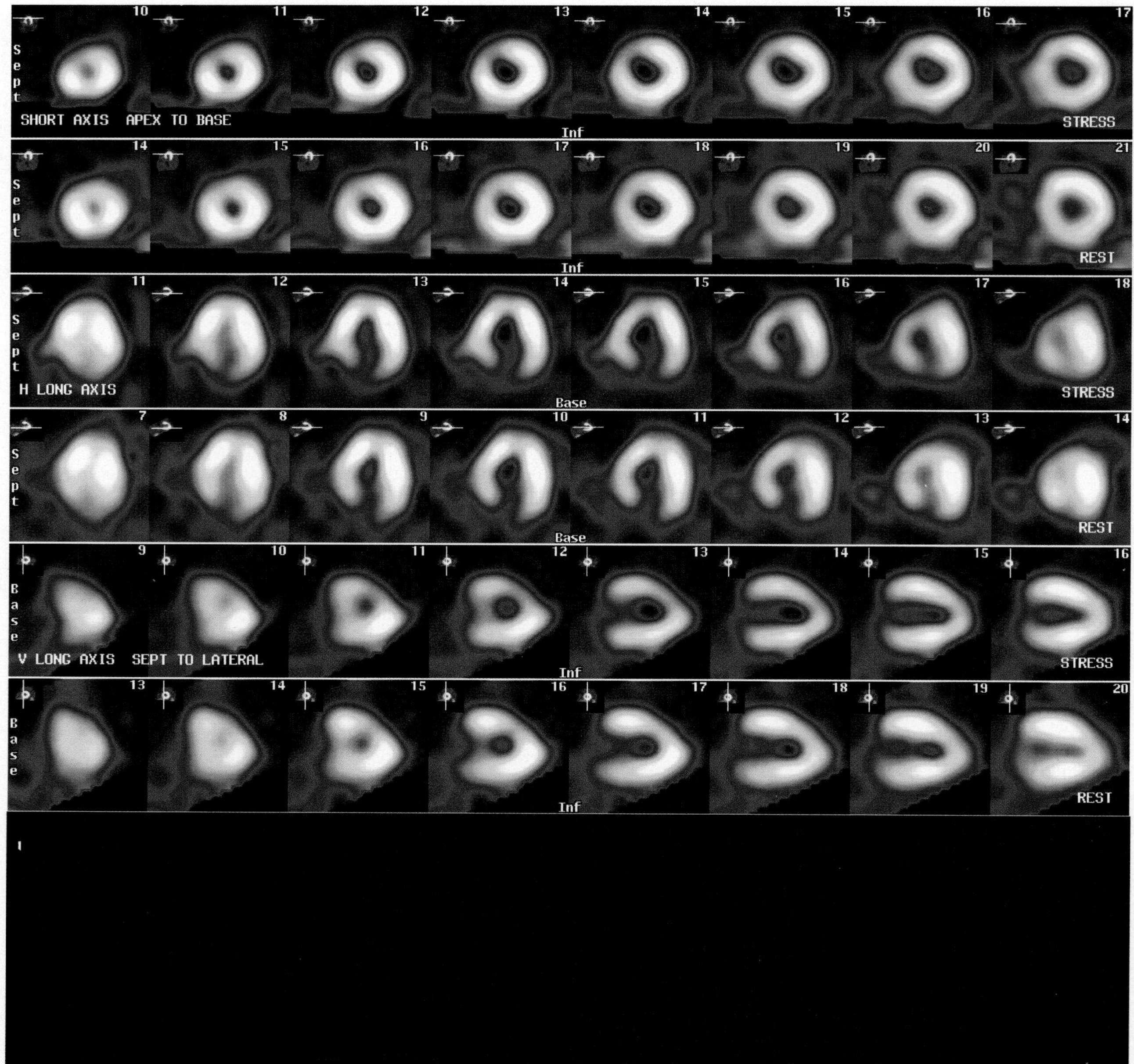

FIGURE 4-6-5 Dipyridamole myocardial perfusion images are displayed, significant for stress images that show a moderately sized area of moderately decreased tracer uptake in the mid-to-distal anteroseptal wall. Rest images show partial redistribution within this defect. Findings are consistent with a small area of infarct accompanied by a small area of peri-infarct ischemia.

is guided by clinical and ECG findings, though echocardiographic parameters suggestive of mechanical dyssynchrony may provide additional evidence to support CRT therapy.

DIAGNOSIS

A prolonged QRS complex is usually the first clue to the presence of dyssynchrony. Any number of echocardiographic signs of dyssynchrony may also be present, although these are not necessary for determining eligibility for CRT. In general, CRT is indicated for patients with an LVEF ≤35% and a QRS duration ≥120 ms. From this heterogeneous group of patients, as stated previously, it remains a challenge to identify those who are likely to benefit.[11]

DIFFERENTIAL DIAGNOSIS

The patient with systolic heart failure may have impaired exercise tolerance for a wide variety of cardiac and noncardiac reasons. Cardiovascular pathologies frequently coexist, such as valvular disease, ischemic heart disease, endothelial dysfunction, and diastolic dysfunction. Pericardial disease, shunts, and orthostasis may also limit exercise. Interventricular dyssynchrony and atrioventricular delay may also contribute to symptoms. Noncardiovascular comorbidities that may directly contribute to exercise intolerance include pulmonary disease, anemia, thyroid disease, and nutritional deficiency.[12]

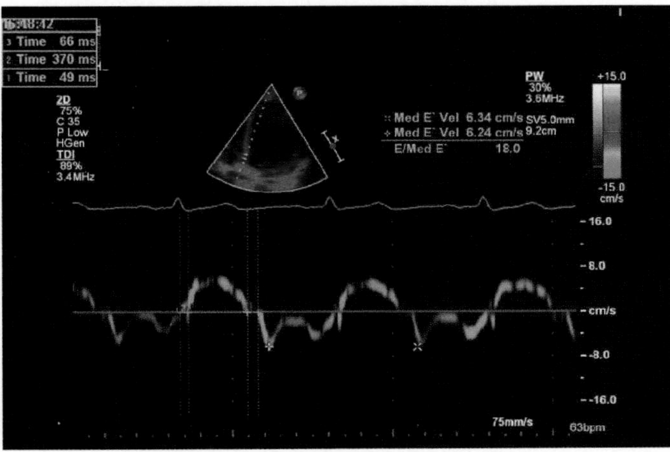

FIGURE 4-6-6 From the patient's echocardiogram, obtained following cardiac resynchronization therapy, a tissue Doppler tracing from the septal mitral annulus is shown. Based on the measured intervals of isovolumic relaxation time (IVRT), isovolumic contraction time (IVCT), and left ventricular ejection time (LVET), the Tei index [(IVRT + IVCT)/LVET] is calculated to be 0.31. The Tei index decreased from 0.9, calculated prior to cardiac resynchronization therapy, and represents improved left ventricular synchrony.

MANAGEMENT

Biventricular pacing, i.e. CRT, is the treatment for dyssynchrony among eligible patients with heart failure. Device implantation is carried out with the patient on optimal medical therapy.

- Prior to CRT, echocardiography is usually obtained to determine eligibility based on LVEF.
- Due to their low sensitivity, echocardiographic parameters of dyssynchrony that are within normal limits should not be used to withhold CRT from a patient.[13]
- Major society guidelines include an LVEF ≤35% and QRS duration >120 ms as indications for CRT. Among these eligible patients with class III CHF, biventricular pacing is more likely to benefit those with a QRS interval >150 ms, LBBB and NYHA class III symptoms.
- Patients with NYHA class IV symptoms who are ambulatory may also derive similar benefits.
- While patients with NYHA class I-II symptoms are less likely to experience relief in symptoms with CRT, they may experience decreased hospital admissions and show improvements in late ventricular remodeling.[11]
- Trials looking at patients with NYHA class I-II symptoms have only shown benefit in those who undergo biventricular pacemaker implantation at the time of ICD placement.[14,15]
- Lead position may influence outcomes in CRT. Among patients with baseline QRS intervals >160 ms, an RV to LV lead distance of at least 100 mm was associated with better clinical response rates.[16] On the other hand, an LV lead placed in the apex was associated with increased mortality.[17] In practice, LV leads are placed along the lateral or inferolateral wall without much guidance from mapping of regional mechanical or electrical dyssynchrony.[3]

FOLLOW-UP

Following CRT, with or without ICD implantation, proper lead placement may be verified by postero-anterior and lateral chest x-rays. In the electrophysiology clinic, adjustment of ventriculoventricular or atrioventricular (AV) delays may improve CRT response. While most patients respond well to simultaneous RV-LV pacing, a subset of patients does better with RV-then-LV sequential activation.[3] As a way to decrease adverse events among CRT non-responders, some studies support a role for enhancing LV filling via echocardiography-guided shortening of the AV delay. An effective AV delay is one in which mitral inflow fusion of E and A waves is reversed without truncating the end of the A wave.[18] During follow-ups, the clinician should also re-appraise his or her own adherence to guideline-directed medical therapy as another way to improve outcomes for his heart failure patients on CRT. Studies show that a significant proportion of heart failure patients are not prescribed the proper target doses of medications such as β-blockers and ACE inhibitors.

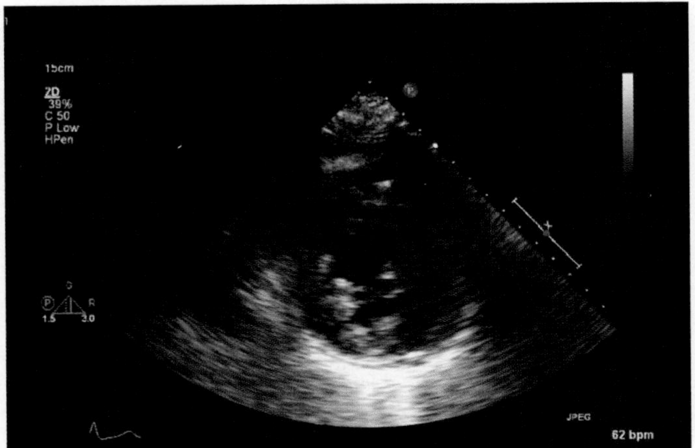

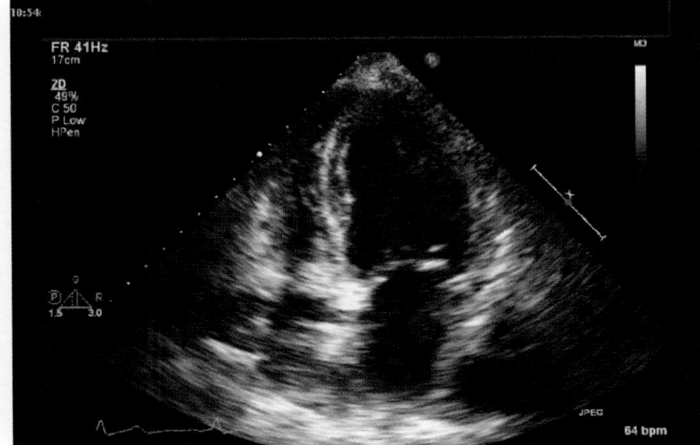

FIGURE 4-6-7 Parasternal short axis (L) and apical four chamber (R) and views from the follow-up echo demonstrating improved LVEF ► (see Videos 4-6-7 L and R).

VIDEO LEGENDS

1. Video 4-6-3 L: Transthoracic echocardiogram in the parasternal short-axis view shows severely depressed left ventricular systolic function and marked dyssynchrony.
2. Video 4-6-3 R: Transthoracic echocardiogram in the apical 4-chamber view shows severely depressed left ventricular systolic function and marked dyssynchrony.
3. Video 4-6-7 L: Following cardiac resynchronization therapy, the transthoracic echocardiogram in the parasternal short-axis view shows marked improvement in the patient's left ventricular systolic function.
4. Video 4-6-7 R: Following cardiac resynchronization therapy, the transthoracic echocardiogram in the apical 4-chamber view shows marked improvement in the patient's left ventricular systolic function.

REFERENCES

1. Sweeney M, Prinzen F. Ventricular pump function and pacing: physiologic and clinical integration. *Circ Arrhythm Electrophysiol*. 2008;1(2):127-139.
2. McAlister FA, Ezekowitz J, Hooton N, et al. Cardiac resynchronization therapy for patients with left ventricular systolic dysfunction: a systematic review. *JAMA*. 2007;297(22):2502-2514.
3. Singh J, Gras D. Biventricular pacing: current trends and future strategies. *Eur Heart J*. 2012;33(3):305-313.
4. Strik M, Ploux S, Vernooy K, Prinzen F. Cardiac resynchronization therapy—refocus on the electrical substrate. *Circ J*. 2011;75(6):1297-1304.
5. Sadaniantz A, Saint Laurent L. Left ventricular Doppler diastolic filling patterns in patients with isolated left bundle branch block. *Am J Cardiol*. 1998;81(5):643-645.
6. Vernooy K, Verbeek X, Peschar M, Prinzen F. Relation between abnormal ventricular impulse conduction and heart failure. *J Interv Cardiol*. 2003;16(6):557-562.
7. Ozdemir K, Altunkeser B, Danis G, et al. Effect of the isolated left bundle branch block on systolic and diastolic functions of left ventricle. *J Am Soc Echocardiogr*. 2001;14(11):1075-1079.
8. Duncan A, Francis D, Henein M, Gibson D. Importance of left ventricular activation in determining myocardial performance (Tei) index: comparison with total isovolumic time. *Int J Cardiol*. 2004;95(2-3):211-217.
9. Miyazaki C, Powell B, Bruce C. Comparison of echocardiographic dyssynchrony assessment by tissue velocity and strain imaging in subjects with or without systolic dysfunction and with or without left bundle-branch block. *Circulation*. 2008;117(20):2617-2625.
10. Salukhe TV, Francis DP, Morgan M, et al. Mechanism of cardiac output gain from cardiac resynchronization therapy in patients with coronary artery disease or idiopathic dilated cardiomyopathy. *Am J Cardiol*. 2006;97(9):1358-1364.
11. Tracy CM, Epstein AE, Darbar D, et al. 2012 ACCF/AHA/HRS focused update of the 2008 guidelines for device-based therapy of cardiac rhythm abnormalities: a report of the American College of Cardiology Foundation/American Heart Association Task Force on Practice Guidelines and the Heart Rhythm Society. *Circulation*. 2012;60(14):1297-1313.
12. Bonow R, Mann D, Zipes D, Libby P. *Braunwald's Heart Disease: A Textbook of Cardiovascular Medicine*, 9th ed. Philadelphia, PA: Elsevier; 2012.
13. Gorcsan J, Abraham T, Agler D, et al. Echocardiography for cardiac resynchronization therapy: recommendations for performance and reporting—a report from the American Society of Echocardiography Dyssynchrony Writing Group. *J Am Soc Echocardiogr*. 2008;21(3):191-213.
14. Moss AJ, Hall WJ, Cannom DS, et al. Cardiac-resynchronization therapy for the prevention of heart-failure events. *N Eng J Med*. 2009;361(14):1329-1338.
15. Linde C, Abraham WT, Gold MR, Sutton M, Ghio S, Daubert C. Randomized trial of cardiac resynchronization in mildly symptomatic heart failure patients and in asymptomatic patients with left ventricular dysfunction and previous heart failure symptoms. *J Am Coll Cardiol*. 2008;52(23):1834-1843.
16. Ariga R, Tayebjee M, Benfield A, Todd M, Lefroy D. Greater three-dimensional ventricular lead tip separation is associated with improved outcome after cardiac resynchronization therapy. *Pacing Clin Electrophysiol*. 2010;33(12):1490-1496.
17. Singh J, Klein H, Huang D, et al. Left ventricular lead position and clinical outcome in the multicenter automatic defibrillator implantation trial—cardiac resynchronization therapy (MADIT-CRT) trial. *Circulation*. 2011;123(11):1159-1166.
18. Mullens W, Grimm R, Verga T, et al. Insights from a cardiac resynchronization optimization clinic as part of a heart failure disease management program. *J Am Coll Cardiol*. 2009;53(9):765-773.
19. Chung R, Sutton R, Henein MY. Beyond dyssynchrony in cardiac resynchronization therapy. *Heart*. 2008;94(8):991-994.

SECTION 7

Echocardiographic Evaluation of Hemodynamics in a Patient With Heart Failure

Gerard P. Aurigemma, MD,
FAHA, FASE, FACC

CLINICAL CASE PRESENTATION

A 79-year-old man is admitted from a nursing home after collapsing and sustaining a concussion. He is somnolent, arousable, but cannot give a history; records accompanying him from the nursing home indicate that he has suffered a heart attack in the past, has the diagnosis of "CHF" as well as hypertension, has undergone prior cardiac surgery, but there are no details. His medications include furosemide, lisinopril, and amlodipine.

On examination, he is a frail older man, febrile to 102° F (38.8° C), with blood pressure 90/60 mm Hg, pulse rate 100 beats/min and irregular, and respirations 20 breaths/min. General exam is notable for a midline sternotomy scar, bilateral carotid endarterectomy scars, and a large scalp laceration. He has diffuse rhonchi, normal first and second heart sounds, and a holosystolic murmur heard at the lower left sternal border. An RV heave is appreciated, and an S_3 gallop is heard. There is mild peripheral edema. The chest x-ray (Figure 4-7-1) shows marked cardiomegaly, and there is likely left ventricular and right atrial enlargement. The lung fields are relatively clear, and there is no evidence for significant pulmonary edema on this film. A 12-lead electrocardiogram is obtained and demonstrated atrial fibrillation with a slow ventricular response, right axis deviation, right ventricular hypertrophy, and right bundle branch block. The white blood cell count was 12,000 with a pronounced left shift. Brain natriuretic peptide level was 917 mg/dL. A comprehensive echocardiogram was subsequently performed, which revealed impaired LVEF and significant mitral regurgitation (MR) as well as evidence of pulmonary hypertension and elevated LA pressure.

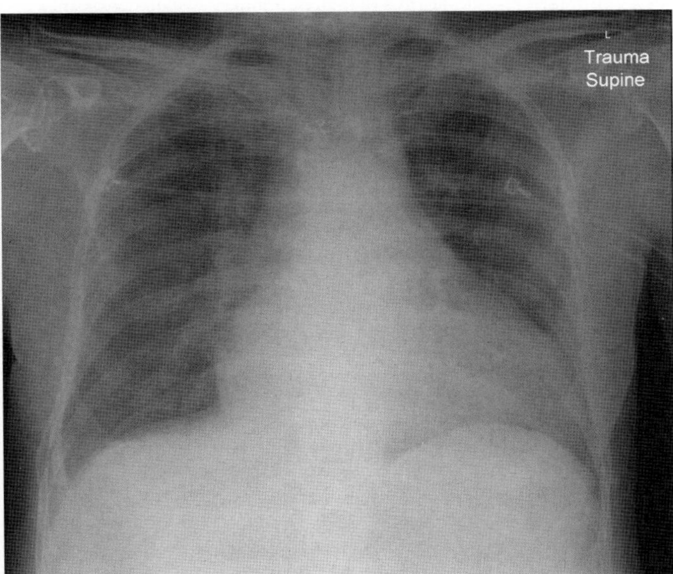

FIGURE 4-7-1 The admission CXR shows marked cardiomegaly. The lung fields are relatively clear, and there is no evidence for significant pulmonary edema on this film. See text for details.

DIAGNOSIS, MANAGEMENT AND DECISION MAKING, AND THE ROLE OF ECHOCARDIOGRAPHY

- This case highlights the many findings on an echocardiogram that can be employed to assess LV structure and function, valvular abnormalities, and hemodynamic parameters, and demonstrates correlation with invasively obtained hemodynamic information.
  - 2-D echocardiogram (Figure 4-7-2)
    - Overall LVEF is moderately reduced, estimated at 35% by biplane method of disks methodology. This study is remarkable for a large area of akinesis and wall thinning seen in the inferior wall and inferolateral wall. These findings are almost assuredly due to a large right coronary artery or left circumflex coronary artery infarction. The wall thinning that is manifest indicates that the infarction is likely old.
    - There is malcoaptation of the mitral leaflets associated with a large jet of mitral regurgitation, directed posteriorly. Other views show that the largest jet area exceeds 40% of the size of the left atrium.
    - There is left atrial enlargement; this is likely due to chronic diastolic dysfunction and mitral regurgitation.
  - Doppler examination (Figures 4-7-3 to 4-7-8):
    - Transmitral flow is illustrated in Figure 4-7-3. There is a single early ("E") wave, due to atrial fibrillation.
    - The pulmonary venous flow (Figure 4-7-4) demonstrates marked dominance of the diastolic wave ("D" dominance).
    - The tissue Doppler profile (Figure 4-7-5), obtained at the lateral mitral annulus shows a relatively preserved tissue Doppler e' wave of 12 cm/s. Thus the E/e' ratio is not elevated.
    - The tricuspid regurgitation spectral profile (Figure 4-7-6) is characterized by a high signal intensity, which provides indirect evidence of severe tricuspid regurgitation. In addition, the upstroke of this profile is more gradual than is normal, indicative of right

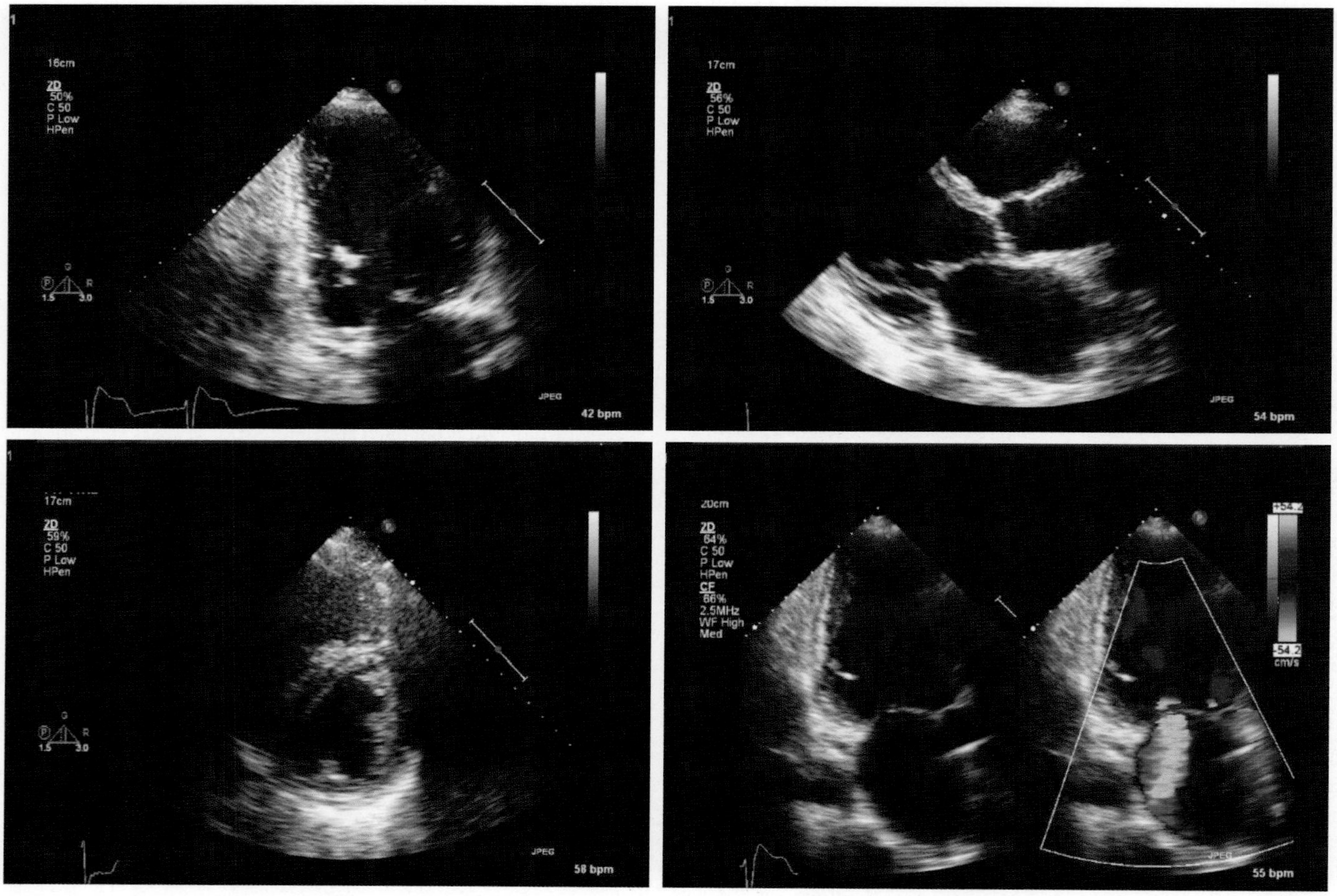

FIGURE 4-7-2 Selected still frames from the 2-D echocardiogram. See text for details. There is a large area of akinesis and wall thinning seen in the inferior wall (upper left panel) and inferolateral wall (upper right panel). The short axis view (lower left panel) demonstrates septal flattening in systole consistent with elevated RV systolic pressure. The lower right panel demonstrates malcoaptation of the mitral leaflets associated with a large jet of mitral regurgitation ▶ (see Videos 4-7-2 A -F).

ventricular systolic dysfunction. The pressure gradient estimated from this tricuspid regurgitation jet is approximately 80 mm Hg, consistent with severe pulmonary hypertension.

- Spectral Doppler (Figure 4-7-7) is obtained with the sample volume at the pulmonary valve. There is a notch in the spectral profile. This is indicative of high pulmonary vascular resistance and is indirect evidence of pulmonary hypertension.
- A 2-D-directed M-Mode through the inferior vena cava (IVC) (Figure 4-7-8) shows a dilated IVC with less than 50% collapse with inspiration. Based on this finding, a value of 15 mm Hg

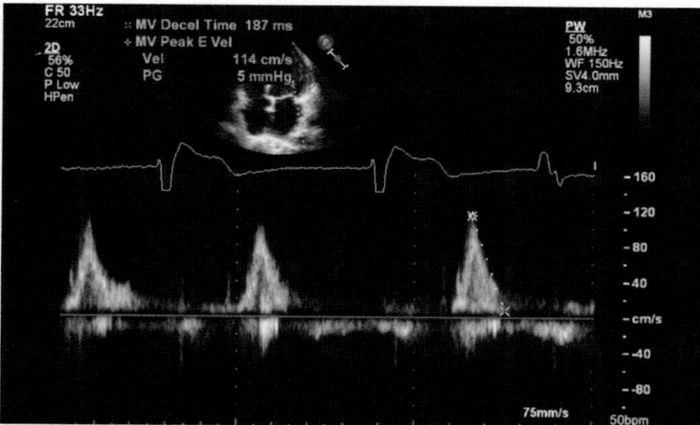

FIGURE 4-7-3 Transmitral flow is illustrated. There is a single early ("E") wave, due to atrial fibrillation.

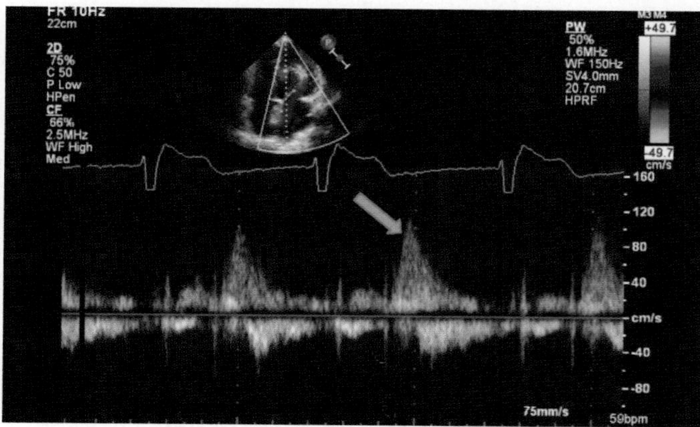

FIGURE 4-7-4 The pulmonary venous flow demonstrates marked dominance of the diastolic wave (arrow).

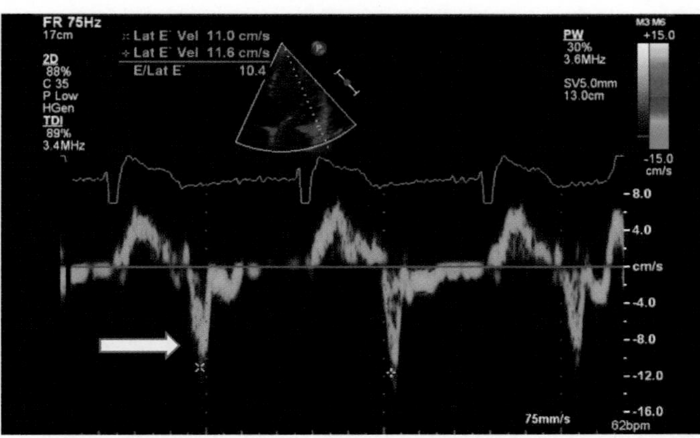

FIGURE 4-7-5 The tissue Doppler profile obtained at the lateral mitral annulus shows a relatively preserved tissue Doppler e′ wave of 12 cm/s (arrow).

should be assigned to be right atrial pressure. Taken in aggregate, then, an estimate of pulmonary artery pressure from this study is 95 mm Hg.

- Cardiac catheterization was performed to assess the etiology of the pulmonary hypertension and to assess his coronary anatomy.
  - Figures 4-7-9 and 4-7-10 highlight the salient points of the right heart catheterization. (There is beat-to-beat variation in all pressures due to the rhythm irregularity.) The RA pressure is estimated at 10 to 12 mm Hg and the mean pulmonary capillary wedge pressure is approximately 22 mm Hg with markedly elevated "v" waves of approximately 50 mm Hg.
  - The pulmonary artery pressure was estimated at 80 mm Hg.
  - The left ventricular end-diastolic pressure was approximately 25 mm Hg.
  - Coronary arteriography was performed and showed patent grafts to his left anterior descending artery, right coronary artery, and circumflex system. His large native right coronary artery showed an ostial occlusion.

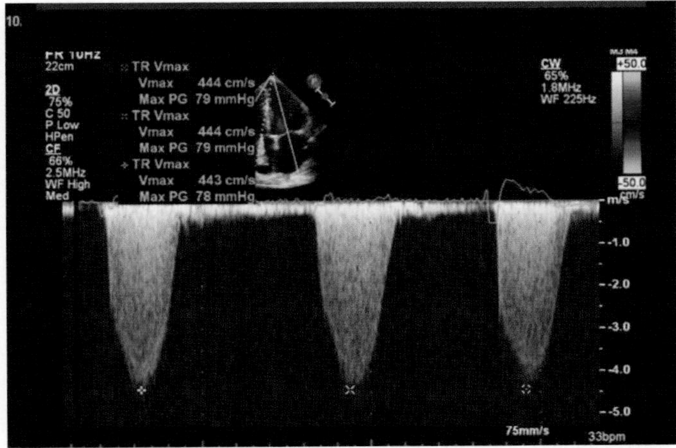

FIGURE 4-7-6 The tricuspid regurgitation spectral profile is characterized by a high signal intensity, gradual upstroke, and a peak velocity of 4.4 m/sec. See text for details.

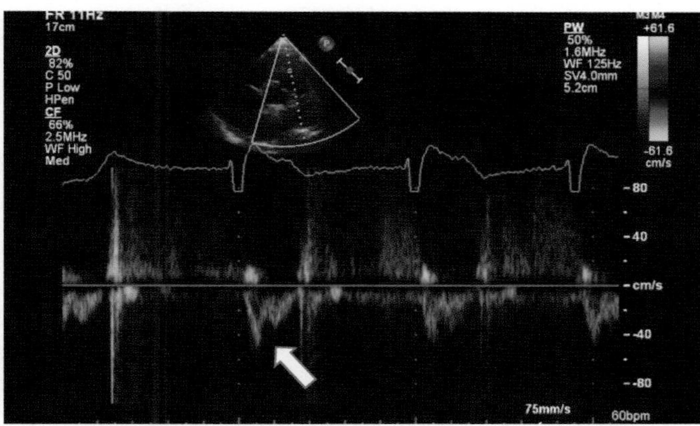

FIGURE 4-7-7 Spectral Doppler of the pulmonary valve flow. There is a notch in the spectral profile (arrow). See text for details.

HEMODYNAMIC CORRELATIONS AND THE ROLE OF ECHOCARDIOGRAPHY

- This case illustrates the role that echocardiography plays in contemporary cardiology in the assessment of a complicated hemodynamic picture. The interested reader can find more details in the references listed that provide further information on the details of the echocardiographic assessment of mitral valve disease, LV systolic and diastolic function, and the echocardiographic assessment of the RV.[1-7]
- Salient points from our current case include:
  - All of the major findings of the echo examination were confirmed at catheterization. However, as is commonly the case, the actual invasive pressures differed somewhat from the echo estimates, most likely due to slight differences in hemodynamics that result from in-hospital treatment and mild conscious sedation.
  - The 2-D echocardiogram demonstrated signs of prior ischemic heart disease with a marked wall motion abnormality in the inferior and inferolateral walls. This had resulted from a complete occlusion of the right coronary artery in the patient with a right dominant coronary circulation.

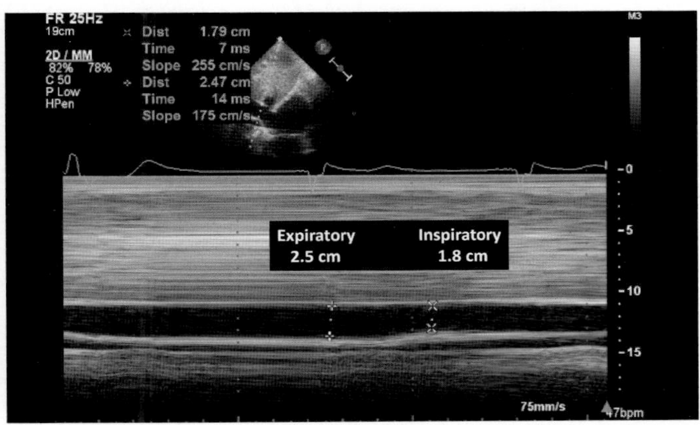

FIGURE 4-7-8 A 2-D–directed M-Mode through the inferior vena cava (IVC) shows a dilated IVC with less than 50% collapse with inspiration. See text for details.

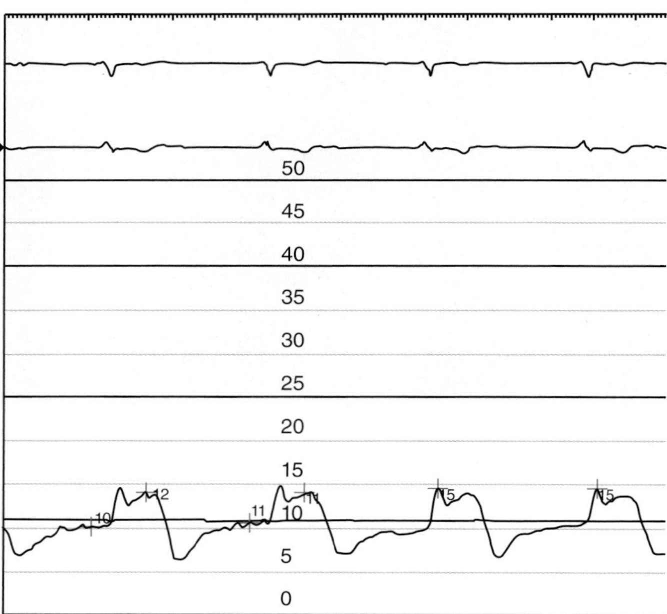

FIGURE 4-7-9 Right atrial pressure tracing taken from the patient's right heart catheterization. See text for details.

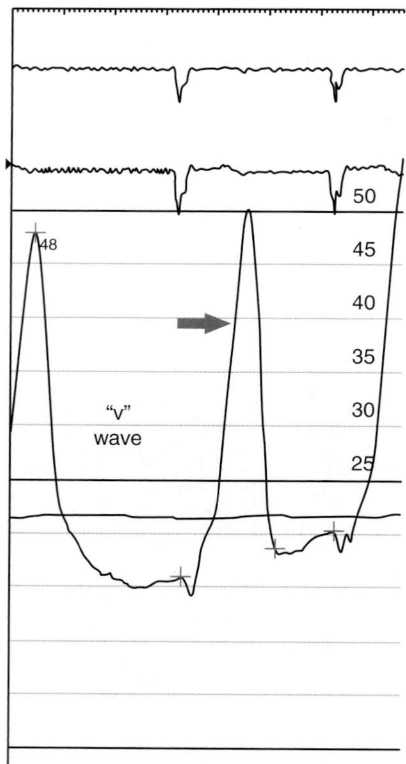

FIGURE 4-7-10 Pulmonary capillary wedge pressure tracing taken from the patient's right heart catheterization. The red arrow points to the large V-wave. See text for details.

- This patient also demonstrated severe mitral regurgitation with the sequellae of left atrial enlargement and a substantial elevation in left atrial pressure. It was concluded that the severe pulmonary hypertension was passive, ie, due to chronically elevated left sided pressure. The echo findings were subsequently confirmed by invasive left and right heart catheterization and hemodynamics.
- The left atrial pressure is elevated as demonstrated by the significant "v" waves seen on the pulmonary capillary wedge tracing. These tall "v" waves are likely a result of the combination of chronic mitral regurgitation and either a stiff left atrium, or an atrium that is operating on the curvilinear portion of its pressure volume relationship (strain-dependent abnormalities in compliance).
- It can be a challenge to reconcile findings from the x-ray examination, which did not demonstrate significant pulmonary congestions and the echo/catheterization findings. In this instance, we hypothesized that the development of severe pulmonary hypertension likely led to an oligemic chest x-ray picture; the lung fields are remarkably clear, belying the chronic elevations in pulmonary capillary wedge pressure. In this instance, the elevated BNP is probably multifactorial, due to myocardial stretch in the left and right ventricles, the latter related to pulmonary hypertension. If the elevations in pulmonary capillary pressure are chronic, as was surely the case here, pulmonary lymphatic drainage may be enhanced, and thus the lung fields can appear clear despite proven elevations in filling pressure.
- One note of caution should be issued for the use of tissue Doppler to estimate left-sided pressures in instances of a focal wall motion abnormality involving the inferior wall, as is the case here. In this situation, the lateral tissue Doppler velocity can be high, and thus one must use caution in computing E/e' ratio in patients with focal wall motion abnormalities involving the septal annulus.
- Finally, the mechanism of the mitral regurgitation should be discussed. The echo demonstrates that there is malcoaptation of the leaflets due, in part, to tethering of posterior leaflet (ischemic MR). Consequently, the anterior leaflet tip coapts against the body of the posterior leaflet. This provides a channel through which regurgitant flow can issue into the left atrium. Simple annular dilation is not the sole mechanism for this mitral regurgitation. Rather, the mechanism, as has been worked out by Levine and colleagues, is related to apical displacement of papillary muscles, and loss of coaptation surface of the mitral leaflets.

HOSPITAL COURSE AND PATIENT FOLLOW-UP

The patient was found to have a urinary tract infection and bacteremia with a gram-negative species. His scalp laceration was sutured. Antibiotic therapy was instituted, and he was also treated for heart failure with intravenous furosemide and improved. He was transitioned to an oral diuretic regimen, and his lisinopril was reinstated once his BP was stable. β-Blocker therapy was not started due to persistent bradycardia. He improved and was discharged to the nursing facility.

Due to his dementia and the desires of his health care proxy, no discussion was entertained concerning surgical or interventional treatment for his mitral regurgitation or advanced therapy for his pulmonary hypertension, beyond continuing his outpatient medications, nor did they want to pursue pacemaker or ICD therapy (which would be a consideration given his ischemic cardiomyopathy and impaired LVEF).

VIDEO LEGENDS

1. Video 4-7-2 A: Parasternal long axis demonstrating inferolateral wall thinning and reduced LVEF. The LA is enlarged.
2. Video 4-7-2 B: Parasternal short axis demonstrating inferior and inferolateral wall thinning and reduced LVEF. There is septal flattening in systole consistent with an elevated RV systolic pressure.
3. Video 4-7-2 C: Apical 4 chamber view demonstrating reduced LVEF with a basal inferior septal and apical wall motion abnormality
4. Video 4-7-2 D: Apical 2 chamber view demonstrating inferior akinesis
5. Video 4-7-2 E: Apical 3 chamber view demonstrating the inferolateral wall motion abnormality and the malcoaption of the MV leaflets
6. Video 4-7-2 F: Apical 2 chamber view with color Doppler demonstrating the MR.

REFERENCES

1. Zoghbi WA, Enriquez-Sarano M., Foster E, et al. Recommendations for evaluation of the severity of native valvular regurgitation with two-dimensional and Doppler echocardiography. *J Am Soc Echocardiogr*. 2003;16(7):777-802.
2. Rudski LG, Lai WW, Afilalo J, et al. Guidelines for the echocardiographic assessment of the right heart in adults: a report from the American Society of Echocardiography endorsed by the European Association of Echocardiography, a registered branch of the European Society of Cardiology, and the Canadian Society of Echocardiography. *J Am Soc Echocardiogr*. 2010;23(7):685-713; quiz 786-688.
3. Otsuji Y, Handschumacher MD, Liel Cohen N, et al. Mechanism of ischemic mitral regurgitation with segmental left ventricular dysfunction: three-dimensional echocardiographic studies in models of acute and chronic progressive regurgitation. *J Am Coll Cardiol* 2001;37(2):641-648.
4. Otsuji Y, Levine RA, Takeuchi M, et al. Mechanism of ischemic mitral regurgitation. *J Cardiol*. 2008;51(3):145-156.
5. Levine RA, Schwammenthal E. Ischemic mitral regurgitation on the threshold of a solution: from paradoxes to unifying concepts. *Circulation*. 2005;112(5):745-758.
6. Nagueh SF, Appleton CP, Gillebert TC, et al. Recommendations for the evaluation of left ventricular diastolic function by echocardiography. *J Am Soc Echocardiogr*. 2009;22(2):107-133.
7. Lam CS, Roger VL, Rodeheffer RJ, et al. Pulmonary hypertension in heart failure with preserved ejection fraction: a community-based study. *J Am Coll Cardiol*. 2009;53(13):1119-1126.

SECTION 8

Left Ventricular Assist Devices

Sitaramesh Emani, MD

CLINICAL CASE PRESENTATION

A 68-year-old man with a history of severe chronic heart failure due to a dilated cardiomyopathy is evaluated for persistent symptoms despite optimal medical therapy. He has experienced a progressive decline in his functional capacity. Due to his advanced age, he was not considered a candidate for cardiac transplantation. He is ultimately referred for permanent mechanical circulatory support (destination therapy) in the form of a left ventricular assist device (LVAD). He successfully undergoes the surgical implant of an LVAD and is discharged. At a follow-up visit 3 months later, he is found to have an improvement in his heart failure symptoms. A routine echocardiogram is ordered to assess his native heart and LVAD function.

CLINICAL FEATURES[1]

The clinical evaluation of an LVAD patient can be difficult, particularly with the use of new generation continuous flow pumps.

- Continuous flow pumps may not produce a palpable peripheral pulse in patients.
- Blood pressure measurements may be inaccurate due to the lack of Korotkoff sounds.
- Cardiac auscultation is often obscured by the continuous mechanical hum of the LVAD.
- Signs of volume overload such as elevated jugular venous pressures and peripheral edema can be seen in LVAD patients.
- LVAD dysfunction is often accompanied by alarms on the controller unit as well as worsening of heart failure symptoms.

- Generalized assessment of functional status are of particular use when evaluating an LVAD patient.

EPIDEMIOLOGY[2]

In the United States, approximately 5 million people are affected with some degree of HF. Of these, approximately 50,000 can be considered end-stage with the potential to benefit from advanced therapies. Since cardiac transplant is a limited option, the use of ventricular assist devices may provide a therapeutic strategy for many of these patients. The use of LVADs as definitive treatment has increased since clinical trials demonstrated survival benefits over medical therapy alone.

ECHOCARDIOGRAPHY[3-6]

Echocardiography is essential in the management of the patient with chronic heart failure, as detailed in other sections of this atlas. Prior to LVAD placement, an echocardiogram is warranted to assess LV and RV function, assess for the presence of intracardiac (atrial level) shunting, LV thrombus, and the presence and severity of pulmonary hypertension, as well as the presence of aortic regurgitation.

In the operating room, intraoperative TEE is used to monitor the patient, document the position of the LVAD cannula, and assess for any immediate complications.

Postprocedure, echocardiography is an essential component of ongoing patient management and evaluation. Echocardiography in the evaluation of an LVAD patient includes several aspects:

- Left ventricular (LV) dimensions can help determine the appropriate settings and function of the LVAD.
- A distended LV may indicate flow through the LVAD is too low.
  - Decreased LVAD flow may result from the LVAD speed being set too low.
  - However, decreased LVAD flow might also indicate LVAD malfunction, particularly in the setting of a thrombus within the device.
- An underfilled or compressed LV may indicate increased flow through the LVAD.
  - LV compression may indicate the LVAD speed is set too high.
  - Increased LVAD flow may result from complications such as hemolysis or anemia.
  - Compressed LVs can physically obstruct flow into the LVAD, causing further malfunction.
- Native cardiac contraction, particularly that of the interventricular septum, can help determine appropriate LVAD settings and should be assessed when possible.
- Opening of the aortic valve should be evaluated to determine the contribution of the native ventricle to cardiac output.
  - Doppler flow across the LV outflow tract and aortic valve can be a useful adjunct.
  - M-mode imaging through the AV is another useful tool (Figure 4-8-1).
  - Generally, optimal LVAD function allows native ejection through the aortic valve approximately once every 3 beats.
  - Caution is advised, however, as the aortic valve is sometimes surgically over sewn to prevent regurgitation. Flow across the valve should not be seen in these instances.

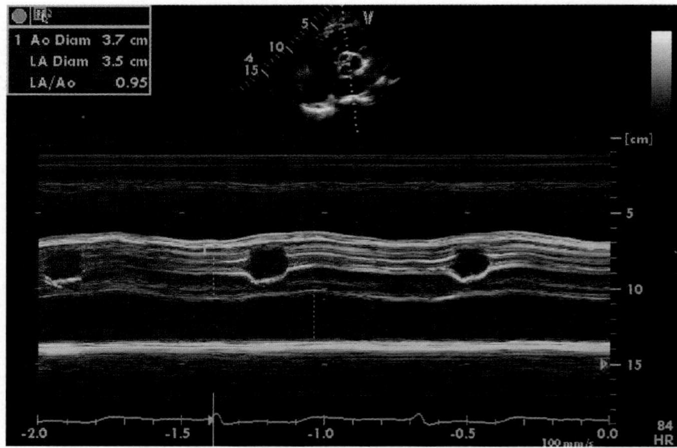

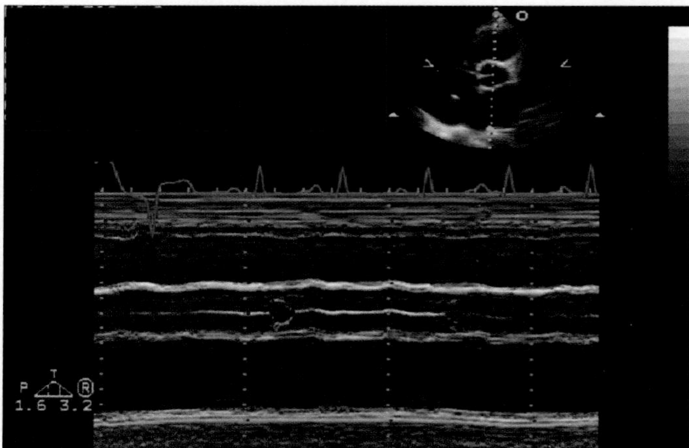

FIGURE 4-8-1 M-mode image through the plane of the AV. Note AV opening with each QRS complex in this case (top panel). In the bottom panel, from another patient, the AV opens intermittently, consistent with LV ejection with some but not all beats.

- Aortic regurgitation can represent "closed loop" circulation and may contribute to recurrent heart failure symptoms post LVAD. Significant AR can result in LV distention. The progression of aortic valve regurgitation is a particularly concerning finding.
- Visualization of the LVAD inflow cannula should be attempted at the LV apex (Figures 4-8-2 to 4-8-4). The presence of a thrombus or vegetation on the cannula is a potentially dangerous finding.
- Likewise, visualization of the LVAD outflow cannula might be possible in the ascending aorta.
- Doppler flows of both the inflow and outflow cannulae are helpful in the evaluation for obstruction such as a thrombus (Figures 4-8-5 and 4-8-6). Increases in Doppler velocities, especially compared to prior evaluations, should raise the suspicion of an obstruction.
- Right ventricular (RV) function assessment is extremely beneficial (systolic and right-sided valvular function). Clinical status can be greatly affected by changes in RV function.
- Figures 4-8-7 to 4-8-11 from other patients demonstrate several other features and potential LVAD complications as seen and evaluated with echocardiography.

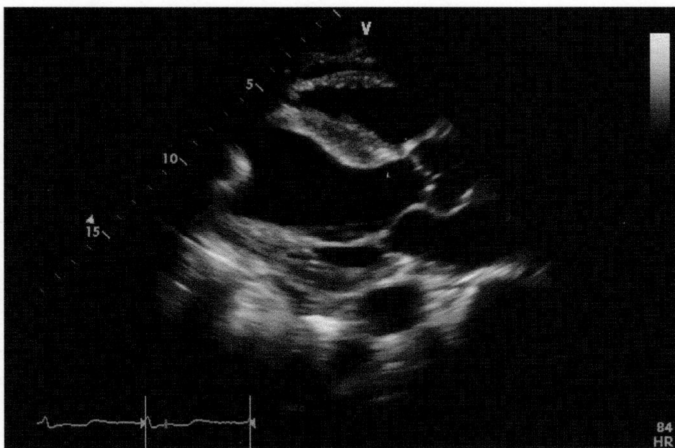

FIGURE 4-8-2 Parasternal long axis view of the LV. The tip of the LVAD cannula can be seen in the apex ▶ (see Video 4-8-2).

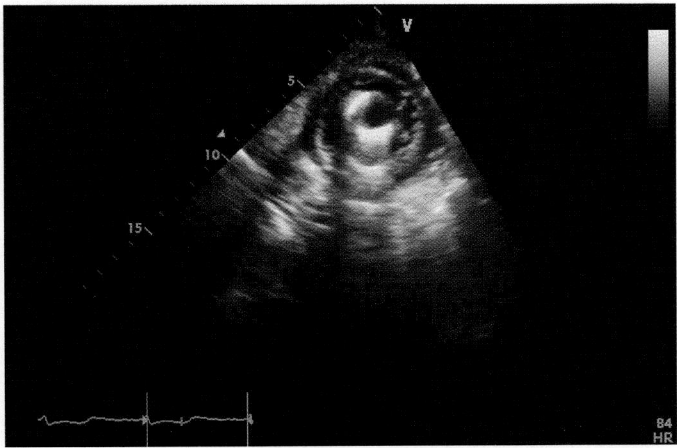

FIGURE 4-8-3 Parasternal short axis view of the LV apex. The concentric ring within the LV is the LVAD cannula ▶ (see Video 4-8-3).

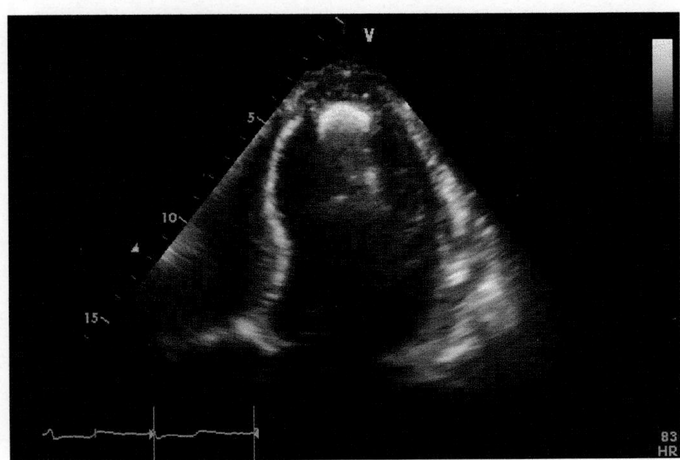

FIGURE 4-8-4 Apical 4 chamber view showing the LVAD cannula in the apex ▶ (see Video 4-8-4).

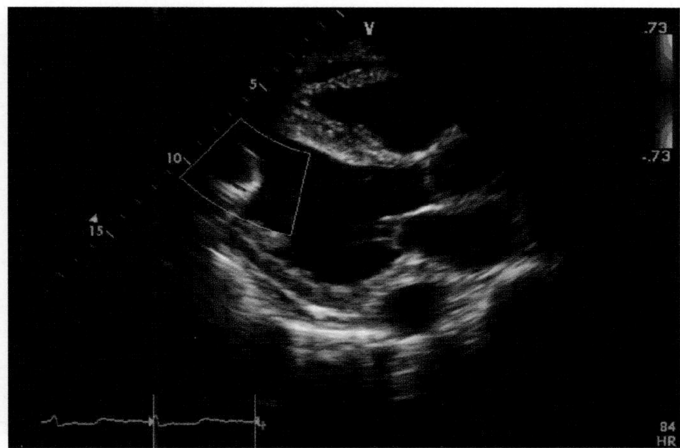

FIGURE 4-8-5 Image of Doppler flow into the LVAD apical cannula in the parasternal long axis view ▶ (see Video 4-8-5).

OTHER TESTS AND PROCEDURES[6]

- Computed tomography (CT scan) is sometimes used to evaluate LVAD positioning.
- Blood work is often a key component when assessing LVAD function. Blood cell counts, renal function, evidence of hemolysis, and anticoagulation levels all play a role in LVAD management.
- Evaluation for LVAD thrombosis can be extremely difficult as no imaging modality can visualize the internal chambers or flow of an LVAD.

MANAGEMENT[6]

Management of LVAD patients is typically done through specific centers experienced with this patient population. Common issues include:

- Maintaining anticoagulation to specified goals, which may vary among patients and types of LVADs.
- Adjusting diuretic doses to maintain volume status.
- Monitoring for complications such as device infection, gastrointestinal bleeding, stroke, renal dysfunction, or hemolysis.

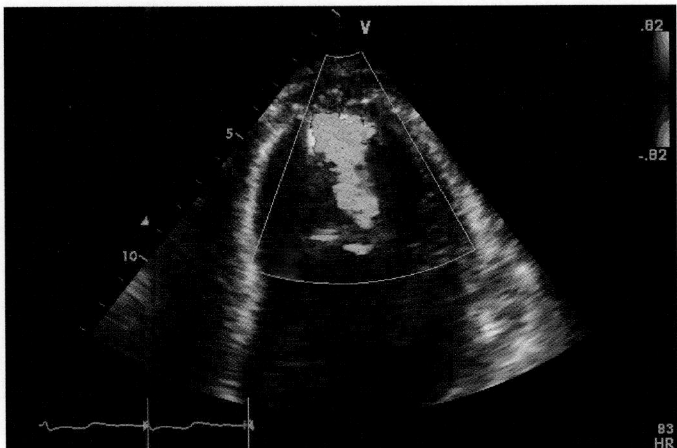

FIGURE 4-8-6 Doppler flow into the LVAD apical cannula in the apical 4 chamber view ▶ (see Video 4-8-6).

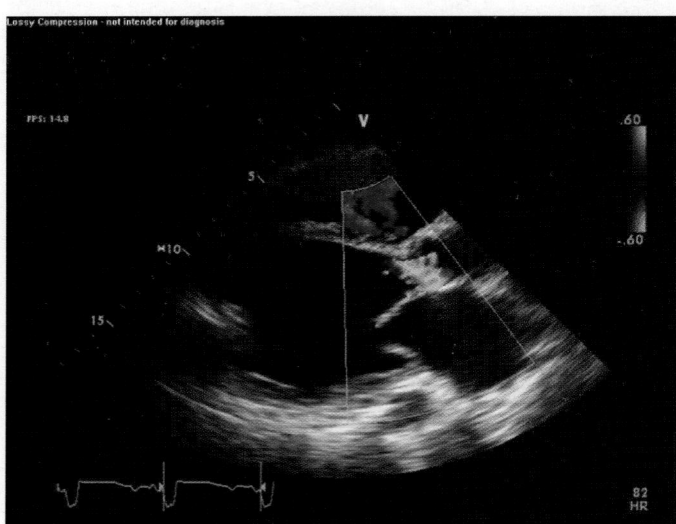

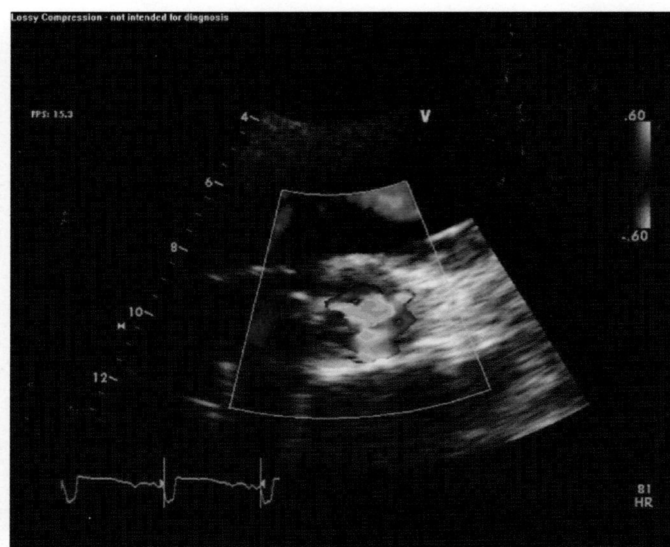

FIGURE 4-8-7 Parasternal long axis (L) and short axis (R) demonstrating severe AR in an LVAD patient who presented with worsening CHF symptoms ▶ (Videos 4-8-7 L and R). He was taken to the operating room, and the AV was sutured closed. Postoperatively, his symptoms improved.

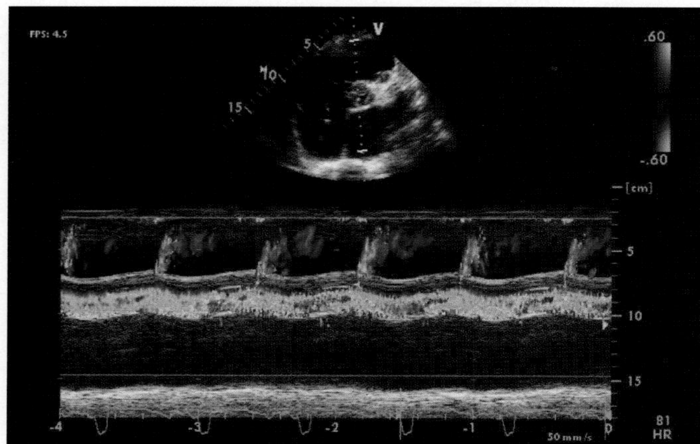

FIGURE 4-8-8 Color M-mode of the patient in Figure 4-8-7 demonstrating severe AR.

VIDEO LEGENDS

1. Video 4-8-2 : Parasternal long axis view of the LV. The tip of the LVAD cannula can be seen in the apex
2. Video 4-8-3: Parasternal short axis view of the LV apex. The concentric ring within the LV is the LVAD cannula
3. Video 4-8-4: Apical four chamber view showing the LVAD cannula in the apex
4. Video 4-8-5: Image of Doppler flow into the LVAD apical cannula in the parasternal long axis view
5. Video 4-8-6: Doppler flow into the LVAD apical cannula in the apical four chamber view
6. Video 4-8-7 L: Parasternal long axis demonstrating severe AR in an LVAD patient who presented with worsening CHF symptoms

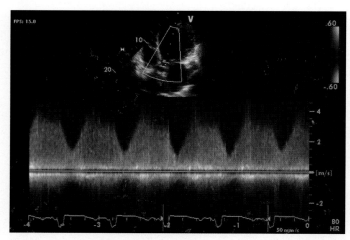

FIGURE 4-8-9 Continuous-wave Doppler across the AV of the patient in Figure 4-8-7. Note the continuous AR. After each QRS, the velocity is decreased consistent with a rise in the LV pressure due to ventricular systole. The LV is not able to generate enough pressure to open the AV, however.

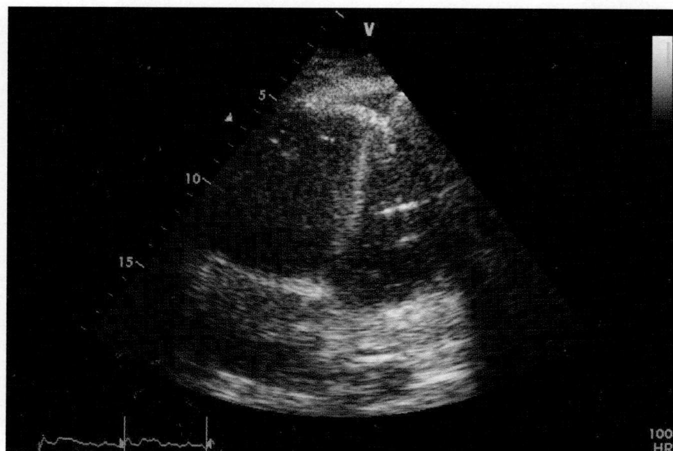

FIGURE 4-8-10 Apical 4 chamber view from a patient with an LVAD who presented with acute dyspnea and hypotension. The patient had evidence of massive pulmonary embolism and expired ▶ (see Video 4-8-10).

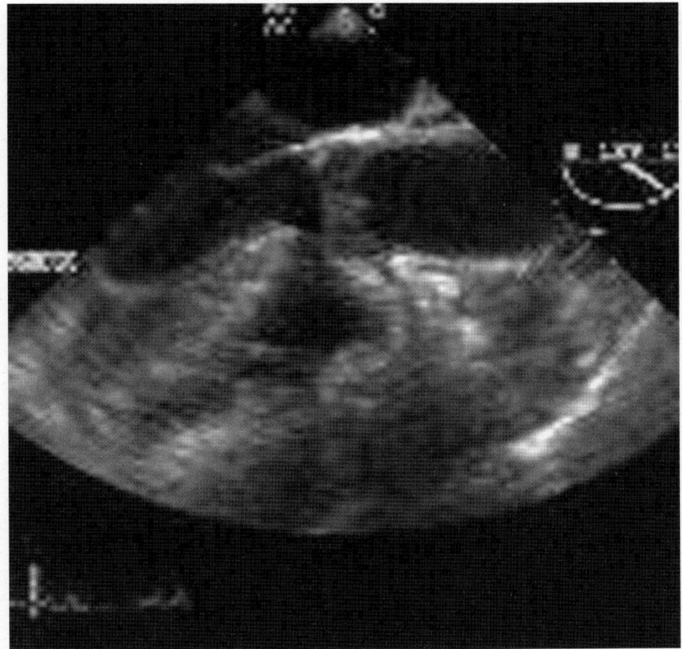

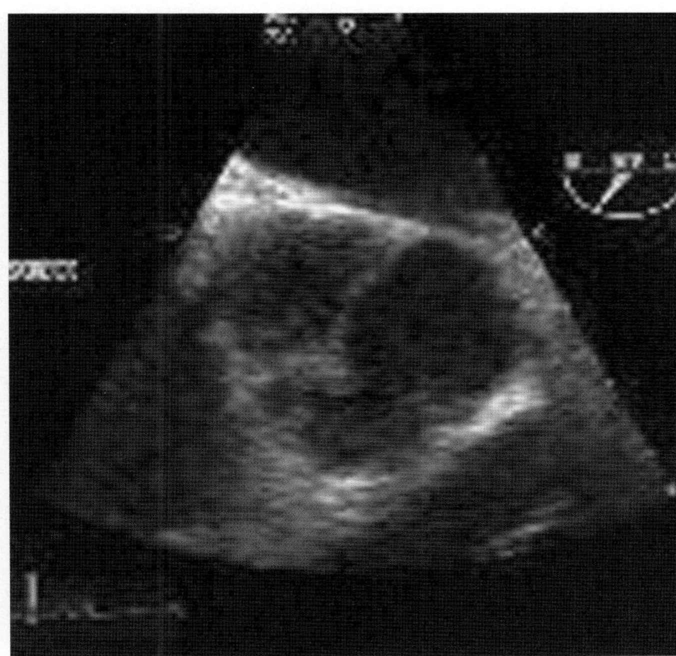

FIGURE 4-8-11 Transesophageal echo images of the AV in a patient with a temporary centrifugal LVAD placed for cardiogenic shock. An AV thrombus developed in this patient who subsequently went to the OR and underwent debridement of the AV thrombus and placement of a continuous flow LVAD. The long axis is seen on the left (A) and the short axis view is seen on the right (B) ► (see Videos 4-8-11 L and R).

7. Video 4-8-7 R: Parasternal short axis demonstrating severe AR in an LVAD patient who presented with worsening CHF symptoms
8. Video 4-8-10: Apical 4 chamber view from a patient with an LVAD who presented with acute dyspnea and hypotension. The patient had evidence of massive pulmonary embolism and expired
9. Video 4-8-11 L: Transesophageal echo image of the AV in a patient with a temporary centrifugal LVAD placed for cardiogenic shock. An AV thrombus developed in this patient who subsequently went to the OR, underwent debridement of the AV thrombus and placement of a continuous flow LVAD. The long axis is seen in this video
10. Video 4-8-11 R: Transesophageal echo image of the AV in a patient with a temporary centrifugal LVAD placed for cardiogenic shock. An AV thrombus developed in this patient who subsequently went to the OR, underwent debridement of the AV thrombus and placement of a continuous flow LVAD. The short axis view is seen in this video

REFERENCES

1. HeartMate II LVAS Clinical Operation & Patient Management. Pleasonton, CA: Thoratec Corp., 2011.
2. Rose EA, Gelijns AC, Moskowitz AJ, et al. Long-term use of a left ventricular assist device for end-stage heart failure. *N Engl J Med*. 2001;345:1435-1443.
3. Uriel N, Morrison KA, Garan AR, et al. Development of a novel echocardiography ramp test for speed optimization and diagnosis of device thrombosis in continuous-flow left ventricular assist devices: the Columbia ramp study. *J Am Coll Cardiol*. 2012;60:1764-1775.
4. Scalia GM, McCarthy PM, Savage RM, Smedira NG, Thomas JD. Clinical utility of echocardiography in the management of implantable ventricular assist devices. *J Am Soc Echocardiogr*. 2000;13:754-763.
5. Mookadam F, Kendall CB, Wong RK, et al. Left ventricular assist devices: physiologic assessment using echocardiography for management and optimization. *Ultrasound Med Biol*. 2012;38:335-345.
6. Feldman D, Pamboukian SV, Teuteberg JJ, et al. The 2013 International Society for Heart and Lung Transplantation Guidelines for mechanical circulatory support: executive summary. *J Heart Lung Transplant*. 2013;32:157-187.

SECTION 9

Cardiac Transplantation and Echocardiography

Sakima Smith, MD, and Sitaramesh Emani, MD

CLINICAL CASE PRESENTATION

A 68-year-old woman was referred for a cardiac transplant evaluation. She had a history of a nonischemic cardiomyopathy possibly due to myxomatous mitral valve disease. She had previously undergone placement of an ICD with CRT therapy as well as treatment with optimal medical therapy including a β-blocker, ACE inhibitor, and spironolactone. During her visit, she stated that she has noted a significant functional decline since her last aborted sudden cardiac death/ventricular tachycardia (VT) episode 3 months ago. Since that time she is easily fatigued and has difficulty with daily activities. She estimated her exercise tolerance being equivalent to 2 to 3 blocks of walking slowly and less than 1 flight of stairs. Given her functional decline despite medical therapy, as well as her history of recurrent VT, it was deemed appropriate to proceed with an evaluation for transplant candidacy. She had severe left ventricular systolic function on her echocardiogram (LVEF <20%) (Figure 4-9-1) and severe reduction in her aerobic capacity (peak functional VO_2 was 12.2 ml/kg/min; 48% predicted). She was listed for cardiac transplantation and several months later received a donor heart. She continues to do well posttransplant with a marked improvement in her quality of life.

EPIDEMIOLOGY

Heart failure (HF) is a global epidemic with a lifetime risk of developing HF of 20%.

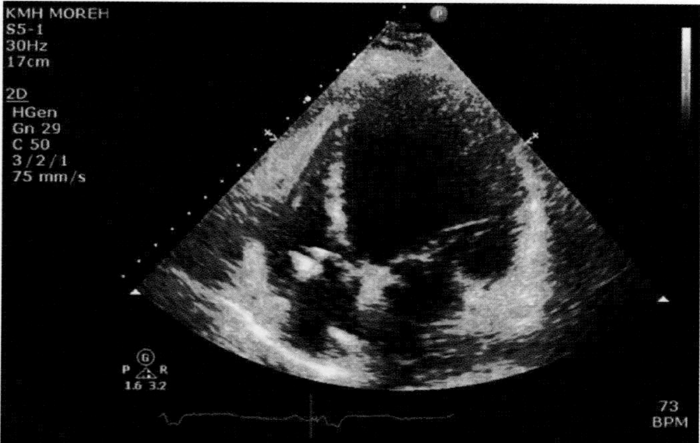

FIGURE 4-9-1 Apical 4 chamber view pretransplant. Note the dilated left ventricle associated with progressive cardiomyopathy. In addition, the CRT device is seen, and the ECG has evidence of biventricular pacing ► (see Video 4-9-1).

- Each year nearly 500,000 new patients are diagnosed with HF, and currently there are over 5 million people in the United States living with HF.[1]
- Heart transplantation is the treatment of choice for end-stage HF, but there is a significant shortage of suitable donors. The Registry of the International Society for Heart and Lung Transplantation (ISHLT) reported 3742 heart transplants worldwide in 2010.
- In the United States, the number of heart transplants performed has been stable at approximately 2300 cases annually.[2]

INDICATIONS[3]

In general, patients must have organic heart disease of sufficient severity to impair functional status and quality of life, as well as objective data to suggest a one-year mortality greater that 50%. Patients will meet one or more of the following criteria:

- Heart failure with NYHA Class III or IV status on maximal medical therapy.
- Objective data would include a reduced left ventricular ejection fraction (usually assessed by echocardiography) and/or severe diastolic dysfunction and a reduced functional capacity (VO_2 <14 ml/kg/min or predicted VO_2 <50% on cardiopulmonary stress testing).
- Inoperable coronary artery disease with intractable anginal symptoms refractory to medical therapy.
- Malignant ventricular arrhythmias unresponsive to medical or surgical therapy.
- Have an expected survival time without transplant of less than 36 months.

CONTRAINDICATIONS[3]

Patients undergo a thorough pretransplant evaluation, usually by a team of cardiologists with expertise in the management of patients with CHF and posttransplant management, as well as cardiothoracic surgeons, a team of nurses, coordinators, and social workers to assess their candidacy for a transplant. Contraindications for a cardiac transplant include:

- Age >70 years, older patients by individual assessment (can vary by institution)
- Severe pulmonary hypertension as evidenced by a fixed pulmonary vascular resistance (PVR) ≥4 Woods units, transpulmonary gradient (TPG) ≥15 mm Hg, or pulmonary artery systolic pressure ≥65 mm Hg (following provocative testing with vasodilators)

- Evidence of severe end organ damage due to diabetes (eg, retinopathy—if not treatable, nephropathy, neuropathy) and/or brittle diabetes mellitus (eg, history of diabetic ketoacidosis)
- Major chronic disabling illness (eg, lupus, severe arthritis, and neurologic diseases)
- Symptomatic severe peripheral vascular or carotid disease
- Active infection (bacterial, viral, fungal, protozoa)
- Excessive obesity (eg, >30% over normal or BMI >35 kg/m^2 [ISHLT guidelines 30 kg/m^2])
- Active substance or tobacco dependence
- Active or recent malignancy
- HIV infection
- Severe pulmonary disease
- Irreversible hepatic disease or dysfunction
- Active gastrointestinal bleeding
- Poor nutrition as evidenced by serum Albumin <2.0, significant weight loss, BMI <18, actual body weight that is 85% or less than IBW
- Chronic narcotic abuse
- Active mental illness or psychosocial instability
- Significant cognitive impairment with lack of adequate support

PATHOPHYSIOLOGY

- The major limitations to survival in the early posttransplant period (first year) are nonspecific graft failure, multiorgan failure, acute rejection, and infection.[2]
- The most recent cohort of patients who received transplants in 2006 through June 2011 had an unadjusted 1-year survival of 84%, and unadjusted mean survival is now more than 10 years.[2]
- Graft failure and organ rejection is complex, and is likely related to immunologic factors, HLA mismatch, T-cell activation, cytokine activation, and humoral factors.[4]

ECHOCARDIOGRAPHIC UTILIZATION AND FEATURES POSTCARDIAC TRANSPLANT

Echocardiography plays a critical role in the evaluation and management of the cardiac transplant patient.

- As we have explored both this chapter and Chapter 5, echocardiography is a critical tool in the evaluation and management of the CHF patient.
- Posttransplantation, echocardiography is employed to monitor cardiac structure and function and assess for potential complications. Serial echocardiography is used to monitor LV/RV function as well as valvular pathology.
- In patients who present with signs and symptoms of CHF posttransplant, echo is appropriate to assess for new/worsening systolic and diastolic dysfunction.
- Surveillance endomyocardial biopsies (employed to detect allograft rejection) are often performed under echocardiographic guidance.
- The chronic management of transplant patients includes evaluation for coronary artery disease and/or coronary allograft vasculopathy. Periodic cardiac testing is performed, which can be in the form of either coronary angiography or echocardiographic stress testing. Dobutamine stress echo is employed in some centers to assess for myocardial ischemia due to transplant vasculopathy.[5]

There are many new changes seen by echocardiography in the posttransplant heart.

- Changes in the atrial structure of the transplanted heart are caused by structural alterations necessitated by surgical implantation. The standard biatrial surgical approach involves anastomosis of the donor heart to retained cuffs of the recipient's left and right atria.[6]
  - This technique results in bilaterally enlarged atria, easily appreciated on the echocardiographic examination as elongation of the longitudinal axis of the right and left atria in the apical views (Figure 4-9-2).
  - Typically, as a result of the surgical anastomosis of the left and right atria, an echodense ridge is visible along the suture line

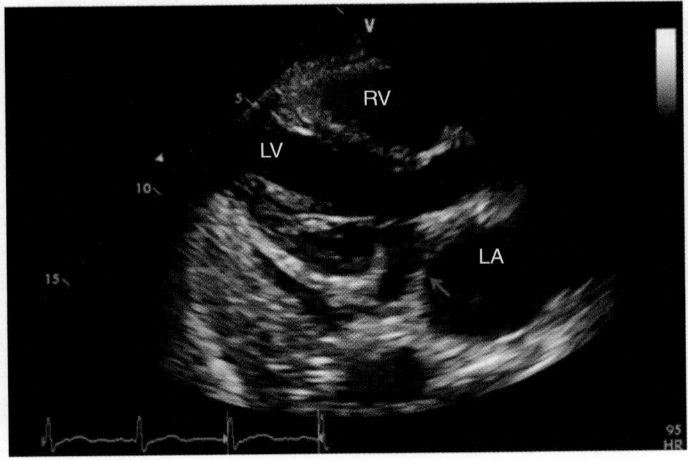

A

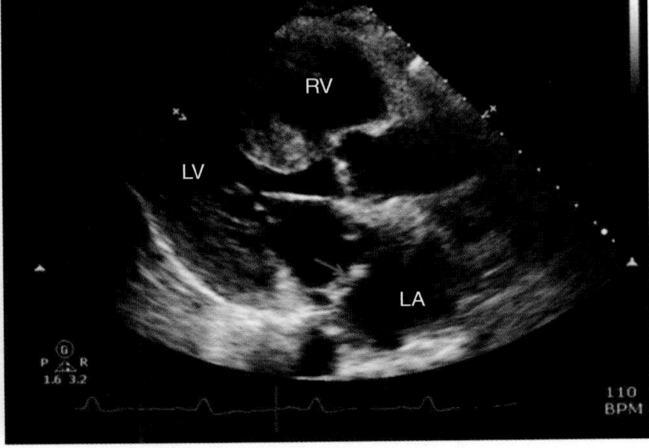

B

FIGURE 4-9-2 Parasternal long-axis view of biatrial posttransplant heart. The left atrium (LA) is enlarged and elongated, consistent with biatrial cardiac transplantation (A and B). The suture line can be seen in the left atrium (red arrows). RV=right ventricle, LV=left ventricle ► (see Video 4-9-2).

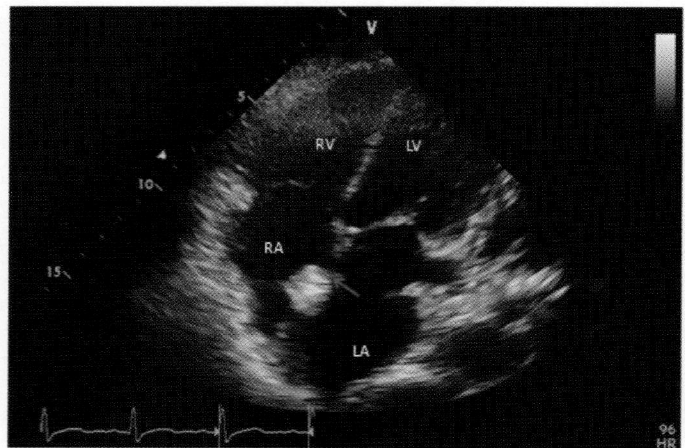

FIGURE 4-9-3 Apical 4 chamber view of posttransplant heart. The red arrow highlights an echodense ridge visible along the suture line, a result of the surgical anastomosis of the left and right atria. There is also RV enlargement and a pericardial effusion, better appreciated on the accompanying video ▶ (see Video 4-9-3). LA=left atrium, RA=right atrium, LV=left ventricle, RV=right ventricle.

(Figure 4-9-3), allowing discrimination between the donor and recipient components (particularly in patients transplanted by way of the biatrial technique).

- An alternative implant technique involves anastamosis of the vena cava (superior and inferior) in the venous circulation instead of a right-atrial anastomosis (bicaval technique).[7] This technique results in normal right atrial size (Figure 4-9-4) but may result in a suture-based stenosis within the cava.

- Pericardial effusions are not uncommon in the first year following transplantation (Figure 4-9-5). One group of investigators found pericardial effusions in 40% at some point during the first year posttransplantation.[8]
- Significant tricuspid regurgitation (Figure 4-9-6) early posttransplantation is likely related to elevated pulmonary vascular resistance in the recipient, and later is likely related to injury to the chordal apparatus caused by endomyocardial biopsy.

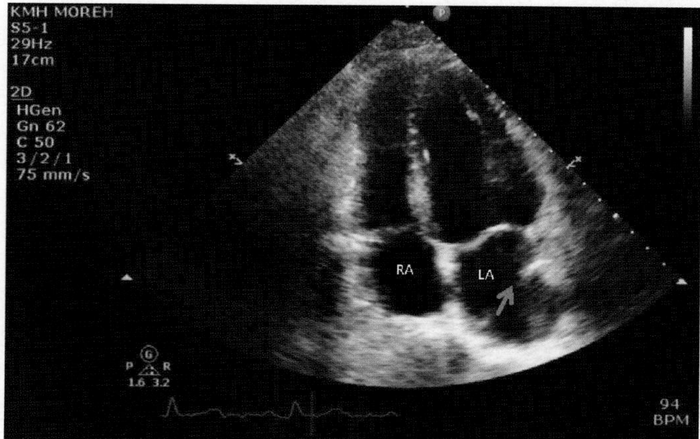

FIGURE 4-9-4 Apical 4 chamber view after transplantation using a bicaval technique. Note the normal sized right atrium (RA). A suture line (red arrow) is seen in the left atrium (LA), which denotes the anastomosis between the donor and recipient left atria ▶ (see Video 4-9-4).

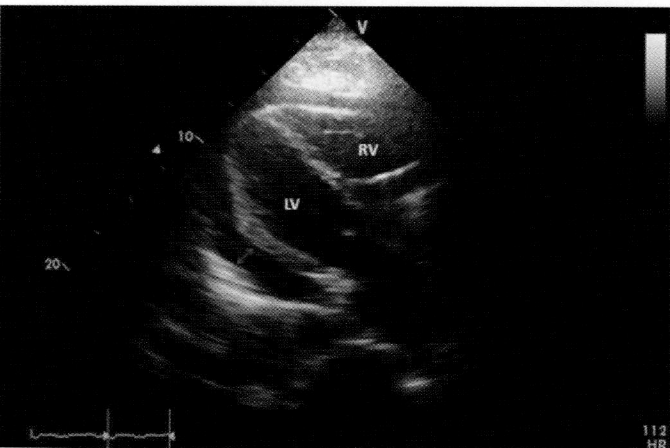

FIGURE 4-9-5 Parasternal long-axis view demonstrating a moderate-sized pericardial effusion posttransplant (red arrow). RV and LV systolic function are normal ▶ (see Video 4-9-5). LV=left ventricle, RV=right ventricle.

LABORATORY STUDIES

Routine laboratory monitoring is required posttransplant. Adequate immunosuppression with specific agents such as calcineurin inhibitors and mTOR inhibitors is monitored via therapeutic drug levels, whereas other immunosuppressive agents such as corticosteroids and antiproliferative agents are monitored clinically. Renal function, electrolyte concentrations, and cell counts can all be affected by various classes of immunosuppression and therefore require close monitoring. Serum monitoring for opportunistic infections (especially cytomegalovirus) is routinely undertaken as well. Direct endomyocardial biopsies, performed at some centers under echo guidance (Figure 4-9-7) are utilized to monitor for rejection of the transplanted heart.

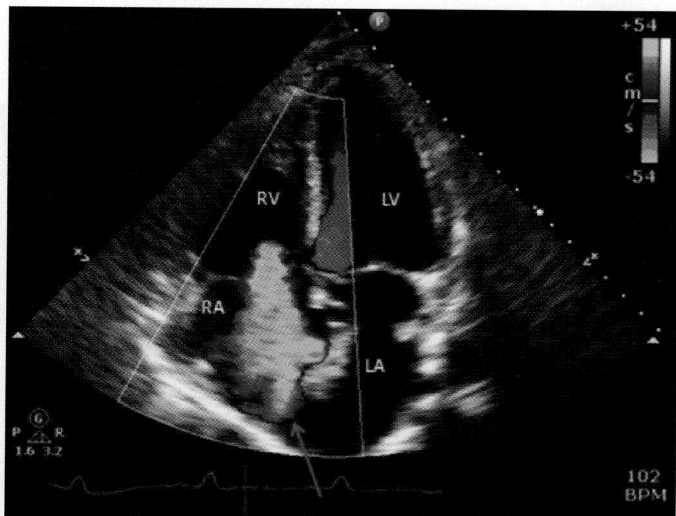

FIGURE 4-9-6 Apical 4 chamber view demonstrating severe tricuspid regurgitation (red arrow) postcardiac transplant. In this patient, the TR was the result of TV chordal disruption resulting in the TR. Some patients may require TV repair or replacement ▶ (see Video 4-9-6) LA=left atrium, RA=right atrium, LV=left ventricle, RV=right ventricle.

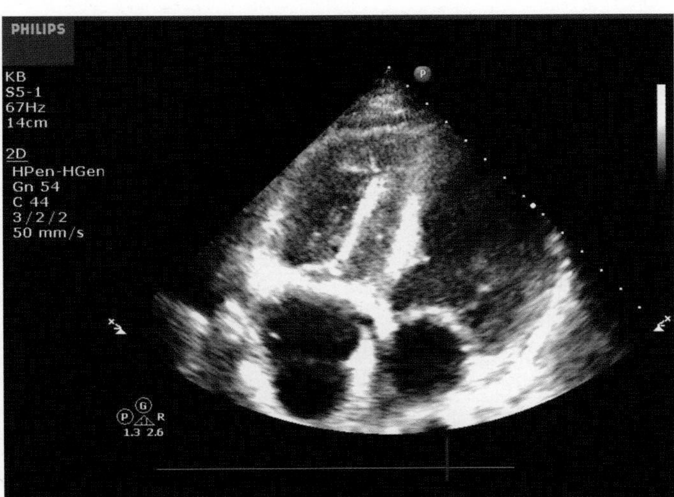

FIGURE 4-9-7 Endomyocardial biopsy performed with echo guidance. The bioptome can be seen in the RV with the sampling forceps directed toward the septum. With echo guidance, immediate complications such as chordal disruption resting in TR and the development of a pericardial effusion can be identified ▶ (see Videos 4-9-7 A and B). In this patient the pericardial effusion was present prior to the procedure.

MANAGEMENT

Postoperative care is primarily provided by a specialized transplant team, which monitors for complications of transplant including rejection, allograft failure, or sequelae of immunosuppression. Many of these patients continue to see their primary care physician as well for ongoing management of other chronic medical conditions as well as for routine evaluations and health screening/immunizations.

PATIENT EDUCATION

If there are signs or symptoms of shortness of breath, fever, rash, oral candidiasis, syncope, or edema then cardiac consultation should be pursued to minimize the risk of serious infections or cardiac rejection.

FOLLOW-UP

The evaluation, care, and management of transplant patients should be done through specialized transplant centers.

VIDEO LEGENDS

1. Video 4-9-1: Apical four-chamber view pre-transplant. Note the dilated left ventricle associated with progressive cardiomyopathy. In addition, the CRT device is seen and the ECG has evidence of bi-ventricular pacing
2. Video 4-9-2: Parasternal long-axis view of biatrial post-transplant heart. The left atrium (LA) is enlarged and elongated, consistent with biatrial cardiac transplantation
3. Video 4-9-3: Apical four-chamber view of post-transplant heart. There is an echodense ridge visible along the suture line, a result of the surgical anastomosis of the left and right atria (better seen on the still image). There is also RV enlargement and a pericardial effusion, appreciated on this video.
4. Video 4-9-4: Apical four-chamber view after transplantation using a bicaval technique. Note the normal sized right atrium (RA). A suture line is seen in the left atrium (LA), which denotes the anastomosis between the donor and recipient left atria.
5. Video 4-9-5: Parasternal long-axis view demonstrating a moderate sized pericardial effusion post-transplant. RV and LV systolic function are normal.
6. Video 4-9-6: Apical four-chamber view demonstrating severe tricuspid regurgitation post-cardiac transplant. In this patient, the TR was the result of TV chordal disruption resulting in the TR.
7. Video 4-9-7 A: Endomyocardial biopsy performed with echo guidance. The bioptome can be seen entering the RV being withdrawn toward the RA. With echo guidance, immediate complications such as chordal disruption resting in TR and the development of a pericardial effusion can be identified. In this patient the pericardial effusion was present prior to the procedure.
8. Video 4-9-7 B: Endomyocardial biopsy performed with echo guidance. The bioptome can be seen in the RV with the sampling forceps directed toward the septum. With echo guidance, immediate complications such as chordal disruption resting in TR and the development of a pericardial effusion can be identified. In this patient the pericardial effusion was present prior to the procedure.

REFERENCES

1. Go AS, Mozaffarian D, Roger VL, et al. Executive summary: heart disease and stroke statistics—2013 update: a report from the American Heart Association. *Circulation*. 2013;127(1):143-52.
2. Lund LH, Edwards LB, Kucheryavaya AY, et al. The Registry of the International Society for Heart and Lung Transplantation: thirtieth official adult heart transplant report—2013; focus theme: age. *J Heart Lung Transplant*. 2013;32:951-964.
3. Costanzo MR, Dipchand A, Starling R, et al. The International Society of Heart and Lung Transplantation Guidelines for the care of heart transplant recipients. *J Heart Lung Transplant*. 2010;29:914-956.
4. Heeger PS, Dinavahi R. Transplant immunology for non-immunologist. *Mt Sinai J Med*. 2012;79:376-387.
5. Derumeaux G, Redonnet M, Mouton-Schleifer D, et al. Dobutamine stress echocardiography in orthotopic heart transplant recipients. VACOMED Research Group. *J Am Coll Cardiol*. 1995;25(7):1665-1672.
6. Yacoub M, Mankad P, Ledingham S. Donor procurement and surgical techniques for cardiac transplantation. *Semin Thorac Cardiovasc Surg*. 1990;2:153-161.
7. Dreyfus G, Jebara V, Mihaileanu S, Carpentier AF. Total orthotopic heart transplantation: an alternative to the standard technique. *Ann Thorac Surg*. 1991;52:1181-1184.
8. Vandenberg BF, Mohanty PK, Craddock KJ, et al. Clinical significance of pericardial effusion after heart transplantation. *J Heart Transplant*. 1988;7:128-134.

5 ECHOCARDIOGRAPHIC ASSESSMENT OF CARDIOMYOPATHIES

Dennis A. Tighe, MD, FACC, FACP, FASE

INTRODUCTION

Broadly defined, the cardiomyopathies are a heterogeneous group of disorders that primarily or secondarily affect the myocardium leading to impairment of systolic and/or diastolic performance. Several schemes have been proposed to classify the cardiomyopathies. While differences in classification exist between the various schemes, the basic approach to the patient with heart muscle disease remains unchanged: a comprehensive history and physical examination and appropriately targeted imaging are required in all patients for appropriate diagnosis and treatment. Echocardiography is usually employed in the initial patient evaluation and is often sufficient to provide an adequate assessment of the heart based on morphology and physiology. Selected patients may qualify for more advanced imaging techniques, invasive biopsy, or genetic testing depending upon individual circumstances. Using a case-based approach, this chapter will review the clinical and imaging features, pathophysiology, and management of the cardiomyopathies.

SECTION I

Ischemic Cardiomyopathy

CLINICAL CASE PRESENTATION

An actively smoking 85-year-old man with a history of previous myocardial infarction, permanent atrial fibrillation, peripheral arterial disease, coronary artery bypass surgery 12 years prior, and an LV ejection fraction of 20% presented to an outside hospital with severe respiratory distress that required endotracheal intubation and mechanical ventilation. He denied having experienced chest discomfort. He was transferred to our institution for further care. On arrival, a 12-lead electrocardiogram (ECG) showed atrial fibrillation with right bundle branch block and lateral ST-segment depressions. Chest radiography revealed cardiomegaly and the presence of bilateral pleural effusions and interstitial edema. A brain natriuretic peptide (BNP) level was >4000 pg/mL; cardiac troponin I levels were within normal limits. Echocardiography demonstrated LV dilatation and evidence of regional wall motion abnormalities with akinesis and thinning in the distributions of the circumflex and right coronary arteries and severe hypokinesis in the distribution of the anterior descending artery. The left atrium was markedly dilated, and LV filling pressures were elevated. Moderate to severe mitral regurgitation (MR) was demonstrated and the pulmonary artery systolic pressure (PASP) was estimated to be about 50 to 55 mm Hg. With aggressive diuresis, the patient was able to be separated from the ventilator within 24 hours. Appropriate guideline-recommended medical therapy was initiated and titrated to tolerance; smoking cessation was stressed. A subsequent SPECT-thallium viability study confirmed the depressed LVEF and documented infarct (scar) involving the entirety of the distributions of the circumflex and right coronary arteries; no evident ischemia was demonstrated in the LAD distribution. After discussion with his primary cardiologist, and taking into consideration his clinical status, a decision not to pursue coronary angiography and prophylactic ICD implantation was made.

CLINICAL FEATURES

As demonstrated by this case vignette, a history of prior coronary heart disease (CHD) is evident in most patients, although some may offer no such history.

- Patients may present with an asymptomatic reduction in left ventricular ejection fraction (LVEF), but most present with symptoms and signs of heart failure, such as fluid retention, exertional dyspnea, fatigue, or exercise intolerance, with or without angina pectoris.
- A history of prior CHD with prior revascularization procedures or myocardial infarction, peripheral artery disease or significant risk factors for CHD is common and should prompt further investigation because in up to two-thirds of cases of heart failure with reduced LVEF the underlying cause is found to be ischemic heart disease.
- In a large retrospective database study of patients undergoing coronary angiography for LVEF ≤40%, three-quarters of the patients with ischemic cardiomyopathy had greater than or equal to 75% stenoses of the left anterior descending artery, and 46% had three-vessel CHD.[1]
- Patients with ischemic cardiomyopathy more often were older, men, and possessed a higher incidence of risk factors for CHD

compared to patients with nonischemic cardiomyopathies. In this database, patients with nonischemic cardiomyopathies had lower LVEFs and longer duration of heart failure symptoms.

- It should be appreciated that as many as one-third of patients with nonischemic cardiomyopathy may complain of chest pain.[1]

EPIDEMIOLOGY

- Currently, it is estimated that 6 million people in the United States live with heart failure; approximately 40% to 50% have preserved LVEF. The remaining individuals have heart failure with impaired systolic function (systolic CHF).
- Coronary heart disease is the leading cause of systolic heart failure in industrialized nations. Among heart failure patients with reduced LVEF, it is estimated that 60% of cases occur secondary to an ischemic etiology.
- About 7% of heart failure patients with previously unexplained cardiomyopathies are subsequently identified to have ischemic heart disease as the cause of LV dysfunction.[2] Among a cohort of patients with myocardial infarction and no previous history of heart failure, approximately 40% developed heart failure (most often with reduced LVEF) over a follow-up period averaging 6.6 years.[3]
- Compared to patients with nonischemic etiology, a lower 5-year survival is found among patients with ischemic cardiomyopathy.[1]

PATHOPHYSIOLOGY

Ischemic cardiomyopathy refers to significantly impaired LV systolic function (ejection fraction ≤35%-40%) resulting from the presence of underlying CHD.

- Impaired systolic function may be due to irreversible loss of myocardium (scarring) with resultant adverse ventricular remodeling, reduced function due to ischemic but still viable myocardium (hibernation and/or repetitive stunning), or a combination of the two. Multivessel CHD with involvement of the left anterior descending artery is common.[1]
- In the presence of extensive scar, revascularization would not be expected to lead to improved LVEF. Targeted revascularization would be expected to improve symptoms and prognosis in the presence of significant amounts of viable myocardium.
- Among patients with CHD, underlying risk factors such as systemic hypertension, diabetes mellitus, and/or LV hypertrophy may also contribute to the observed ventricular dysfunction.

ECHOCARDIOGRAPHY

For patients presenting with new onset heart failure symptoms, echocardiography has a Class I indication in the initial evaluation.[4] Recently published appropriate use criteria would consider use of echocardiography as "appropriate" for this clinical indication.[5] While the history, physical examination, and ECG often help identify heart failure patients with ischemic etiology, the echocardiographic picture may not always be quite so clear.

- It may be difficult to distinguish an ischemic from a nonischemic dilated cardiomyopathy on the basis of echocardiography alone. Findings common to both conditions include the presence of a dilated, hypocontractile LV cavity with evidence for reduced systolic and diastolic performance.
  - Wall thickness may be normal or reduced.
  - With advanced disease, a more spherical LV geometry may be seen in both conditions.
  - Dilatation of the left atrium, right atrium, and/or right ventricle (RV) may be present. The RV may display reduced (systolic) performance due to an imposed afterload (such as increased PA systolic pressure or pulmonary vascular resistance) and/or pathological involvement.
  - Intracavitary thrombus may be seen coincident with areas of akinesis (Figure 5-1-1). Similar to findings that may be encountered with nonischemic dilated cardiomyopathy, the M-mode examination may show an increased E-point-septal separation distance (indicative of reduced LV stroke volume), a B-bump (interrupted A-C closure) indicating elevated LV end diastolic (and LA)

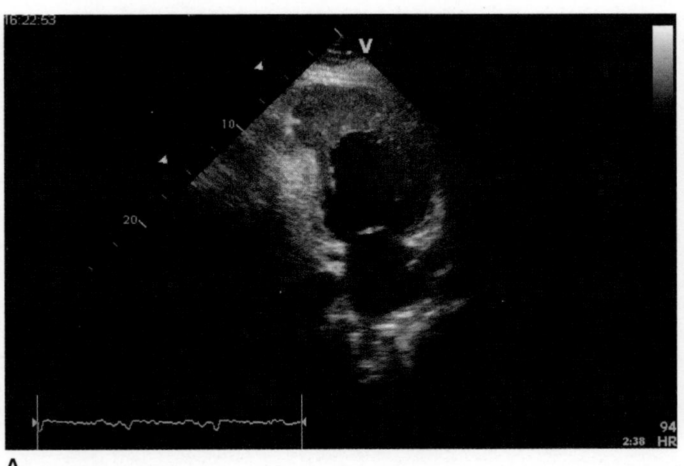

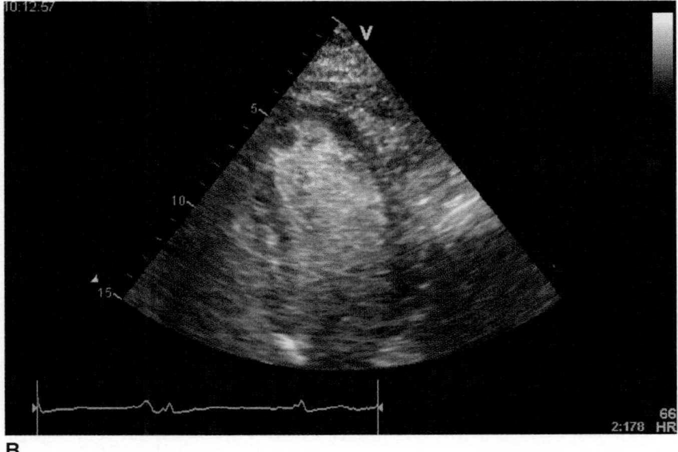

FIGURE 5-1-1 (A) Apical 2 chamber view recorded in a patient with prior myocardial infarction and a large left ventricular apical aneurysm. Echodensity consistent with thrombus fills the anuerysmal area ▶ (see Video 5-1-1 A). (B) Microbubble contrast-enhanced apical 4 chamber view showing a protruding, rounded filling defect adjacent to the apical portion of the septum. In the presence of a focal wall motion abnormality in this segment, thrombus is highly likely as the etiology ▶ (see Video 5-1-1 B).

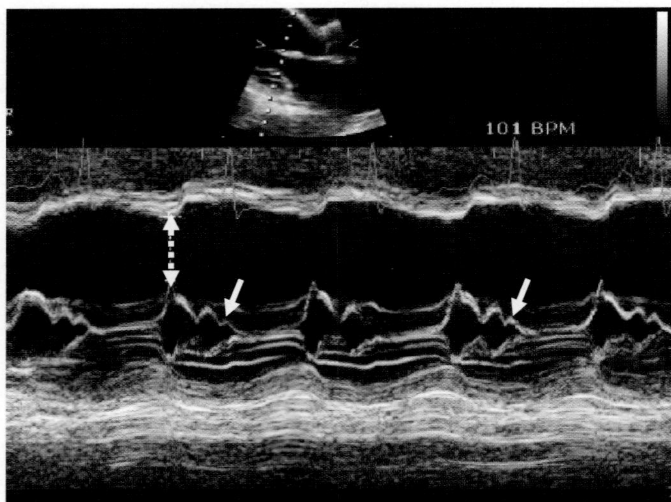

FIGURE 5-1-2 M-mode recording made through the mitral valve demonstrating increased E-point septal separation distance (stippled arrow) and interrupted A-C closure (B-bump) [solid arrows]. The presence of an increased E-point septal separation distance is indicative of reduced stroke volume while a B-bump is indicative of increased left ventricular end-diastolic pressure.

pressure, and gradual closure of the aortic valve echo during systole (Figures 5-1-2 and 5-1-3).

- Doppler assessment of diastolic function, including the E/A ratio, E/e' ratio, deceleration time, and analysis of the pulmonary vein spectral profile, rarely is normal among patients with advanced ischemic or nonischemic cardiomyopathies.
- Increased pulmonary artery systolic pressures and mild or greater functional mitral regurgitation can be observed occur in the majority of patients.

• The hallmark of ischemic heart disease is the presence of regional wall motion abnormality in the distribution of known coronary artery territories.

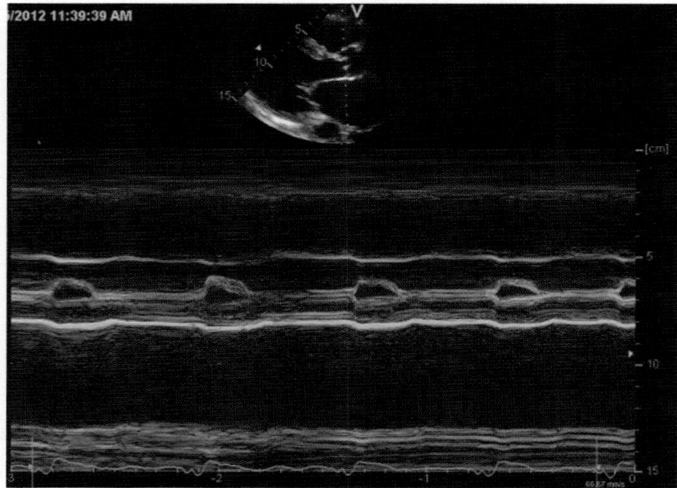

FIGURE 5-1-3 M-mode recording of the aortic valve in systole demonstrating that after initial opening the leaflets drift to closure gradually rather than exhibiting the usual "boxcar-like" configuration. This finding is indicative of reduced stroke volume.

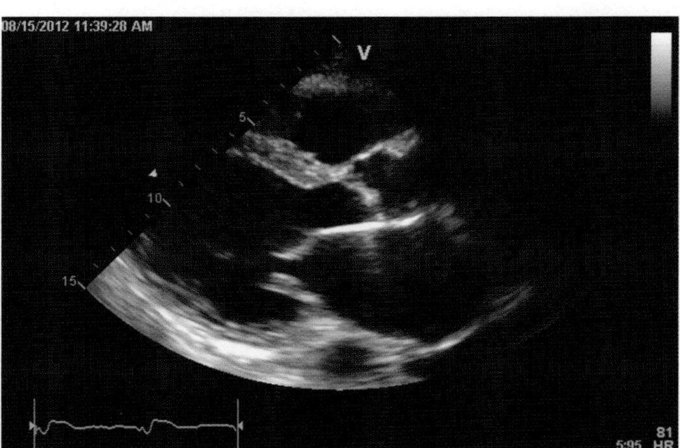

FIGURE 5-1-4 Parasternal long-axis image showing a dilated left ventricular cavity with thinning and akinesis of the visualized portion of the inferolateral wall. The interventricular septum is hypokinetic. The excursion of the mitral valve is reduced due to the low stroke volume ► (see Video 5-1-4).

- Among patients with dilated cardiomyopathy, regional wall motion abnormalities must be interpreted with caution as regional variation in systolic function may be seen in nonischemic cardiomyopathies.
- When a substantial area of scar (thinning [<6 mm wall thickness] with increased echo-reflectivity) (Figures 5-1-4 and 5-1-5) corresponding to the known distribution of a coronary artery territory is present or an LV aneurysm (apical or inferobasal) is observed, the likelihood of ischemic etiology is increased.
- Functional studies, such as dobutamine stress echocardiography, myocardial perfusion imaging, or positron emission tomographic imaging may be useful in making this distinction. In many instances, however, another imaging modality, such as cardiac magnetic resonance with gadolinium enhancement or coronary angiography (most commonly), will be required.

• Deformation (strain/strain rate) imaging can provide an objective measure of both global and regional myocardial function and

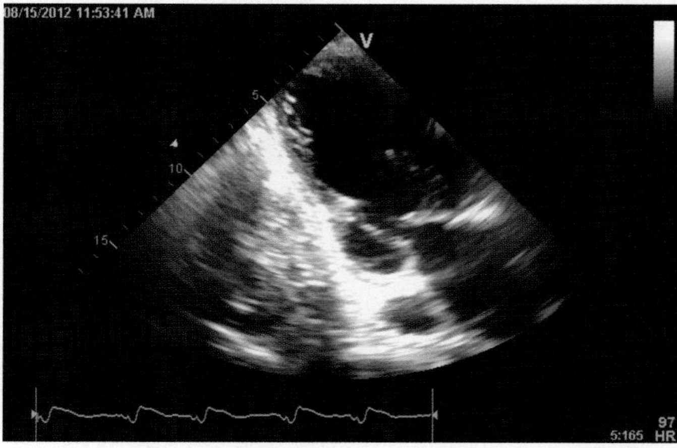

FIGURE 5-1-5 Apical 2 chamber image demonstrating akinesis and thinning of the inferior wall. A left pleural effusion is present ► (see Video 5-1-5).

thus may offer additional information in distinguishing myocardial infarction from ischemic but viable tissue.

- Deformation imaging can help distinguish between passive motion (such as with tethering of infarcted tissue by adjacent segments) and active contraction characteristic of viable tissue and may be predictive of the transmural extent of infarction.
- Postsystolic shortening has been reported to be a specific marker of ischemic tissue, and indexed post-systolic stain rates may help define transmural extent of infarction.[6]

OTHER DIAGNOSTIC TESTS AND PROCEDURES

- Electrocardiography: The ECG finding of pathological Q waves should strongly raise the suspicion of an ischemic etiology. The ECG, however, may be nonspecific in the absence of diagnostic Q waves; findings such as sinus tachycardia, nonspecific ST/T abnormalities, bundle-branch block, and conduction defects may be observed.
- Chest radiography is often nonspecific. The finding of cardiomegaly, with or without interstitial edema, is often observed. Pleural effusions may be observed in more advanced disease.
- Other imaging modalities that may be employed include nuclear medicine studies to evaluate for ischemia/viability, cardiac MRI, and cardiac PET. Cardiac catheterization is appropriate to define coronary artery anatomy and evaluate the patient for potential revascularization.

DIFFERENTIAL DIAGNOSIS

The clinical presentation of ischemic cardiomyopathy is relatively straightforward as the majority of patients have a prior history of CHD and frequently present with angina pectoris. The main differential is that of a dilated, nonischemic cardiomyopathy. Two points must be emphasized.

- The presence of asymptomatic, nonobstructive CHD does not prove causality unless prior infarction or significant hibernating/stunned myocardium is documented.
- Patients with nonischemic cardiomyopathies often present with chest pain symptoms that can resemble angina pectoris.
- Any number of other conditions can cause dilated cardiomyopathy. The history should focus on identification of specific etiologies (Table 5-1-1).
- The physical examination often reveals signs of heart failure. In some cases, discovery of an underlying systemic disease may be aided by the physical examination. In addition, the physical examination may help to exclude other potential causes of heart failure such as valvular heart disease or pericardial disease.
- In the setting of rapid supraventricular tachycardia or atrial fibrillation or flutter, a diagnosis of a tachycardia-mediated cardiomyopathy should be entertained.

DIAGNOSIS

- The diagnosis is made on the basis of clinical features, ECG findings, recognition of regional wall motion abnormalities and assessment of LVEF by echocardiography, and results of coronary angiography.

TABLE 5-1-1 Causes of Dilated Cardiomyopathy

Toxins
Ethanol, cocaine
Chemotherapeutic agents
Medications
Trace elements
Metabolic
Nutritional
Infectious
Inflammatory
Neuromuscular disorders
Familial/genetic
Idiopathic
Ischemic
Stress-induced
Peripartum
Tachycardia-induced
LBBB dyssynchrony

- Most patients present with a history of known CHD.
- While noninvasive testing may strongly suggest the diagnosis, coronary angiography is recommended for definitive diagnosis among patients with angina or significant ischemia potentially eligible for revascularization (Class I, LOE B).[7] The extent of disease found at angiography is a better indicator of prognosis than is the clinical diagnosis of ischemic cardiomyopathy.[1]
- It must be reemphasized that in patients with reduced LVEF chest pain alone is not a sufficient diagnostic criterion since as many as one-third of patients with nonischemic cardiomyopathies may complain of this symptom. For this group of patients, coronary angiography is suggested due to common occurrence of false-positive findings on noninvasive testing.

MANAGEMENT

- Treatment with antiplatelet agents is recommended for all patients without contraindications.
- ACE-inhibitors and β-blockers are recommended for all patients with LV dysfunction (LVEF ≤40%). Management of patients with heart failure should follow that which is detailed in published guidelines.[7]
- While risk factor modification is recommended for all patients with ischemic heart disease and heart failure, the role of statins among patients with systolic heart failure (including those with ischemic cardiomyopathy) is less clear. The two largest randomized trials to date addressing this issue[8,9] showed that initiating therapy with a HMG Co-A reductase-inhibitor was not useful among patients

with systolic heart failure regardless of whether or not CHD was present.

- Per guideline recommendations, placement of ICDs is indicated for patients with appropriate indications.[7]
- Until recently, the role of coronary artery bypass grafting (CABG) surgery among patients receiving contemporary medical therapy was uncertain. In the recently published STITCH trial,[10] patients with ischemic cardiomyopathy (LVEF <35%) and CHD amenable to bypass surgery were randomized to strategies that compared best medical therapy to surgical revascularization along with medical therapy. After a median follow-up of 56 months there was no difference in all cause mortality; patients undergoing CABG experienced lower rates of death from cardiovascular causes and hospitalizations for cardiac-related causes. A second publication from the STITCH group[11] addressed the issue of whether or not surgical revascularization improved survival among patients with chronic ischemic LV dysfunction when viable myocardium is documented. This investigation has shown no survival benefit from revascularization in this population. It should be appreciated that patients with left main-stem disease or acute coronary syndromes were excluded from further analysis.
- Symptomatic patients with angina pectoris despite optimal medical therapy should be considered for revascularization. A trial of medical therapy may be appropriate in all other patients with revascularization held in reserve for those with progressive symptoms despite optimal medical therapy.

FOLLOW-UP

Patients should be followed regularly by a cardiologist to assess for adequacy of therapy and progression of underlying disease processes. Consultation with a heart failure specialist is prudent with significant disease progression despite adequate medical/device therapy and when more advanced therapies are being considered.

VIDEO LEGENDS

1. Video 5-1-1 A: Apical 2-chamber view recorded in a patient with prior myocardial infarction and a large left ventricular apical aneurysm. Echodensity consistent with thrombus fills the aneurysmal area.
2. Video 5-1-1 B: Microbubble contrast-enhanced apical 4-chamber view showing a protruding, rounded filling defect adjacent to the apical portion of the septum. In the presence of a focal wall motion abnormality in this segment, thrombus is highly likely as the etiology.
3. Video 5-1-4: Parasternal long-axis image showing a dilated left ventricular cavity with thinning and akinesis of the visualized portion of the inferolateral wall. The interventricular septum is hypokinetic. The excursion of the mitral valve is reduced due to the low stroke volume.
4. Video 5-1-5 : Apical 2-chamber image demonstrating akinesis and thinning of the inferior wall. A left pleural effusion is present.

REFERENCES

1. Bart BA, Shaw LK, McCants CB Jr, et al. Clinical determinants of mortality in patients with angiographically diagnosed ischemic or nonischemic cardiomyopathy. *J Am Coll Cardiol.* 1997;30:1002-1008.
2. Felker GM, Thompson RE, Hare JM, et al. Underlying causes and long-term survival in patients with initially unexplained cardiomyopathy. *N Engl J Med.* 2000;342:1077-1084.
3. Hellermann JP, Jacobsen SJ, Redfield MM, Reeder GS, Weston SA, Roger VL. Heart failure after myocardial infarction: clinical presentation and survival. *Eur J Heart Fail.* 2005;7:119-125.
4. Cheitlin MD, Armstrong WF, Aurigemma GP, et al. ACC/AHA/ASE 2003 guideline update for the clinical application of echocardiography: summary article: a report of the American College of Cardiology/American Heart Association Task Force on Practice Guidelines (ACC/AHA/ASE Committee to Update the 1997 Guidelines for the Clinical Application of Echocardiography). *Circulation.* 2003;108:1146-1162.
5. Douglas PS, Garcia MJ, Haines DE, et al. ACCF/ASE/AHA/ASNC/HFSA/ HRS/SCAI/SCCM/ SCCT/SCMR 2011 appropriate use criteria for echocardiography: a report of the American College of Cardiology Foundation Appropriate Use Criteria Task Force, American Society of Echocardiography, American Heart Association, American Society of Nuclear Cardiology, Heart Failure Society of America, Heart Rhythm Society, Society of Cardiovascular Angiography and Interventions, Society of Critical Care Medicine, Society of Cardiovascular Computed Tomography, and Society of Cardiovascular Magnetic Resonance. *J Am Coll Cardiol.* 2011;57(9):1126-1166.
6. Gorcsan J 3rd, Tanaka H. Echocardiographic assessment of myocardial strain. *J Am Coll Cardiol.* 2011;58:1401-1413.
7. Yancy CW, Jessup M, Bozkurt B, et al. 2013 ACCF/AHA guideline for the management of heart failure: a report of the American College of Cardiology Foundation/American Heart Association Task Force on Practice Guidelines. *J Am Coll Cardiol.* 2013;62:e147–239. This document is available on the World Wide Web sites of the American College of Cardiology (www.cardiosource.org) and the American Heart Association (my.americanheart.org).
8. Kjekshus J, Apetrei E, Barrios V, et al. Rosuvastatin in older patients with systolic heart failure. *N Engl J Med.* 2007;357:2248-2261.
9. GISSI-HF investigators. Effect of rosuvastatin in patients with chronic heart failure (the GISSI-HF trial): a randomised, double-blind, placebo-controlled trial. *Lancet.* 2008;372:1231-1239.
10. Velazquez EJ, Lee KL, Deja MA, et al. STICH Investigators. Coronary-artery bypass surgery in patients with left ventricular dysfunction. *N Engl J Med.* 2011;364:1607-1616.
11. Bonow RO, Maurer G, Lee KL, et al. STICH Trial Investigators. Myocardial viability and survival in ischemic left ventricular dysfunction. *N Engl J Med.* 2011;364:1617-1625.

SECTION 2

Nonischemic Cardiomyopathy

CLINICAL CASE PRESENTATION

A 41-year-old man with Becker muscular dystrophy was referred for evaluation of cardiac performance due to progressively worsening dyspnea on exertion and bilateral lower extremity edema. Two years prior he was seen at an outside institution for evaluation of fatigue and cough. At that time, he was found to be in atrial fibrillation and to have a dilated LV, severe mitral regurgitation (MR), and an LVEF of 30%. Coronary angiography showed nonobstructive disease. He underwent electrical cardioversion, and an appropriate medical program was initiated. Subsequently, he developed episodes of nonsustained ventricular tachycardia, and an ICD was implanted. He denied paroxysmal nocturnal dyspnea and orthopnea and did not complain of chest pain. He did not complain of palpitations and had experienced no ICD discharges. Due to insurance issues, he could not afford several of his medications. He noted an approximate 10-pound weight gain since his last visit with a physician. An older brother died several years earlier from noncardiac complications of Becker muscular dystrophy. He did not smoke, consume alcohol, or use illicit drugs. He held part-time employment as a librarian. Echocardiography showed a dilated and hypocontractile LV (end-diastolic dimension 80 mm and end-systolic dimension 70 mm) with inferolateral akinesis and wall thinning; the LVEF was estimated to be 20%. The LA was dilated, and severe functional MR was present. The PA systolic pressure was estimated to be 60 mm Hg. The RV was dilated and hypokinetic.

CLINICAL FEATURES AND PRESENTATION

- Patients with nonischemic cardiomyopathies often present with manifestations of heart failure such as progressive exertional dyspnea, exercise intolerance, PND or orthopnea, or fluid retention/edema.
- Other symptoms such as chest pain, atrial or ventricular arrhythmias, conduction disturbances, thromboembolic events, or sudden cardiac death may also lead to clinical presentation.
- Patients with advanced disease can present with clinical features consistent with a low cardiac output syndrome that may include fatigue, anorexia, hepatic congestion, edema, cool extremities, and tachycardia.
- Patients may present with asymptomatic LV dysfunction discovered as cardiomegaly on chest imaging or a low LVEF on echocardiography obtained for another clinical indication.
- The physical examination may show signs of cardiac dysfunction such as narrowed pulse pressure, resting tachycardia, pulsus alternans, jugular venous distention, pulmonary rales, displaced apical impulse, gallop rhythm, and peripheral edema. A low cardiac output state is likely when a narrow pulse pressure (<25 mm Hg), cool extremities due to peripheral vasoconstriction, diaphoresis, and resting (sinus) tachycardia are found.

EPIDEMIOLOGY

- The estimated incidence of nonischemic dilated cardiomyopathy is 5 to 8 cases/100,000 persons per year. The prevalence is estimated to be 36 cases/100,000 population. Preclinical heart failure may be present in up to 50% patients with LV dysfunction.[1]
- The diagnosis is made most often among persons 20 to 60 years old, but individuals of any age can be affected. A slight male predominance is observed.
- Up to 20% to 35% of first-degree relatives may be affected (most subclinical), suggesting an underlying genetic susceptibility to disease.

PATHOPHYSIOLOGY AND ETIOLOGY

- Diverse causes of dilated cardiomyopathy are recognized (see Table 5-1-1).
- After excluding an ischemic etiology, almost 50% of cases are considered idiopathic.[2] Other potential etiologies of nonischemic cardipomyopathy include a variety of infectious, toxic/metabolic, nutritional, genetic, and miscellaneous causes.
- Dilated cardiomyopathy is the most common form of cardiomyopathy. It is characterized by enlargement and impairment of systolic performance (ejection fraction ≤40%) of one or both ventricles.
  - Often the LV assumes a more spherical geometry leading to papillary muscle displacement and functional MR.
  - Dilatation of the mitral annulus along with impaired LV systolic performance may also contribute to the occurrence of functional MR.
  - Concomitant diastolic dysfunction is common.
  - Intracavitary thrombus (often layered and located at the LV apex) is seen frequently on postmortem examinations, but less often is documented by echocardiography.
- On histology, myocyte hypertrophy and interstitial fibrosis are characteristic findings. Infiltration with lymphocytes or giant cells may be observed with myocarditis.
- Survival is dependent on the etiology of the underlying disease process along with disease-independent factors such as LVEF, NYHA class, 6-minute walk distance, and maximal oxygen consumption on cardiopulmonary exercise testing.

ECHOCARDIOGRAPHY

The hallmark of a dilated cardiomyopathy is the presence of a dilated LV cavity with reduced systolic (and diastolic) performance (Figures 5-2-1 and 5-2-2).

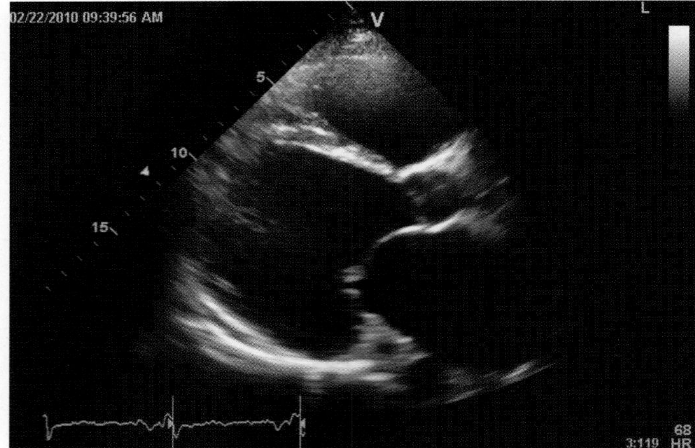

FIGURE 5-2-1 Parasternal long-axis view showing a massively dilated and diffusely hypocontractile LV in a patient with an advanced nonischemic cardiomyopathy ▶ (see Video 5-2-1). As illustrated by this example, a regional wall motion abnormality is demonstrated; however, the majority of patients with nonischemic dilated cardiomyopathies do not manifest such a focal finding. Also note that both the left atrium and right ventricle are dilated, mitral leaflet excursion is reduced, and the coronary sinus is prominent.

- In comparison to an ischemic cardiomyopathy, LV systolic dysfunction often manifests in a pattern of global rather than regional wall motion abnormality.
- However, with nonischemic cardiomyopathies, regional variation in contraction can be observed commonly; often the basal inferolateral wall shows relatively preserved contractility in comparison to other wall segments. As illustrated by this case example, regional wall motion abnormalities may be seen in certain cases.
- An accurate assessment of LVEF is mandatory (biplane Simpson's method or 3-D echocardiography are preferred) as patients with persisting LVEF <35% despite adequate medical therapy are candidates for prophylactic ICD placement.
    - Wall thickness may be normal or reduced.

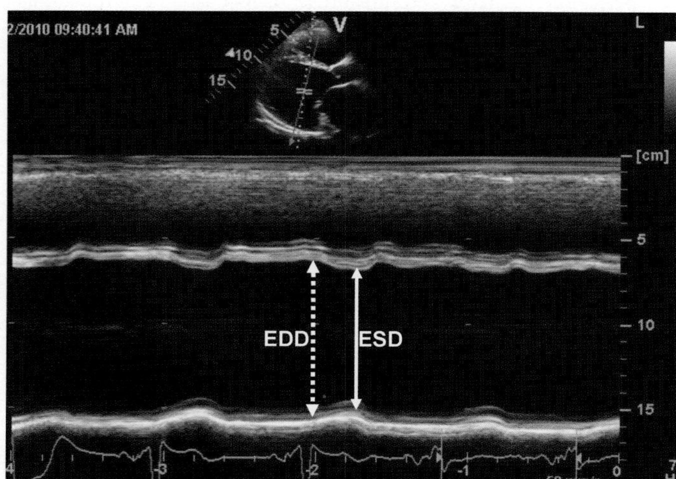

FIGURE 5-2-2 M-mode recording demonstrating the findings of a dilated and hypocontractile LV. EDD = end-diastolic dimension; ESD = end-systolic dimension.

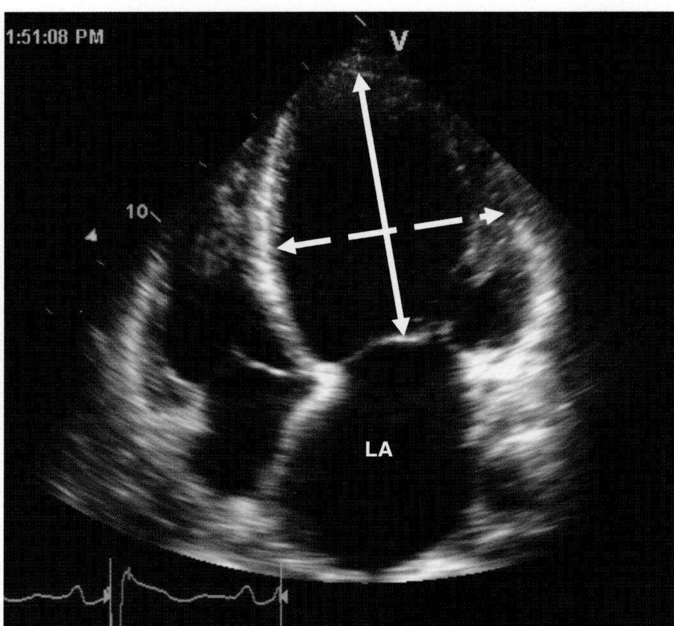

FIGURE 5-2-3 Apical 4 chamber view illustrating adverse geometric remodeling in a patient with nonischemic cardiomyopathy. The LV has assumed a more spherical geometry as illustrated by a reduced sphericity index, ratio of major-axis dimension (solid arrow) to minor-axis dimension (stippled arrow), of 1.33 in this example. Note also the dilatation of the left atrium (LA).

- With advanced disease, a more spherical LV geometry (ratio of long-axis/minor axis <1.5) may be seen (Figure 5-2-3).
- Dilatation of the LA, RV, and/or RV may be present.
- The LV apex should be scanned carefully for the presence of thrombus.
- The RV may exhibit reduced systolic performance due to imposed afterload (such as increased PA systolic pressure or pulmonary vascular resistance) and/or pathological involvement.
- The M-mode examination may show an increased E-point-septal separation distance (corresponding with reduced LV stroke volume), a B-bump (interrupted A-C closure) indicative of elevated LV end-diastolic (and LA) pressure, and gradual closure of the aortic valve echo during systole.
- Doppler assessment of diastolic function rarely is normal among patients with advanced nonischemic cardiomyopathies.
- Increased pulmonary artery systolic pressures and functional mitral regurgitation (Figures 5-2-4 and 5-2-5) are present in the majority of patients.
- Indicators of adverse prognosis on echocardiography include increased end-diastolic and end-systolic volumes, LVEF <40%, sphericity index <1.5, LV dp/dt <600 mm Hg/s, abnormal myocardial performance index (>0.4), a restrictive filling pattern, and increased left atrial volume index.

OTHER DIAGNOSTIC TESTS AND PROCEDURES

- As a number of conditions may potentially result in a nonischemic cardiomyopathy, the history should focus on identification of specific etiologies (see Table 5-1-1).

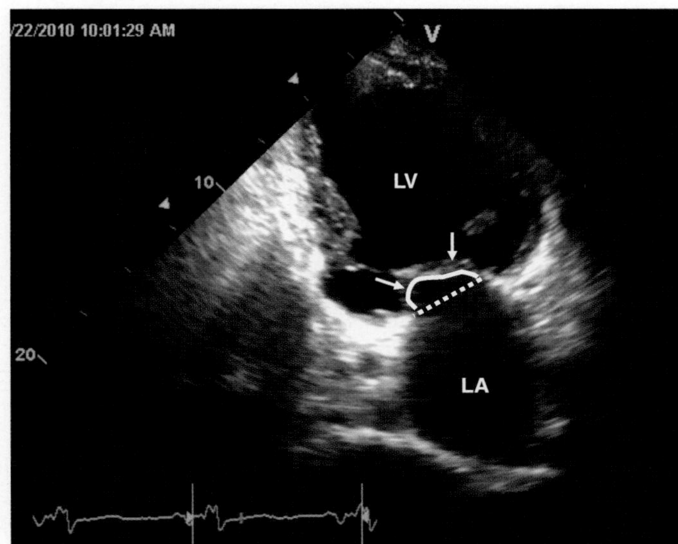

FIGURE 5-2-4 Apical 2 chamber view recorded in systole illustrating adverse LV geometrical remodeling that results in papillary muscle displacement and failure of the mitral leaflets to coapt at the plane of the mitral annulus (dotted line). This apical displacement ("tenting") of the leaflets (arrows) can be quantified by assessing the area encompassed between the solid line and the annular plane.

- The physical examination often reveals signs of heart failure. In some cases, discovery of an underlying systemic disease may be aided by the physical examination. In addition, the physical examination may help to exclude other potential causes of heart failure such as valvular heart disease or pericardial disease.
- Appropriate biochemical tests and serologies should be obtained as indicated.
- The ECG is often non-specific; findings such as sinus tachycardia, non-specific ST/T abnormalities, bundle-branch blocks, and conduction defects may variably be observed. A finding of pathological Q waves should raise the suspicion of possible ischemic etiology.

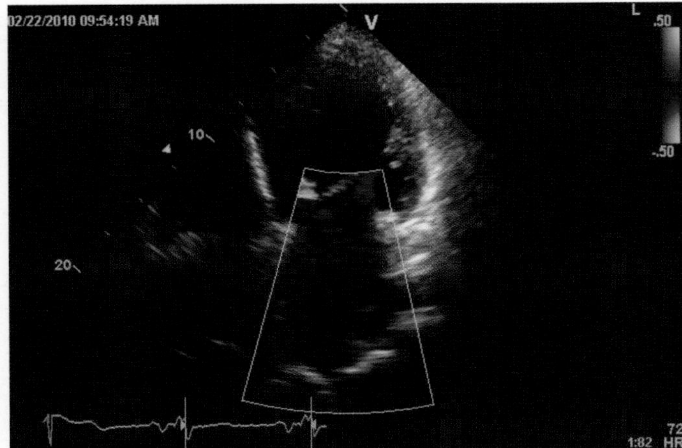

FIGURE 5-2-5 This apical 4 chamber view illustrates the presence of severe functional mitral regurgitation due to papillary muscle displacement occurring as consequence of the adverse LV remodeling ► (see Video 5-2-5).

- In the setting of supraventricular tachycardia or atrial fibrillation or flutter, a diagnosis of a tachycardia-mediated cardiomyopathy should be entertained.
- Chest radiography findings are often nonspecific. Cardiomegaly, with or without interstitial edema, may be observed. Pleural effusions are often observed in more advanced disease.
- Other imaging procedures such as myocardial perfusion imaging to assess for possible ischemia and viability and CMR to evaluate for entities such as arrhythmogenic right ventricular cardiomyopathy/dysplasia (ARVC/D), myocarditis, or sarcoidosis should be employed as indicated.
- Coronary arteriography should be used to exclude CHD when complaints of chest pain exist, with the finding of regional wall motion abnormalities suggestive of ischemic heart disease on echocardiography, or with findings suggestive of an ischemic etiology on stress perfusion imaging.
- Endomyocardial biopsy is not routinely recommended. In general, this procedure is reserved for patients with dilated cardiomyopathy and new onset heart failure associated with hemodynamic compromise or electrical instability. Specific instances where cardiac biopsy may prove useful include distinguishing lymphocytic from giant cell myocarditis, grading the severity of anthracycline-induced cardiomyopathy, and in diagnosing disorders such as amyloidosis and sarcoidosis.

DIAGNOSIS

The diagnosis is usually made on the basis of clinical history, findings on physical examination, and comprehensive echocardiography. In some cases, additional testing such as coronary angiography or CMR may be required. Endomyocardial biopsy may be required for definitive diagnosis in highly selected cases.

MANAGEMENT

- For patients with symptomatic heart failure (ACC/AHA stages C and D), provision of standard heart failure therapy as detailed in the ACC/AHA HF guideline[3] is indicated.
- For patients with CHD, valvular heart disease, or uncorrected congenital defects, percutaneous intervention or surgery as appropriate is indicated.
- Patients with alcohol-induced cardiomyopathy should abstain from alcohol completely.
- Medical therapy and/or ablation of atrial arrhythmias are indicated for patients with tachycardia-induced cardiomyopathy.
- Device therapy (CRT, ICD) should be used when appropriate clinical indications exist.
- For selected patients with advanced disease, mechanical support, as a temporizing measure or destination therapy, or cardiac transplantation may be indicated.
- For patients with asymptomatic LV dysfunction (LVEF ≤40%), ACC/AHA Stage B heart failure, attention should be paid to reducing the risk of disease progression by modifying risk factors for development of cardiovascular disease. Administration of

ACE-inhibitors and/or β-blocker is indicated in the absence contraindications to their use.

FOLLOW-UP

Close follow-up with a clinical cardiologist or heart failure specialist is suggested depending upon the stage of the disease. Clinical screening of first-degree family members of patients with idiopathic dilated cardiomyopathy is suggested as 20% to 35% of these family members may be affected.[4]

VIDEO LEGENDS

1. Video 5-2-1: Parasternal long-axis view showing a massively dilated and diffusely hypocontractile LV in a patient with an advanced non-ischemic cardiomyopathy
2. Video 5-2-5: This apical 4-chamber view illustrates the presence of severe functional mitral regurgitation due to papillary muscle displacement occurring as consequence of the adverse LV remodeling

REFERENCES

1. Redfield MM, Jacobsen SJ, Burnett JC Jr, Mahoney DW, Bailey KR, Rodeheffer RJ. Burden of systolic and diastolic ventricular dysfunction in the community: appreciating the scope of the heart failure epidemic. *JAMA*. 2003;289:194-202.
2. Felker GM, Thompson RE, Hare JM, et al. Underlying causes and long-term survival in patients with initially unexplained cardiomyopathy. *N Engl J Med*. 2000;342:1077-1084.
3. Yancy CW, Jessup M, Bozkurt B, et al. 2013 ACCF/AHA guideline for the management of heart failure: a report of the American College of Cardiology Foundation/American Heart Association Task Force on Practice Guidelines. *J Am Coll Cardiol*. 2013;62:e147–239. This document is available on the World Wide Web sites of the American College of Cardiology (www.cardiosource.org) and the American Heart Association (my.americanheart.org).
4. Hershberger RE, Siegfried JD. Update 2011: clinical and genetic issues in familial dilated cardiomyopathy. *J Am Coll Cardiol*. 2011;57:1641-1649.

SECTION 3

Peripartum Cardiomyopathy

CLINICAL CASE PRESENTATION

A previously healthy 37-year-old woman presented to hospital with complaints of increasing fatigue and having had progressive orthopnea and paroxysmal nocturnal dyspnea over the prior 2 weeks. About 12 weeks earlier, she delivered a healthy child after an uncomplicated full-term delivery. In the emergency department she was found to have a blood pressure of 70/40 mm Hg, pulse rate of 120 beats/min, and respiratory rate of 20 breaths/min; she was afebrile. Jugular venous distention was present along with decreased bibasilar breath sounds and crepitant pulmonary rales. Her heart rhythm was regular, and biventricular gallop sounds were heard. A grade II/VI holosystolic murmur was heard at the apex, and a grade II/VI holosystolic murmur was heard at the left lower sternal border. Bilateral ankle edema was present. A 12-lead ECG showed sinus tachycardia with frequent ventricular premature contractions. Chest radiography demonstrated cardiomegaly, bilateral pleural effusions, and intersti tial edema. A lactate level was measured at 5.1 mmol/L (upper limit of normal = 2.4 mmol/L). Her BNP level was 2540 pg/mL. Cardiac troponin I levels were in the normal range. Thyroid function tests were normal. Two-dimensional echocardiography (Figure 5-3-1) showed severe biventricular dysfunction with an estimated LVEF of 18%, biatrial enlargement, moderate mitral regurgitation, moderate to severe tricuspid regurgitation, a PASP estimated to be 30 mm Hg plus right atrial pressure, and a dilated inferior cava. Supportive care, including furosemide, dopamine, and milrinone drips, was started. Over the ensuing 48 hours she experienced improved hemodynamic status and excellent urine output. The intravenous medications were able to be weaned off, and she was started on an appropriate oral heart failure regimen. On follow-up echocardiography performed 3 months following hospital dismissal, her LVEF was 40% to 45%; echocardiography performed at 18 months (Figure 5-3-2) showed her LVEF to be 55% and the valvular insufficiency had resolved. She remains on an ACE-inhibitor and β-blocker.

CLINICAL FEATURES

Peripartum cardiomyopathy (PPCM) is a cause of pregnancy-associated heart failure occurring among women without previously known cardiovascular disease.

- Most patients present with heart failure symptoms and reduced LVEF (<45%) that develop in the last month of pregnancy, or more commonly, within the first 5 to 6 months following delivery (about 78% present with symptoms within 4 months of delivery).
- A more encompassing definition of this syndrome has been proposed recently by the Heart Failure Association of the European Society of Cardiology Working Group on PPCM.[1]
- This condition often presents insidiously; a high-index of suspicion is required as ankle edema, shortness of breath, and fatigue are frequent complaints occurring in the peripartum period.

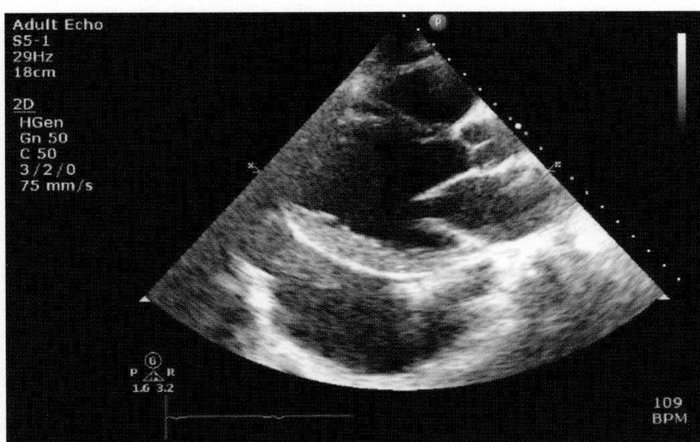

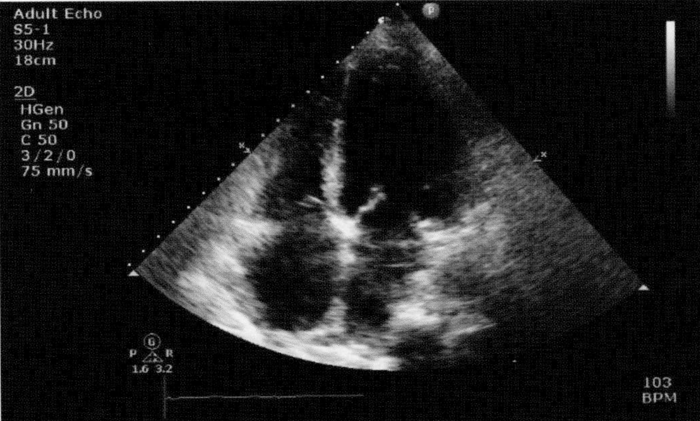

FIGURE 5-3-1 Parasternal long-axis (top panel) and apical 4 chamber (bottom panel) views of echocardiography performed on the day of presentation in the patient described in the case vignette. Note the presence of diffuse, severe hypokinesis of the LV, reduced RV function, and biatrial enlargement. A large left pleural effusion is seen on parasternal long-axis imaging ▶ (see Videos 5-3-1 A and B).

- Other presenting complaints may include cough, PND, orthopnea, hemoptysis, abdominal discomfort due to liver congestion, palpitations, and dizziness. Patients most often present with NYHA Class III or IV symptoms.[1]
- Systemic or pulmonary embolism may bring a patient to clinical attention as thromboembolism is more frequent with PPCM than with dilated cardiomyopathies of other etiologies.
- The physical examination is similar to that of other dilated cardiomyopathies.
- The clinical course can be highly variable; spontaneous and complete recovery of LV function may occur (45%-78% by 6 months); however, some may be left with persisting LV dysfunction. Rapid progression with marked hemodynamic instability, ventricular arrhythmia, and development of end-stage heart failure may be an outcome in a subset of patients.

EPIDEMIOLOGY

As emphasized by the European Working Group, little is known about the true incidence of PPCM.[1]

- The incidence appears to vary by geographical locale ranging from 1:300 live births in Haiti to 1:1500-4350 live births in the United States.[1,2]

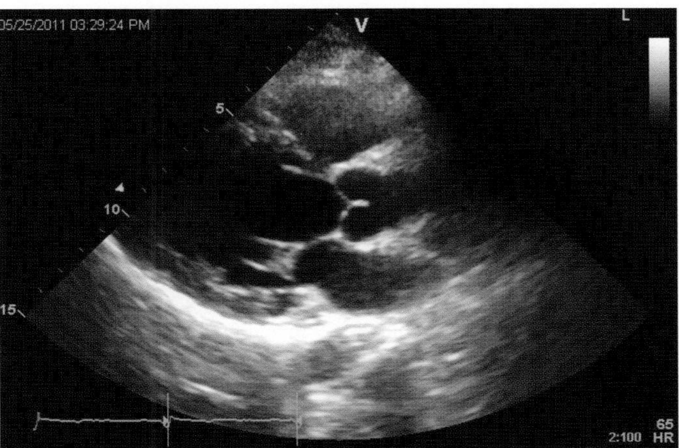

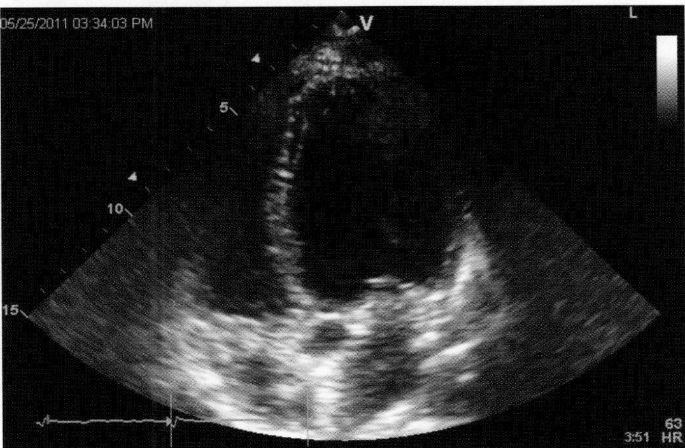

FIGURE 5-3-2 Parasternal long-axis (top panel) and apical 4 chamber (bottom panel) views from follow-up echocardiography obtained about 21 months after initial presentation. Normalization of LV and RV systolic function and atrial sizes is demonstrated ▶ (see Videos 5-3-2 A and B).

- Over time, the incidence of PPCM in the United States appears to be rising and may be tied to factors such as increasing maternal age, increased incidence of multi-fetal pregnancy, and increased disease recognition.[2]
- In the United States, the incidence of PPCM is reported to be highest among African American women and lowest in Latinas.
- The annual incidence of PPCM in the United States is estimated to be about 1350 cases.[2]

PATHOPHYSIOLOGY AND ETIOLOGY

The underlying mechanism of disease remains unknown. Several putative processes have been postulated as contributing factors in the pathogenesis.

- Pregnancy-related factors (age, multiparity, multifetal pregnancy).
- Presence of established risk factors for cardiovascular disease.
- Viral myocarditis, inflammation, and autoimmune responses.
- Genetic susceptibility and environmental risk factors are postulated to also play a role.
- Recent research has identified enhanced oxidative stress leading to activation of cathepsin D in cardiomyocytes and subsequent

cleavage of the hormone prolactin into an angiostatic and pro-apoptotic 16 kDa fragment.[3]

- Suppression of prolactin production by bromocriptine has been shown to prevent the onset of PPCM in a mouse model.[3]

ECHOCARDIOGRAPHY

Echocardiography is an essential tool in helping establish the diagnosis of PPCM and excluding other possible diagnoses of myocardial dysfunction. By definition, the LVEF should be <45% and/or the fractional shortening (FS) should <30%.[4] In addition, the LV end-systolic dimension should be >2.7 cm/m^2.

- In a recent study, the mean LVEF on presentation was 29±11%.[5]
- Fractional shortening <20% and LV end-diastolic diameter >60 mm has been associated with a greater than 3-fold risk for persistent LV dysfunction.[6]
- Diastolic function abnormalities are the norm, and a restrictive filling pattern is common.
- Abnormal RV systolic performance and dilatation may be present and are encountered with greater frequency in PPCM compared to other causes of dilated cardiomyopathy.[7]
- Other findings may include dilatation of the atria, functional MR and TR, and pericardial effusions.
- Ventricular thrombus is reported to be present in 10% to 17% of cases.[2]

OTHER DIAGNOSTIC TESTING AND PROCEDURES

- Electrocardiography often exhibits nonspecific findings, but is rarely normal in PPCM. Sinus tachycardia, nonspecific ST/T abnormalities, voltage criteria for LVH, left bundle-branch block, and LA enlargement can be observed.
- The chest x-ray typically shows cardiomegaly and pulmonary congestion/edema. Pleural effusions may be present.
- Levels of NT-proBNP are reported to be markedly elevated in patients with PPCM on presentation and significantly higher in the patients who did not improve LV function at 6 months.[8]
- Cardiac magnetic resonance imaging has had limited study in patients with PPCM. In addition to a dilated and hypocontractile LV, other findings may include the presence of mural thrombus and evidence of fibrosis. While some reports have documented the occurrence of late gadolinium enhancement in PPCM, others have not.[9] Guidelines recommend that gadolinium be avoided during pregnancy and that breast feeding not be performed for 24 hours after IV administration.[10]
- Other diagnostic tests and procedures such as right and left heart catheterization, endomyocardial biopsy, and assessment of viral titers are generally not indicated.

DIFFERENTIAL DIAGNOSIS

The diagnosis of PPCM is one of exclusion. The diagnosis is suggested by a carefully performed history and physical examination and often confirmed on the basis of increased BNP levels and echocardiography while excluding other potential causes of LV dysfunction in this patient population.

- Important alternative diagnoses to consider include aggravation or unmasking of a preexisting dilated cardiomyopathy, structural heart diseases such as preexisting congenital heart disease, valvular heart disease, or hypertensive heart disease, HIV/AIDS cardiomyopathy, pulmonary vascular disease, coronary heart disease, and pulmonary embolism.

MANAGEMENT

As the majority of patients present with NYHA Class III/IV symptoms, initial therapy is often directed at treating acute decompensated heart failure.

- Standard heart failure therapies, including administration of diuretics, renin-angiotensin-aldosterone modifying agents, and β-blockers, are indicated.
- For patients yet to deliver use of ACE-inhibitors and ARBs is contraindicated; hydralazine and nitrates can be used safely during pregnancy.
- Among patients with severe LV dysfunction (LVEF <30%), the use of anticoagulants should be considered due to the substantial risk of the presence of LV/RV thrombus.
- Coordination of care with a specialist in high-risk obstetrics is advised for pregnant patients (about 9% of patients with PPCM).[1]
- For patients with severe hemodynamic compromise, positive inotropic and/or pressor agents should used as dictated by the prevailing hemodynamics. Support with an intraaortic balloon counterpulsation device (IABP) may be required in selected cases. Inotropic agent or IABP-dependent patients may require further support with a ventricular assist device. Cardiac transplantation may be required if these therapies prove ineffective.
- An emerging, still experimental treatment is the addition of bromocriptine to standard heart failure therapy.[1,11]

PROGNOSIS

It should be noted that prognosis appears to vary by geographical location.[1]

- In the United States, recovery of LV function (LVEF ≥50%) is reported to occur in 45% to 78% of patients within 6 months.[2]
- Recovery of LV function may be lower among African American women compared with Caucasians.[2]
- Predictors of recovery include an LVEDD <55 mm, LVEF >30% to 35%, absence of LV thrombus, lower NT-pro BNP levels, and non-African American ethnicity.
- Mortality among US patients with PPCM is reported to range from 0% to 19%.[2]

FOLLOW-UP

As stated above, many US patients experience recovery of LV function within 6 months of diagnosis.

- Patients with residual LV dysfunction require ongoing follow-up and treatment with standard heart failure therapies per the ACC/AHA heart failure guideline recommendations.[12]
- Controversy exists over whether or not to withdraw heart failure medications among patients who experience recovery of LV function.[2]

Limited data exist to give formal recommendations regarding future pregnancy.

- It is clearly advised that patients with persisting LV dysfunction be strongly advised against future pregnancy.[1,2,13]
- Given limited data, the risk of future pregnancy among patients who recover LV function cannot be predicted accurately. It is recommended that these patients should be advised that future pregnancy may cause detrimental effects on cardiac function with attendant risks of worsening heart failure and possibly maternal and/or fetal death.[13]

VIDEO LEGENDS

1. Video 5-3-1 A: Parasternal long-axis of echocardiography performed on the day of presentation in the patient described in the case vignette. Note the presence of diffuse, severe hypokinesis of the LV and left atrial enlargement. A large left pleural effusion is seen.
2. Video 5-3-1 B: Apical 4-chamber view of echocardiography performed on the day of presentation in the patient described in the case vignette. Note the presence of diffuse, severe hypokinesis of the LV, reduced RV function, and biatrial enlargement.
3. Video 5-3-2 A: Parasternal long-axis from follow-up echocardiography obtained about 21 months after the initial presentation. Normalization of LV systolic function is demonstrated.
4. Video 5-3-2 B: Apical 4-chamber view from follow-up echocardiography obtained about 21 months after the initial presentation. Normalization of LV and RV systolic function and atrial sizes is demonstrated.

REFERENCES

1. Sliwa K, Hilfiker-Kleiner D, Petrie MC, et al. Heart Failure Association of the European Society of Cardiology Working Group on Peripartum Cardiomyopathy. Current state of knowledge on aetiology, diagnosis, management, and therapy of peripartum cardiomyopathy: a position statement from the Heart Failure Association of the European Society of Cardiology Working Group on peripartum cardiomyopathy. *Eur J Heart Fail*. 2010;12:767-778.
2. Elkayam U. Clinical characteristics of peripartum cardiomyopathy in the United States: diagnosis, prognosis, and management. *J Am Coll Cardiol*. 2011;58:659-670.
3. Hilfiker-Kleiner D, Kaminski K, Podewski E, et al. A cathepsin D-cleaved 16 kDa form of prolactin mediates postpartum cardiomyopathy. *Cell*. 2007;128:589-600.
4. Hibbard JU, Lindheimer M, Lang RM. A modified definition for peripartum cardiomyopathy and prognosis based on echocardiography. *Obstet Gynecol*. 1999;94:311-316.
5. Elkayam U, Akhter MW, Singh H, et al. Pregnancy-associated cardiomyopathy: clinical characteristics and a comparison between early and late presentation. *Circulation*. 2005;111:2050-2055.
6. Chapa JB, Heiberger HB, Weinert L, Decara J, Lang RM, Hibbard JU. Prognostic value of echocardiography in peripartum cardiomyopathy. *Obstet Gynecol*. 2005;105:1303-1308.
7. Karaye KM. Right ventricular systolic function in peripartum and dilated cardiomyopathies. *Eur J Echocardiogr*. 2011;12:372-374.
8. Forster O, Hilfiker-Kleiner D, Ansari AA, et al. Reversal of IFN-gamma, oxLDL and prolactin serum levels correlate with clinical improvement in patients with peripartum cardiomyopathy. *Eur J Heart Fail*. 2008;10:861-868.
9. Mouquet F, Lions C, de Groote P, et al. Characterisation of peripartum cardiomyopathy by cardiac magnetic resonance imaging. *Eur Radiol*. 2008;18:2765-2769.
10. Webb JA, Thomsen HS, Morcos SK. Members of Contrast Media Safety Committee of European Society of Urogenital Radiology (ESUR). The use of iodinated and gadolinium contrast media during pregnancy and lactation. *Eur J Radiol*. 2005;15:1234-1240.
11. Sliwa K, Blauwet L, Tibazarwa K, et al. Evaluation of bromocriptine in the treatment of acute severe peripartum cardiomyopathy: a proof-of-concept pilot study. *Circulation*. 2010;121:1465-1473. Erratum in: *Circulation*. 2010;121:e425.
12. Yancy CW, Jessup M, Bozkurt B, et al. 2013 ACCF/AHA guideline for the management of heart failure: a report of the American College of Cardiology Foundation/American Heart Association Task Force on Practice Guidelines. *J Am Coll Cardiol*. 2013;62:e147-239. This document is available on the World Wide Web sites of the American College of Cardiology (www.cardiosource.org) and the American Heart Association (my.americanheart.org).
13. Elkayam U, Tummala PP, Rao K, et al. Maternal and fetal outcomes of subsequent pregnancies in women with peripartum cardiomyopathy. *N Engl J Med*. 2001;344:1567-1571 Erratum in: *N Engl J Med*. 2001;345:552.

SECTION 4

Stress-Induced ("Tako-Tsubo") Cardiomyopathy

CLINICAL CASE PRESENTATION

A 74-year-old woman with hypothyroidism presented to an outside hospital after experiencing a single episode of syncope. She was active and otherwise healthy; she had never before experienced syncope. On the day of presentation she felt a sense of generalized weakness and lightheadedness and then passed out while taking a shower. She recovered consciousness quickly, and a witness did not observe any seizure-like activity. She suffered bruising to her right knee. The patient denied chest discomfort, shortness of breath, nausea or vomiting, diaphoresis, or palpitation. Upon further questioning, she expressed concern about a recent economic downturn and its impact on her family-run business.

At the outside hospital, a 12-lead ECG showed ST-segment elevations in leads I, avL, and V1-V3. She was transferred for consideration of emergent coronary intervention. Her cardiac troponin I (cTnI) was 3.8 ng/mL (normal <0.03) and CK-MB was 18.7 ng/dL (normal <4.4). Prior to angiography, an urgent echocardiogram showed evidence of severe LV dysfunction; the basal segments of all walls showed preserved to increased contractility while the midapical segments of all walls were akinetic. The LVEF was estimated visually as being 30%.

Coronary angiography showed only minor luminal irregularities throughout the coronary tree. Appropriate heart failure medications were initiated. Over the ensuing 24 hours, the cTnI peaked at 9.3 ng/mL. Follow-up ECG revealed resolution of the ST-segment elevations with development of new T wave inversions in the anterolateral leads along with QT interval prolongation. The patient remained asymptomatic, and no rhythm disturbances were documented while she was monitored.

Echocardiography prior to hospital dismissal showed only mild mid-to-apical anteroseptal hypokinesis. Within 2 weeks of discharge her LV function normalized fully, and by 2 months the ECG abnormalities resolved. She has had no recurrent symptoms over the past several years.

CLINICAL FEATURES

Stress-induced (tako-tsubo) cardiomyopathy is a clinical syndrome characterized by transient and often severe LV systolic dysfunction that frequently is presaged by concomitant physical or emotional stressors.

- An identifiable "trigger" may not be apparent in 11% to 30% of cases.
- While this syndrome most commonly occurs in postmenopausal women, recent reports reveal men and younger (premenopausal) women may account for 10% to 30% of cases.
- The presentation can be quite similar to that of an acute coronary syndrome with chest pain and ECG abnormalities that mimic acute myocardial infarction.[1] Other presenting complaints may include dyspnea or syncope.
- This syndrome occurs most commonly among post-menopausal women and is reported to account for up to 2% of urgent coronary angiography performed for presumed acute coronary syndromes.[2]
- Coronary angiography typically shows minimal disease or disease that cannot explain the diffuse nature of the wall motion abnormalities seen on echocardiography or contrast ventriculography.
- As described originally,[3] wall motion abnormalities involving the mid-distal LV while sparing the basal segments led to development of a peculiar ventricular morphology (Figure 5-4-1) resembling that of a "tako-tsubo" (Japanese octopus trap).
- Recent reports, however, show that variants of this syndrome with wall motion abnormalities involving only the midventricluar wall segments or the basal-midventricle with sparing of the apex ("inverted tako-tsubo") occur in 18% to 25% of cases.[4]
- Involvement of the RV is seen in about one-third of cases[5] (Figure 5-4-2).
- In addition to patients presenting with symptoms mimicking acute coronary events, this syndrome in our experience often occurs in critically ill patients in intensive care units and may manifest as heart failure, ECG abnormalities, and mild elevations of cardiac biomarkers.
- The majority of patients experience a relatively benign in-hospital course, and rapid recovery of LV function is expected. Delay in recovery of LVEF for up to 12 months is reported to occur in about 5% of patients.[6]
- Ventricular cavitary thrombus may be seen in 5% of patients.[6]
- Some patients may experience severe heart failure symptoms requiring intravenous diuretics.
- A subset of patients presents with severe hemodynamic compromise due to pump dysfunction, ventricular arrhythmias, or LV outflow tract obstruction can be seen. Such patients may require supportive therapy with mechanical ventilation, inotropic or vasopressor agents, IABP, or antiarrhythmic agents depending upon the clinical circumstances.
- The in-hosptial mortality rate is reported to be about 2%.

ECHOCARDIOGRAPHY

The classic finding is that of wall motion abnormalities not confined to a single epicardial coronary artery territory, typically involving the mid-distal LV. Variants of the "classic" pattern of apical ballooning

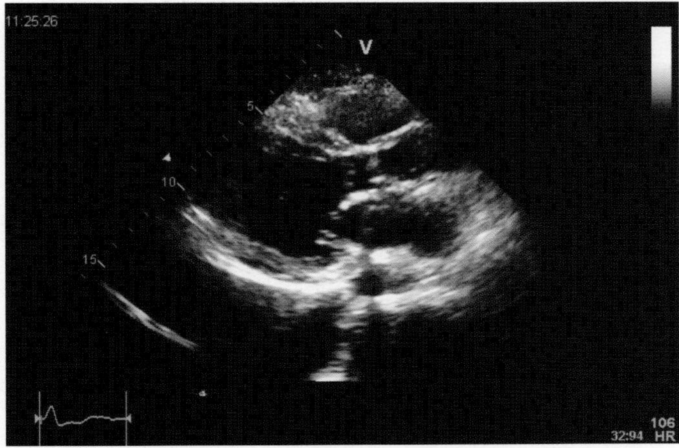

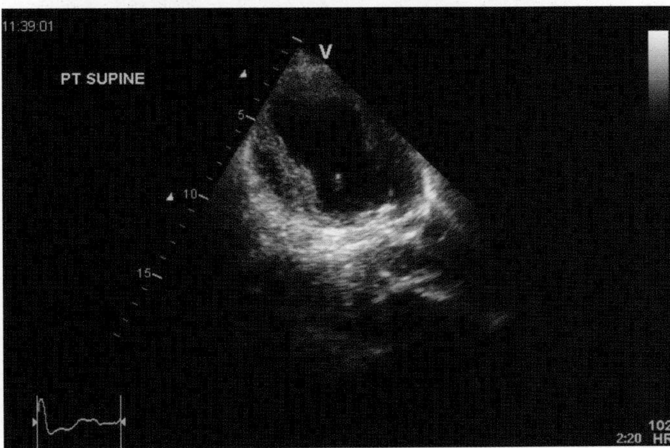

FIGURE 5-4-1 Parasternal long-axis (top panel) and apical 4 chamber (bottom panel) views in a patient with the classic form of stress-induced ("Tako-tsubo") cardiomyopathy ▶ (see Videos 5-4-1 A and B). In this example, only the basal segments of the left ventricular (LV) walls contract; the remaining walls segments are shown to be akinetic. The extensive nature of the LV wall motion abnormality observed is not consistent with involvement of a single coronary artery flow distribution.

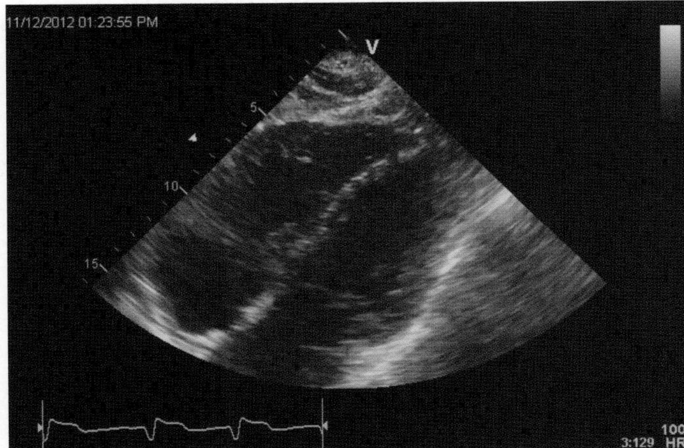

FIGURE 5-4-2 Subcostal 4 chamber view demonstrating akinesis of the mid and distal portions of the diaphragmatic wall of the right ventricle (RV) in a patient with stress-induced cardiomyopathy ▶ (see Video 5-4-2). Approximately 25% to 30% of patients with stress cardiomyopathy are shown to have RV involvement.

can be recognized (Figure 5-4-3) readily. The typical findings on echocardiography can be seen with other imaging modalities such as contrast ventriculography or CMR.

- Echocardiography may also reveal other findings including valvular dysfunction such as mitral regurgitation, intracavitary thrombus located in proximity to akinetic wall segments, and evidence of RV involvement.
- An important application of echocardiography in this syndrome is assessment of the patient with hemodynamic compromise. While poor pump function accounts for the majority of such patients, recognition of LV outflow tract obstruction due to systolic anterior motion of the anterior mitral leaflet (10%-15% of such patients) is important and may prompt an alteration in the therapeutic plan.
- Because of its utility in performing serial evaluation, echocardiography is ideally suited for follow-up of these patients in order to document resolution of LV dysfunction.

OTHER DIAGNOSTIC TESTING

Coronary Angiography

- Patients often undergo urgent catheterization as their clinical presentation, and ECG findings often mimic an acute coronary syndrome. The diagnosis is often apparent after excluding significant epicardial CAD on coronary angiography.

Electrocardiography

- May show a spectrum of findings ranging from initially normal ECG to ST-segment elevation (most common presentation), nonspecific ST/T abnormalities, Q waves, and diffuse T-wave inversion with prolonged QT interval.
- During recovery, greater than 80% of patients manifest diffuse T-wave inversion.[7]

Cardiac troponin levels are increased, but less so than with acute myocardial infarction.

CMR has been used to aid in making this diagnosis:

- Similar to other imaging modalities, wall motion abnormalities in a distribution not explained by that of single epicardial coronary artery involvement are observed.
- In a recent study, Eitel et al.,[5] reported that 82% of patients with stress cardiomyopathy exhibited the "classic" pattern of apical ballooning, 17% had involvement limited to midventricular wall segments, and 1% had basal-only involvement ("reverse tako-tsubo").
- In addition to defining wall motion abnormalities, CMR late gadolinium enhancement is usually absent with stress cardiomyopathy in comparison to acute myocardial infarction.
- Myocardial edema may be found in patients with stress cardiomyopathy, but this is a nonspecific finding also seen with myocarditis or acute myocardial infarction.

PATHOPHYSIOLOGY/ETIOLOGY

The precise etiologic mechanism remains unknown.

- Most episodes are preceded by an identifiable physical or emotional stressor.

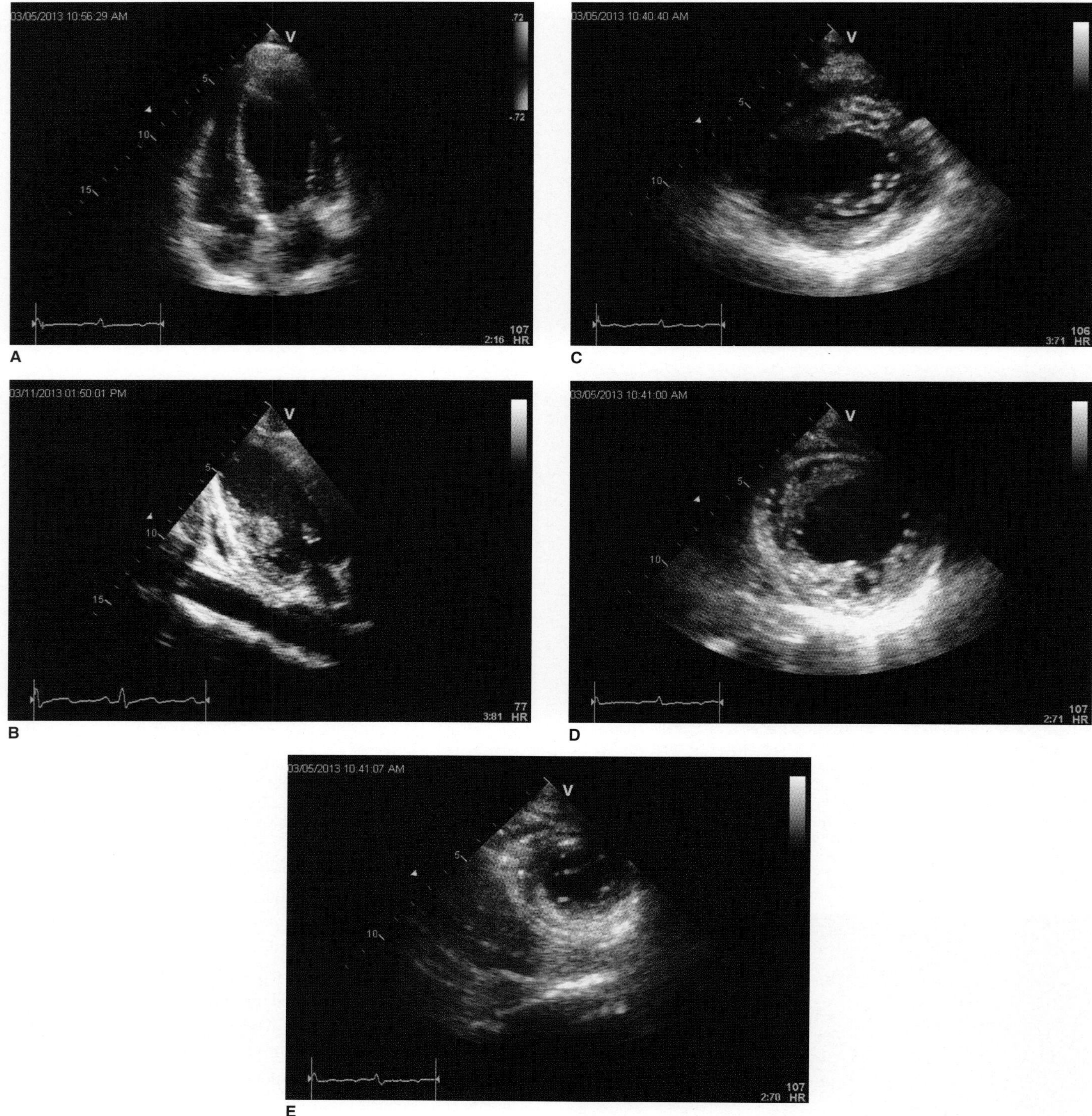

FIGURE 5-4-3 Mid-ventricular variant form of stress-induced cardiomyopathy. In this example, imaging in the apical 4 (A) and 2 chamber (B) planes demonstrates preserved contractility of the apical and basal portions of the LV with akinesis of the mid segments of the ventricular walls. Short-axis slices at the basal (C), mid (D), and apical (E) portions of the left ventricle further demonstrate the distinct regionality of wall motion abnormality in this variant form of stress-induced cardiomyopathy ▶ (see Videos 5-4-3 A to E).

- At present, catecholaminergic excess, either by causing direct myocardial toxicity or microvascular spasm, appears to be the most plausible mechanism. Catecholamoine levels in patients with stress cardiomyopathy have been documented to be higher than in patients with acute myocardial infarction in Killip class III.[8]
- Endomyocyocardial biopsy results obtained in a small number of patients with stress cardiomyopathy revealed changes consistent with a direct catecholamine effect on the myocardium.
- It must be emphasized that stress cardiomyopathy appears to be a heterogeneous clinical syndrome and likely no single mechanism can be advanced as an explanation for all cases.

The predilection for mid-apical LV cavity involvement is also not explained.

- A number of mechanisms such as multivessel coronary artery spasm, LAD plaque rupture, and microvascular dysfunction have been postulated as causes of this syndrome, but these purported mechanisms find little support.

DIAGNOSIS

The diagnosis is usually made by recognition of the clinical setting (often occurring among postmenopausal women with antecedent physical or emotional stress) and by exclusion of an acute coronary syndrome given that presentation with chest pain and ECG changes is common. Most patients undergo coronary angiography and contrast ventriculography. The recognition of substantial wall motion abnormalities not in the typical distribution of a coronary supply territory and with nonobstructive disease suggests the diagnosis. Typically, the rise in biomarkers of myocardial injury (cardiac troponin) is relatively minor given the extent of ECG changes and wall motion abnormality observed. Diagnostic criteria have been proposed by investigators at the Mayo Clinic.[1]

- Transient LV wall motion abnormalities involving the apical and/or midventricular myocardial segments with wall motion abnormality extending beyond a single epicardial coronary distribution.
- Absence of obstructive epicardial CAD or angiographic evidence of plaque rupture that could be responsible for the wall motion abnormality.
- New ECG abnormalities.
- Absence of other causes of transient LV dysfunction (such as acute myocarditis, pheochromocytoma, or intracranial bleeding).

DIFFERENTIAL DIAGNOSIS

- The differential diagnosis includes any process that may cause acute, reversible LV dysfunction. Conditions to consider include ischemic heart disease, myocarditis of any etiology, coronary vasospasm/Prinzmetal's angina, pheochromocytoma, intracranial bleeding/trauma, afterload excess states, cocaine abuse, and cardiac syndrome X.

MANAGEMENT

The most important aspect of management is recognition of this syndrome and appreciation of its often transient nature. For most patients, therapy is both supportive and expectant. At present, there exists no randomized or controlled clinical trial data to define the optimal management strategy.

- As these patients present with LV systolic dysfunction, they often exhibit heart failure symptoms. Treatment with ACE-inhibitors or ARBs, β-blockers, and diuretics is indicated.
- For patients with LV or RV thrombus observed on imaging studies, warfarin anticoagulation is recommended for a period of time until the wall motion abnormalities have resolved. Some investigators recommend anticoagulation for extensive LV apical wall motion abnormality independent of the presence of thrombus seen on an imaging study.
- For patients with severely compromised hemodynamic status, LV outflow tract obstruction (present in 10%-15% of such cases) should be excluded by echocardiography.
    - For those without obstruction, inotropic support is indicated; an IABP may be required in select cases.
    - For those with documented LV outflow tract obstruction, inotropic agents should be withdrawn, and gentle administration of fluids along with cautious use of β-blockers is suggested; refractory hypotension may require support with a pure α-agonist such as phenylephrine.

FOLLOW-UP

Stress-induced cardiomyopathy is a most often a transient disorder, and the vast majority of patients make a prompt, full recovery usually within 1 to 4 weeks (Figure 5-4-4).

- A minority of patients (about 5%) show delayed recovery of LV function over a period of 2.5 to 12 months.[6]
- Controversial at present is whether or not to continue with ACE-inhibitors and/or β-blockers once LV function has recovered fully.

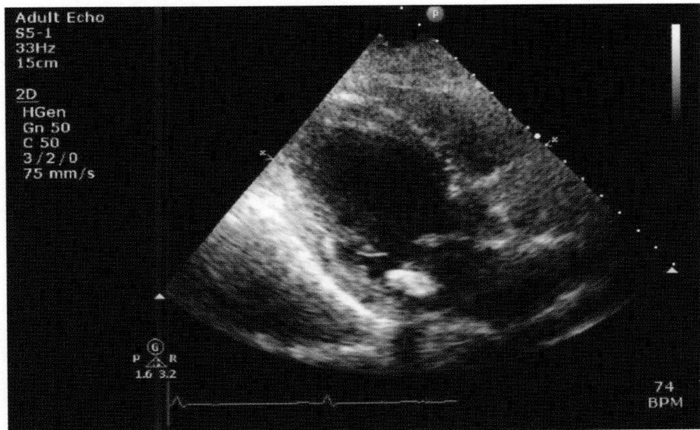

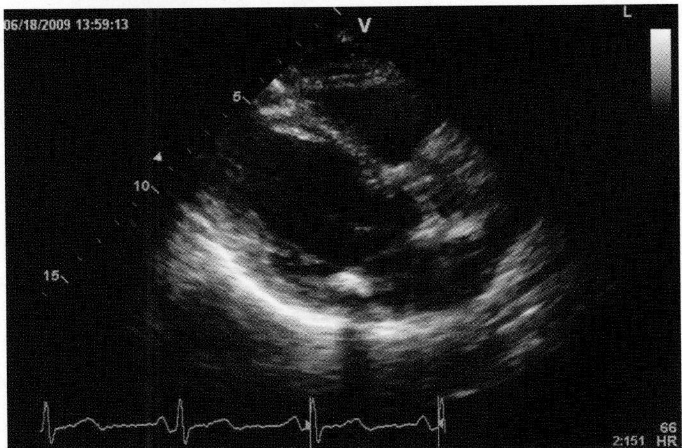

FIGURE 5-4-4 Parasternal long-axis images of the patient described in the case vignette. The image obtained on presentation (top panel) shows hyperkinetic contraction of the basal portions of the septum and inferolateral walls with akinesis of the remaining segments. Note involvement of the right ventricular free wall. In a follow-up image obtained 10 days later (bottom panel), LV systolic function has returned to normal ► (see Videos 5-4-4 A and B).

- In a retrospective study with a mean follow-up of 4.4 years, 11.4% of patients experienced a recurrence within 4 years.[9] Survival in this study was not different to compared to an age- and gender-matched population.
- Another group of investigators has reported that survival was reduced in comparison with an age- and gender-matched population; however, the excess mortality was due to noncardiac diseases and often occurred within the first year following the index hospitalization. A second study[6] reported a recurrence rate of 5%.

VIDEO LEGENDS

1. Video 5-4-1 A: Parasternal long-axis view in a patient with the classic form of stress-induced ("Tako-tsubo") cardiomyopathy. In this example, only the basal segments of the left ventricular (LV) walls contract; the remaining wall segments are shown to be akinetic. The extensive nature of the LV wall motion abnormality observed is not consistent with involvement of a single coronary artery flow distribution.
2. Video 5-4-1 B: Apical 4-chamber view in a patient with the classic form of stress-induced ("Tako-tsubo") cardiomyopathy. In this example, only the basal segments of the left ventricular (LV) walls contract; the remaining wall segments are shown to be akinetic. The extensive nature of the LV wall motion abnormality observed is not consistent with involvement of a single coronary artery flow distribution.
3. Video 5-4-2: Subcostal 4-chamber view demonstrating akinesis of the mid and distal portions of the diaphragmatic wall of the right ventricle (RV) in a patient with stress-induced cardiomyopathy.
4. Video 5-4-3 A: Mid-ventricular variant form of stress-induced cardiomyopathy. In this example, imaging in the apical 4-chamber view demonstrates preserved contractility of the apical and basal portions of the LV with akinesis of the mid segments of the ventricular walls.
5. Video 5-4-3 B: Mid-ventricular variant form of stress-induced cardiomyopathy. In this example, imaging in the apical 2-chamber plane demonstrates preserved contractility of the apical and basal portions of the LV with akinesis of the mid segments of the ventricular walls.
6. Video 5-4-3 C: Mid-ventricular variant form of stress-induced cardiomyopathy. Short-axis slices at the basal portion of the left ventricle further demonstrate the distinct regionality of wall motion abnormality in this variant form of stress-induced cardiomyopathy.
7. Video 5-4-3 D: Mid-ventricular variant form of stress-induced cardiomyopathy. Short-axis slices at the mid portions of the left ventricle further demonstrate the distinct regionality of wall motion abnormality in this variant form of stress-induced cardiomyopathy.
8. Video 5-4-3 E: Mid-ventricular variant form of stress-induced cardiomyopathy. Short-axis slices at the apical portion of the left ventricle further demonstrate the distinct regionality of wall motion abnormality in this variant form of stress-induced cardiomyopathy.
9. Video 5-4-4 A: Parasternal long-axis image of the patient described in the case vignette obtained on presentation shows hyperkinetic contraction of the basal portions of the septum and inferolateral walls with akinesis of the remaining segments. Note involvement of the right ventricular free wall.
10. Video 5-4-4 B: Parasternal long-axis images of the patient described in the case vignette. This image was obtained at follow-up 10 days later. The LV systolic function has returned to normal.

REFERENCES

1. Bybee KA, Kara T, Prasad A, et al. Systematic review: transient left ventricular apical ballooning: a syndrome that mimics ST-segment elevation myocardial infarction. *Ann Intern Med.* 2004;141:858-865.
2. Bybee KA, Prasad A. Stress-related cardiomyopathy syndromes. *Circulation.* 2008;118:397-409.
3. Tsuchihashi K, Ueshima K, Uchida T, et al. Transient left ventricular apical ballooning without coronary artery stenosis: a novel heart syndrome mimicking acute myocardial infarction. Angina Pectoris-Myocardial Infarction Investigations in Japan. *J Am Coll Cardiol.* 2001;38:11-18.
4. Eitel I, von Knobelsdorff-Brenkenhoff F, Bernhardt P, et al. Clinical characteristics and cardiovascular magnetic resonance findings in stress (tako-tsubo) cardiomyopathy. *JAMA.* 2011;306:277-286.
5. Fitzgibbons TP, Madias C, Seth A, et al. Prevalence and clinical characteristics of right ventricular dysfunction in transient stress cardiomyopathy. *Am J Cardiol.* 2009;104:133-136.
6. Sharkey SW, Windenburg DC, Lesser JR, et al. Natural history and expansive clinical profile of stress (tako-tsubo) cardiomyopathy. *J Am Coll Cardiol.* 2010;55:333-341.
7. Sharkey SW, Lesser JR, Menon M, Parpart M, Maron MS, Maron BJ. Spectrum and significance of electrocardiographic patterns, troponin levels, and thrombolysis in myocardial infarction frame count in patients with stress (tako-tsubo) cardiomyopathy and comparison to those in patients with ST-elevation anterior wall myocardial infarction. *Am J Cardiol.* 2008;101:1723-1728.
8. Wittstein IS, Thiemann DR, Lima JA, et al. Neurohumoral features of myocardial stunning due to sudden emotional stress. *N Engl J Med.* 2005;352:539-548.
9. Elesber AA, Prasad A, Lennon RJ, Wright RS, Lerman A, Rihal CS. Four-year recurrence rate and prognosis of the apical ballooning syndrome. *J Am Coll Cardiol.* 2007;50:448-452.

SECTION 5

Hypertensive Heart Disease

CLINICAL CASE PRESENTATION

A 58-year-old man originally from Ghana presented for evaluation of shortness of breath. Over the past several months prior to clinical presentation, he noted gradual onset of exertional dyspnea with activities such as climbing 1 to 2 flights of stairs. He has not experienced resting dyspnea, PND, or orthopnea. He did not complain of chest discomfort or intermittent claudication. He has never smoked cigarettes.

The patient has a history of long-standing, relatively poorly controlled essential hypertension (HTN) for which multiple classes of medications have been prescribed previously. The patient admits to not following a DASH (Dietary Approaches to Stop Hypertension)-type diet and to not taking the prescribed antihypertensive medications regularly. He does not monitor home blood pressures with any regularity. Four years prior to this visit he weighed 225 pounds; he now weighed 236 pounds (BMI = 40.3 kg/m^2). Several family members also have systemic HTN. He does not drink alcohol and denied use of NSAIDs. A formal sleep study had not been performed.

His blood pressure was 170/110 mm Hg in the left arm and 170/105 mm Hg in the right arm. The pulse rate was 80 beats/min and the rhythm was regular. Waist circumference was 44 inches. No signs of occular HTN were found on fundoscopy. No JVD was present. The carotid upstrokes were normal, no vascular bruits were heard, and no radial-femoral delay was appreciated. The lungs were clear. The PMI was non-displaced. The first and second heart sounds were normal, and there was no S_3. An S_4 was heard. No murmur was heard. The abdomen was soft and non-tender, no bruits were heard, and the abdominal aorta could not be palpated. No lower extremity edema was present. The lower extremity pulses were 2+ bilaterally.

The electrolytes, BUN, and creatinine were within normal limits; the eGFR was >60 mL/min. A urinalysis showed no protein. The LDL-C was 91 mg/dL, and the HDL-C was 45 mg/dL. The HbA1C was 6.9%.

A 12-lead ECG showed sinus rhythm, LA enlargement, and LVH with strain pattern. Echocardiography (Figure 5-5-1) showed severe concentric LVH (LV mass index 138 g/m^2, relative wall thickness (RWT) 1, LVEF of 70%-75%, LA enlargement (LAVI = 62 mL/m^2), and the PASP was estimated to be 40 mm Hg. The averaged E/e' ratio was 19 (Figure 5-5-2), indicating that mean LA pressure was elevated. No significant valvular heart was identified.

CLINICAL FEATURES

This case vignette describes a classic presentation of a patient with hypertensive heart disease. This patient with long-standing, poorly controlled systemic HTN presented with exertional dyspnea.

- There was evidence of end-organ effects on the heart: concentric LVH (increased LV mass and RWT), diastolic dysfunction, and elevated LV filling pressures and PASP.
- Patients with hypertensive heart disease also may come to clinical attention due to the consequences of uncontrolled systemic HTN such as atrial fibrillation, ventricular arrhythmias, coronary heart disease, renal insufficiency, aortic dissection, stroke, intracerebral hemorrhage, and cerebrovascular disease.
- Some patients with hypertensive heart disease develop impaired LVEFs.[1] A recent study found that about 13% of patients with a normal LVEF and concentric LVH progressed to systolic dysfunction over a follow-up period of 3 years. Risk factors for reduced LVEF included interval myocardial infarction, QRS duration >120 ms, and elevated arterial impedance.[2]

EPIDEMIOLOGY

Systemic hypertension is a very common disease, estimated to affect approximately 30% (65 million individuals) of the adult US population.[3] While recent statistics show increased control of blood pressure in the general population, only 50% of contemporary patients achieve adequate control. Prevalent hypertension is greater among individuals age 60 years or older compared with younger individuals and is greater in blacks as compared to whites and Latinos.[3]

PATHOPHYSIOLOGY/ETIOLOGY

Left ventricular hypertrophy is defined as an increase in LV mass.

- It can be characterized as being either concentric (normal cavity dimensions, RWT ≥0.42) or eccentric (RWT <0.42).
- The partition points for defining increased LV mass as defined by the ASE[4] are gender-dependent; >95 g/m^2 in women and >115 g/m^2 in men. An LV mass >225 g (>131 g/m^2) among men and >193 g (>113 g/m^2) in women is considered as being severely abnormal.

With systemic HTN, the increased LV mass (either concentric or eccentric hypertrophy) appears to result in large part from a chronic increase in ventricular afterload, although genetic, racial, neurohormonal, and environmental components are also recognized as contributing to the development of LVH. Pertinent to this case is that HTN is more common and often more severe among blacks, and greater LV mass is noted to be a more common finding.[5] Risk factors may include ingestion of a more sodium-rich diet and lower socioeconomic status.

Histologically, an increase in the number and/or size of the sarcomeres is found.

- Myocardial fibrosis, particularly common among HTN patients with diabetes mellitus, may be present.[6] This interstitial fibrosis correlates directly with heart weights and contributes to increased chamber stiffness and diastolic heart failure.
- Abnormalities of the intramyocardial coronary vasculature, including medial hypertrophy and perivascular fibrosis, are also found.[1,7]

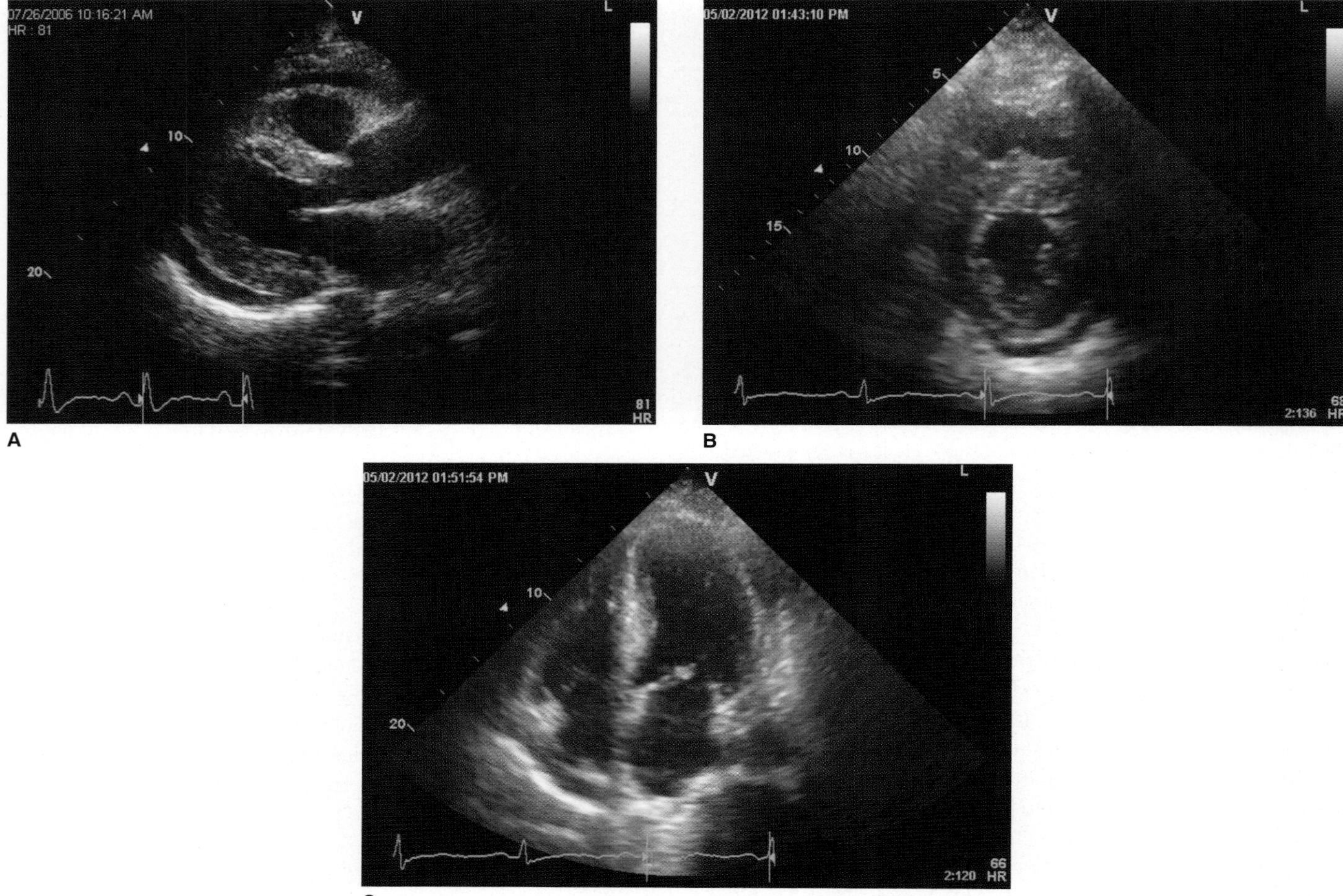

FIGURE 5-5-1 (A) Parasternal long-axis, (B) parasternal short-axis, and (C) apical 4 chamber views in the patient described in the case vignette. Severe concentric left ventricular hypertrophy with preserved ejection fraction is demonstrated. A small pericardial effusion is also present ▶ (see Videos 5-5-1 A to C).

Cardiac complications associated with hypertensive heart disease include increased risks for cardiac events such as fatal and nonfatal myocardial infarction, heart failure (systolic or diastolic), ventricular arrhythmias, sudden death, increased CV mortality, aortic dilatation/dissection, and atrial fibrillation.

- The increased risk of cardiovascular events may be related to small vessel ischemia, reduced capillary density, impaired vasodilator reserve, and altered electrical substrate.
- Patients with hypertensive heart disease are also at increased of ischemic stroke and end-stage renal disease.
- Regression of LVH has been associated with reduced risk of adverse CV events.[8]

ECHOCARDIOGRAPHY

Patients with hypertensive heart disease often present with complaints of exertional dyspnea. Echocardiography is the test of choice to evaluate patients with HF complaints and enables the clinician to assess LV systolic (and diastolic) function, wall thickness, and LV mass (LV geometry).[9] In addition, valvular abnormalities and the pericardium can be assessed.

- According to the 2005 ASE Chamber Quantification document,[4] it is recommended that the standard linear measurements be made at the level of the minor axis at end-diastole and end-systole.
  - The most important parameters to be measured include the septal wall thickness, posterior wall thickness, and the end-diastolic and end-systolic chamber dimensions.
  - Using these linear measurements, the RWT and the LV mass can be calculated.[4,10]
  - Among patients with hypertensive heart disease, the most common LV geometries encountered are concentric remodeling and concentric hypertrophy.[4] Both findings have prognostic implications in patients with HTN.[11]
  - Recently, 3-D echocardiography has been shown to be more accurate than 2-D echocardiography for assessment of LV mass[12] when CMR is used as the reference method.
- Given the underlying pathophysiology of hypertensive heart disease, LV diastolic dysfunction and diastolic heart failure are common.[13]
- A subset of patients will develop systolic dysfunction with reduced LVEF and a picture of dilated cardiomyopathy.[1]

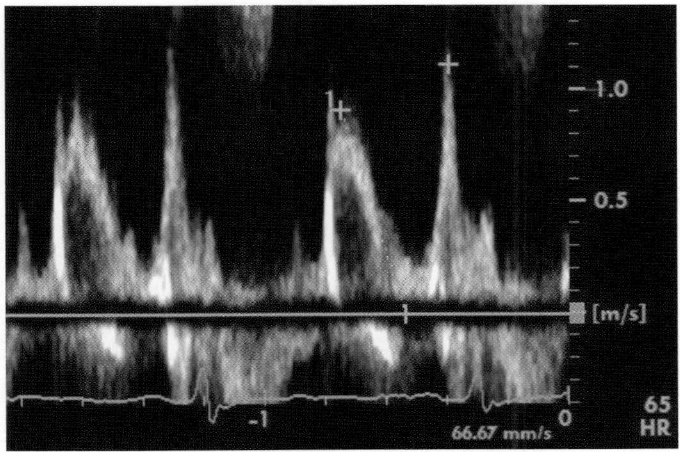

Trans-mitral flow

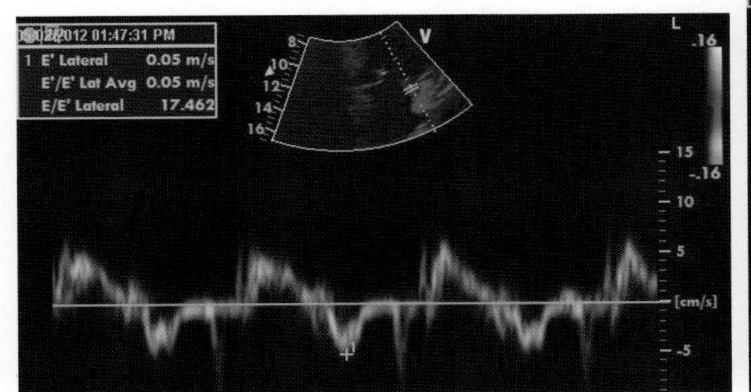

Lateral annulus

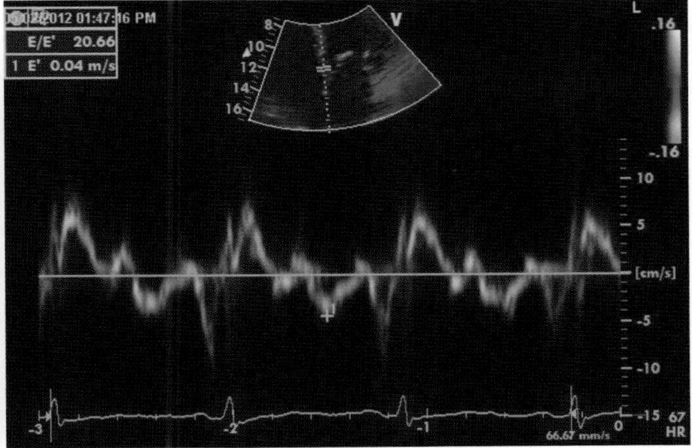

Medial annulus

FIGURE 5-5-2 Trans-mitral flow velocities and tissue Doppler imaging velocities at the lateral and medial mitral annular locations of the patient described in the case vignette. The average E/e′ ratio is 19.

- Echocardiographic findings in addition to hypertrophy or concentric remodeling include increased LA volume index, increases in pulmonary artery systolic pressures, and abnormalities in Doppler flow patterns such as alterations in transmitral inflows, pulmonary venous spectral pattern, and tissue Doppler imaging at the mitral annulus.
- An approach to diagnosing diastolic function abnormalities based on these findings is detailed in a recently released guideline statement.[13]
- While considered experimental, speckle ("feature") tracking 2-D echocardiography has shown that patients with hypertensive heart disease exhibit abnormalities in rates of longitudinal and circumferential deformation and twist/untwist parameters compared to patients without LVH.[14]

OTHER DIAGNOSTIC TESTING AND PROCEDURES

A 12-lead ECG is most frequently the first test obtained to evaluate cardiac status in such patients and may show evidence of LVH. The ECG exhibits high specificity but low sensitivity for the detection of LVH.[15] Evidence of dysrhythmias and atrial enlargement may also be seen.

For patients with suspected HF, use of biomarkers such as BNP or NT-proBNP may be helpful for diagnosis; they have shown limited utility in screening general populations for the presence of LVH or LV systolic dysfunction.[16]

CMR is considered the gold-standard noninvasive test for determination of LV mass. CMR may help to distinguish hypertrophy caused by hypertension from hypertrophic cardiomyopathy. In general, however, CMR is not routinely needed for management of hypertensive heart disease.

Ambulatory blood pressure monitoring may be employed to assess hypertension control in "resistant" cases and for complaints of hypotensive symptoms while taking blood pressure lowering medications.

- For patients with resistant HTN, a review of the history and physical examination is mandatory.
- Compliance with an adequately crafted regimen should be stressed, and medications or ingestions that can raise blood pressure should be discontinued if possible.
- Assessment for sleep apnea is mandatory, and evaluation for potential secondary causes of HTN is indicated.

DIAGNOSIS

The diagnosis of hypertensive heart disease is made by the combination of clinical features along with findings on ECG and echocardiography. Other specific tests for secondary causes of HTN, as guided by clinical suspicion, should be obtained.

DIFFERENTIAL DIAGNOSIS

The differential diagnosis includes other disease processes that present with LVH such as hypertrophic cardiomyopathy, restrictive cardiomyopathies, Fabry disease, diabetes mellitus, obesity, valvular heart disease (aortic stenosis, aortic regurgitation), congenital heart disease (subaortic or supravalvular stenosis; coarctation of the aorta), and athlete's heart.

MANAGEMENT

Treatment of HTN, consisting of institution of therapeutic lifestyle changes in all patients and administration of pharmacological agents in most patients to achieve a BP goal of <140/90 mm Hg is indicated.

- Regression of LVH has been documented to occur with several classes of antihypertensive agents; an exception appearing to be the direct-acting vasodilators.
- Diuretics and β-blockers appear to be less successful in reducing LV mass compared to renin-angiotensin system modifying agents and calcium channel blockers.[17]
- Maximum regression of LVH may take up to 3 years and has been associated with reductions in LA size and improvements in diastolic function.[18]
- For those with reduced LVEF, an appropriate regimen to treat systolic heart failure should be initiated.

Risk factors for progression of cardiac disease (such as obesity, diabetes mellitus, dyslipidemia, and the metabolic syndrome) commonly coexist.

- Aggressive treatment of these risk factors is indicated.

FOLLOW-UP

Regular follow-up with a physician is indicated to assess for adequacy of blood pressure control and identification of complications of systemic hypertension. The choice of blood pressure-controlling agents should be tailored to existing co-morbidities. Patients should be encouraged to participate actively in the treatment of their hypertension; home blood pressure monitoring is an essential component of follow-up care.

VIDEO LEGENDS

1. Video 5-5-1 A: Parasternal long-axis view in the patient described in the case vignette. Severe concentric left ventricular hypertrophy with preserved ejection fraction is demonstrated. A small pericardial effusion is also present.
2. Video 5-5-1 B: Parasternal short-axis views in the patient described in the case vignette. Severe concentric left ventricular hypertrophy with preserved ejection fraction is demonstrated. A small pericardial effusion is also present.
3. Video 5-5-1 C: Apical 4-chamber view in the patient described in the case vignette. Severe concentric left ventricular hypertrophy with preserved ejection fraction is demonstrated.

REFERENCES

1. Drazner MH. The progression of hypertensive heart disease. *Circulation*. 2011;123:327-334.
2. Milani RV, Drazner MH, Lavie CJ, Morin DP, Ventura HO. Progression from concentric left ventricular hypertrophy and normal ejection fraction to left ventricular dysfunction. *Am J Cardiol*. 2011;108:992-996.
3. Egan BM, Zhao Y, Axon RN. US trends in prevalence, awareness, treatment, and control of hypertension, 1988-2008. *JAMA*. 2010;303:2043-2050.
4. Lang RM, Bierig M, Devereux RB, et al. Chamber Quantification Writing Group; American Society of Echocardiography's Guidelines and Standards Committee; European Association of Echocardiography. Recommendations for chamber quantification: a report from the American Society of Echocardiography's Guidelines and Standards Committee and the Chamber Quantification Writing Group, developed in conjunction with the European Association of Echocardiography, a branch of the European Society of Cardiology. *J Am Soc Echocardiogr*. 2005;18:1440-1463.
5. Drazner MH, Dries DL, Peshock RM, et al. Left ventricular hypertrophy is more prevalent in blacks than whites in the general population: the Dallas Heart Study. *Hypertension*. 2005;46:124-129.
6. van Hoeven KH, Factor SM. A comparison of the pathological spectrum of hypertensive, diabetic, and hypertensive-diabetic heart disease. *Circulation*. 1990;82:848-855.
7. Raman SV. The hypertensive heart. An integrated understanding informed by imaging. *J Am Coll Cardiol*. 2010;55:91-96.
8. Pierdomenico SD, Cuccurullo F. Risk reduction after regression of echocardiographic left ventricular hypertrophy in hypertension: a meta-analysis. *Am J Hypertens*. 2010;23:876-881.
9. Douglas PS, Garcia MJ, Haines DE, et al. ACCF/ASE/AHA/ASNC/HFSA/HRS/SCAI/SCCM/SCCT/SCMR 2011 Appropriate use criteria for echocardiography: a report of the American College of Cardiology Foundation Appropriate Use Criteria Task Force, American Society of Echocardiography, American Heart Association, American Society of Nuclear Cardiology, Heart Failure Society of America, Heart Rhythm Society, Society of Cardiovascular Angiography and Interventions, Society of Critical Care Medicine, Society of Cardiovascular Computed Tomography, and Society of Cardiovascular Magnetic Resonance. *J Am Coll Cardiol*. 2011;57(9):1126-1166.doi:10.1016/j.jacc.2010.11.002.
10. Devereux RB, Casale PN, Kligfield P, et al. Performance of primary and derived M-mode echocardiographic measurements for detection of left ventricular hypertrophy in necropsied subjects and in patients with systemic hypertension, mitral regurgitation and dilated cardiomyopathy. *Am J Cardiol*. 1986;57:1388-1393.
11. Verdecchia P, Schillaci G, Borgioni C, et al. Adverse prognostic significance of concentric remodeling of the left ventricle in hypertensive patients with normal left ventricular mass. *J Am Coll Cardiol*. 1995;25:871-878.

12. Caiani EG, Corsi C, Sugeng L, et al. Improved quantification of left ventricular mass based on endocardial and epicardial surface detection with real time three dimensional echocardiography. *Heart*. 2006;92:213-219.

13. Nagueh SF, Appleton CP, Gillebert TC, et al. Recommendations for the evaluation of left ventricular diastolic function by echocardiography. *J Am Soc Echocardiogr*. 2009;22:107-133.

14. Goebel B, Gjesdal O, Kottke D, et al. Detection of irregular patterns of myocardial contraction in patients with hypertensive heart disease: a two-dimensional ultrasound speckle tracking study. *J Hypertens*. 2011;29:2255-2264.

15. Levy D, Labib SB, Anderson KM, Christiansen JC, Kannel WB, Castelli WP. Determinants of sensitivity and specificity of electrocardiographic criteria for left ventricular hypertrophy. *Circulation*. 1990;81:815-820.

16. de Lemos JA, McGuire DK, Khera A, et al. Screening the population for left ventricular hypertrophy and left ventricular systolic dysfunction using natriuretic peptides: results from the Dallas Heart Study. *Am Heart J*. 2009;157:746-753.

17. Klingbeil AU, Schneider M, Martus P, Messerli FH, Schmieder RE. A meta-analysis of the effects of treatment on left ventricular mass in essential hypertension. *Am J Med*. 2003;115:41-46.

18. Franz IW, Tönnesmann U, Müller JF. Time course of complete normalization of left ventricular hypertrophy during long-term antihypertensive therapy with angiotensin converting enzyme inhibitors. *Am J Hypertens*. 1998;11:631-639.

SECTION 6

Athlete's Heart

CLINICAL CASE PRESENTATION

A 23-year-old man was seen by his primary care physician for a routine physical examination. The patient is an endurance athlete participating actively in college athletics. He runs an average of 50 to 70 miles per week. He offered no specific complaint, and his physical examination was unremarkable except that his pulse rate was 46 beats/min. His physician ordered an ECG that showed sinus bradycardia, LVH by voltage criteria, and T-wave inversions in leads III and avF. Due to these ECG findings and suspicion of possible hypertrophic cardiomyopathy he was referred for an echocardiogram that showed normal LV size (EDD 53 mm), upper normal wall thickness (11 mm septal and posterior wall thickness), and an LVEF estimated to be 70%. The LA was normal in size; however, the RV and RA were dilated. The PASP was estimated to be 25 to 30 mm Hg. Mild tricuspid regurgitation was present. The inferior vena cava was dilated (27 mm), but showed normal collapse to a sniff. The flow velocities across the pulmonary outflow compared to the aortic outflow were not increased. No obvious atrial septal defect was identified; a saline contrast study revealed a very small number of bubbles in the left heart following Valsalva release. He was referred to see an outside cardiologist who recommended that he reduce his level of exertion in response to the abnormal ECG and echocardiogram. The patient sought a second opinion because he did not want to interrupt his training routine. His history and physical examination were reviewed along with the prior imaging studies. A CMR was recommended to exclude atrial septal defect/anomalous pulmonary venous drainage, to assess RV size and function, wall thickness, and chamber volumes, and to assess LV morphology. The CMR confirmed several of the echo findings. The RV was dilated (EDV 228 ml), and the estimated RVEF was 49%. Other than the dilatation, no other pathological RV findings were noted. The LV was morphologically normal and no pathological hypertrophy was identified. No defect in the atrial septum was identified, and the pulmonary veins drained normally to the LA. The findings were felt to be consistent with an athletic training effect on the heart. The patient continues to run regularly without limitations.

CLINICAL FEATURES

This case highlights some of the anatomic findings that can be encountered in the spectrum of cardiac remodeling associated with athletic training.

- It is estimated that up to 50% of trained athletes exhibit a variety of structural alterations including changes in ventricular dimensions, atrial dilatation, and increases in wall thickness.[1]
- The type of training may influence the pattern of cardiac remodeling; endurance training (rowing, cycling, swimming, long-distance running) has been associated with a volume overload pattern while strength training (weight lifting, American football) has been associated with pressure overload and a greater impact on wall thickness than cavity size.[1,2]
- In most cases, absolute wall thickness does not exceed 13 mm; a maximum wall thickness of 16 mm in young trained athletes is considered to represent the upper limit of physiological LV hypertrophy.
- Regression of LVH may be induced by periods of discontinuation of training, a recommendation that most athletes would be reluctant to consider.
- Dilatation of the aortic root in conditioned athletes (≥40 mm in men and ≥34 mm in women) is not believed to be a physiological consequence of training and more likely represents a pathological condition.[4]

In addition to the structural and functional remodeling seen with training, "distinctly abnormal" ECG findings can be encountered in large number of highly trained athletes.

- These ECG abnormalities are rarely found to represent structural disorders and have been correlated with the remodeling induced by athletic training.[5]
- Arrhythmias associated with heightened vagal tone are encountered commonly.
- Ventricular arrhythmias (VPCs, couplets, runs of NSVT) may also be encountered with frequency; their presence has not been associated with adverse events, and they may be abolished by periods of deconditioning.[1]

EPIDEMIOLOGY

The overall incidence of athlete's heart is difficult to define as the vast majority of US athletes are asymptomatic and undergo minimal screening. It is estimated that some form of cardiac remodeling occurs in about 50% of highly trained athletes.[3]

PATHOPHYSIOLOGY/ETIOLOGY

The athlete's heart refers to the structural, functional, and electric changes which occur with exercise training. It is recognized that different forms of conditioning place differing loads on the heart and vasculature.

- Endurance training increases cardiac output through increases in stroke volume and heart rate; blood pressure rises modestly, and peripheral arterial resistance is lowered. The net effect is a predominant volume load being placed on the ventricle.
- Strength training, in contrast, is associated with greater increases in blood pressure and peripheral vascular resistance and lesser increases in heart rate and stroke volume—changes which place a predominant pressure load on the ventricle.
- Most sports incorporate both types of training to varying degrees, and thus most highly trained athletes have both pressure and volume load imposed by training.
    - These loads imposed by training induce structural changes in approximately 50% of trained athletes.
    - Compared to nonathletic controls, increased ventricular mass (concentric or eccentric hypertrophy) and cavity size are observed regardless of the type of training[6]; an LVEDD >60 mm is reported to occur in about 15% of trained athletes.[3]
    - Among endurance athletes, RV dilatation and increased mass have been observed, and atrial dilatation is a common finding.[6]
    - The LVEF is reported to be similar to that of nontrained individuals; an exception may be among endurance athletes where more dilated ventricles and larger stroke volumes are found.[6]
    - Diastolic function has been demonstrated to be preserved.
- Recently published guidelines[7] describe the spectrum of ECG findings considered to be commonly related to training effects; sinus bradycardia, first-degree AV delay, early repolarization, incomplete RBBB, and voltage criteria for LVH are considered to be normal findings related to training.
- The molecular mechanisms associated with changes induced by athletic training ("physiological hypertrophy") are believed to be different from those caused by pathological conditions; however, exact definition of these mechanisms remains ill-defined.[6]

ECHOCARDIOGRAPHY

The principle findings on echocardiography relate to alterations in chamber dimensions, ventricular hypertrophy and altered function (Figures 5-6-1 and 5-6-2). These changes in morphology and function appear to relate to the type of training.

- Dilatation of the LV and/or RV and the atria may be seen, and wall thickness may be increased. About 15% of athletes have a LVEDD ≥60 mm, 20% exhibit a LA transverse diameter ≥40 mm, and 2% have a maximum wall thickness >13 mm.[8]
- Diastolic filling properties are not pathologically altered.[9]
- In comparison to patients with HCM, LV end-diastolic cavity dimensions among patients with athlete's heart are not reduced (<45 mm), the pattern of hypertrophy is symmetric, and diastolic function is not impaired.

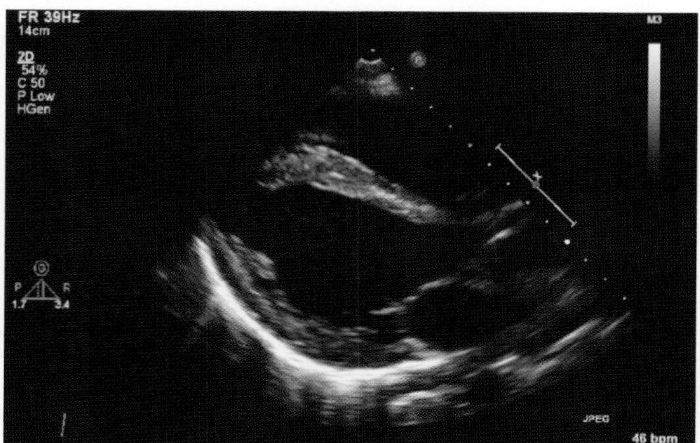

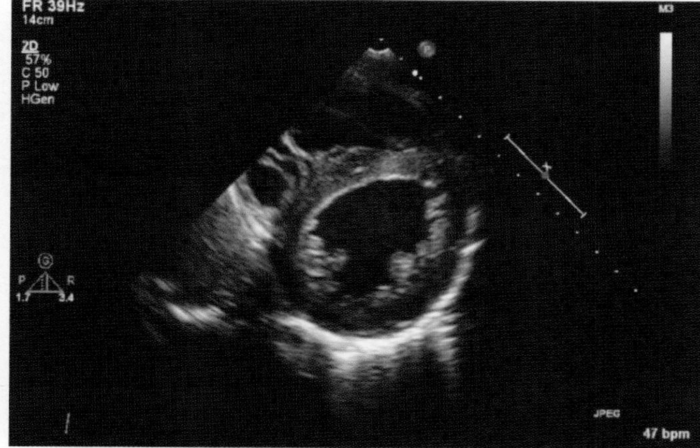

FIGURE 5-6-1 Parasternal long- (left panel) and short-axis (right panel) images of the patient described in the case vignette. Left ventricular (LV) systolic function is normal. Note the presence of increased posterior wall thickness with normal cavity size ► (see Videos 5-6-1 A and B). Sinus bradycardia is present.

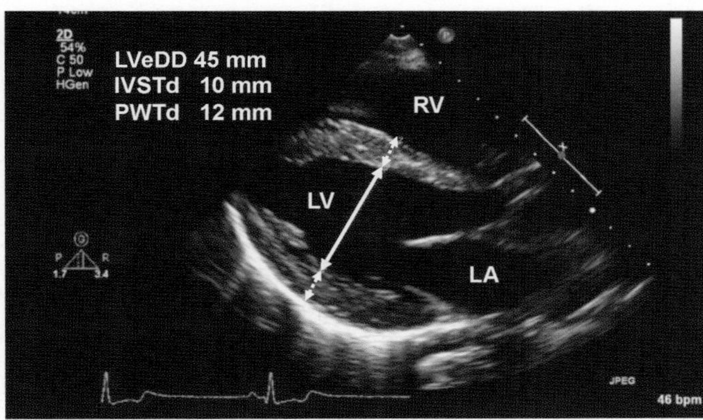

FIGURE 5-6-2 Still frame in the parasternal long-axis view showing the dimensions of the LV cavity and wall thicknesses. The LV end-diastolic dimension (long, white, double-headed arrow) is 45 mm, the posterior wall thickness (PWTd) is 12 mm, and the thickness of the interventricular septum (IVSTd), taking care not to include the RV contribution, is 10 mm.

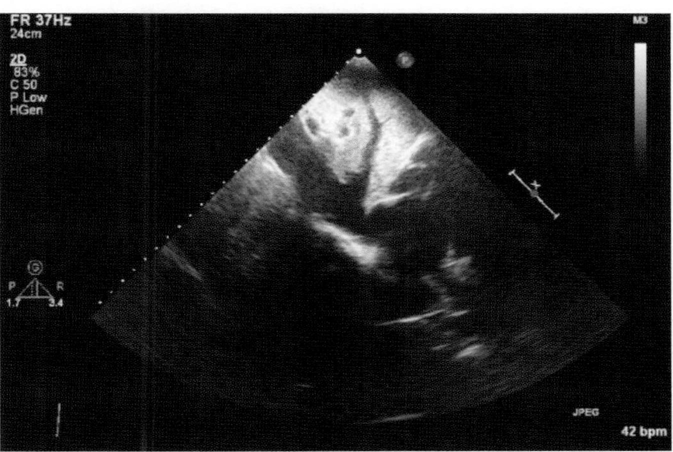

FIGURE 5-6-4 Subcostal imaging of the inferior vena cava. The IVC is frequently found to be dilated in endurance athletes; it often collapses >50% with a sniff (not shown). Also note spontaneous echo-contrast material seen in the IVC and large hepatic vein ▶ (see Video 5-6-4).

- Using 3-D echocardiography, it has been demonstrated that athletes have higher LV end-diastolic volumes and LV mass compared to controls.
- Gender and type of training were determinants of LV remodeling; male gender and endurance training were associated with greatest effects on LV end-diastolic volume and LV mass.[10]
- Dilatation and hypertrophy of the RV (Figure 5-6-3) and dilation of the inferior vena cava (Figure 5-6-4) may be prominent findings encountered among endurance athletes.

OTHER DIAGNOSTIC TESTING AND PROCEDURES

The ECG frequently displays abnormalities associated with increased vagal tone (sinus bradycardia, first-degree AV delay, Mobitz-type 1 second-degree AV block), incomplete RBBB, and voltage criteria for LVH.[7] Other findings may include the presence of repolarization abnormalities, Q waves, and atrial enlargement.[10] Ambulatory ECG monitoring, in addition to documenting intermittent conduction abnormalities, may show episodes of ventricular arrhythmias including frequent isolated VPCs, couplets, and runs of NSVT.

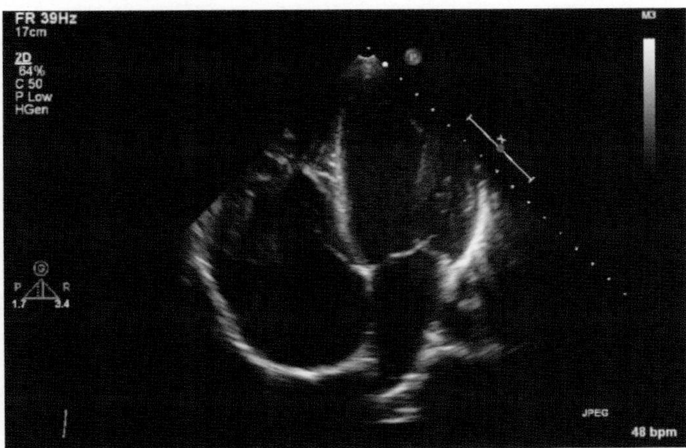

FIGURE 5-6-3 Apical 4 chamber image showing significant remodeling (enlargement) of the right ventricle and right atrium in this endurance athlete ▶ (see Video 5-6-3).

CMR is an important test when differentiation of athlete's heart from HCM by history and echocardiography cannot be firmly established. Specifically, CMR can measure wall thickness, assess LV mass, characterize the distribution of hypertrophy, and assess for myocardial fibrosis with administration of gadolinium. CMR is also a useful test to provide additional information when ARVC/D is considered.

Cardiopulmonary exercise testing may be employed as a tool to separate patients with pathological hypertrophy from well-trained athletes with excess physiological wall thickening. In general, athletes attain high peak MVO_2 values (often ≥70 ml/kg-min) while patients with HCM often have lower peak MVO_2 values (<40-45 ml/kg-min).

In selected cases, genetic testing for mutations associated with HCM may be indicated.

DIFFERENTIAL DIAGNOSIS

The differential diagnosis includes a number of structural heart diseases such as HCM, dilated cardiomyopathy, ARVC/D, and myocarditis.

- For patients with increased wall thickness (>13-15 mm) and relatively nondilated LV cavities, HCM must be considered strongly. Differential points favoring the diagnosis of HCM include a family history of HCM, evidence of abnormal LV diastolic filling properties, the presence of asymmetric LVH, late gadolinium enhancement on CMR, impaired exercise capacity, and lack of reduction in LV wall thickness with periods of deconditioning.
- When a dilated LV with mildly reduced or low-normal LVEF is found, dilated cardiomyopathy should be considered. Preserved exercise capacity, augmentation of LVEF with exercise, and preserved diastolic function on echocardiography favors the presence of athlete's heart. In selected cases, CMR with gadolinium may be indicated.
- With excessive RV enlargement, ARVC/D should be a diagnostic consideration. The diagnosis is often difficult to make and requires consideration of multiple factors including the family history,

the presence of abnormalities affecting depolarization and repolarization on ECG, arrhythmia, suggestive structural findings on echocardiography and/or CMR, and tissue characterization.[11]

- The presence of complex ventricular arrhythmia should prompt a consideration of the diagnosis of myocarditis.

DIAGNOSIS

The diagnosis is suggested by an appropriate history and physical examination along with findings on ECG and echocardiography compatible with an athlete's heart. In some cases, CMR, cardiopulmonary exercise testing, or a period of deconditioning (to document regression of the echocardiographic and ECG abnormalities) may be required to establish the diagnosis.

MANAGEMENT

The most important aspect of management is recognition of this entity and reassuring the patient that the observed structural remodeling is physiological. In appropriate situations, as discussed above, separating an athlete's heart from pathological conditions causing hypertrophy and/or chamber dilatation is essential as these conditions often preclude athletic participation and are associated with increased morbidity and mortality.

FOLLOW-UP

The long-term effects of intense athletic training are not fully known, but to date no proof exists that the morphological changes of the athlete's heart lead to adverse cardiac outcomes.

- In a study of 114 Olympic athletes, continuous endurance training over periods of time up to 17 years was not associated with deterioration of LV function, significant changes in LV morphology, or occurrence of cardiovascular symptoms or events.[12]
- Following periods of long-term (1-13 years) detraining in elite athletes, significant reductions in LV cavity size and normalization of wall thickness were observed. Substantial LV dilatation (≥60 mm) may persist in about 20% of athletes.[13]

VIDEO LEGENDS

1. Video 5-6-1 A: Parasternal long axis image of the patient described in the case vignette. Left ventricular (LV) systolic function is normal. Note the presence of increased posterior wall thickness with normal cavity size.
2. Video 5-6-1 B: Parasternal short-axis image of the patient described in the case vignette. Left ventricular (LV) systolic function is normal. Note the presence of increased posterior wall thickness with normal cavity size.
3. Video 5-6-3: Apical 4-chamber image showing significant remodeling (enlargement) of the right ventricle and right atrium in this endurance athlete.
4. Video 5-6-4: Subcostal imaging of the inferior vena cava (IVC). The IVC frequently is found to be dilated in endurance athletes; it often collapses >50% with a sniff (not shown). Also note spontaneous echo-contrast material seen in the IVC and large hepatic vein

REFERENCES

1. Maron BJ, Pelliccia A. The heart of trained athletes. Cardiac remodeling and the risks of sports, including sudden death. *Circulation*. 2006;114:1633-1644.
2. Oxborough D, Sharma S, Shave R, et al. The right ventricle of the endurance athlete: the relationship between morphology and deformation. *J Am Soc Echocardiogr*. 2012;25:263-271.
3. Pelliccia A, Maron BJ, Spataro A, Proschan MA, Spirito P. The upper limit of physiological hypertrophy in highly trained elite athletes. *N Engl J Med*. 1991;324:295-301.
4. Pelliccia A, Di Paolo FM, De Blasiis E, et al. Prevalence and clinical significance of aortic root dilation in highly trained competitive athletes. *Circulation*. 2010;122:698-706.
5. Pelliccia A, Maron BJ, Culasso F, et al. Clinical significance of abnormal electrocardiographic patterns in trained athletes. *Circulation*. 2000;102:278-284.
6. Prior DL, La Gerche A. The athlete's heart. *Heart*. 2012;98:947-955.
7. Corrado D, Pelliccia A, Heidbuchel H, et al. Section of Sports Cardiology, European Association of Cardiovascular Prevention and Rehabilitation. Recommendations for interpretation of 12-lead electrocardiogram in the athlete. *Eur Heart J*. 2010;31:243-259.
8. Pelliccia A, Maron MS, Maron BJ. Assessment of left ventricular hypertrophy in a trained athlete: differential diagnosis of physiologic athlete's heart from pathologic hypertrophy. *Prog Cardiovasc Dis*. 2012;54:387-396.
9. Vinereanu D, Florescu N, Sculthorpe N, Tweddel AC, Stephens MR, Fraser AG. Differentiation between pathologic and physiologic left ventricular hypertrophy by tissue Doppler assessment of long-axis function in patients with hypertrophic cardiomyopathy or systemic hypertension and in athletes. *Am J Cardiol*. 2001;88:53-58.
10. Caselli S, Di Paolo FM, Pisicchio C, et al. Three-dimensional echocardiographic characterization of left ventricular remodeling in Olympic athletes. *Am J Cardiol*. 2011;108:141-147.
11. Marcus FI, McKenna WJ, Sherrill D, et al. Diagnosis of arrhythmogenic right ventricular cardiomyopathy/dysplasia: proposed modification of the task force criteria. *Circulation*. 2010;121:1533-1541.
12. Pelliccia A, Kinoshita N, Pisicchio C, et al. Long-term clinical consequences of intense, uninterrupted endurance training in olympic athletes. *J Am Coll Cardiol*. 2010;55:1619-1625.
13. Pelliccia A, Maron BJ, De Luca R, Di Paolo FM, Spataro A, Culasso F. Remodeling of left ventricular hypertrophy in elite athletes after long-term deconditioning. *Circulation*. 2002;105:944-949.

SECTION 7

Hypertrophic Cardiomyopathy

CLINICAL CASE PRESENTATION

A 60-year-old man originally from China presented for evaluation of mitral regurgitation in the setting of progressive effort intolerance. An outside cardiologist recommended mitral valve replacement after he determined that severe regurgitation was present. The patient was referred to a cardiac surgeon for evaluation. Following this visit, he sought a second opinion about his cardiac status. The patient noticed the development of ankle swelling, a 19-pound weight gain, and worsening exertional dyspnea over the preceding 1 year. He denied PND or orthopnea, and he had not experienced chest discomfort or palpitation. He denied having had syncope or near-syncope. There was no family history of sudden death and no apparent history of cardiomyopathy. He does not have a history of HTN and never smoked. His past medical history was otherwise unremarkable. His only medication was metoprolol tartrate 25 mg twice daily. The physical examination was remarkable for the presence of an irregularly-irregular heart rhythm at a rate of 62 beats/min. His blood pressure was 144/84 mm Hg. Jugular venous distention at 8 cm was found, and HJR was present. The carotid upstrokes were normal without bruit or transmitted sounds. The breath sounds were decreased at both lung bases without evidence of consolidation, and fine crackles were heard to the mid-lung fields bilaterally. The first heart sound was variable, S_2 was normal, and a third heart sound was heard. A grade 4/6 holosytolic murmur was best heard at the apex radiating to the axilla; the murmur was accentuated in the upright position following a squat. The abdominal exam was nonrevealing. The peripheral pulses were full bilaterally, and 1-2+ pitting edema involving the lower extremities extending up to the mid-portion of the calves bilaterally was present.

A 12-lead ECG showed atrial fibrillation with a controlled ventricular response and LVH with strain. Chest radiography showed blunting of both costophrenic angles and mild interstitial edema.

Review of prior echocardiography showed the presence of a small LV cavity (LVEDD 36 mm) and asymmetric septal hypertrophy (IVSTd 16 mm, PWTd 11 mm) with systolic anterior motion of the anterior mitral leaflet. An eccentric, posterior-directed jet of mitral regurgitation was present. The LA was massively dilated (LAVI = 96 mL/m^2), and the RA was dilated. The aortic valve appeared normal for age. At rest, a late peaking systolic profile with peak instantaneous gradient of 25 mm Hg that increased to 75 mm Hg with Valsalva maneuver was found where the anterior mitral leaflet contacted the IVS causing obstruction of the LV outflow tract. The PASP was estimated to be 37 mm Hg plus the RA pressure. The patient was in sinus rhythm at the time of the echocardiogram.

CLINICAL FEATURES

This case study illustrates several of the presenting features and potential complications that may be encountered among patients with symptomatic hypertrophic obstructive cardiomyopathy (HCM). The disease exhibits a marked heterogeneity of symptoms, structural findings, and risk for sudden death.

- Most patients with HCM experience no or only minimal clinical symptoms and may come to attention only because of a family history of disease, auscultation of a murmur, or an abnormal ECG.
- Because of the heterogeneous nature of this disease, a variety of clinical presentations among symptomatic patients may occur.
  - The most common presenting symptoms are exertional dyspnea and chest pain.[1]
  - Other presenting symptoms may include fatigue, palpitation, near-syncope, syncope, or sudden death.
  - A number of mechanisms, alone or in concert, including diastolic dysfunction, left ventricular outflow tract obstruction, microvascular disease, mitral regurgitation, atrial fibrillation, and ventricular arrhythmia may account for symptoms.

PHYSICAL EXAMINATION

- Among patients with minimal disease, the physical examination may be within normal limits.
- As approximately 25% to 30% of patients have an outflow tract gradient at rest or provoked on echocardiography; a distinctive murmur that can be influenced by dynamic auscultation will be heard. Classically, the murmur of dynamic LV outflow tract obstruction is a harsh, systolic murmur heard best at the left lower sternal border or apex; typically it does not radiate to the neck. As illustrated by the clinical case, maneuvers such as standing after a squat, performing a Valsalva maneuver, or administration of amyl nitrate can increase the intensity of the murmur allowing separation from other causes of a systolic murmur such as aortic stenosis and mitral regurgitation.
- Additional findings on physical examination may include a forceful apical impulse, an S_4 (with sinus rhythm), a bifid cartotid pulse contour, and an apical holosystolic murmur of mitral regurgitation.

RISK STRATIFICATION

Individuals with HCM are at increased risk for sudden cardiac death.

- Important prognostic indicators for sudden death include a personal history of ventricular arrhythmia, a family history of sudden cardiac death, wall thickness ≥30 mm, episodes of nonsustained ventricular tachycardia on ambulatory monitoring, abnormal blood pressure responses to exercise, and a history of syncope.[2]
- The LV outflow tract gradient is not closely correlated with risk of sudden death.

PATHOPHYSIOLOGY/ETIOLOGY

HCM is a genetic disease of the cardiac sarcomere with autosomal dominant inheritance pattern characterized by a non-dilated ventricle and LVH in the absence of conditions that impose a pressure load on the heart.

- Sarcomere mutations are found in 60% to 70% of cases; the most common involve myosin heavy chain and myosin binding protein C. Phenotypic expression and penetrance are variable.[1]
- Histologically, HCM is characterized by myocardial fiber disarray and variable amounts of interstial fibrosis.

The pathophysiology of obstructive HCM is complex and involves multiple factors including LV outflow tract obstruction, diastolic dysfunction, mitral regurgitation, myocardial ischemia, and atrial and ventricular arrhythmias.[2]

- LV outflow tract obstruction is mechanistically caused by systolic anterior motion (SAM) of the mitral valve and its contact with the hypertrophied proximal septum. Factors such as displacement of the mitral apparatus, mitral leaflet elongation, and slack also contribute to the pathophysiology of SAM.[3] Systolic anterior motion is related to a "flow-drag" phenomenon in early systole and after mitral septal contact to increasing cavitary pressure gradient across the outflow tract ("pushing").[3]
- Outflow tract obstruction increases LV pressure leading to a variety of deleterious effects on ventricular systolic and diastolic performance, myocardial ischemia, and mitral regurgitation. Factors such as reduced LV afterload, increased contractility, use of vasodilators, and reduced LV chamber volumes contribute to increased severity of LV outflow obstruction.
- Diastolic dysfunction, caused by impaired relaxation secondary to several factors and increased chamber stiffness due to hypertrophy and ischemia, is an important cause of symptoms in patients with HCM.
- Myocardial ischemia is usually not the result of significant epicardial CHD but more often secondary to increased demand due to hypertrophy and small vessel disease.
- Mitral regurgitation occurs commonly and most often is secondary to a distortion of the valve caused by systolic anterior motion associated with LV outflow tract obstruction.
- Other variants, including apical variant, mid-cavity hypertrophy with mid-ventricular obstruction, and free wall hypertrophy, are recognized as not being associated with LV outflow tract obstruction.

EPIDEMIOLOGY

The estimated prevalence in the general population is 0.2%.[2] Although most disease expression begins during childhood and adolescence, HCM is found in patients of all ages. Many patients with genetic disease often are not identified clinically. The risk for complications associated with HCM is age-related; complications occur infrequently among patients >60 years old.[4] Patients with resting LVOT obstruction are at greater risk for HCM-related complications than those without obstruction. The estimated annual risk for sudden cardiac death is approximately 1%, with the peak incidence occurring in adolescence and young adulthood.[1]

ECHOCARDIOGRAPHY

Transthoracic echocardiography is recommended as an initial diagnostic test in all patients with suspected HCM (Class I, LOE B).

Other class I indications for echocardiography include screening of first-degree relatives of genotype positive family members, patients with a change in clinical status, periodic monitoring of children of affected patients, and guidance and follow-up of therapeutic procedures.[2]

Echocardiography is used to identify the presence, extent, and distribution of hypertrophy, document the presence and site of a resting or provoked LV outflow tract gradient, evaluate systolic and diastolic function, quantify the severity of mitral regurgitation, document the LA size, and estimate the pulmonary artery systolic pressures. Another goal should be to evaluate for other potential causes of ventricular hypertrophy (see Differential Diagnosis).

- Historically, asymmetric septal hypertrophy was defined using M-mode echocardiography as a ratio of septal-to-posterior wall thickness ≥1.3:1.
- At present, 2-D echocardiography is the primary imaging modality used; identification of wall thickness ≥15 mm in a nondilated ventricle is the morphologic expression of HCM (Figure 5-7-1).
- About one-third of patients have evidence of LV outflow tract obstruction at rest (defined as a peak instantaneous gradient ≥30 mm Hg). About another one-third of patients have outflow tract gradients of ≥30 mm Hg that develop using provocative manuevers (such as Valsalva maneuver or administration of amyl nitrate); the remaining one-third of subjects are judged to have nonobstructive disease (gradients <30 mm Hg at rest and with provocation).[2]
- Two-dimensional imaging in patients with obstruction shows SAM of the mitral valve with septal contact (Figure 5-7-2); an area of echo-brightness, representing scar, may be seen at the site of frequent leaflet contact with the septum (Figure 5-7-3).
- Color-flow Doppler characteristically shows turbulent flow at the point of leaflet-septal contact (see Figure 5-7-2).
- The continuous-wave Doppler spectral profile typically shows the dynamic nature of this LV outflow tract obstruction as a late peaking systolic profile with a "dagger-shaped" morphology (Figure 5-7-4).
- Treadmill stress echocardiography can be used to determine functional capacity and response to therapy, assess ECG and blood pressure responses to exercise, and provoke dynamic LVOT obstruction among patients without significant resting gradients.
- M-mode echocardiography can identify outflow tract obstruction and its hemodynamic effects.
  - Obstruction is identified by observing SAM of the mitral valve (Figure 5-7-5) with septal contact. A longer duration of septal contact has been associated with more severe LV outflow tract obstruction.
  - Observation of early systolic closure and subsequent reopening of the aortic valve is another sign of the presence of LV outflow tract obstruction (Figure 5-7-6).
- A subset of patients may show evidence of wall thinning, LV dilatation, and reduced LVEF. This "burned-out" phase is estimated to occur in 5% of patients with HCM and appears to be more common among those with severe wall thickening (>30 mm) on initial presentation.[5]
- Mitral regurgitation of variable severity may be found. In the presence of LV outflow tract obstruction, the jet is often eccentric in nature and occurs predominantly in mid-to-late systole.
- Diastolic dysfunction is present in the vast majority of patients with HCM. Use of traditional Doppler variables has shown weak

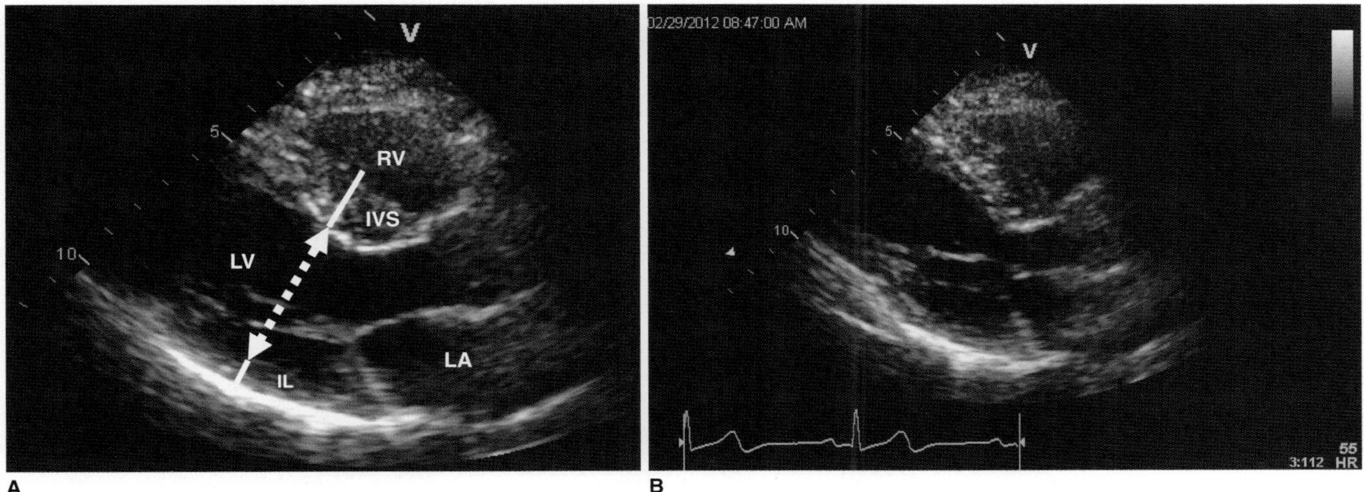

FIGURE 5-7-1 Parasternal long-axis still (A) and moving (B) images demonstrating asymmetric septal hypertrophy in a patient with obstructive hypertrophic cardiomyopathy ► (see Video 5-7-1). Note the increased thickness of the interventricular septum (IVS) in relation to the basal segment of the inferolateral (IL) wall. In this case, the septal thickness in diastole measured 16 mm. The video also demonstrates SAM of the MV. The stippled arrow corresponds to the left ventricular (LV) end-diastolic dimension. LA = left atrium; RV = right ventricle.

correlations with LV filling pressures.[6] The early diastolic (e') velocity at the mitral annulus is reduced in patients with HCM; however, the E/e' ratio has been shown to correlate only modestly with invasive measurements of LA pressures.[7]

- Left atrial enlargement may reflect chronically increased diastolic filling pressures, the presence of significant mitral regurgitation, or an associated atrial myopathy.
- With tissue Doppler imaging (TDI), systolic annular velocities (s') have been shown to be reduced and related to the degree of hypertrophy.[8] In addition, use of TDI may help to distinguish pathological causes of hypertrophy from physiological hypertrophy.[9]
- Using speckle tracking echocardiography, investigators have shown abnormalities in myocardial strain and twist mechanics in patients with HCM.[10,11]

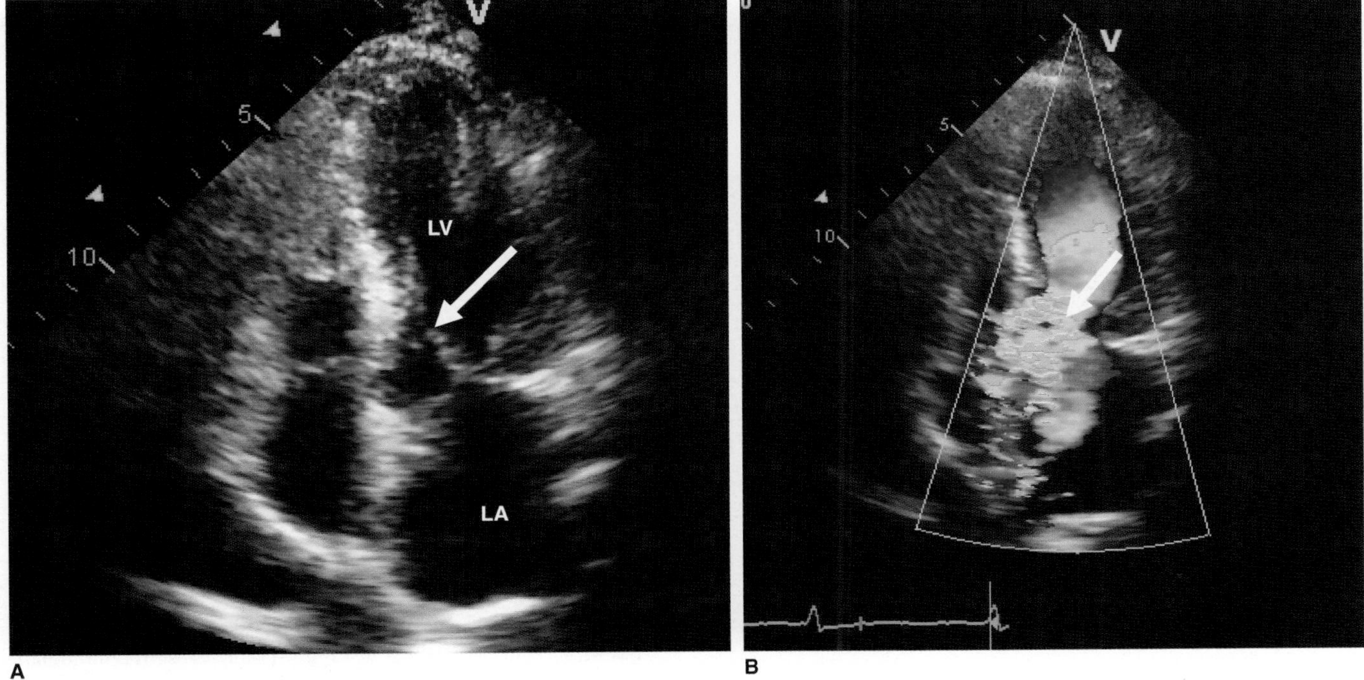

FIGURE 5-7-2 Apical 4 chamber images showing septal contact (white arrow) by the anterior leaflet of the mitral valve (A) and turbulent flow (white arrow) occurring at this site of left ventricular (LV) outflow tract obstruction as shown with color-flow Doppler (B). In real-time, the leaflet-septal contact is demonstrated using the regional expansion mode (C) ► (see Videos 5-7-2 A- C). LA = left atrium.

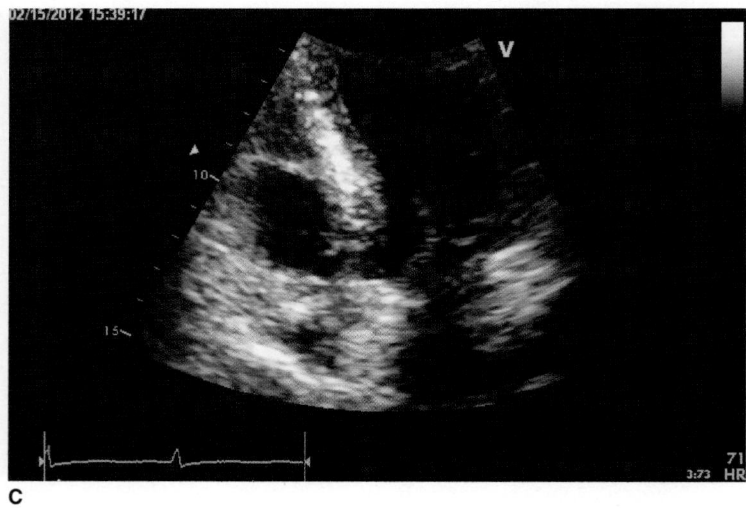

C

FIGURE 5-7-2 (*Continued*)

- Variants of HCM can be recognized with echocardiography.
  - Diagnostic findings of the apical variant include distal ventricular and apical hypertrophy with sparing of the base, apical obliteration during systole, and narrowed apical outflow with turbulence on color-flow Doppler. This variant of HCM easily can be missed on routine 2-D imaging and misinterpreted as apical hypokinesis unless clinical suspicion leads to dedicated apical imaging with a high frequency transducer and zoom-magnified low-Nyquist color ventriculography (Figure 5-7-7). Administration of a transpulmonary contrast agent for LV opacification (Figure 5-7-8) may also help to identify this variant and an associated apical aneurysm.[12]
  - It is also important to recognize that the midventricular variant can be associated with an akinetic apical chamber which must be diligently searched for when performing echocardiography due to its adverse prognostic implications.[3,13]
- Transesophageal echocardiography can be used for assessment of HCM when TTE is nondiagnostic. Its primary utility, however, is in guidance of interventional procedures such as alcohol septal ablation to assess the perfusion territory of the septal perforators or following surgical myectomy to judge the adequacy of the surgery, assess severity of mitral and/or aortic regurgitation, and detect ventricular septal defect occurring as a complication of surgery.

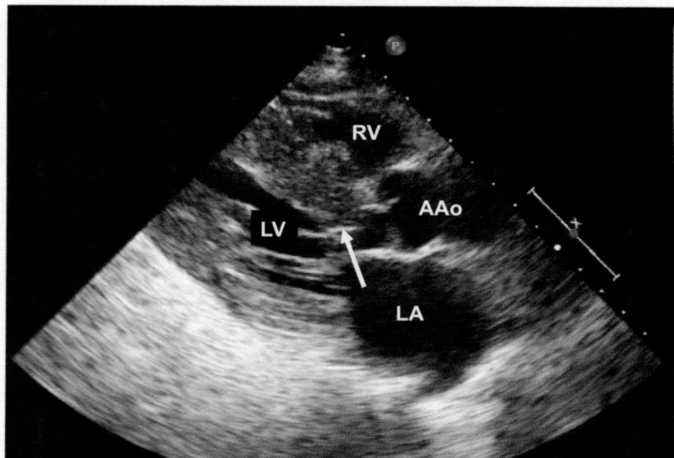

FIGURE 5-7-3 Parasternal long-axis image showing an echo-bright region involving the endocardium of the proximal interventricular septum at the site of repeated mitral leaflet-septal contact (arrow). AAo = ascending aorta; LA = left atrium; LV = left ventricle; RV = right ventricle.

OTHER DIAGNOSTIC TESTS

Electrocardiography

- A "normal" ECG is an uncommon occurrence.
- Frequent findings on 12-lead electrocardiography include increased LV voltage and ST-segment and T-wave abnormalities.
- With the apical variant, "giant" negative T waves in the mid-precordial leads may be observed (Figure 5-7-9). Other abnormalities potentially found on ECG can include LA enlargement, Q waves in the inferior and lateral leads (pseudo-MI), and the presence of atrial fibrillation.

Ambulatory ECG monitoring is indicated initially and at 1 to 2 year intervals in patients with HCM (Class I, LOE B).[2]

- This test can identify atrial and ventricular arrhythmias. Nonsustained ventricular tachycardia has been associated with increased risk of sudden death and its discovery may help make a more informed decision regarding ICD placement in certain subsets of patients.

Exercise stress testing/stress echocardiography may provide important diagnostic and prognostic information.

- Failure to augment systolic blood pressure (≥20 mm Hg) or a decline in blood pressure with exercise (>20 mm Hg) have been associated with increased risk of sudden death.[14]
- Stress echo/Doppler studies are helpful to document significant stress-induced LV outflow tract obstruction or the development of mitral regurgitation that was not present at rest in symptomatic patients.

Cardiac MR is indicated for patients with suspected HCM when echocardiography is nondiagnostic (Class I, LOE B) and when more

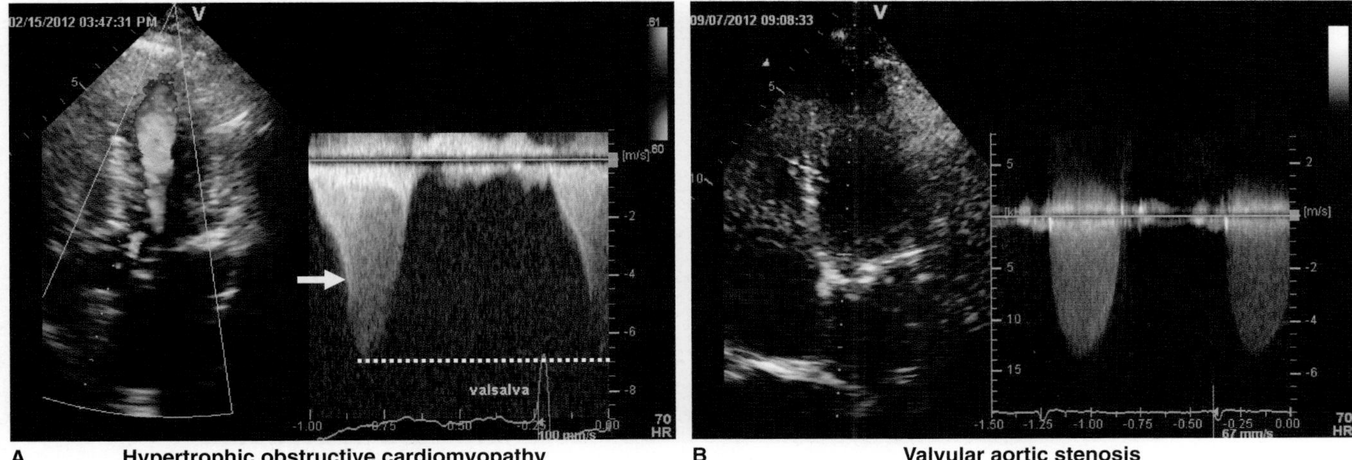

FIGURE 5-7-4 Continuous wave spectral profiles of a patient with hypertrophic obstructive cardiomyopathy (A) and another with severe valvular aortic stenosis (B). The spectral profile of obstructive HCM is dagger-shaped (arrow) and late-peaking in comparison to severe aortic stenosis in which the profile is mid-peaking and rounded. Also note the very high peak velocity (approximately 7 m/sec) associated with this HCM profile.

information about the extent and distribution of hypertrophy is clinically important.[2]

- A particularly useful application of CMR is to visualize hypertrophy involving the anterolateral wall and to diagnose apical HCM and/or aneurysm when echocardiography is inadequate.[2,12]
- Documentation of late gadolinium enhancement (LGE) identifies HCM patients with myocardial fibrosis and possibly increased risk for adverse outcomes.[2] The presence and distribution pattern of LGE may suggest alternative diagnoses provoking LVH, and lack of LGE may suggest the presence of athlete's heart in the appropriate clinical setting.

Cardiac catheterization is rarely required to make/confirm the diagnosis due to the availability of echocardiography and CMR. Coronary angiography is indicated for patients presenting with chest pain and intermediate to high likelihood of CHD. A "spade-like" configuration of the LV on contrast ventriculography is a characteristic finding in the apical variant.

Genetic testing is recommended (Class IIa, LOE B) as being reasonable in the index patient to help in identification of first-degree relatives at risk for developing HCM.[2]

DIFFERENTIAL DIAGNOSIS

The differential diagnosis includes the various conditions that produce ventricular hypertrophy.

- In younger, physically active individuals, physiological remodeling (athlete's heart) must be considered strongly. In the vast majority of cases of athlete's heart, wall thickness does not exceed 15 mm, the LV (and other chambers) may be dilated, and a period of deconditioning may lead to regression of LVH. "Sigmoid septum" in the elderly may mimic the presence of HCM.
- Among older individuals with systemic HTN, hypertensive heart disease must be a strong consideration.
- Conditions leading to pressure load hypertrophy, such valvular aortic stenosis or regurgitation or discreet subvalvular stenosis, should be considered.

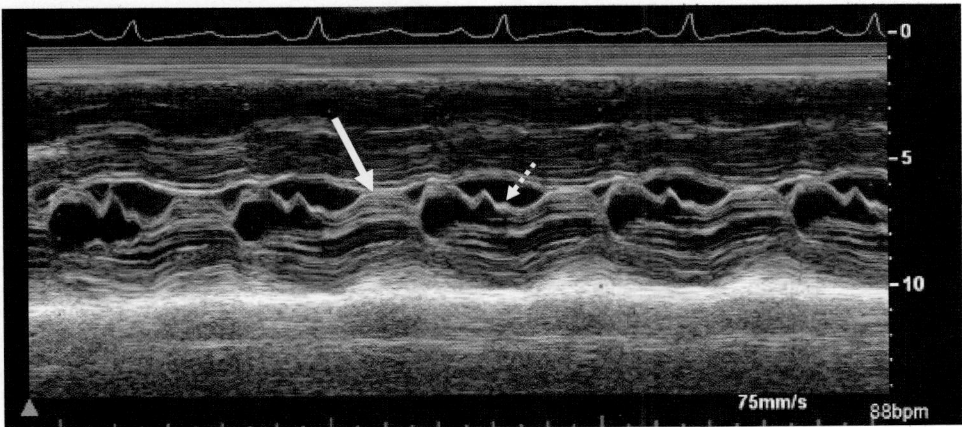

FIGURE 5-7-5 M-mode recording of the mitral valve in a patient with hypertrophic obstructive cardiomyopathy demonstrating systolic anterior motion of the anterior mitral leaflet with septal contact (large arrow). An interrupted A-C closure ("b-notch") is also seen (stippled arrow).

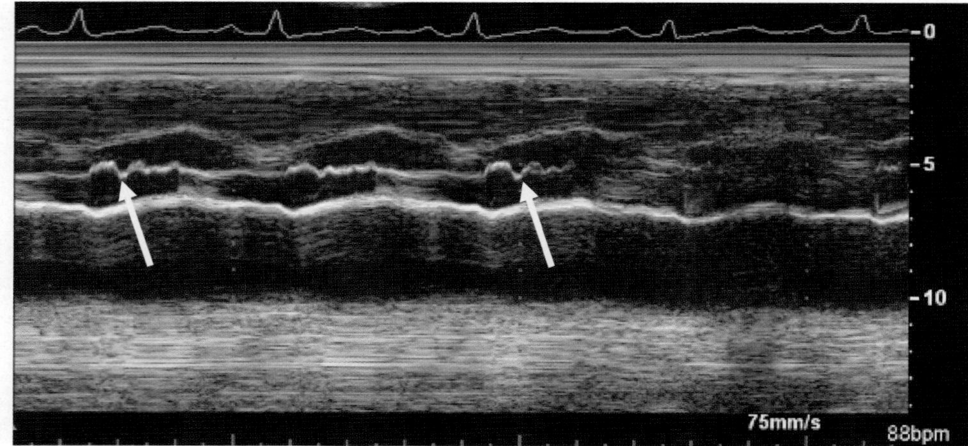

FIGURE 5-7-6 M-mode recording of the aortic valve from the patient shown in Figure 5-7-4 demonstrating mid-systolic closure (arrows) and reopening of the valve.

- Other pathological causes of LVH associated with restrictive cardiomyopathies and infiltrative diseases (amyloidosis, Fabry disease, Pompe's disease) must also be considered in the differential diagnosis.
- Isolated LV noncompaction may produce thickening of the apex and distal portions of the LV.
- With end-stage HCM, systolic dysfunction and chamber dilatation may occur producing the clinical picture of a dilated cardiomyopathy.

DIAGNOSIS

The diagnosis is made on the basis of the history, physical examination, and results of cardiac imaging. Echocardiography is the most commonly used imaging modality and typical findings, as previously described, are often sufficient to make the diagnosis. In some instances, as when echocardiography is nondiagnostic or incomplete, CMR with gadolinium administration will be diagnostic. Genetic testing plays a role in screening of first-degree family members without phenotypic evidence of disease.

MANAGEMENT

Management focuses on 3 key components: management of symptoms, risk stratification for sudden death, and counseling/family screening of first-degree relatives.[1,2]

- For patients with symptoms such as angina, exertional dyspnea, or palpitation, pharamacological therapy is indicated.[2]
  - β-Blockers are the mainstay of therapy due to their negative inotropic and chronotropic effects (Class I, LOE B).
  - For patients intolerant of β-blockers or with persisting symptoms, non-dihydropyrindine calcium channel blockers (verapamil preferred) are recommended (Class I, LOE B). Some patients may require both classes of medications to achieve symptomatic relief.
  - If symptoms are not relieved using these agents in appropriate dosages, addition of disopyramide to the therapeutic regimen may bring symptomatic benefit (Class IIa, LOE B).
  - Diuertics should be used cautiously, and dihyropyridine-type calcium channel blockers should be avoided.

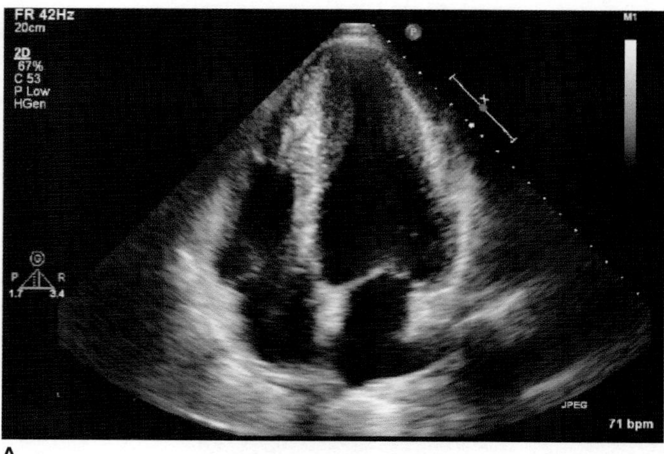

A

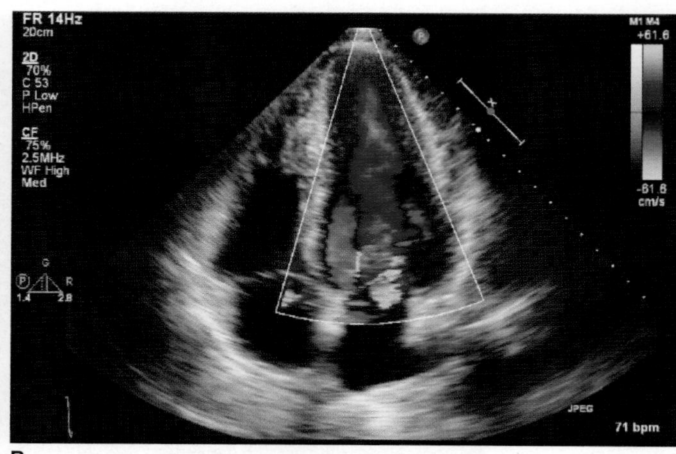

B

FIGURE 5-7-7 Apical 4 chamber views demonstrating findings in a patient with the apical variant of hypertrophic cardiomyopathy. Diagnostic findings include distal ventricular and apical hypertrophy with sparing of the base and apical obliteration during systole (A); narrowed apical outflow with turbulence on color-flow Doppler is demonstrated (B) ► (see Videos 5-7-7 A and B).

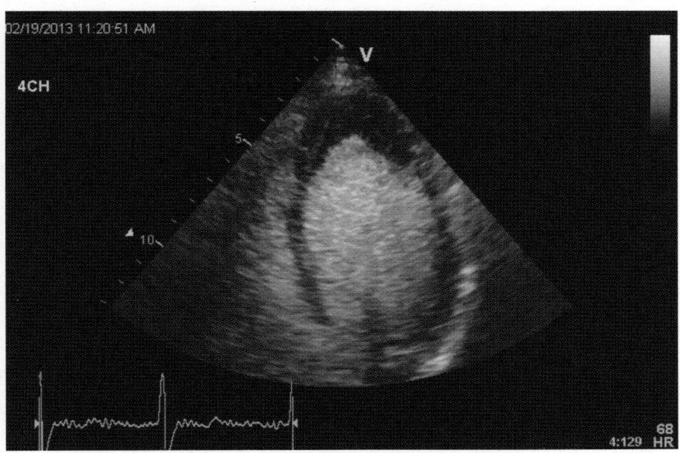

FIGURE 5-7-8 Adminstration of a microbubble echo contrast agent demonstrating the characteristic morphological findings in the apical variant of hypertrophic cardiomyopathy. Contrast use should be considered when the 2-dimensional and Doppler findings are nondiagnostic ► (see Video 5-7-8).

- Septal reduction therapies (septal myectomy, alcohol septal ablation) are recommended in cases of drug-refractory symptoms in association with LVOT gradients >50 mm Hg at rest or when provoked (Class IIa, LOE B).
- Permanent DDD pacing as a means to reduce the LVOT gradient is recommended only if drug therapy has failed and patient characteristics render them suboptimal for a septal reduction therapy (Class IIb, LOE B).

For patients with severe systolic dysfunction, guideline-based therapy as recommended for patients with LV dysfunction is indicated; some patients with refractory symptoms may be candidates for heart transplantation.

Atrial fibrillation should be treated aggressively as it contributes to symptomatic status and places the patient at increased risk for thromboembolic complications. Using a rate-control or rhythm-control strategy depends upon individual patient circumstances. Due to heightened risk of thromboembolism, therapeutic anticoagulation is recommended.[2]

In patients with prior cardiac arrest, ventricular fibrillation, or hemodynamically important ventricular tachycardia, placement of an ICD should be recommended. In addition, ICD placement should be recommended as a primary prevention measure in patients with significant risk factors for sudden cardiac death as listed previously.

As HCM is a genetic disease transmitted with autosomal dominant inheritance, clinical evaluation of first-degree relatives and genetic counseling is recommended (Class I, LOE B). For patients who undergo genetic testing (expensive, may not be covered by insurance), consultation with a knowledgeable genetic counselor is recommended.[2]

FOLLOW-UP

For asymptomatic patients, general measures to promote cardiovascular health should be reinforced. While competitive athletics should be avoided, regular lower-intensity aerobic exercise is permissible. Annual follow-up is suggested.[2]

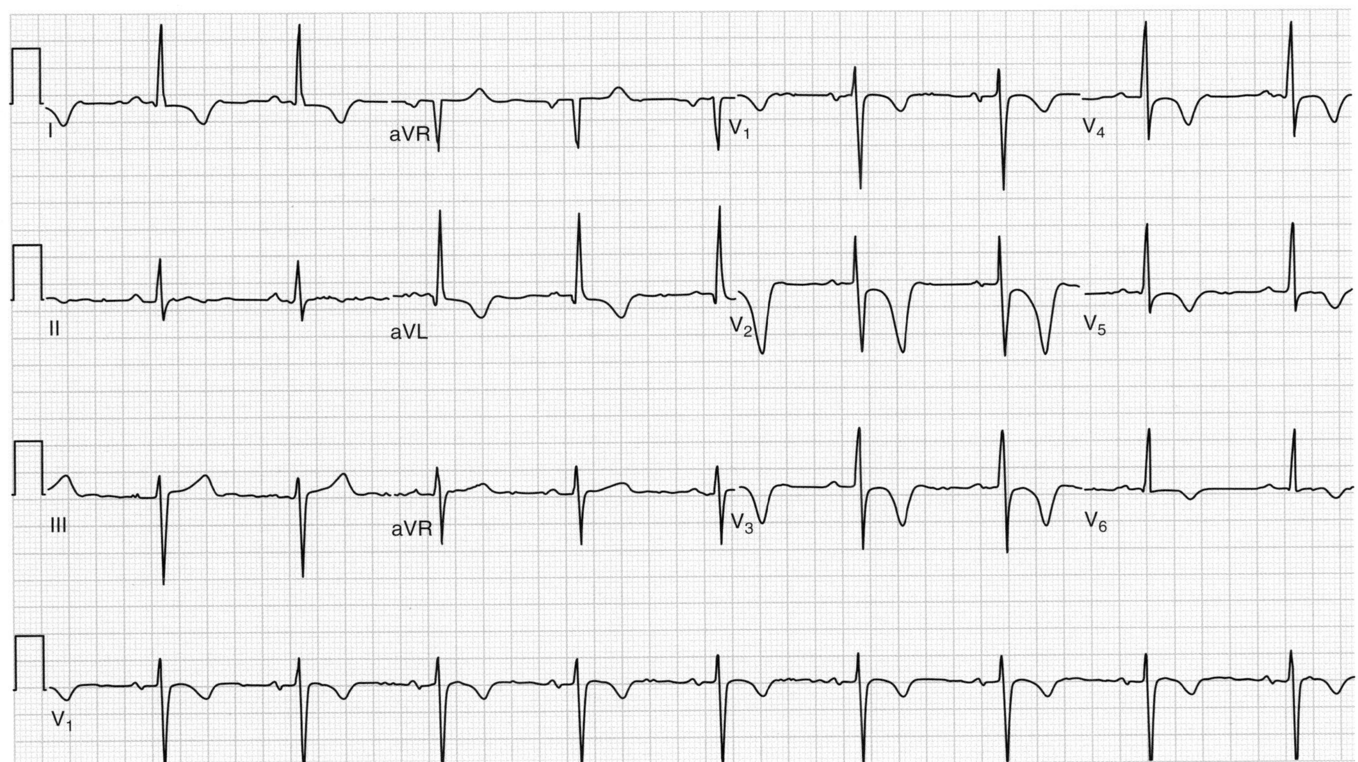

FIGURE 5-7-9 12-lead ECG from a patient with apical variant hypertrophic cardiomyopathy. Note the "giant" negative T waves in the mid-precordial leads.

Periodic assessment with Holter ECG monitoring and echocardiography as recommended by professional guidelines is indicated.[2] For patients with symptomatic disease, regular clinical follow-up with a cardiologist is recommended. For patients with advanced disease not responding to standard therapies, appropriate referral to specialized centers is recommended.

VIDEO LEGENDS

1. Video 5-7-1: Parasternal long-axis video image demonstrating asymmetric septal hypertrophy in a patient with obstructive hypertrophic cardiomyopathy. Note the increased thickness of the interventricular septum (IVS) in relation to the basal segment of the inferolateral (IL) wall.
2. Video 5-7-2 A: Apical 4/5 chamber view demonstrating turbulent flow occurring at the site of left ventricular (LV) outflow tract obstruction as shown with color-flow Doppler.
3. Video 5-7-2 B: Apical 3 chamber view demonstrating turbulent flow occurring at the site of left ventricular (LV) outflow tract obstruction as shown with color-flow Doppler
4. Video 5-7-2 C: The leaflet-septal contact is demonstrated using the regional expansion mode.
5. Video 5-7-7 A: Apical 4-chamber view demonstrating findings in a patient with the apical variant of hypertrophic cardiomyopathy. Diagnostic findings include distal ventricular and apical hypertrophy with sparing of the base and apical obliteration during systole
6. Video 5-7-7 B: Apical 4-chamber view demonstrating findings in a patient with the apical variant of hypertrophic cardiomyopathy. Note the narrowed apical outflow with turbulence demonstrated with color-flow Doppler
7. Video 5-7-8: Administration of a microbubble echo contrast agent demonstrating the characteristic morphological findings in the apical variant of hypertrophic cardiomyopathy.

REFERENCES

1. Ho CY. Hypertrophic cardiomyopathy in 2012. *Circulation*. 2012;125:1432-1438.
2. Gersh BJ, Maron BJ, Bonow RO, et al. American College of Cardiology Foundation/American Heart Association Task Force on Practice Guidelines. 2011 ACCF/AHA Guideline for the Diagnosis and Treatment of Hypertrophic Cardiomyopathy: a report of the American College of Cardiology Foundation/ American Heart Association Task Force on Practice Guidelines. Developed in collaboration with the American Association for Thoracic Surgery, American Society of Echocardiography, American Society of Nuclear Cardiology, Heart Failure Society of America, Heart Rhythm Society, Society for Cardiovascular Angiography and Interventions, and Society of Thoracic Surgeons. *J Am Coll Cardiol*. 2011;58:e212-260.
3. Sherrid MV, Arabadjian M. Echocardiography to individualize treatment for hypertrophic cardiomyopathy. *Prog Cardiovasc Dis*. 2012;54:461-476.
4. Maron BJ, Braunwald E. Evolution of hypertrophic cardiomyopathy to a contemporary treatable disease. *Circulation*. 2012;126:1640-1644.
5. Thaman R, Gimeno JR, Reith S, et al. Progressive left ventricular remodeling in patients with hypertrophic cardiomyopathy and severe left ventricular hypertrophy. *J Am Coll Cardiol*. 2004;44:398-405.
6. Nagueh SF, Appleton CP, Gillebert TC, et al. Recommendations for the evaluation of left ventricular diastolic function by echocardiography. *J Am Soc Echocardiogr*. 2009;22:107-133.
7. Geske JB, Sorajja P, Nishimura RA, Ommen SR. Evaluation of left ventricular filling pressures by Doppler echocardiography in patients with hypertrophic cardiomyopathy: correlation with direct left atrial pressure measurement at cardiac catheterization. *Circulation*. 2007;116:2702-2708.
8. Matsumura Y, Elliott PM, Virdee MS, Sorajja P, Doi Y, McKenna WJ. Left ventricular diastolic function assessed using Doppler tissue imaging in patients with hypertrophic cardiomyopathy: relation to symptoms and exercise capacity. *Heart*. 2002;87:247-251.
9. Vinereanu D, Florescu N, Sculthorpe N, Tweddel AC, Stephens MR, Fraser AG. Differentiation between pathologic and physiologic left ventricular hypertrophy by tissue Doppler assessment of long-axis function in patients with hypertrophic cardiomyopathy or systemic hypertension and in athletes. *Am J Cardiol*. 2001;88:53-58.
10. Sun JP, Stewart WJ, Yang XS, et al. Differentiation of hypertrophic cardiomyopathy and cardiac amyloidosis from other causes of ventricular wall thickening by two-dimensional strain imaging echocardiography. *Am J Cardiol*. 2009;103:411-415.
11. Garceau P, Carasso S, Woo A, Overgaard C, Schwartz L, Rakowski H. Evaluation of left ventricular relaxation and filling pressures in obstructive hypertrophic cardiomyopathy: comparison between invasive hemodynamics and two-dimensional speckle tracking. *Echocardiography*. 2012;29:934-942.
12. Maron MS, Finley JJ, Bos JM, et al. Prevalence, clinical significance, and natural history of left ventricular apical aneurysms in hypertrophic cardiomyopathy. *Circulation*. 2008;118:1541-1549.
13. Minami Y, Kajimoto K, Terajima Y, et al. Clinical implications of midventricular obstruction in patients with hypertrophic cardiomyopathy. *J Am Coll Cardiol*. 2011;57:2346-2355.
14. Sadoul N, Prasad K, Elliott PM, Bannerjee S, Frenneaux MP, McKenna WJ. Prospective prognostic assessment of blood pressure response during exercise in patients with hypertrophic cardiomyopathy. *Circulation*. 1997;96:2987-2991.
15. Spirito P, Bellone P, Harris KM, Bernabo P, Bruzzi P, Maron BJ. Magnitude of left ventricular hypertrophy and risk of sudden death in hypertrophic cardiomyopathy. *N Engl J Med*. 2000;342:1778-1785.

SECTION 8

Restrictive Cardiomyopthy (Cardiac Amyloidosis)

CLINICAL CASE PRESENTATION

An 81-year-old woman with well-controlled systemic hypertension, paroxysmal atrial fibrillation, and sick sinus syndrome with permanent pacemaker insertion 2 years prior presented to an outside hospital with worsening shortness of breath and reduced urine output. The patient described several months of gradually worsening shortness of breath, anorexia, and fatigue to the point where she was unable to carry on the majority of her activities of daily living. She was told that she had "diastolic heart failure," and it was suggested that her pacemaker needed to be upgraded to a biventricular device. Recent echocardiography reportedly showed LVEF of 50% with biatrial enlargement and mild to moderate mitral and tricuspid regurgitation. The dose of her daily diuretic medicine was increased. Her "baseline" serum creatinine was 1.7 mg/dL. On presentation to the outside hospital, her blood pressure was observed to be 70/40 mm Hg and the heart rate was 110 beats/min. Jugular venous distention was noted along with bilateral lower extremity edema. Evaluation included a chest x-ray showing bilateral pleural effusions, an ECG documenting an AV-sequential paced rhythm, creatinine of 2.26 mg/dL, and white cells in the urine. The initial impression was septic shock; a central venous line was placed, and she was started on intravenous dopamine and transferred subsequently to the medical ICU at our institution for further care. On arrival, she remained hypotensive despite dopamine infusion; other vasoactive agents were added to the regimen, and bedside echocardiography was obtained. Echocardiography showed that the LV and RV walls were thickened with high relative wall thickness, a "granular" appearance of the myocardium, LVEF of 35% with diffuse hypokinesis, reduced RV systolic function, severe biatrial dilatation, moderate to severe MR and severe TR, evidence of increased filling pressures, and the presence of bilateral pleural effusions. The cardiac troponin I was 0.32 ng/mL and BNP was 3092 pg/mL. She was transferred to the CCU for further care. Blood and urine cultures revealed no growth. Over the next several days, pressor agents were able to be weaned, and her serum creatinine decreased to 1.4 mg/dL with adequate diuresis being achieved; however, low-dose inotropic support with dobutamine could not be weaned off. Subsequent serum and urinary electrophoresis and immunofixation showed evidence of IgG kappa-type monoclonal free light chains. A tissue biopsy was not pursued due to poor prognosis. The patient was discharged to home hospice where she expired about 2 weeks later.

CLINICAL FEATURES

This case vignette illustrates the clinical features and course of a patient with advanced AL-type amyloidosis with cardiac involvement.

The restrictive cardiomyopathies are a diverse group of diseases characterized primarily by progressive diastolic cardiac dysfunction with a small- or normal-sized LV cavity and biatrial enlargement. Overt systolic dysfunction (reduced EF) may occur in the latter stages of the disease process.

- Idiopathic restrictive cardiomyopathy is rare.
- Other causes of restrictive cardiomyopathy, such as infiltrative processes like cardiac amyloidosis, iron-overload, and sarcoidosis, will be encountered more frequently.
- Disorders such as endomyocardial fibroelastosis, radiation toxicity, and scleroderma may also cause restrictive cardiomyopathy.[1]

The presentation of patients with the various types of restrictive cardiomyopathy will vary depending upon etiology and stage of the disease.

- In general, the clinical features may include symptoms such as exertional dyspnea, effort intolerance, fatigue, weakness, fluid retention, and palpitation. These symptoms can mimic those seen with constrictive pericarditis.
- With advanced disease, as illustrated by this case study, significant jugular venous distention, which may be accompanied by prominent y-descents and Kussmaul sign, is often present.
- Other features may include a prominent third heart sound, soft murmurs of A-V valve regurgitation, peripheral edema, hepatomegaly and ascites, and reduced breath sounds due to pleural effusions.

The discussion that follows focuses primarily on the cardiac amyloidoses as these are the most commonly encountered causes of restrictive cardiomyopathy. With the amylodoses, clinical presentation varies depending upon the type of amylodosis.

- Cardiac involvement is frequent with AL-type amyloidosis and uncommon with secondary (AA) amyloidosis. Prognosis is related to the presence of cardiac involvement and the degree of systemic involvement.
- As illustrated by this case study, cardiac involvement with AL-type amyloidosis is characterized by an often rapidly progressive clinical course. Senile and familial amyloidoses more often follow a more indolent course.
- AL-type amyloidosis is a systemic disease; its manifestations can include autonomic and peripheral neuropathy, syncope, renal insufficiency, carpal tunnel syndrome, easy bruising, purpura (may be periorbital), macroglossia, atrial fibrillation, conduction-system disease and intracardiac thrombosis. Angina, due to small vessel involvement, may be a presenting symptom.
- With the hereditary transthyretin-related form, neuropathy and nephropathy can be prominent clinical features.
- Among patients with "senile" amyloidosis, a significant elderly male predominance is observed.[2]

PATHOPHYSIOLOGY/ETIOLOGY

The amyloidosis are characterized by the interstitial deposition of a fibillary proteinaceous material (amyloid) leading to disruption of tissue architecture and, in some cases, toxic injury to myocardial cells. Amyloid deposits are caused by misfolding of precursor proteins.

The characteristic wall thickening observed on cardiac imaging studies is not due to hypertrophy per se, as the disease process is characterized by infiltration of the myocardium and not myocyte hypertrophy.

- Pathologically, the heart is observed to be thickened with normal to small size ventricular cavities and biatrial enlargement.
- Thickening of the cardiac valves and interatrial septum may be present.
- Intracardiac thrombus is a common finding and is especially prevalent with AL-type amyloidosis.

The diagnosis should be confirmed on biopsy of an affected tissue. The classic finding is demonstration of amyloid protein with Congo-red staining. Once amyloidosis is diagnosed, special staining techniques are indicated to determine the specific type of amyloid as the prognosis and treatment differ among the varying forms of this disease.

- Several types of amyloidosis are recognized.
  - With AL-type amyloidosis, suspected in the case study presented, a plasma cell dyscrasia accounts for production of the amyloid derived from monoclonal immunoglobulin light chains.
  - Mutations of the liver-synthesized transport protein transthyretin lead to the production of abnormal protein and its deposition in the hereditary ("familial") transthyretin-related form.
  - Senile amyloidosis is related to deposition of wild-type transthyretin produced in the liver.
  - Systemic AA amyloidosis occurs as a result of marked increase in production of the protein serum amyloid-A seconadry to sustained acute-phase response.

EPIDEMIOLOGY

AL-type amyloidosis is the most commonly recognized form. About 2000 to 2500 cases are diagnosed annually in the United States.

- The median age at diagnosis is 55 to 60 years old.
- In up to 90% of cases the heart is affected; diastolic heart failure is the presenting symptom in about 50% of cases.
- Among patients with AL-type amyloidosis, the presence of cardiac involvement is often marked by rapidly progressive cardiac dysfunction; in the presence of heart failure the median survival is 4 to 6 months.
- Death in AL-type amyloidosis is often due to progressive heart failure or electromechanical dissociation.[3]
- Systemic involvement is frequent.

Patients with the hereditary transthyretin-related form often are younger than patients with AL-type or senile-type amyloidoses.

- Neurological involvement is frequent, and carpal tunnel syndrome is reported to be a common presenting complaint.[4]
- Among African Americans, approximately 4% are heterozygous for a particular mutation characterized by a valine-isoleucine substitution at position 122, and this variant is reported to cause 23% of cases of cardiac amyloidsis in African Americans.[5] In this particular group of patients, the disease is characterized by prominent cardiac manifestations with onset in the late 60s with less neurological involvement and more common involvement among women.

Senile amyloidosis is reported to be exceptionally rare in patients <60 years-old; its prevalence is estimated to be about 25% to 36% in those >80 years-old.[5]

- The disease frequently involves the heart and predominantly is found in men; the male to female ratio is reported to be about 20:1.[3]
- Compared to AL amyloidosis, the senile-type is characterized by more prominent LV wall thickening and a more favorable prognosis.

ECHOCARDIOGRAPHY

Several of the salient echocardiographic features of amyloid cardiomyopathy are illustrated by this case study. Echocardiography provides anatomical and functional information to suggest the diagnosis and also may provide important prognostic information. It is important to emphasize, however, that most of the "classic" echocardiographic manifestations associated with amyloid cardiomyopathy are seen in advanced stages of the disease and definitive diagnosis requires biopsy of involved tissue.

- The most common and prominent findings on 2-dimensional echocardiography include increased wall thickeness, normal or small-sized LV cavity dimensions, and atrial dilatation (Figures 5-8-1 and 5-8-2).
- Increased wall thickness is a nonspecific finding as other processes that produce myocardial hypertrophy or which infiltrate the heart may lead to wall thickening. In the presence of low-voltage on ECG, an infiltrative process is more likely.
- Atrial size is often related to the severity and chronicity of elevation of diastolic filling pressures.
- Early in the disease process, LV and RV ejections fractions often are preserved; however, as illustrated by the case study, impaired biventricular systolic function may occur with advanced disease.
- Other findings on 2-dimensional echocardiography may include the presence of increased myocardial echogenicity ("granular" or "sparkling" appearance), thickening of the heart valves, thickening of the interatrial septum (Figue 5-8-3), the presence of pericardial and pleural effusions (see Figure 5-8-1), plethora of the inferior vena cava, functional mitral and tricuspid regurgitation, and atrial thrombus.
- Granular appearance of the myocardium is both a nonspecific and insensitive marker of amyloid infiltration. Other disease entities associated with hypertrophy may cause a similar appearance, and it must be appreciated that this finding was described with the use of fundamental imaging; tissue harmonic imaging tends to cause a generalized increase of myocardial echogenicity.
- In isolation, individual 2-dimensional findings provide limited diagnostic accuracy; consideration of the findings in totality along with

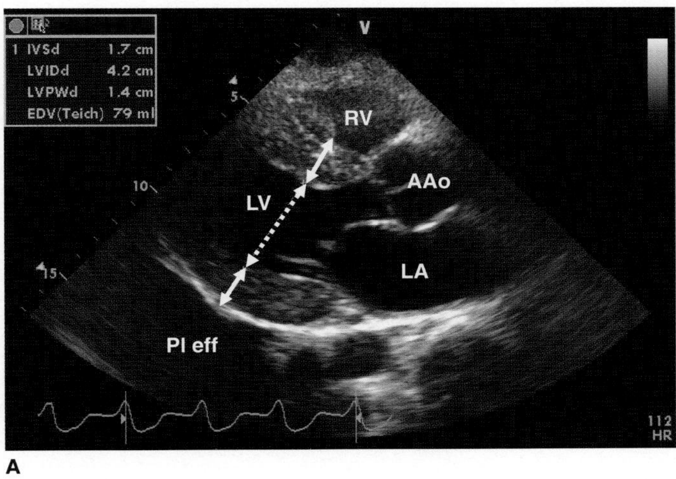

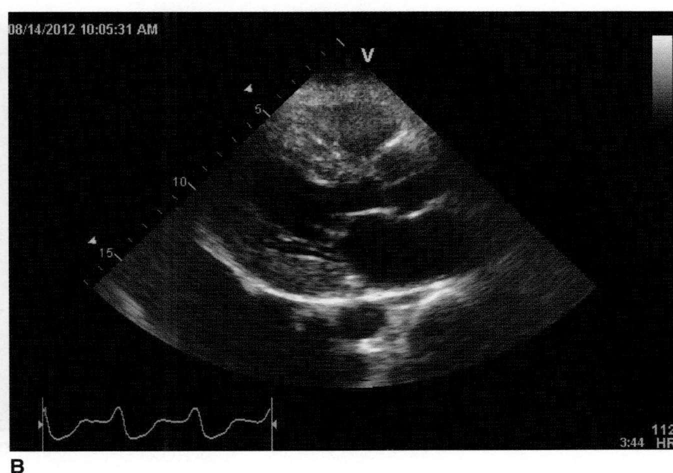

FIGURE 5-8-1 Parasternal long-axis images in a patient with AL-type amyloidosis and heart failure ▶ (see Video 5-8-1). Left ventricular (LV) systolic function is reduced, and the left atrium (LA) is dilated. Note the presence of wall thickening with a relatively small LV cavity (relative wall thickness 0.67). Increased echogenicity of the myocardium is present. A left pleural effusion (Pl eff) is present. AAo = ascending aorta; RV = right ventricle.

the information provided by Doppler echocardiography increases the diagnostic power of echocardiography.

- Doppler echocardiography is an important component in the evaluation of such patients. Diastolic dysfunction is the hemodynamic hallmark of restrictive cardiomyopathies. With progression of the disease process, a transmitral inflow pattern of impaired relaxation may transition to one of restrictive filling. Previous work has shown that the presence of restrictive filling with a rapid deceleration time (<150 msec) is associated with reduced survival in cardiac amyloidosis[6]; however, more recent studies have called this association into question.[7]
- Tissue Doppler imaging of the mitral annulus characteristically reveals reduced e' and a' velocities; an e' velocity <8 cm/s has been shown to be a good discriminator between restrictive cardiomyopathy and constrictive pericarditis.[8] The E/e' ratio characteristically is increased in restrictive cardiomyopathy (Figure 5-8-4).
- Advanced techniques (strain and strain rate imaging) have been shown to be valuable to identify preclinical disease, identify systolic dysfunction, offer prognostic information, and separate cardiac amyloidosis from other etiologies of ventricular wall thickening such as hypertrophic cardiomyopathy and secondary LVH.[9,10] All 3 components of strain (longitudinal, cicunferential, and radial) have been shown to be decreased significantly in patients with cardiac amyloidosis[10] compared to normal subjects and those with other causes of hypertrophy.

OTHER DIAGNOSTIC TESTS AND PROCEDURES

Clinical evaluation of the patient with suspected cardiac amyloidosis should include a thorough history and physical examination with attention to the features previously described.

A 12-lead ECG may offer important information.

- Low QRS voltage (<5 mm in all limb leads or <10 mm in all precordial leads) is present in about 50% of patients.
- A pseudo-infarction pattern may be observed in about 50% of patients.

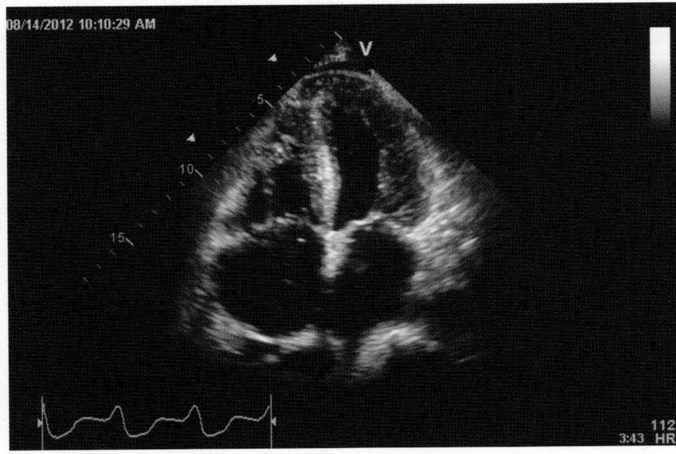

FIGURE 5-8-2 Apical 4 chamber image showing biatrial enlargement and biventricular systolic dysfunction ▶ (see Video 5-8-2).

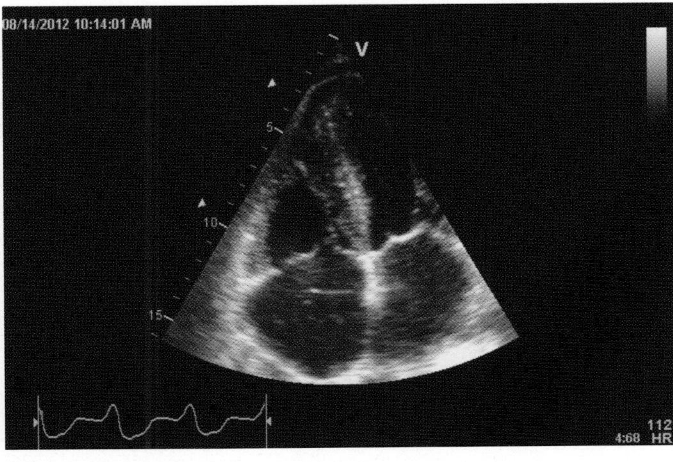

FIGURE 5-8-3 Right ventricular (RV) focused view demonstrating reduced RV systolic function, dilatation of the right atrium, and thickening of the interatrial septum ▶ (see Video 5-8-3).

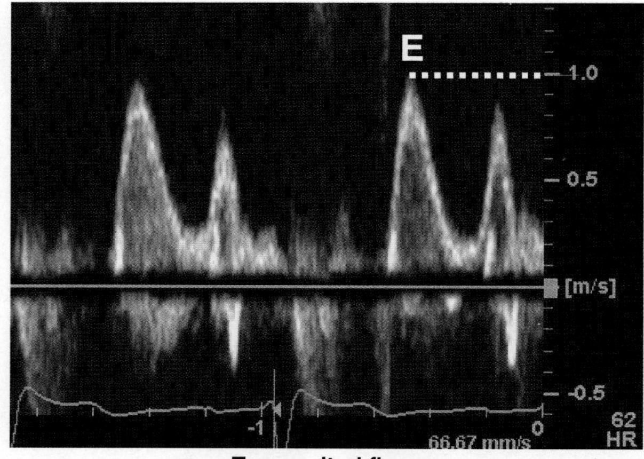

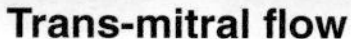

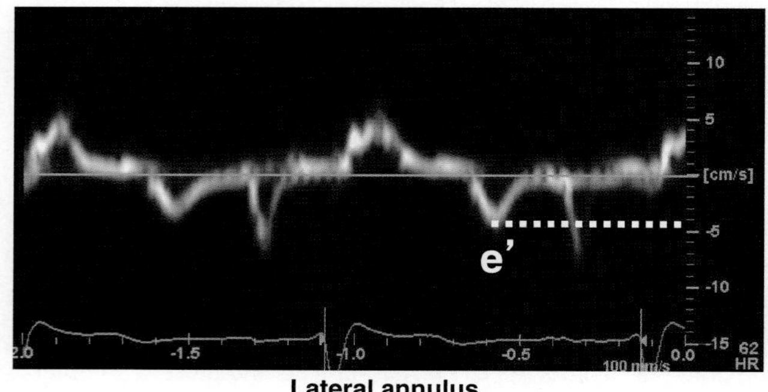

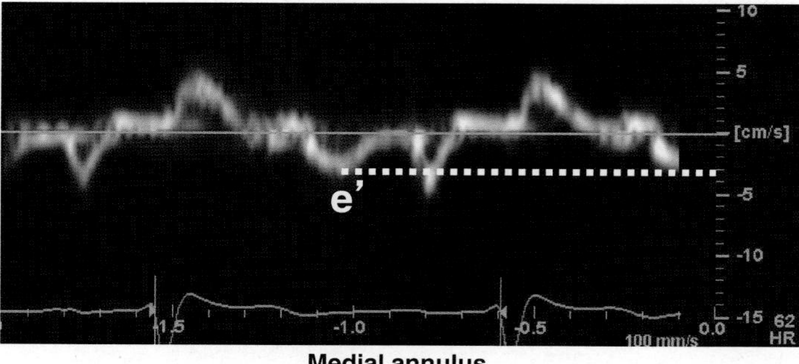

FIGURE 5-8-4 Trans-mitral flow velocities and tissue Doppler imaging velocities at the lateral and medial mitral annular locations. Consistent with the presence of a restrictive cardiomyopathy, the e' values are reduced significantly (<8 cm/sec). In this case, the average E/e' ratio exceeds 20.

- Other findings may include first-degree AV delay, atrial fibrillation or flutter, and second or third-degree AV block.
- ECG-LVH may be present in patients with cardiac amyloidosis, thus its presence should not be used to exclude the diagnosis.
- When low ECG voltage is combined with the finding of increased wall thickness on echocardiography, the diagnosis of cardiac amyloidosis is more likely.[5]

Chest radiography may show evidence of pulmonary congestion and pleural effusions. As constrictive pericarditis should be considered in the differential diagnosis, the finding of pericardial calcification (uncommon) would make this latter diagnosis more likely.

Biomarkers, such as caradic troponins and natriuretic peptides, offer prognostic information. Increased cardiac troponins and NT-proBNP levels have been identified as markers of poor prognosis in AL-type amyloidosis.

Cardiac magnetic resonance (CMR) may be a useful test when cardiac amyloidosis is suspected and echocardiography is suboptimal or nondiagnostic. A pattern of global transmural or subendocardial late gadolinium enhancement (LGE) along with abnormal myocardial gadolinium kinetics is considered characteristic of cardiac amyloidosis.[11,12] This pattern is distinct from other conditions that cause interstitial expansion such as myocardial infarction and HCM. In addition, the pattern and extent of LGE is associated with the amount of amyloid deposition on biopsy specimens and other clinical and imaging markers of prognosis in cardiac amyloidosis.[12]

Serum and urinary protein electrophoresis and immunofixation should be obtained and may help to suggest a diagnosis of AL-type amyloidosis if a monoclonal paraprotein is found. Caution is suggested as monoclonal gammopathy of undetermined significance may also be present; thus these tests should not be used to "confirm" a diagnosis of AL-amyloidosis.

Tissue biopsy remains the gold standard for diagnosis of cardiac amyloidosis and is important when distinction between AL-type and the hereditary transthyretin-related form of amylodosis is required as potential treatment regimens differ substantially.

DIFFERENTIAL DIAGNOSIS

Disease entities that cause increased wall thickness with normal LV chamber dimensions along with diastolic dysfunction and symptoms of right heart failure should be considered in the differential diagnosis.[13]

- The entities most commonly encountered among adults in clinical practice include hypertensive heart disease and hypertrophic cardiomyopathy.
- Other causes of restrictive cardiomyopathy such iron-overload states, sarcoidosis, endomyocardial fibroelastosis, radiation toxicity, and scleroderma should also be considered.

- In adolescents and young adults, infiltrative conditions such as Fabry disease, Danon disease, Friedrich ataxia, the mucopolysaccharidoses, and cardiac oxalosis are potential causes of restrictive cardiomyopathy.
- Idiopathic restrictive cardiomyopathy is a rare entity.

An important consideration in the differential diagnosis is constrictive pericarditis; this entity may present with quite similar clinical findings to a restrictive cardiomyopathy. This condition can often be differentiated from cardiac amyloidosis by a careful history and physical examination. Often echocardiography is diagnostic; evidence of preserved longitudinal function on tissue Doppler imaging and demonstration of enhanced LV/RV interaction favors the diagnosis of constrictive pericarditis. In cases where echocardiography is not diagnostic, CMR and/or simultaneous left and right heart catheterization may be required.[14]

DIAGNOSIS

The diagnosis is made on the basis of a thorough history and physical examination along with appropriately targeted laboratory studies (assessment for proteinuria, serum and urinary protein electrophoresis, and immunofixation), ECG, and cardiac imaging (echocardiography and/or CMR). While noninvasive assessment may strongly suggest the diagnosis, confirmation of disease and the specific type of amyloid should be obtained from a biopsy of involved tissue.

MANAGEMENT

Cardiac involvement in amyloidosis is often associated with poor prognosis, but this can vary with the particular type of amyloidosis and response to therapy. In general, management centers on two important strategies: supportive care for heart failure and interruption of the process accounting for formation and deposition of the abnormal amyloid proteins.

As patients with cardiac amyloidosis have a restrictive cardiomyopathy, diuretic agents are often the mainstay of therapy. Care must be exercised to balance fluid status so that adequate blood pressure is maintained.

- Some patients may require administration of an α-agonist (midodrine) to maintain blood pressure and allow for adequate diuresis.
- Due to possible underlying autonomic neuropathy, agents such as ACE-inhibitors and ARBs should be used with caution as often blood pressure is dependent on angiotensin II.
- β-Blockers may also lead to hypotension and have not been shown to favorably impact outcome in amyloid cardiomyopathy.[3]
- Digoxin and certain calcium channel blockers bind to amyloid fibrils leading to toxicity and worsening of heart failure, thus these agents should be avoided in patients with amyloid cardiomyopathy.
- Pacemakers may be required for symptomatic bradycardia or heart block; in general, if pacing is required, a biventricular device would be favored.
- Some experts do not recommend implanation of an ICD unless symptomatic ventricular tachycardia has been documented as arrhythmic death in patients with amyloid cardiomyopathy is most often due to electromechanical dissociation.[2]
- Anticoagulation is strongly recommended for patients with atrial fibrillation and when intracardiac thrombus is seen on cardiac imaging studies.

Management of the underlying process causing amyloid production depends highly on the type of amyloidosis.

- Among patients with AL-type amyloidosis, therapy is targeted at the plasma cell dyscrasia causing production of the monoclonal immunoglobulin light chains. Specific description of these chemotherapeutic regimens is beyond the scope of this discussion, but the interested reader is referred to recent reviews on this topic.[2,5,15]
- Stem cell transplantation following high dose chemotherapy has led to treatment successes, but treatment-related mortality remains high. It must be recognized that many patients do not qualify for such therapy due to the advanced nature of their disease. Cardiac transplantation has been offered to highly selected patients, but outcomes are documented to be inferior compared to other indications for transplantation.[2]

As the liver is the main source of mutant transthyretin in patients with the hereditary transthyretin-related form of amylodosis, liver transplantation is a recommended therapy used to eliminate the source of the abnormal protein. In selected patients with cardiac involvement, combined liver and heart transplantation has been performed.

Among patients with senile amyloidosis, prognosis is better than with AL-amyloidosis,[4] and heart failure appears to be more amenable to medical therapies.[3] Organ transplantation is rarely recommended in this population.

Treatment of secondary (AA) amyloidosis centers on suppressing the inflammatory disease process responsible for the production of the amyloid fibrils.

FOLLOW-UP

For patients with cardiac amyloidosis and advanced disease, follow-up with a heart failure specialist is indicated. Patients with AL-amyloidosis and extensive cardiac and systemic involvement have a particularly poor prognosis, and recommendations for care of patients with ACC/AHA stage D heart failure symptoms are indicated. In contrast, senile-type amyloidosis is associated with better prognosis and response to standard heart failure therapies. For patients with AL-amyloidosis and limited cardiac and systemic involvement, referral to a center that specializes in the cardiac and hematological aspects of this disease is indicated.

VIDEO LEGENDS

1. Video 5-8-1: Parasternal long-axis images in a patient with AL-type amyloidosis and heart failure. Left ventricular (LV) systolic function is reduced and the left atrium (LA) is dilated.
2. Video 5-8-2: Apical 4-chamber image showing biatrial enlargement and biventricular systolic dysfunction.
3. Video 5-8-3: Right ventricular (RV) focused view demonstrating reduced RV systolic function, dilatation of the right atrium, and thickening of the interatrial septum

REFERENCES

1. Nihoyannopoulos P, Dawson D. Restrictive cardiomyopathies. *Eur J Echocardiogr*. 2009;10:iii23-iii33.
2. Falk RH, Dubrey SW. Amyloid heart disease. *Prog Cardiovasc Dis*. 2010;52:347-361.
3. Falk RH. Cardiac amyloidosis. A treatable disease, often overlooked. *Circulation*. 2011;124:1079-1085.
4. Rapezzi C, Merlini G, Quarta CC, et al. Systemic cardiac amyloidoses: disease profiles and clinical courses of the 3 main types. *Circulation*. 2009;120:1203-1212.
5. Selvanayagam JB, Hawkins PN, Paul B, Myerson SG, Neubauer S. Evaluation and management of the cardiac amyloidosis. *J Am Coll Cardiol*. 2007;50:2101-2110.
6. Klein AL, Hatle LK, Taliercio CP, et al. Prognostic significance of Doppler measures of diastolic function in cardiac amyloidosis. A Doppler echocardiography study. *Circulation*. 1991;83:808-816.
7. Koyama J, Falk RH. Prognostic significance of strain Doppler imaging in light-chain amyloidosis. *JACC Cardiovasc Imaging*. 2010;3:333-342.
8. Ha JW, Ommen SR, Tajik AJ, et al. Differentiation of constrictive pericarditis from restrictive cardiomyopathy using mitral annular velocity by tissue Doppler echocardiography. *Am J Cardiol*. 2004;94:316-319.
9. Tsang W, Lang RM. Echocardiographic evaluation of cardiac amyloid. *Curr Cardiol Rep*. 2010;12:272-276.
10. Sun JP, Stewart WJ, Yang XS, et al. Differentiation of hypertrophic cardiomyopathy and cardiac amyloidosis from other causes of ventricular wall thickening by two-dimensional strain imaging echocardiography. *Am J Cardiol*. 2009;10:411-415.
11. Maceira AM, Joshi J, Prasad SK, et al. Cardiovascular magnetic resonance in cardiac amyloidosis. *Circulation*. 2005 Jan 18;111(2):186-193.
12. Syed IS, Glockner JF, Feng D, et al. Role of cardiac magnetic resonance imaging in the detection of cardiac amyloidosis. *JACC Cardiovasc Imaging*. 2010;3:155-164.
13. Seward JB, Casaclang-Verzosa G. Infiltrative cardiovascular diseases. Cardiomyopathies that look alike. *J Am Coll Cardiol*. 2010;55:1769-1779.
14. Talreja DR, Nishimura RA, Oh JK, Holmes DR. Constrictive pericarditis in the modern era: novel criteria for diagnosis in the cardiac catheterization laboratory. *J Am Coll Cardiol*. 2008;51:315-319.
15. Dubrey SW, Comenzo RL. Amyloid diseases of the heart: current and future therapies. *QJ Med*. 2012;105:617-631.

SECTION 9

Chemotherapy-Induced Cardiomyopathy

CLINICAL CASE PRESENTATION

A 32-year-old woman presented to her local physician with complaints of shortness of breath and fatigue. Several weeks earlier she reported a loss of consciousness, which was ascribed to a seizure. About 10 years prior to this presentation, she was diagnosed with non-Hodgkin lymphoma; she received chemotherapy with several cycles of the CHOP (cytoxan, adriamycin, oncovin, and prednisone) regimen that reportedly cured her disease. No radiation therapy was delivered. She did not follow-up regularly after completing therapy, and a study to assess cardiac function following completion of therapy was not obtained. She was referred initially to an electrophysiologist for evaluation of a possible cardiac cause of syncope. As part of the evaluation echocardiography was performed (Figure 5-9-1). The evaluation showed the presence of mild to moderate global LV hypokinesis, normal chamber dimensions, and normal valvular function. The LVEF was estimated to be 35% to 40%. There was no personal history of hypertension, and none of the other standard risk factors for premature cardiac disease were present. The patient denied a familial history of cardiomyopathy, and she did not consume alcohol or use illicit drugs. There was no history of palpitations, and she could not recall any recent viral illness. She delivered a healthy baby more than 1 year prior to presentation and experienced no complications during or early after her pregnancy. Her only medication was clonazepam as needed. The physical examination revealed a regular tachycardia at 120 beats/min, blood pressure of 90/60 mm Hg, and respirations of 16/min. The jugular venous pulsation was estimated to be at 5 cm above the sternal angle. Bibasilar rales were noted and an S_3 was heard. No dependent edema was noted, and there was adequate peripheral perfusion. A 12-lead ECG showed sinus tachycardia with normal intervals. Thyroid function testing was normal as were a complete blood count and basic metabolic panel. Subsequently, she presented to hospital after having experienced another seizure. Several more seizures were observed in-hospital, none of which was accompanied by loss of consciousness or arrhythmia. She was initiated on a cardiac regimen consisting of a diuretic, ACE-inhibitor, and β-blocker. Follow-up echocardiography has shown reduced but stable LVEF, and the patient has not had any subsequent heart failure-related hospital admissions.

CLINICAL FEATURES

Chemotherapy-induced cardiomyopathy may present with heart failure symptoms as exemplified by the case study.

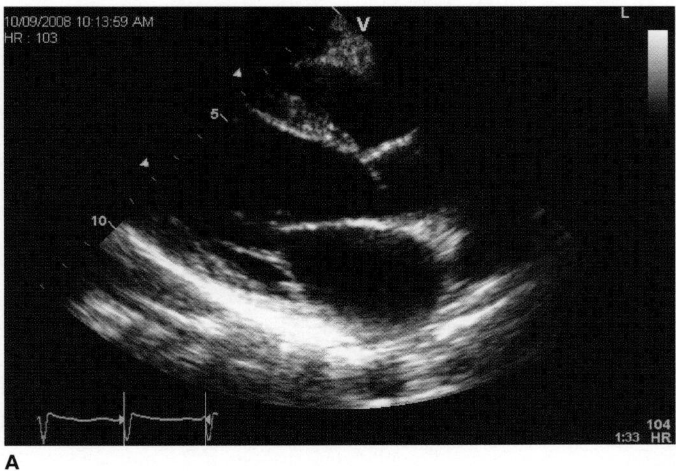

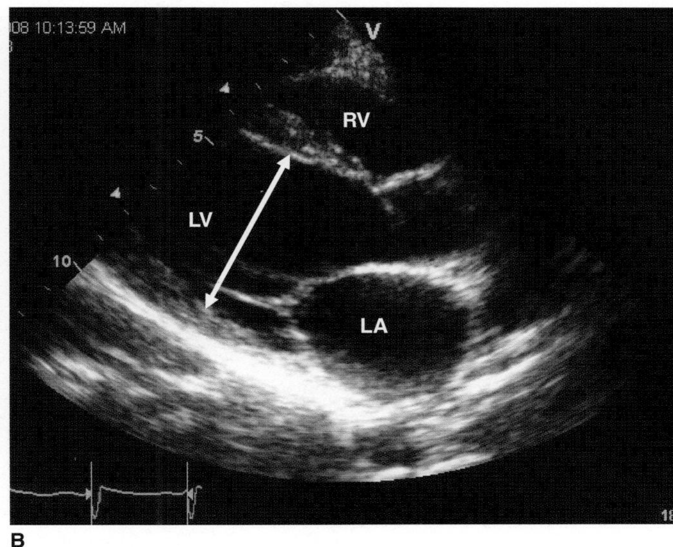

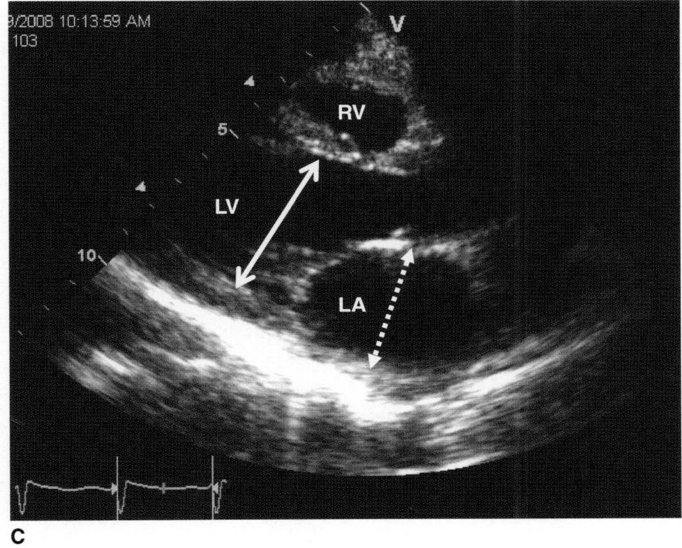

FIGURE 5-9-1 Parasternal long-axis images of the patient described in the case vignette. The moving image (A) ► (see Video 5-9-1) demonstrates poor contractile function with relatively preserved thickening of the basal segment of the inferolateral wall. End-diastolic (B) and end-sytsolic (C) images show the left ventricle (LV) to be dilated with reduced systolic function. The LVEF, as estimated by the biplane method of discs, was 38%. In addition, note the increased anterior-posterior dimension of the left atrium (LA) in the systolic frame (stippled arrow, C). The LA volume index was 36 mL/m^2. RV = right ventricle.

- Such presentations may occur within a few weeks to months following completion of a chemotherapeutic regimen.
- Increasingly recognized is the fact that subclinical LV dysfunction may lead to delayed presentations, sometimes occurring years later.
- The risk of development of heart failure depends upon the particular chemotherapeutic agent(s) and the cumulative doses administered, whether or not radiation therapy was prescribed, and several other clinical factors.
- Most patients present with a picture of a nonischemic dilated cardiomyopathy; asymptomatic LV dysfunction and arrhythmia may also lead to clinical presentation.
- When symptoms appear soon after completion of chemotherapy, the diagnosis is often secure; however, with delayed presentations the multiple other causes for nonischemic cardiomyopathy must be considered.

PATHOPHYSIOLOGY/ETIOLOGY

A classification scheme has been proposed to differentiate agents that lead to irreversible myocyte destruction (so-called "type-1" agents) from those that do not ("type-2" agents) as their predominant mechanism.

- Anthracylines (doxorubicin, daunorubicin, epirubicin) and mitoxantrone (structurally related to anthracyclines) are considered prototypical type-1 agents.
  - The anthracyclines are widely used in the treatment of breast cancer, lymphomas, leukemias, and sarcomas.

- These agents may cause early reversible toxicities such as tachycardia and other dysrhythmias, pericarditis, ECG changes, and (rarely) myocarditis.
- The most feared side effect of these agents is development of cardiac dysfunction and heart failure.
- Although the mechanism of anthracycline-induced cardiotoxicity has not been fully elucidated, it is believed that production of toxic free radicals and increased oxidative stress leads to cardiac injury and ultimately cell death.[1]
- Clinical factors increasing the risk of anthracycline-induced cardiomyopathy include cumulative dose administered (increased with doxorubicin dose >300 mg/m^2), concomitant cardiac irradiation, aged >65 years, preexisting heart disease, and presence of coronary disease.[1]
- Similar to the anthracyclines, mitoxantrone use is associated with a cumulative dose-related cardiac toxicity. Ultrastructural alterations in cardiac architecture seen with mitoxantrone are reported to be identical to those seen in anthracycline-induced cardiac injury.

• Cyclophosphamide (Cytoxan), also considered a type-1 agent, causes cardiac injury by inducing hemorrhagic necrosis. In contrast to anthracycline-induced cardiac toxicity, a cumulative dose effect is not observed.[1]

• Trastuzumab (Herceptin) is considered the prototypical type-2 agent. This IgG_1 monoclonal antibody directed against the human epidermal growth factor receptor tyrosine kinase HER2 (erbB-2) is used clinically in patients with breast cancers that express this cell surface marker (about 25%-30% of patients with breast cancer).
  - Early reports[2] suggested that a significant increase in cardiac dysfunction was associated with this therapy. Subsequent reports have shown that trastuzumab cardiotoxicity does not induce changes on cardiac biopsy and is largely associated with reversible cardiac dysfunction.
  - Carditoxicity is increased markedly with concomitant use of anthracyclines.[3]
  - Other purported risk factors for trastuzumab-associated cardiotoxicity include low normal LVEF, systemic hypertension requiring drug-therapy, advanced age, and body-mass index >25 kg/m^2.[3]

• The use of the tyrosine-kinase inhibitors sunitinib, laputinib, and imatinib has been associated with increased risk of LV dysfunction.

EPIDEMIOLOGY

• Early reports suggested that the incidence of doxorubicin-associated cardiomyopathy was 2.2%.[4]

• More recent analysis revealed that the incidence is approximately 5.1% with the majority of events occurring at cumulative doses exceeding 500 mg/m^2.[5] Furthermore, this study estimated that the cumulative percentage of patients with heart failure was 5% at a cumulative dose of 400 mg/m^2, 16% at a dose of 500 mg/m^2, and 48% at a dose of 700 mg/m^2. Another finding of this study was that heart failure could occur (albeit infrequently) at relatively low cumulative doses (<300 mg/m^2).

• In addition to cumulative dose, risk factors for anthracycline-induced cardiotoxicity include age at exposure (very young and very old have increased risk), concomitant administration of other chemotherapeutic agents (taxanes, trastuzumab), cardiac irradiation, bolus dosing, and preexisting cardiac disease (systemic hypertension, CAD).

ECHOCARDIOGRAPHY

Echocardiography is indicated to monitor patients receiving potentially cardiotoxic chemotherapy and to evaluate cardiac symptoms in those who have received such therapy.

• While monitoring protocols for patients receiving anthracyclines and trastuzumab have been proposed[6,7] and the FDA label suggests monitoring of LVEF periodically, no formally adopted guidelines exist. It must be emphasized that LVEF is an insensitive parameter of early cardiac injury.

• Two-dimensional and Doppler echocardiography is indicated to evaluate new or changing symptoms in patients with suspected LV dysfunction. Outside of expected findings with a nonischemic cardiomyopathy, no individual finding is specific for chemotherapy-induced cardiac dysfunction.

• Recent attention has focused on use of refined techniques such as tissue Doppler imaging (TDI) and speckle tracking-derived strain imaging to detect early signs of chemotherapy-associated cardiotoxicity. These data are preliminary, and how this information would be used in the clinical setting has yet to be determined.
  - In a recent study conducted in human subjects with breast cancer treated with anthracyclines and trastuzumab, altered radial and global longitudinal strain imaging parameters, and reduced TDIs' values were shown to be predictive of subsequent cardiotoxicity.[8]
  - A second study conducted in a similar cohort, reduced systolic longitudinal strain along with increased levels of ultrasensitive cardiac troponin I predicted subsequent cardiotoxicity.[9]

OTHER DIAGNOSTIC TESTS AND PROCEDURES

A complete history and physical examination to elicit symptoms and signs of LV dysfunction is imperative. In addition to performance of comprehensive echocardiography, other diagnostic tests may be helpful.

• An ECG is indicated in all patients with cardiac disease; however, findings such as non-specific ST-segment and T-wave changes and low QRS voltage are nondiagnostic.

• Chest radiography may reveal cardiomegaly and signs of pulmonary vascular congestion.

• Although rarely obtained today due to radiation exposure and ready availability of echocardiography, radionuclide ventriculography historically has been used to monitor LVEF during chemotherapy and to assess suspected LV dysfunction.

• Measurement of cardiac biomarkers is indicated when certain clinical circumstances exist. Cardiac troponin levels can be used to assess for acute injury with administration of anthracyclines. In addition, elevated levels of cardiac troponins during or following chemotherapy may be predictive of cardiotoxicity.

• Natriuretic peptide levels, such as BNP or NT-proBNP, increase with conditions leading to increased ventricular wall stress (such as in heart failure). Some studies suggest that increased levels of these natriuretic peptides may predict cardiac subsequent dysfunction in anthracylcine-treated patients.

- Cardiac magnetic resonance imaging may be helpful in assessing LV structure and function when images obtained with echocardiography are suboptimal or when the study is nondiagnostic.
- Endomyocardial biopsy is considered to be the most accurate method to assess possible anthracycline-associated cardiotoxicity. This invasive procedure requires expertise in performance and interpretation. As with any invasive intracardiac procedure, serious complications may occur. In order to obtain an adequate sample of tissue multiple specimens should be obtained. Due to its invasive nature, this procedure is recommended only when noninvasive evaluation fails to provide the necessary information.

DIAGNOSIS

The diagnosis is made on the basis of the history, physical examination, and findings on echocardiography. As stated previously, other potential causes of nonischemic cardiomyopathy should be considered.

DIFFERENTIAL DIAGNOSIS

The differential diagnosis is primarily that of nonischemic cardiomyopathy.

- Among older patients and those with preexisting cardiac disease, etiologies such as ischemic heart disease and valvular heart disease should be entertained.
- For patients who have received cardiac irradiation, manifestations of radiation-induced cardiac dysfunction including pericardial constriction, pericardial effusion, restrictive cardiomyopathy, coronary artery disease, and radiation-induced valve disease should be considered.
- Lastly, recurrence of cancer and its effects on the heart such as with pericardial and/or myocardial involvement or direct tumor invasion must be considered.

MANAGEMENT

The management of chemotherapy-related cardiotoxicity importantly begins with measures that identify risk factors that may lead to potential cardiac injury.

- For the anthracyclines, efforts to limit cumulative dose, following continuous infusion protocols, use of liposomal delivery systems, and administration of cardioprotective agents (such as dexrazone) may limit the cardiotoxicity associated with these agents.[1]
- Small studies have shown some benefit for use of enalapril[10] or carvedilol[11] to prevent adverse cardiac events in anthracycline-treated patients.
- Surveillance programs for patients receiving anthracyclines that assess LVEF before therapy and monitor it during treatment have been proposed; to date no scheme has been independently validated.

Once chemotherapy-associated cardiomyopathy has occurred, treatment is primarily that suggested for LV systolic dysfunction per established guidelines.[12]

- One small trial[13] has shown that treatment with enalapril and carvedilol in anthracycline-treated patients with LVEF ≤45% reduced cardiac events when treatment was initiated soon after the discovery of LV dysfunction.
- Among selected patients with advanced disease not responding to standard heart failure therapies, cardiac transplantation has been performed.

FOLLOW-UP

- The risk of anticancer therapy-induced cardiotoxicity depends upon the presence of underlying cardiac risk factors and the type(s) of therapy administered.
- Early diagnosis of impaired cardiac performance and being able to predict those more likely to suffer cardiotoxicty are important goals of follow-up in order to limit or prevent development of chronic heart failure.
- Collaboration between medical oncology and cardiology in the care of these patients is of paramount importance.
- For patients at greatest risk of cardiotoxicity, regular follow-up with history and physical examination is suggested.
- At present, the determination of LVEF during therapy is the primary means utilized in various management schemes[1,3,7] to assess for declines in cardiac performance and determine if further therapy should be administered. It should be recognized that determination of LVEF is a rather insensitive marker of early cardiac dysfunction; while other more-refined methods offer the potential to identify sub-clinical disease, at present these methods remain investigational.
- Follow-up after completion of anticancer therapy for patients at risk of developing heart failure is suggested since LV dysfunction may manifest months to years following completion of therapy.[13] For patients with established heart failure, regular follow-up with a cardiologist/heart failure specialist is suggested.

VIDEO LEGEND

1. Video 5-9-1: Parasternal long-axis images of the patient described in the case vignette. The image demonstrates poor contractile function with relatively preserved thickening of the basal segment of the inferolateral wall.

REFERENCES

1. Ewer MS, Ewer SM. Cardiotoxicity of anticancer treatments: what the cardiologist needs to know. *Nat Rev Cardiol.* 2010;7:564-575.
2. Slamon DJ, Leyland-Jones B, Shak S, et al. Use of chemotherapy plus a monoclonal antibody against HER2 for metastatic breast cancer that overexpresses HER2. *N Engl J Med.* 2001;344:783-792.
3. Suter TM, Ewer MS. Cancer drugs and the heart: importance and management. *Eur Heart J.* 2013;34(15):1102-1111.
4. Von Hoff DD, Layard MW, Basa P, et al. Risk factors for doxorubicin-induced congestive heart failure. *Ann Intern Med.* 1979;91:710-717.

5. Swain SM, Whaley FS, Ewer MS. Congestive heart failure in patients treated with doxorubicin: a retrospective analysis of three trials. *Cancer*. 2003;97:2869-2879.

6. Takemura G, Fujiwara H. Doxorubicin-induced cardiomyopathy from the cardiotoxic mechanisms to management. *Prog Cardiovasc Dis*. 2007;49:330-352.

7. Geiger S, Lange V, Suhl P, Heinemann V, Stemmler HJ. Anticancer therapy induced cardiotoxicity: review of the literature. *Anticancer Drugs*. 2010;21:578-590.

8. Fallah-Rad N, Walker JR, Wassef A, et al. The utility of cardiac biomarkers, tissue velocity and strain imaging, and cardiac magnetic resonance imaging in predicting early left ventricular dysfunction in patients with human epidermal growth factor receptor II-positive breast cancer treated with adjuvant trastuzumab therapy. *J Am Coll Cardiol*. 201;57:2263-2270.

9. Sawaya H, Sebag IA, Plana JC, et al. Assessment of echocardiography and biomarkers for the extended prediction of cardiotoxicity in patients treated with anthracyclines, taxanes, and trastuzumab. *Circ Cardiovasc Imaging*. 2012;5:596-603.

10. Cardinale D, Colombo A, Sandri MT, et al. Prevention of high-dose chemotherapy-induced cardiotoxicity in high-risk patients by angiotensin-converting enzyme inhibition. *Circulation*. 2006;114:2474-2481.

11. Kalay N, Basar E, Ozdogru I, et al. Protective effects of carvedilol against anthracycline-induced cardiomyopathy. *J Am Coll Cardiol*. 2006;48:2258-2262.

12. Yancy CW, Jessup M, Bozkurt B, et al. 2013 ACCF/AHA guideline for the management of heart failure: a report of the American College of Cardiology Foundation/American Heart Association Task Force on Practice Guidelines. *J Am Coll Cardiol*. 2013;62:e147–239. This document is available on the World Wide Web sites of the American College of Cardiology (www.cardiosource.org) and the American Heart Association (my.americanheart.org).

13. Cardinale D, Colombo A, Lamantia G, et al. Anthracycline-induced cardiomyopathy: clinical relevance and response to pharmacologic therapy. *J Am Coll Cardiol*. 2010;55:213-220.

SECTION 10

Left Ventricular Noncompaction Cardiomyopathy

CLINICAL CASE PRESENTATION

A 60-year-old woman with systemic hypertension, dyslipidemia, left bundle branch block and asthma was referred to the electrophysiology clinic for evaluation of palpitations. On further questioning, she described progressive effort intolerance such that she could no longer climb a flight of stairs without having to stop. One year prior she could ambulate without limitation. She denied having chest discomfort, paroxysmal nocturnal dyspnea, or orthopnea. She reports that recently she has noticed her pulse rate has been about 100 beats/min. She experienced an episode of syncope 1 year prior. Physical examination revealed a blood pressure of 120/80 mm Hg with a regular pulse rate of 112 beats/min. Jugular venous distention was present, and the carotid upstrokes were normal. The lungs were clear to auscultation; no audible wheezing was present. The point of maximal impulse was displaced inferolaterally. An LV S_3/S_4 gallop sound was heard along with a grade II/VI holosystolic murmur at the apex. No peripheral edema was present. A 12-lead ECG showed sinus tachycardia (110/min) with unifocal VPCs and left bundle branch block. She was referred for echocardiography (Figure 5-10-1). This study revealed the presence of a dilated LV (LVeDD 62 mm) with severely reduced LVEF (25%) with global hypokinesis. The RV was normal in size and systolic function. The LA was dilated. The LV filling pressures were increased, and the PASP was estimated to be 45 to 50 mm Hg. Moderate functional MR was present. At the apical-third of the LV cavity, prominent trabeculations with increased ratio of noncompacted to compacted myocardium along with deep intratrabecular sinusoids communicating with the LV cavity were demonstrated. Subsequent

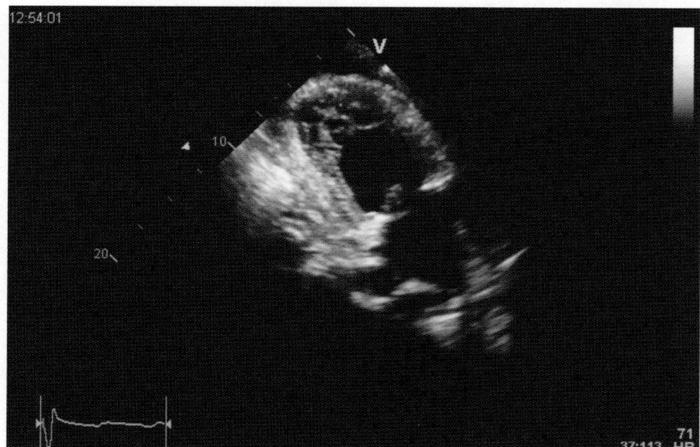

FIGURE 5-10-1 Apical 2 chamber view demonstrating prominent trabeculations and deep recesses located adjacent to the inferoapical portion of the ventricle in this patient with left ventricular noncompaction cardiomyopthy ► (see Video 5-10-1).

coronary angiography, ventriculography, and right heart catheterization showed nonobstructive coronary artery disease and confirmed the presence of increased filling pressures, increased PASP, and the severely reduced LVEF.

CLINICAL FEATURES

This case vignette illustrates some of the features that may lead to clinical presentation among patients with advanced forms of left ventricular noncompaction (LVNC).

- Symptomatic patients may present with heart failure, chest pain, arrhythmias (particularly ventricular in origin), thromboembolism, or sudden death.[1,2] The incidence of atrial fibrillation among patients with LVNC is reported to be 7% to 26%.[3]
- The spectrum of disease appears to be wide, and patients may be diagnosed at an asymptomatic stage as part of screening or when echocardiography is obtained for another clinical indication.
- Especially important is the recognition of report bias existing in the medical literature. Similar to that seen with hypertrophic cardiomyopathy, early reports included highly symptomatic patients evaluated at referral centers; it is likely that adverse outcomes and clinical symptoms are seen less commonly than previously reported.[1,2]
- While LVNC may occur in isolation, this cardiomyopathy has been reported in association with several neuromuscular disorders, genetic syndromes, and congenital cardiac defects.[1,2]
- Predictors of adverse outcome in adolescents and adults include presentation with a cardiac complication (decompensated heart failure, embolic event, or sustained ventricular arrhythmia) or NYHA Class III/IV symptoms. LV dilatation and reduced LVEF appear to be less strong predictors of adverse outcome.[4]

PATHOPHYSIOLOGY/ETIOLOGY

- LVNC is hypothesized to occur as a result of arrest of normal ventricular compaction that is often completed in the early fetal period.[1,3] The exact mechanism underlying the arrested LV maturation is unknown at present. Other investigators have raised the issue that some cases may develop post-natally as a result of genetic mutations involving sarcomere protein genes.[1]
- LVNC is classified as a distinct, genetic form of cardiomyopathy by the American Heart Association. This disorder is genetically heterogenous with sporadic and familial forms being recognized. Autosomal dominant inheritance is believed to be more common than X-linked and autosomal recessive inheritance. Familial involvement is estimated to occur in 18% to 50% of cases.[1]

EPIDEMIOLOGY

The true prevalence of LVNC remains unknown. Among patients referred for echocardiography, the prevalence of disease is reported to be between 0.014% and 0.24%.[3] Among patients attending a heart failure clinic, a prevalence of 12.1% to 18.6%, depending on the diagnostic criteria used, has been reported.[5] Men are more often affected than women.

ECHOCARDIOGRAPHY

The diagnosis is most often made by echocardiography.

- Characteristic features include the presence of a thickened myocardium with noncompacted and compacted layers, prominent LV trabeculations, and deep intertrabecular recesses perfused from the LV cavity (as documented with color flow Doppler examination or LV opacification with contrast microbubbles) and not by the epicardial coronary circulation (Figures 5-10-2, 5-10-3, and 5-10-4).
- These findings primarily involve the distal portions of the LV (the apical region is the final portion of the LV to undergo compaction); the apicolateral segment has the greatest predilection for involvement.[2]
- Among symptomatic patients, abnormalities of systolic and diastolic function are common.
- LV thrombus may be visualized, but most patients suffering a cerebral or peripheral embolism often have other concomitant conditions such as atrial fibrillation, systolic dysfunction, or atherosclerosis that may predispose to such clinical events.[6]

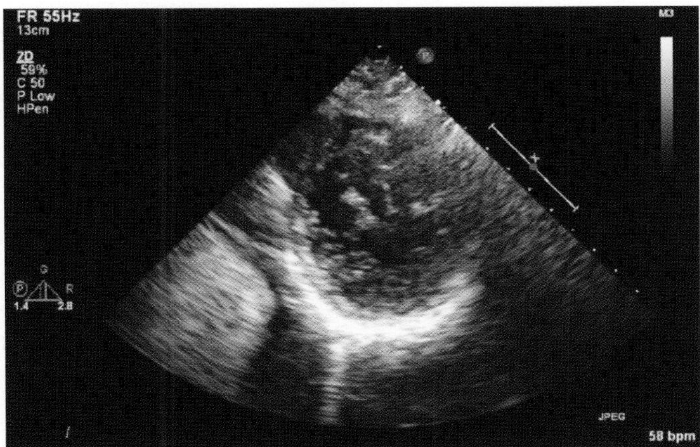

A

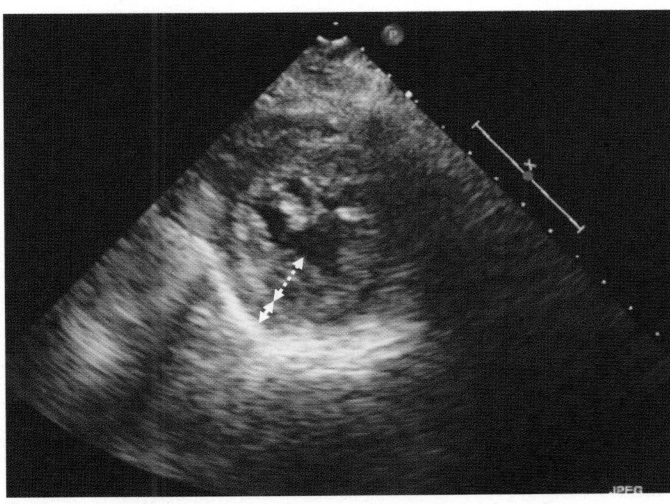

B

FIGURE 5-10-2 Apical short-axis image (A) demonstrating prominent trabeculations with intertrabecular recesses ► (see Video 5-10-2). In panel B, the ratio of noncompacted (stippled arrow) to compacted (solid arrow) myocardium assessed at end-systole excceds 2.0.

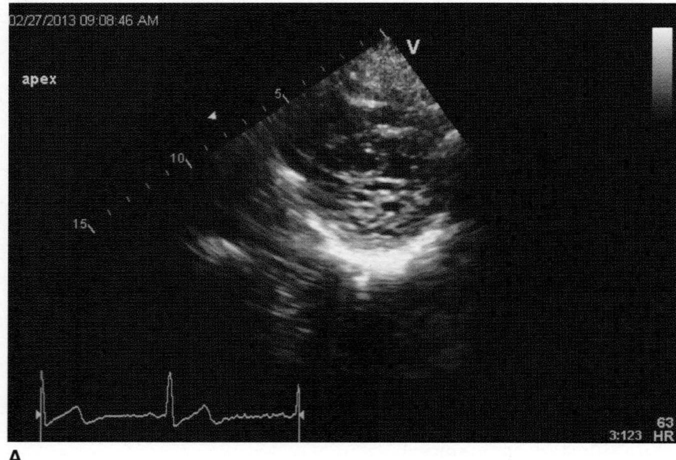

A

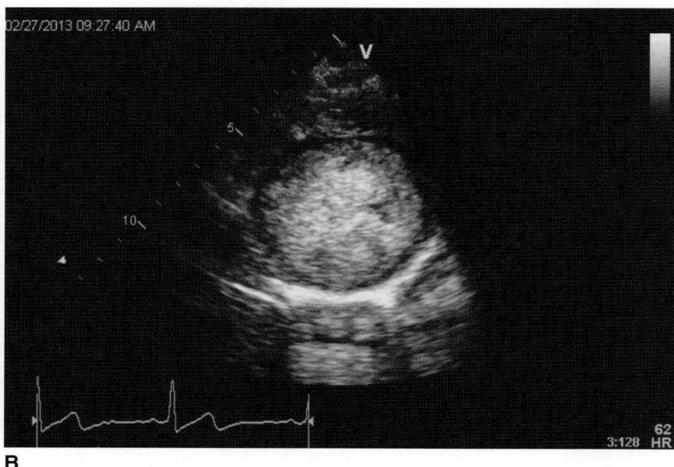

B

FIGURE 5-10-3 Short-axis images recorded at the left ventricular apex. Note the presence of extensive trabeculation involving this portion of the chamber (A). Following injection of a perfluten microbubble contrast agent to achieve LV opacification (B), the presence of deep intertrabecular recesses being perfused from the cavity is demonstrated ▶ (see Videos 5-10-3 A and B).

While diagnosis currently rests on the morphological appearance of the LV, the ability to confirm the diagnosis is somewhat confounded by the existence of several varying diagnostic criteria.

- The most widely applied criteria[7-9] are listed in Table 5-10-1. Paterick et al.,[2] have proposed that the ratio of noncompacted to compacted myocardium measured on short-axis LV views at end-diastole be considered as diagnostic; however; this proposal awaits validation.
- When these established diagnostic criteria are applied to adult patients attending a heart failure clinic and controls, a poor correlation was found between the various echocardiographic definitions of LVNC.[5] This study also suggested that current diagnostic criteria were overly sensitive and resulted in overdiagnosis of LVNC in this cohort of patients; a finding that appeared to be even more common among blacks.[5]
- A recent study has reported poor reproducibility in diagnosing LVNC when current criteria are applied.[10]
- In assessing the morphology of LV, one must take into consideration the prevalence and location of LV trabeculations in normal hearts. Trabeculations are a common finding; however, >3 trabeculations are found in only 4% of normal hearts and >5 trabeculations are not reported.[11]
- Newer techniques such as tissue Doppler imaging, strain and strain rate imaging, and twist mechanics via speckle tracking have been employed to identify abnormalities of myocardial function in LVNC.[12,13]

OTHER DIAGNOSTIC TESTS AND PROCEDURES

Findings on ECG may include intraventricular conduction disturbances, such as LBBB, LVH, and repolarization abnormalities. The ECG may be normal in 13% of patients. No particular ECG finding is reported to be specific for the diagnosis of LVNC.[14]

Cardiac magnetic resonance (CMR) has been used to characterize ventricular morphology among patients with LVNC.

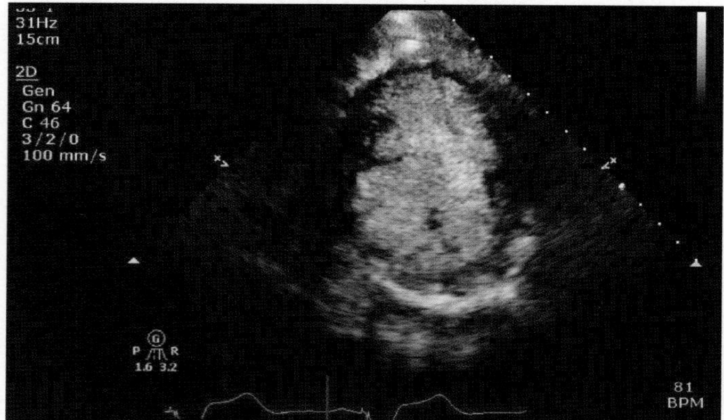

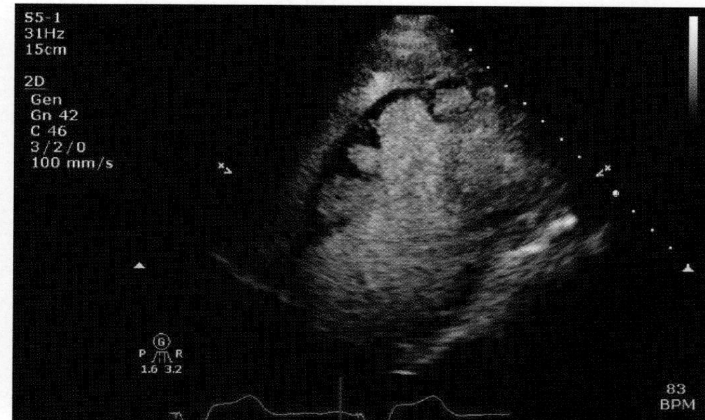

FIGURE 5-10-4 Parasternal short axis (L) and apical (R) images from a different patient with noncompaction cardiomyopathy. The deep trabeculations are well demonstrated with the use of a transpulmonic contrast agent. This patient also has evidence of severe left ventricular dysfunction ▶ (see Videos 5-10-4 L and R). Note the presence of a biventricular paced rhythm on the ECG in this patient who has a CRT-D device in place.

TABLE 5-10-1 Various Diagnostic Criteria for LVNC by Echocardiography

Chin, et al.
X-to-Y ratio (≤0.5) that decreases from the level of the papillary muscles to the apex. X represents the distance between the epicardial surface and the trough of trabeculation; Y represents the distance between the epicardial surface and the peak of the trabeculation. Measurements are made at end-diastole.
Jenni, et al.
Bilayered structure of the myocardium with ratio of noncompacted layer to compacted layer >2 as measured at end-systole on short-axis imaging of the LV.
Demonstration of a trabecular meshwork with deep intramyocardial recesses perfused from the LV cavity.
Predominant localization to mid-lateral and mid-inferior areas of the LV.
Lack of other coexisting cardiac abnormalities.
Stöllberger, et al.
Presence of >3 trabeculations within 1 imaging plane located apically from the insertion of the papillary muscles.
Intertrabecular spaces perfused from the ventricular cavity.

- Similar to echocardiography, multiple diagnostic criteria exist. Petersen et al,[15] have reported that a noncompacted to compacted ratio of >2.3 in diastole accurately separated those with LVNC from healthy controls and those with other pathological conditions.
- Jacquier and colleagues[16] have reported that the finding of a trabeculated LV mass >20% of the global LV mass accurately separated patients with LVNC from healthy controls and those with dilated and hypertrophic cardiomyopathies.
    - A recent study[17] has shown that 43% of subjects in the MESA cohort who were without cardiac disease or hypertension had a noncompacted to compacted ratio >2.3 in at least 1 myocardial segment on CMR; these findings call into question the proposed morphological criteria for diagnosis of LVNC by CMR.
- Delayed contrast enhancement indicative of myocardial fibrosis has been shown to occur in 70% of cases and was not limited to areas of morphological noncompaction.[18]

Similar to echocardiography and CMR, contrast ventriculography and CT angiography can show the characteristic prominent trabeculations with deep intratrabecular recesses.[2]

DIAGNOSIS

The diagnosis may be suspected on the basis of the clinical presentation; however, it rests on the results of cardiac imaging. At present, most cases are identified using echocardiography as detailed previously. With nondiagnostic echocardiography, findings on CMR may help establish the diagnosis. Careful attention to detail with avoidance of overdiagnosis cannot be emphasized enough.[2]

DIFFERENTIAL DIAGNOSIS

The differential diagnosis is wide and must take into account patterns of normal LV trabeculation[11] and the presence of false chords/tendons. Important pathological conditions to consider include the apical variant of hypertrophic cardiomyopathy, dilated cardiomyopathies, endocardial fibroelastosis, apical thrombus, various cardiac tumors, and eosinophilic heart disease.

MANAGEMENT

No randomized/controlled trials exist among patients with LVNC to inform clinical decision-making specific to this group of patients.

- Heart failure is often present among symptomatic patients. It is suggested that the guideline-recommended therapies for management of patients with heart failure be applied.[19] Similarly, use of ICDs and biventricular pacing (CRT) is recommended for appropriate clinical indications. Anticoagulation should be targeted to patients with atrial fibrillation[20] and possibly to those with LV systolic dysfunction (LVEF <40%).[1]

FOLLOW-UP

Symptomatic patients are at high risk of experiencing adverse clinical events; thus close clinical follow-up is suggested. Patients who are asymptomatic with normal LV systolic function at the time of diagnosis appear to experience a more benign clinical course[21]; periodic clinical follow-up with a cardiologist is suggested. As LVNC is a genetic disorder, familial screening with echocardiography, and possibly genetic testing, is recommended for first-degree relatives.[22]

VIDEO LEGENDS

1. Video 5-10-1: Apical 2-chamber view demonstrating prominent trabeculations and deep recesses located adjacent to the inferoapical portion of the ventricle in this patient with left ventricular noncompaction cardiomyopathy
2. Video 5-10-2: Apical short-axis image demonstrating prominent trabeculations with intertrabecular recesses
3. Video 5-10-3 A: Short-axis images recorded at the left ventricular apex. Note the presence of extensive trabeculation involving this portion of the chamber
4. Video 5-10-3 B: Short-axis images recorded at the left ventricular apex following injection of a perfluten microbubble contrast agent to achieve LV opacification. Note the presence of deep intertrabecular recesses being perfused from the cavity.
5. Video 5-10-4 L: Parasternal short axis image from a different patient with non-compaction cardiomyopathy. The deep trabeculations are well demonstrated with the use of a transpulmonic contrast agent. This patient also has evidence of severe left ventricular dysfunction.
6. Video 5-10-4 R: Apical image from a different patient with non-compaction cardiomyopathy. The deep trabeculations are well demonstrated with the use of a transpulmonic contrast agent. This patient also has evidence of severe left ventricular dysfunction

REFERENCES

1. Oechslin E, Jenni R. Left ventricular non-compaction revisited: a distinct phenotype with genetic heterogeneity? *Eur Heart J*. 2011;32:1446-1456.
2. Paterick TE, Umland MM, Jan MF, et al. Left ventricular noncompaction: a 25-year odyssey. *J Am Soc Echocardiogr*. 2012;25:363-375.
3. Sarma RJ, Chana A, Elkayam U. Left ventricular noncompaction. *Prog Cardiovasc Dis*. 2010;52:264-273.
4. Greutmann M, Mah ML, Silversides CK, et al. Predictors of adverse outcome in adolescents and adults with isolated left ventricular noncompaction. *Am J Cardiol*. 2012;109:276-281.
5. Kohli SK, Pantazis AA, Shah JS, et al. Diagnosis of left-ventricular non-compaction in patients with left-ventricular systolic dysfunction: time for a reappraisal of diagnostic criteria? *Eur Heart J*. 2008;29:89-95.
6. Stöllberger C, Blazek G, Dobias C, Hanafin A, Wegner C, Finsterer J. Frequency of stroke and embolism in left ventricular hypertrabeculation/noncompaction. *Am J Cardiol*. 2011;108:1021-1023.
7. Chin TK, Perloff JK, Williams RG, Jue K, Mohrmann R. Isolated noncompaction of left ventricular myocardium. A study of eight cases. *Circulation*. 1990;82:507-513.
8. Jenni R, Oechslin E, Schneider J, Attenhofer Jost C, Kaufmann PA. Echocardiographic and pathoanatomical characteristics of isolated left ventricular non-compaction: a step towards classification as a distinct cardiomyopathy. *Heart*. 2001;86:666-671.
9. Stollberger C, Finsterer J, Blazek G. Left ventricular hypertrabeculation, noncompaction and association with additional cardiac abnormalities and neuromuscular disorders. *Am J Cardiol*. 2002;90:899–902.
10. Saleeb SF, Margossian R, Spencer CT, et al. Reproducibility of echocardiographic diagnosis of left ventricular noncompaction. *J Am Soc Echocardiogr*. 2012;25:194-202.
11. Boyd MT, Seward JB, Tajik AJ, Edwards WD. Frequency and location of prominent left ventricular trabeculations at autopsy in 474 normal human hearts: implications for evaluation of mural thrombi by two-dimensional echocardiography. *J Am Coll Cardiol*. 1987;9:323-326.
12. Niemann M, Liu D, Hu K, et al. Echocardiography quantification of regional deformation helps to distinguish isolated left ventricular non-compaction from dilated cardiomyopathy. *Eur J Heart Fail*. 2012;14:155-161.
13. Attenhofer Jost CH, Connolly HM. Left ventricular non-compaction: dreaming of the perfect diagnostic tool. *Eur J Heart Fail*. 2012;14:113-114.
14. Steffel J, Kobza R, Oechslin E, Jenni R, Duru F. Electrocardiographic characteristics at initial diagnosis in patients with isolated left ventricular noncompaction. *Am J Cardiol*. 2009;104:984-989.
15. Petersen SE, Selvanayagam JB, Wiesmann F, et al. Left ventricular non-compaction: insights from cardiovascular magnetic resonance imaging. *J Am Coll Cardiol*. 2005;46:101-105.
16. Jacquier A, Thuny F, Jop B, et al. Measurement of trabeculated left ventricular mass using cardiac magnetic resonance imaging in the diagnosis of left ventricular non-compaction. *Eur Heart J*. 2010;31:1098-1104.
17. Kawel N, Nacif M, Arai AE, et al. Trabeculated (noncompacted) and compact myocardium in adults: the Multi-Ethnic Study of Atherosclerosis. *Circ Cardiovasc Imaging*. 2012;5:357-366.
18. Dursun M, Agayev A, Nisli K, et al. MR imaging features of ventricular noncompaction: emphasis on distribution and pattern of fibrosis. *Eur J Radiol*. 2010;74:147-151.
19. Yancy CW, Jessup M, Bozkurt B, et al. 2013 ACCF/AHA guideline for the management of heart failure: a report of the American College of Cardiology Foundation/American Heart Association Task Force on Practice Guidelines. *J Am Coll Cardiol*. 2013;62:e147–239. This document is available on the World Wide Web sites of the American College of Cardiology (www.cardiosource.org) and the American Heart Association (my.americanheart.org).
20. Fuster V, Rydén LE, Cannom DS, et al. 2011 ACCF/AHA/HRS focused updates incorporated into the ACC/AHA/ESC 2006 Guidelines for the management of patients with atrial fibrillation: a report of the American College of Cardiology Foundation/American Heart Association Task Force on Practice Guidelines developed in partnership with the European Society of Cardiology and in collaboration with the European Heart Rhythm Association and the Heart Rhythm Society. *J Am Coll Cardiol*. 2011;57:e101-198.
21. Stanton C, Bruce C, Connolly H, et al. Isolated left ventricular noncompaction syndrome. *Am J Cardiol*. 2009;104:1135-1138.
22. Hoedemaekers YM, Caliskan K, Michels M, et al. The importance of genetic counseling, DNA diagnostics, and cardiologic family screening in left ventricular noncompaction cardiomyopathy. *Circ Cardiovasc Genet*. 2010;3:232-239.

6 ECHOCARDIOGRAPHIC ASSESSMENT OF PERICARDIAL DISEASE

Sakima A. Smith , MD, and
David A. Orsinelli, MD, FACC, FASE

INTRODUCTION

Echocardiography remains the principal imaging method to assess pericardial disease, especially in the acute setting, and it is the imaging method of choice to diagnose the presence of pericardial effusions. In fact, one of the initial descriptions of the use of echocardiography in the United States was a seminal paper by Dr. Harvey Feigenbaum in 1965 describing the use of cardiac ultrasound to detect pericardial fluid.[1]

While other imaging techniques have provided improved assessment of pericardial anatomy, such as pericardial thickness, calcification, and congenital pericardial abnormalities, echocardiography is the modality of choice employed to evaluate the hemodynamic consequences of pericardial fluid (tamponade) and to assess (noninvasively) for pericardial constriction. The use of echocardiography is a Class 1 indication for the evaluation of many clinical scenarios in which pericardial involvement is suspected.[2] In the recently revised appropriate use criteria for echocardiography,[3] echocardiography is deemed appropriate in a variety of clinical scenarios, including: possible pericardial effusion after severe trauma (indication 32); suspected pericardial conditions (indication 59); reevaluation of known effusions to guide therapy (indication 61); and guidance of percutaneous pericardiocentesis (indication 62).

Both cardiac CT and MRI do play a role in the evaluation of patients with pericardial disease. The recently published guidelines for multimodality imaging of patients with pericardial disease emphasize the primary role of echocardiography in this patient population, but also highlight the secondary roles of CT and MRI.[4] This document provides a comprehensive review of imaging in these patients.

In this chapter, we will explore the use of echocardiography in a variety of clinical settings, including its role the evaluation of acute pericarditis, its role in the evaluation and management of idiopathic or chronic pericardial effusions, the assessment of cardiac tamponade and constriction, and its role in the acute setting of suspected cardiac perforation as a complication of invasive cardiac procedures.

SECTION 1

Malignant Pericardial Effusion

David A. Orsinelli, MD, FACC, FASE

CLINICAL CASE PRESENTATION

The patient is a young man who was recently diagnosed with stage IV non-small cell lung carcinoma. He also has a history of COPD. He presented to the emergency room with worsening dyspnea for approximately 2 weeks. He had been treated with inhalers without improvement in his symptoms. He also noted increasing cervical adenopathy and generalized upper and lower extremity swelling. He had initially presented (3 months prior to this presentation) with dyspnea, and further workup demonstrated a left upper lobe mass as well as significant mediastinal adenopathy. He was treated with radiation therapy with plans for further chemotherapy, which had not been started.

On physical examination he was found to be tachycardic. He did not have significant neck vein distention. Cardiac exam revealed that he was tachycardiac with no murmurs, gallops, or rubs. He had trace lower extremity edema. Given his physical exam findings and hypoxia there was concern that he could have a pulmonary embolism, and therefore a CT pulmonary embolism study was performed. This demonstrated no evidence of pulmonary embolism but did demonstrate a pericardial effusion. A transthoracic echocardiogram was requested. The echocardiogram demonstrated a large pericardial effusion with evidence of tamponade (Figures 6-1-1 to 6-1-5).

The patient underwent open drainage with creation of a pericardial window. Pathology did not reveal any tumor. A subsequent chest CT demonstrated no pericardial fluid. He was subsequently discharged with plans for institution of outpatient chemotherapy.

CLINICAL FEATURES AND NATURAL HISTORY

- Patients with pericardial involvement due to a malignancy may present with an asymptomatic effusion (detected during imaging for other reasons) or may present with symptoms of pericarditis such as chest pain, cardiac tamponade, or pericardial constriction.

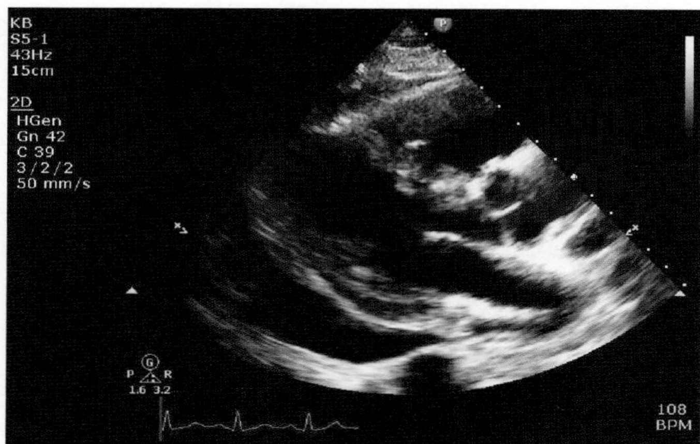

FIGURE 6-1-1 Parasternal long axis demonstrating a large pericardial effusion with evidence of right ventricular collapse ► (see Video 6-1-1).

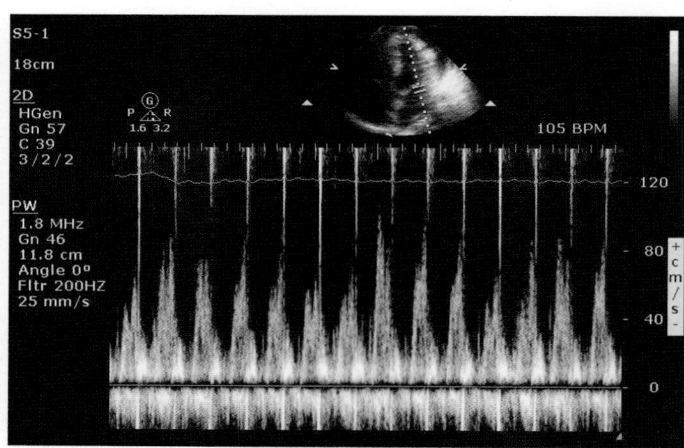

FIGURE 6-1-4 Pulse wave Doppler demonstrating respiratory variation of mitral inflow, a sign of cardiac tamponade.

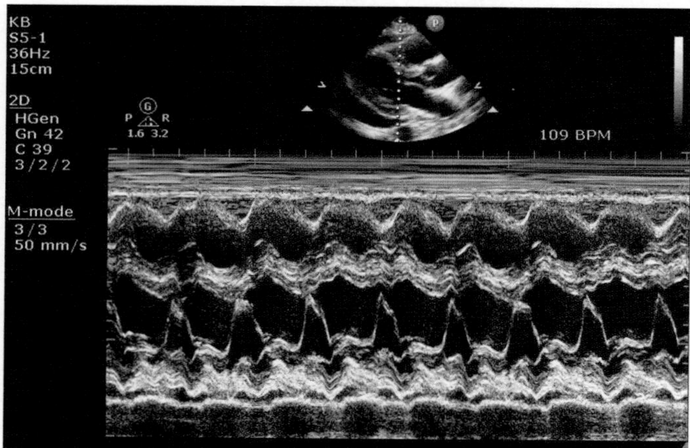

FIGURE 6-1-2 Two-dimensional guided M-mode demonstrating RV diastolic collapse.

- Signs and symptoms may include chest pain, dyspnea, tachycardia, hypotension, and edema.
- Once any acute hemodynamic issues related to pericardial involvement are addressed, such as treatment of cardiac tamponade (Figures 6-1-6 and 6-1-7), the natural history and prognosis are usually driven by the underlying malignancy. Pericardial involvement usually portends a poor prognosis.[5]

EPIDEMIOLOGY[6,7]

- Pericardial involvement due to malignancy is not uncommon, occurring in up to 20% of patients depending on the malignancy.[6]
- The differential diagnosis of pericardial effusions is extensive. Several etiologies are explored in more detail in other sections of this chapter.
- The etiology of a large pericardial effusion will vary depending on the patient population studied. Obvious causes may be determined by history (eg, chest trauma, post cardiac surgery, post myocardial infarction, or post cardiac procedure). In a large cancer centers, malignancies may predominate. Case series report varying

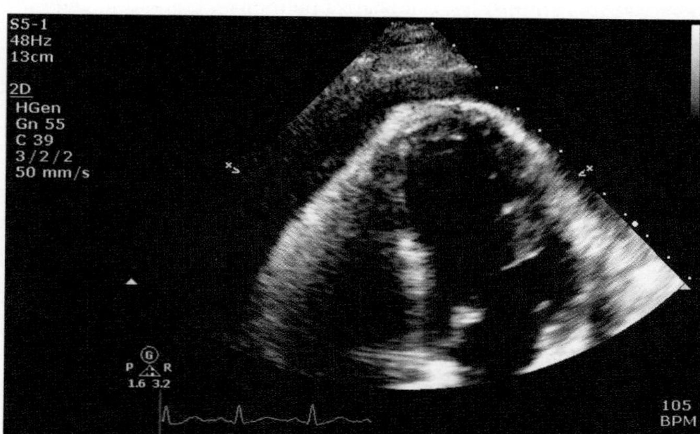

FIGURE 6-1-3 Apical 4 chamber view demonstrating a large pericardial effusion with visceral pericardial thickening and right atrial collapse ► (see Video 6-1-3).

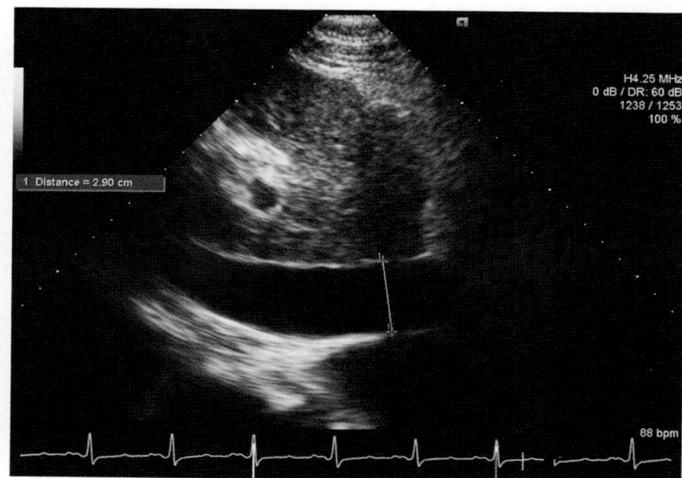

FIGURE 6-1-5 Subcostal view demonstrating a dilated inferior vena cava.

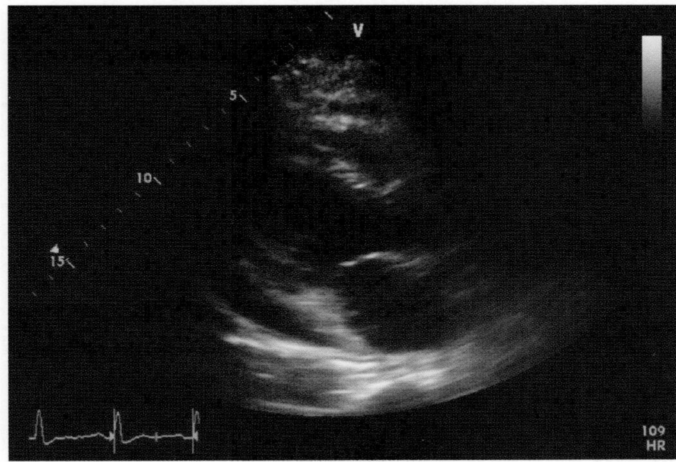

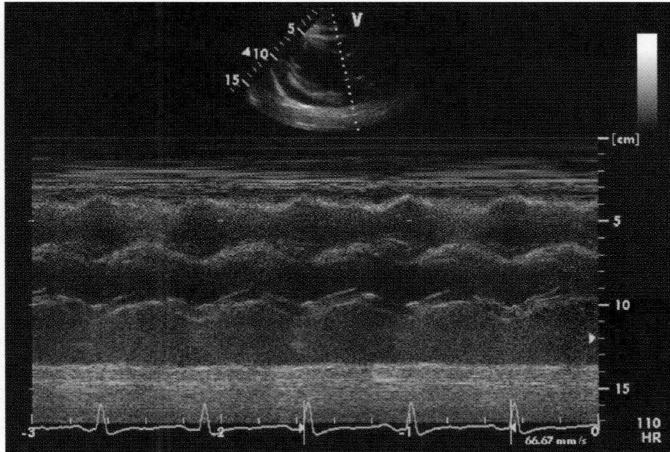

FIGURE 6-1-6 Moderate-sized pericardial effusion in a different patient with RV collapse (left) ▶ (see Video 6-1-6). The M-mode demonstrates RV diastolic collapse (right).

etiologies. In one series of 322 patients,[7] in which 37% of the patients had cardiac tamponade, the etiology of the effusion was as follows: idiopathic, 20%; iatrogenic, 16%; malignancy, 13%; chronic idiopathic effusion, 9%; post myocardial infarction, 8%; uremia, 6%; collagen vascular disease, 5%; infection, 6%; hypothyroidism, 2%; miscellaneous, 15%.

- Table 6-1-1 provides broad categories in the differential diagnosis of pericardial effusion. This is certainly not an exhaustive list, but it references the more common etiologies in each category.[8]
- In patients without a known underlying malignancy, pericardial disease as the first manifestation of cancer is uncommon. This is especially true if the effusion is small. In one series of patients with acute pericarditis or small effusions, 5% were ultimately diagnosed with a malignancy.[9]
- In the population of patients presenting with large effusions or cardiac tamponade and in whom the etiology is not evident after a basic evaluation, malignancy is not an uncommon etiology. Nearly 20% of such patients in one series were found to have an underlying malignancy.[10]

PATHOPHYSIOLOGY AND ETIOLOGY OF MALIGNANT PERICARDIAL EFFUSIONS

- The pathophysiology of pericardial involvement in malignancy may be due to direct extension into the pericardium (eg, lung cancer, esophageal cancer).
- Alternatively, metastatic spread to the pericardium via the hematogenous route or the lymphatic system may occur. Primary pericardial malignancy is quite rare.
- Among the various primary malignancies, lung, breast and esophageal cancers, malignant melanoma as well as leukemias and lymphomas most commonly affect the pericardium[5,11] (Table 6-1-2).
- Cardiac tamponade, as was seen in this case, results from extrinsic compression of the heart as fluid accumulates in the semi-rigid pericardium. Once intrapericardial pressure exceeds the intracardiac pressure, cardiac filling is limited, and the patient may develop hypotension and tachycardia. On physical examination, the neck veins may be elevated with prominent x descents, and a pulsus paradoxus may be appreciated.

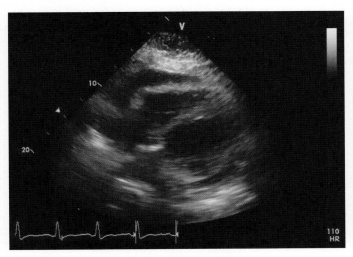

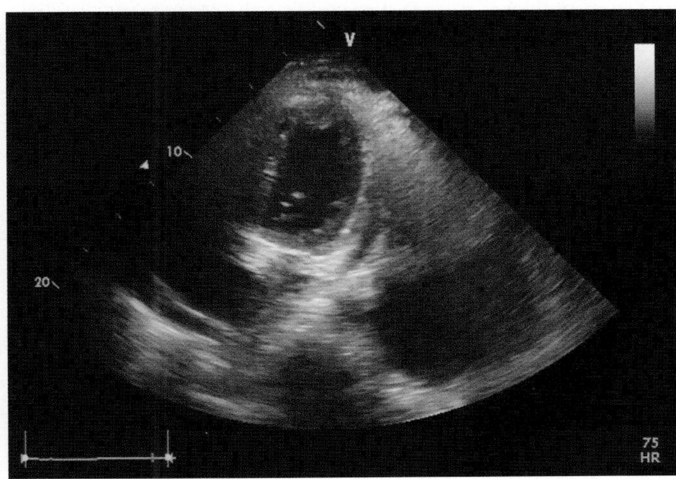

FIGURE 6-1-7 Pre- (left) and post- (right) echocardiogram from the patient in Figure 6-1-6 demonstrating resolution of the pericardial effusion post-pericardiocentesis ▶ (see Videos 6-1-7).

TABLE 6-1-1 Differential Diagnosis of Pericardial Effusion

- Idiopathic
- Viral
  - Multiple organisms, including HIV, cocsackie, influenza
- Malignant
- Metabolic (eg, uremic, dialysis-related, hypothyroidism)
- Bacterial (purulent) pericarditis
- Tuberculous pericarditis
- Other infections (eg, fungal, parasitic)
- Connective tissue diseases/vasculitis
  - eg, systemic lupus, rheumatoid arthritis, scleroderma
- Mediastinal radiation
- Postcardiac surgery
- Cardiac injury as a complication of cardiac procedures
- Postmyocardial infarction
- Aortic dissection
- Chest trauma (blunt/penetrating)
- Drugs/toxins

Adapted with permisison from Spodick, DH. Pericardial Diseases. In: *Heart Disease: A Textbook of Cardiovascular Medicine*, Braunwald E, Zipes D, Libby P (Eds). New York, NY: Saunders; 2001. Page 1823.[8]

ECHOCARDIOGRAPHY[12]

- Echocardiography is the diagnostic test of choice to assess for the presence, size, and physiologic consequences of pericardial effusion.
- Pericardial fluid appears as an echo free space between the parietal and visceral pericardium. Small effusions are usually seen posterior to the heart, frequently in the atrioventricular groove. As the size of the effusion increases, fluid can be seen around the left and right ventricles, around the right atrium and posterior to the left atrium.

TABLE 6-1-2 Common Malignancies with Pericardial Involvement

- Lung
- Breast
- Esophageal
- Melanoma
- Lymphoma
- Leukemia
- Mesothelioma

- Echocardiographic features of cardiac tamponade reflect the increase in intrapericardial pressure as compared to the intracardiac pressure (chamber collapse), elevated intracardiac pressure (IVC findings), and the effects of respiration (mitral and tricuspid filling patterns, caval flow).
- A variety of echocardiographic features support the diagnosis of pericardial tamponade.
  - Right atrial inversion/collapse can be seen with both 2-dimensional and M-mode imaging. M-mode provides better temporal resolution and can be helpful in timing events as they relate to the cardiac cycle.
  - Right ventricular collapse: Typically seen in the RVOT, the free wall of the RV may also be compressed and demonstrate chamber collapse in diastole.
  - Since RA pressure is lower than RV pressure, RA collapse tends to occur earlier (more sensitive) in the spectrum of tamponade than RV collapse. RV collapse is a more specific sign of tamponade.
  - Respiratory variation of mitral and tricuspid inflow.
  - IVC plethora.

OTHER DIAGNOSTIC TESTING AND PROCEDURES

- Echocardiography is the principal imaging modality for the diagnosis and follow-up of pericardial effusions.
- The chest x-ray may demonstrate cardiomegally.
- With a large effusion, the ECG voltage may be low, and electrical alternans may be present.
- Both chest computed tomography CT and magnetic resonance imaging (MRI) may detect pericardial fluid incidentally (as was the case on our patient). Cardiac CT and MRI may be useful in further evaluating the pericardial anatomy/thickness and assessing contiguous structures in the chest.
- In patients with equivocal findings for tamponade and to help in the diagnostic assessment of the hemodynamic consequences of an effusion, cardiac catheterization with hemodynamic assessment may be warranted.
- Basic laboratory investigation to assess for other potential etiologies would include renal function, thyroid function, a complete blood count, and selected markers for connective tissue disease.

DIFFERENTIAL DIAGNOSIS

- As has been explored in this section, the differential diagnosis of a pericardial effusion is quite broad.
- In a patient with a known malignancy, especially a malignancy with a predilection for cardiac involvement, malignancy must be entertained. If the patient has undergone chest radiation with the heart/pericardium in the radiation field, radiation-induced pericardial involvement is possible. Some chemotherapeutic agents may also cause pericardial effusions. In immunocompromised subjects, an infectious etiology must be considered.
- Etiologies of pericardial effusion not related to the malignancy or its treatment must also be considered. A careful history is imperative to explore other systemic signs/symptoms that may lead to an alternative diagnosis.

DIAGNOSIS

- Diagnosing the presence and extent of pericardial effusion is usually straightforward.
- In many cases, the hemodynamic/clinical impact of the effusion may be difficult to ascertain. Patients with malignancy may have other causes for their symptoms. For example, a patient with lung cancer and dyspnea may be short of breath due to the malignancy, concomitant COPD, pneumonia, etc. Infections and other clinical factors such as volume depletion may be the etiology of tachycardia and hypotension, rather than the effusion.
- Diagnosing a malignant effusion can be difficult. Standard fluid analysis (cell count, glucose, protein, and lactate dehydrogenase) should be performed. The diagnostic yield of cytology of the pericardial fluid is frequently unrewarding. Reported sensitivities for the diagnostic yield of cytology vary from 51% to 92%.[10,13]
- A pericardial biopsy may be needed to make the diagnosis.

MANAGEMENT

- The management of malignant pericardial effusions is somewhat controversial. Patients with hemodynamic compromise require removal of the fluid. In many cases, this must be performed emergently to prevent hemodynamic collapse. This is best accomplished with percutaneous drainage, often with echocardiographic guidance.
- In less urgent situations, several options exist. Some experts advocate open pericardial drainage, as was performed in this case, with or without pericardiectomy or the creation of a pericardial window. Others advocate simple percutaneous pericardiocentesis to remove the fluid or percutaneous pericardial drainage with prolonged catheter drainage.[14]
- Malignant effusions not infrequently reaccumulate, depending on the initial therapeutic approach, the underlying malignancy, and its response to therapy. Simple pericardiocentesis may result in fluid reaccumulation within 48 hours. Extended catheter drainage appears to be more effective in preventing recurrence (12%) compared to simple drainage (36%). Surgical management is more effective (0%), albeit with more potential morbidity/mortality.[14]

FOLLOW-UP

- Following therapy (either open drainage or percutaneous drainage), documentation of improvement/resolution of the effusion, usually with a repeat echocardiogram, is appropriate.
- Patients with a malignant pericardial effusion require ongoing follow-up with oncology for their underlying malignancy and its response to therapy.
- Pericardial involvement usually portends a poor prognosis, and the presence of malignant cells in the fluid worsens the prognosis. In one series, patients with a malignancy associated effusion on average survived 15.1 weeks. Those with positive cytology had a median survival of 7.3 weeks, compared to 29.7 weeks in patients without a positive cytology.[5]
- If recurrent signs or symptoms of cardiac/pericardial involvement develop, repeat echocardiography to assess for the recurrence of the effusion or the development of constrictive physiology is warranted.

VIDEO LEGENDS

1. Video 6-1-1: Parasternal long axis view demonstrating a large pericardial effusion with evidence of right ventricular collapse
2. Video 6-1-3: Apical 4 chamber view demonstrating a large pericardial effusion with visceral pericardial thickening and right atrial collapse
3. Video 6-1-6: Moderate sized pericardial effusion in a different patient with RV collapse
4. Video 6-1-7 L: Pre tap echocardiogram from the patient in Video 6-1-6 demonstrating the pericardial effusion.
5. Video 6-1-7 R: Post tap echocardiogram from the patient in Video 6-1-7 L demonstrating resolution of the pericardial effusion post pericardiocentesis

REFERENCES

1. Feigenbaum H, Waldhausen JA, Hyde LP. Ultrasound diagnosis of pericardial effusion. *JAMA.* 1965;191:711-714.
2. Cheitlin MD, Armstrong WF, Aurigemma GP, et al. ACC/AHA/ASE 2003 guideline update for the clinical application of echocardiography- summary article A report of the American College of Cardiology/American Heart Association Task Force on practice guidelines. (ACC/AHA/ASE 2003 Committee to Update the 1997 Guidelines for the Clinical Application of Echocardiography). *J Am Coll Cardiol.* 2003;42:954-970.
3. Douglas PS, Garcia MJ, Haines DE, et al. ACCF/ASE/AHA/ASNC/HFSA/HRS/SCAI/SCCM/SCCT/SCMR 2011 appropriate use criteria for echocardiography: a report of the American College of Cardiology Foundation Appropriate Use Criteria Task Force, American Society of Echocardiography, American Heart Association, American Society of Nuclear Cardiology, Heart Failure Society of America, Heart Rhythm Society, Society of Cardiovascular Angiography and Interventions, Society of Critical Care Medicine, Society of Cardiovascular Computed Tomography, and Society of Cardiovascular Magnetic Resonance. *J Am Coll Cardiol.* 2011;57(9):1126-1166. doi: 10.1016/jacc.2010.11.002.
4. Klein AL, Abbara S, Agler DA, et al. American Society of Echocardiography clinical recommendations for multimodality cardiovascular imaging of patients with pericardial disease: endorsed by the Society for Cardiovascular Magnetic Resonance and Society of Cardiovascular Computed Tomography. *J Am Soc Echocardiogr.* 2013;26:965-1012.
5. Gornik HL, Gerhard-Herman M, Beckman JA. Abnormal cytology predicts poor prognosis in cancer patients with pericardial effusion. *J Clin Oncol.* 2005;23:5211-5216.
6. Maisch B, Ristic A, Pankuweit S. Evaluation and management of pericardial effusion in patients with neoplastic disease. *Prog Cardiovasc Dis.* 2010;53:157-163.
7. Sangrista-Saluda J, Merce J, Parmanyer-Miralda G, Soler-Soler J. Clinical clues to the causes of large pericardial effusions. *Am J Med.* 2000;109:95-101.

8. Spodick, DH. Pericardial Diseases. In: Braunwald E, Zipes D, Libby P, eds. *Heart Disease: A Textbook of Cardiovascular Medicine.* New York, NY: Saunders; 2001:1823-1876.
9. Imazio M, Cecchi E, Demichelis B, et al. Indicators of poor prognosis of acute pericarditis. *Circulation.* 2007;115: 2739-2744.
10. Ben-Horin S, Bank I, Guetta V, Livneh A. Large symptomatic pericardial effusion as the presentation of unrecognized cancer: a study in 173 consecutive patients undergoing pericardiocentesis. *Medicine.* 2006;85:49-53.
11. Abraham KP, Reddy V, Gattuso P. Neoplasms metastatic to the heart: review of 3314 consecutive autopsies. *Am J Cardiovasc Pathol.* 1990;3:195-198.
12. Wann S, Passen E. Echocardiography in pericardial disease. *J Am Soc Echocardiogr.* 2008;21:7-13.
13. Meyers DG, Meyers RE, Prendergast TW. The usefulness of diagnostic tests on pericardial fluid. *Chest.* 1997;111:1213-1221.
14. Tsang TSM, Seward JB, Barnes ME, et al. Outcomes of primary and secondary treatment of pericardial effusion in patients with malignancy. *Mayo Clin Proc.* 2000;75:248-253.

SECTION 2

Acute Pericarditis

Peter M. Bittenbender, MD

CLINICAL CASE PRESENTATION

A 33-year-old man presents to the emergency department after the subacute onset of a sharp, substernal chest pain. This pain developed over the course of 2 to 3 hours. The pain is worse when he is laying flat and when he takes a deep breath. The pain improves when he is sitting upright. He has no significant past medical history, has had no prior surgeries, and takes no regularly scheduled medications. He is a lifelong nonsmoker and has no family history of cardiac disease.

In the emergency department, his blood pressure is 124/82 mm Hg, and his pulse is 110 beats/minute. He is mildly tachypneic and is sitting forward in bed. Auscultation of his heart reveals a tachycardic, but regular, rate. He has a normal S_1 and S_2, and a soft pericardial friction rub. An electrocardiogram (ECG) done in the emergency department is shown in Figure 6-2-1. An echocardiogram was also ordered by the ED staff. It demonstrated no significant pericardial fluid (Figure 6-2-2). He was admitted to the hospital, treated with ibuprofen and colchicine, and discharged after a brief period of observation. His symptoms resolved quickly, and he has had no clinical recurrence.

EPIDEMIOLOGY

- Acute pericarditis is the most common disorder involving the pericardium.
- The exact incidence and prevalence of acute pericarditis is not known, but as many as 5% of patients presenting to the emergency department with chest pain (without myocardial infarction) are thought to be due to acute pericarditis,[1] and 1% of ST elevations on ECG are found to be due to acute pericarditis.[2]
- Acute pericarditis can occur at any age, but it is most prevalent in men aged 20 to 50 years.

ETIOLOGY AND PATHOPHYSIOLOGY

- Roughly 70% to 80% of cases of acute pericarditis are idiopathic. Most of these are presumed to be of a viral etiology.[3]
- Other causes include infections (viral, tuberculosis, bacterial), neoplastic, uremic, radiation induced, or autoimmune.
- Irritation from the underlying condition causes the pericardial serosa to become acutely inflamed, which leads to the infiltration of polymorphonuclear cells and the overproduction of pericardial fluid.
- This inflammation leads to pain, and the overproduction of pericardial fluid can lead to pericardial effusion (usually mild to moderate in size).
- Acute pericarditis only rarely presents with effusions large enough to cause tamponade.
- Chronic inflammation can lead to fibrosis of the pericardium and can cause constrictive pericarditis.

DIAGNOSIS

- The diagnosis of acute pericarditis is made on clinical grounds by suggestive history and physical exam. Electrocardiographic findings can help support the diagnosis.
- Echocardiography may demonstrate a pericardial effusion, a common complication of acute pericarditis. It is important to note that the absence of an effusion does not preclude the diagnosis, nor does the presence of a pericardial effusion confirm the diagnosis of acute pericarditis.
- Caution should be paid as acute pericarditis has presenting factors and electrocardiographic findings that can overlap with life-threatening conditions such as acute myocardial infarction and pulmonary embolism (see Differential Diagnosis).

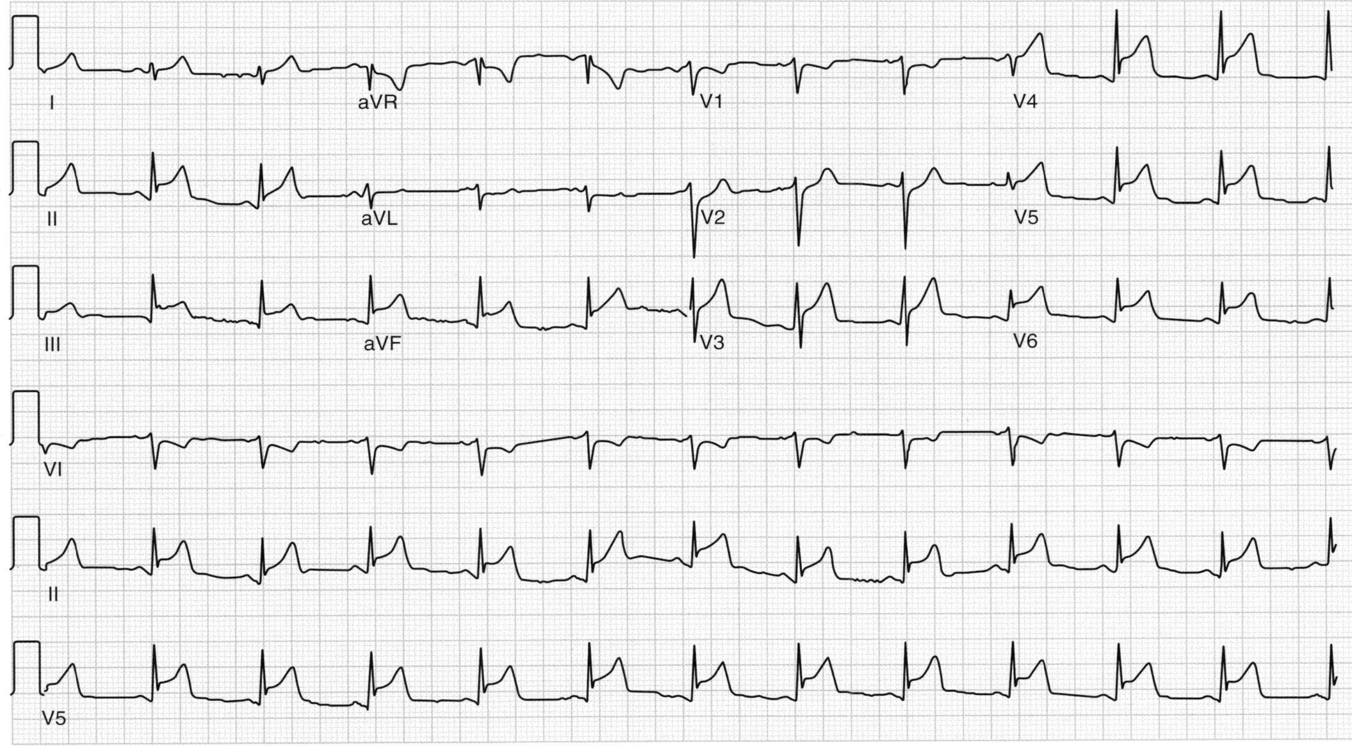

FIGURE 6-2-1 Electrocardiogram (ECG) of a patient with acute pericarditis. This ECG shows classic findings of pericarditis, including diffuse ST elevation, PR depression (best seen in lead aVF), as well as ST depression and PR elevation in aVR.

- The diagnosis of acute pericarditis is made by the presence of two or more of the following:
  - Typical chest pain.
  - A pericardial friction rub.
  - Typical ECG changes.
  - A new, or worsening pericardial effusion by echocardiography provides further evidence of an acute pericardial process (Figures 6-2-3 and 6-2-4).

CLINICAL FEATURES

- Greater than 95% of cases of acute pericarditis present with substernal chest pain.[4]
- Chest pain is usually burning or stabbing in quality and usually develops over minutes or hours.
- The chest pain is generally worse when lying flat, or with deep inspiration, and improves with sitting upright and/or leaning

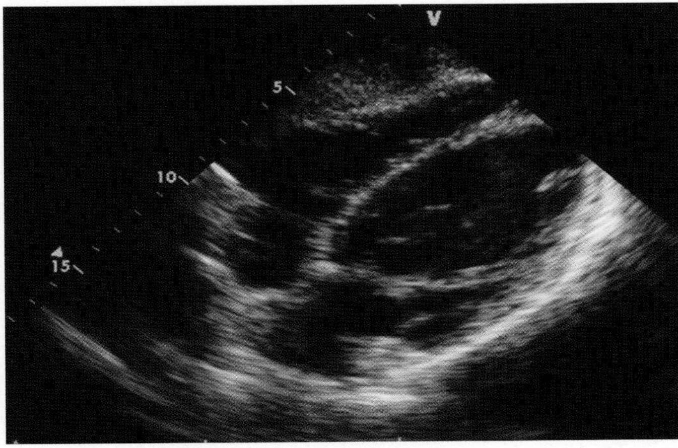

FIGURE 6-2-2 Echocardiogram of the patient described in the text presenting with acute pericarditis. Note the absence of any pericardial effusion in the subcostal view.

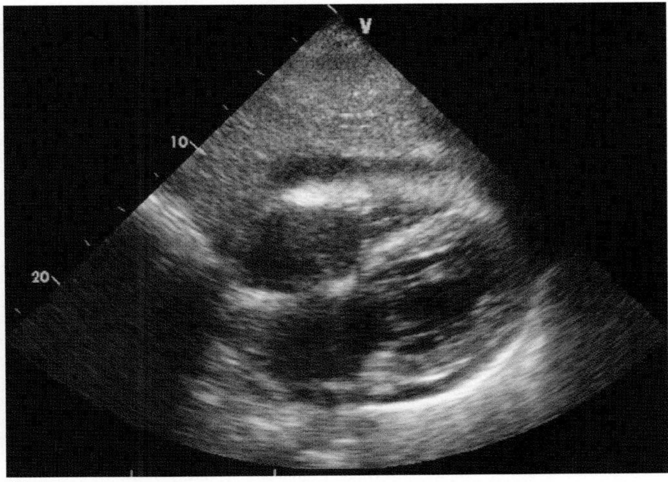

FIGURE 6-2-3 Acute pericarditis in a different patient with a small to moderate pericardial effusion.

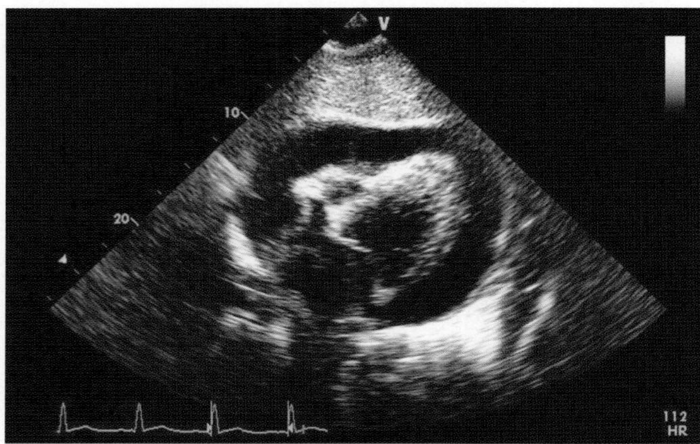

FIGURE 6-2-4 Subcostal view of another patient who presented with fever, chest pain, and hypotension. His ECG was consistent with pericarditis. The echocardiogram demonstrated evidence of cardiac tamponade. He was diagnosed with aortic valve endocarditis with an abscess and underwent emergent surgery with AV replacement.

forward, as the pericardial sac hangs away from the vertebral column in this position.

- Fever can be the initial presentation, or can be present in addition to chest pain.
- Patients are usually tachycardic and can also be tachypnic.
- A pericardial friction rub is present in about 35% of presenting cases.[4]

LABORATORY EVALUTION

- Patients can have high sedimentation rates and high C-reactive protein levels due to the presence of inflammation. Inflammatory markers are very sensitive, but they are also very nonspecific for acute pericarditis.
- Some patients can have elevated troponin levels suggesting some degree of concomitant myocarditis, but this test is also very nonspecific.

ELECTROCARDIOGRAPHY

- An electrocardiogram (ECG) of a patient with acute pericarditis is shown in Figure 6-2-1. Classic ECG findings for acute pericarditis include diffuse ST elevation, diffuse PR depression (especially in the inferior leads), and PR elevation in aVR. Tachycardia is frequently present. While pericarditis usually affects the ECG diffusely, local ECG changes can be seen when pericardial inflammation is isolated to a small portion of the pericardium.

ECHOCARDIOGRAPHY

- Patients with acute pericarditis will often have a normal echocardiogram, or will have abnormalities unrelated to acute pericarditis.
- The most common echocardiographic abnormality associated with acute pericarditis is a pericardial effusion (Figure 6-2-3), which is present in about 60% of cases of acute pericarditis.[4] The absence of a pericardial effusion (as in the present case) does not exclude the possibility of acute pericarditis, but the presence of a pericardial effusion can be helpful in supporting the diagnosis.

OTHER DIAGNOSTIC MODALITIES

- Computed tomography (CT) scan and cardiac magnetic resonance imaging (MRI) can both show thickening of the pericardium in chronic pericardial disease, but have not been evaluated for clinical utility in the evaluation of acute pericarditis.

DIFFERENTIAL DIAGNOSIS

- Acute myocardial infarction resulting from complete or incomplete obstruction of a coronary artery resulting in ischemia or infarction. It can present with chest pain and localized ECG changes. The chest discomfort is usually acute in onset, is usually characterized as a heavy sensation, and usually does not change in intensity with positional changes. When considering the diagnosis of acute pericarditis, one must convincingly exclude the diagnosis of a myocardial infarction, as this can be acutely life-threatening.
- Pulmonary embolism due to venous thromboembolism to the pulmonary arteries causing respiratory compromise, with or without chest pain, is usually acute (or subacute) in onset and can have signs of RV strain on ECG and by echocardiography. Again, when considering the diagnosis of acute pericarditis one must convincingly exclude the diagnosis of a pulmonary embolism, as this can be acutely life threatening.
- Pneumonia is usually more subacute in onset and generally presents with pleuritic chest pain, dyspnea, as well as signs or symptoms of infection such as fever and a productive cough. A chest x-ray may confirm this diagnosis.
- Pneumothorax due to partial or complete collapse of a lung and usually presents acutely with chest pain and dyspnea. A pneumothorax is more likely in patients with underlying lung disease, or as a result of trauma.
- Gastroesophageal reflux disease (GERD) is irritation of the lining of the esophagus by the presence of gastric contents above the lower esophageal sphincter. GERD is usually chronic and episodic. Chest pain is usually of burning quality and commonly occurs after a meal, or when the patient is lying down.
- Costochondritis or musculoskeletal chest pain is due to inflammation of the costrochondral cartilage or chest wall muscles due to irritation or injury. Costochondritis is usually subacute in nature. The pain can usually be reproduced by palpation or body positioning.

MANAGEMENT

- The goal of management in acute pericarditis is to decrease inflammation and treat symptoms (pain).
- Most patients presenting with acute pericarditis are initially admitted to the hospital, are usually discharged after symptom control, and complete a medical regimen at home. Recent data suggests that patients with pericarditis, without high-risk features, can safely be treated on an outpatient basis.[4]

- Non-steroidal anti-inflammatory medications are the standard of care for an initial presentation of acute pericarditis. Commonly used regimens include ibuprofen 300 to 800 mg three times daily or indomethacin 50 mg daily.[5] Treatment continues until symptom resolution and then is slowly tapered over the course of several weeks.
- Some research supports adding colchicine 0.5 mg twice daily to the initial regimen. This data suggests quicker symptom resolution and a decreased rate of recurrent pericarditis.[6] Colchicine is commonly added in recurrent pericarditis.
- Older regimens included systemic glucocorticoids; however, more recent data has suggested that this can increase the risk of recurrent pericarditis and is now usually restricted to cases refractory to standard therapy, or cases caused by autoimmune disease.[7]
- Cases of acute pericarditis rarely require pericardiocentesis or surgical pericardiectomy. The exceptions are those with suspected bacterial (or tuberculous) pericarditis, and those with multiple episodes of recurrent pericarditis or constrictive pericarditis.

PATIENT EDUCATION

- Pericarditis refers to inflammation of the pericardium, the sac (or lining) of the heart. In the majority of cases, an etiology is never found and is thought to be due to a viral infection.
- The acute or subacute onset of chest pain, with or without fever, should prompt presentation to a medical professional.
- Initial work-up will likely include an ECG, an echocardiogram, and blood work.
- Treatment of pericarditis usually includes a regimen of nonsteroidal anti-inflammatory medications.
- Strict adherence to, and completion of, the prescribed medication regimen can help prevent recurrence.
- Only rarely does acute pericarditis warrant a more invasive treatment strategy.

REFERENCES

1. Troughton RW, Asher CR, Klein AL. Pericarditis. *Lancet.* 2004; 363:717-727.
2. Brady WJ, Perron AD, Martin ML, et al. Cause of ST-segment abnormality in ED chest pain patients. *Am J Emerg Med.* 2001;19:25-28.
3. LeWinter MM. Pericardial Disease. In: Braunwald E, Libby P, eds. *Heart Disease: A Textbook of Cardiovascular Medicine.* 8th ed. Philadelphia, PA: Saunders & Co; 2008:1829-1853.
4. Imazio M, Demichelis B, Parrini I, et al. Day-Hospital Treatment of Acute Pericarditis. *J Am Coll Cardiol.* 2004;43(6):1042-1046.
5. Maisch B, Seferović PM, Ristić AD, et al. Guidelines on the diagnosis and management of pericardial disease executive summary; the task force on the diagnosis and management of pericardial disease of the European Society of Cardiology. *Eur Heart J.* 2004;25(7):587-610.
6. Imazio M, Bobbio M, Cecchi E, et al. Colchicine in addition to conventional therapy for acute pericarditis: results of the COlchicine for Acute PEricarditis (COPE) Trial. *Circulation.* 2005;112(13):2012-2016.
7. Imazio M, Bobbio M, Cecchi E, et al. Colchicine as first-choice therapy for recurrent pericarditis; results of the CORE (COlchicine for RE current pericarditis) Trial. *Arch Intern Med.* 2005;165:1987-1991.

SECTION 3

Idiopathic Pericardial Effusion

Sakima A. Smith, MD

CLINICAL CASE PRESENTATION

A 52-year-old female with a history of depression and a recent episode of bronchitis treated with antibiotics presents to a local emergency department with left-sided "tingling" chest pain for one week. An ECG there was normal, but she was told that she had an enlarged heart on a chest radiogram. She followed up with her primary care physician who then prescribed a second course of antibiotics and inhalers. She continued to have dyspnea on exertion for 2 weeks. She was only able to walk approximately 20 feet at a time before feeling fatigued and short of breath. She also reported subjective fevers and night sweats. Her primary physician then ordered an echocardiogram, which showed a large pericardial effusion with evidence of early tamponade physiology, and she was admitted to the hospital (Figure 6-3-1). At the time of admission, she did not show clinical evidence of tamponade, and she was initially treated medically. Despite nonsteroidal anti-inflammatory drugs (NSAIDS) and colchicine, she remained symptomatic with chest discomfort and dyspnea on exertion, and developed a pulsus paradoxus on physical examination. Therefore, she underwent a pericardiocentesis where 560 mL of blood-colored pericardial fluid was removed, and her symptoms improved significantly (Figure 6-3-2). This fluid was negative for malignant cells or evidence of infection. The findings were consistent

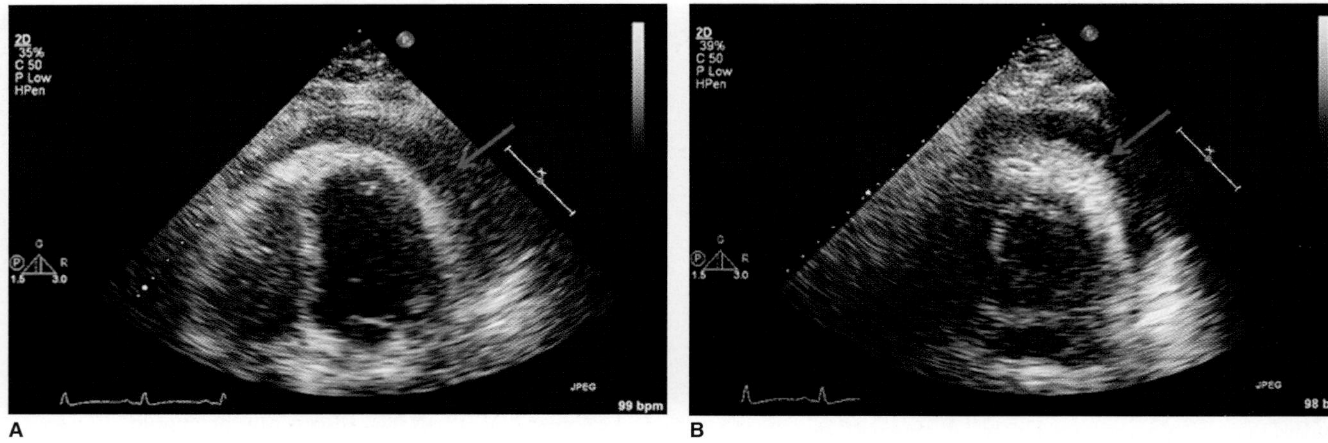

FIGURE 6-3-1 Transthoracic echo in our patient demonstrating a large effusion in the 4 chamber view (A) and short axis view (B) ► (see Videos 6-3-1).

with an inflammatory process and the presence of red blood cells. She tolerated this procedure quite well, and after removal of the pericardial drain, she was ambulating without difficulties and was discharged with a short course of NSAIDS and colchicine with follow-up scheduled with a cardiologist.

EPIDEMIOLOGY

Idiopathic Pericardial Effusion:

- The cause of pericarditis is not defined in up to 30% of patients.[1]
- A prevalence of around 1% in autopsy studies suggests that pericarditis might frequently be subclinical.[1]
- Overt cardiac tamponade may occur in nearly 30% of patients with chronic idiopathic effusions.[2]
- The prevalence of large chronic idiopathic effusions may be around 2.2%.[2]

PATHOPHYSIOLOGY

- The pericardium provides mechanical protection of the heart, reduces the friction between the heart and surrounding structures, and limits the distention of the heart contributing to diastolic coupling of the ventricles.
- Normally, this function is achieved via the presence of a small amount of pericardial fluid (25-50 mL) produced by the visceral pericardium, and intrapericardial pressure is equal to intrapleural pressure.
- Infectious and noninfectious insults are usually responsible for inflammation of pericardial layers leading to increased production of pericardial fluid as exudates.[3]

DIAGNOSIS

Echocardiography provides a rapid, accurate, noninvasive assessment of pericardial and cardiac morphology, the physiological importance

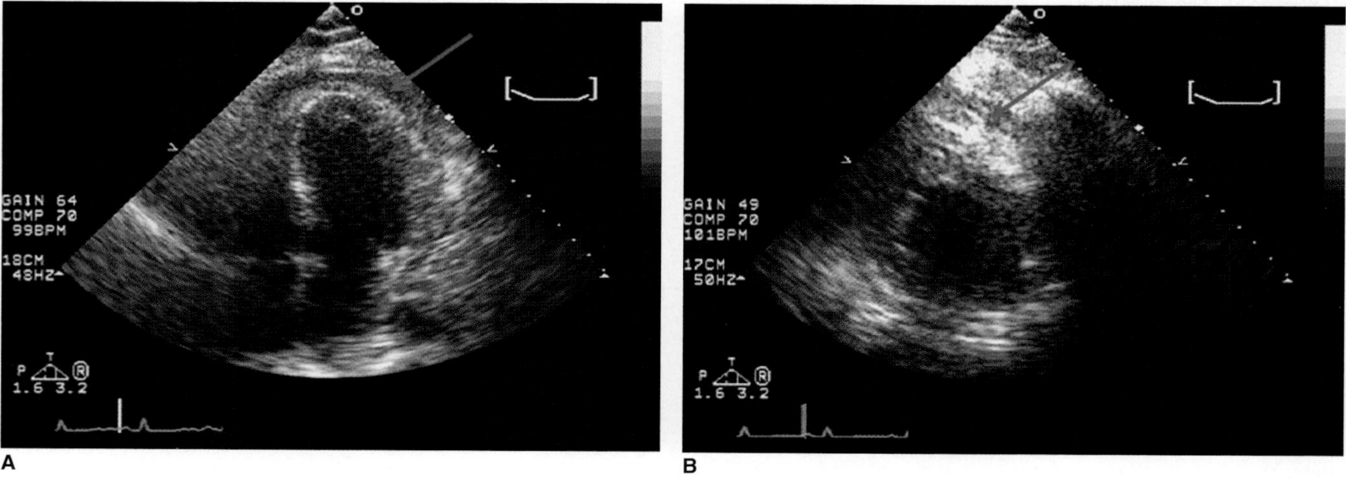

FIGURE 6-3-2 Transthoracic echo post pericardiocentesis demonstrating reduction in the size of the effusion in the 4 chamber view (A) and short axis view (B).

of complications, and an overall assessment of the relative amount of pericardial fluid and its hemodynamic consequences.

- Large idiopathic chronic pericardial effusion criteria:
  - The cause of effusion is not apparent after a thorough evaluation that includes examination of pericardial fluid or tissue.
  - The sum of anterior and posterior echo-free spaces exceeded 20 mm at end diastole.
  - There is no progression of disease during the observation period, and the effusion persists for more than three months.[2]
- Chest radiography is frequently normal, but cardiomegaly can be seen in patients who have substantial pericardial effusion. More than 250 mL fluid is needed to enlarge the cardiac outline.
- The electrocardiogram may show low voltage in the limb and precordial leads.

CLINICAL FEATURES

- Acute pericarditis classically presents with progressive, frequently severe chest pain that is sharp and pleuritic. The pain is generally worse when lying supine and is relieved by sitting (see Section II, Acute Pericarditis).
- In contrast, most patients with chronic idiopathic effusions are asymptomatic, and the effusion is found incidentally.
- If the effusion accumulates rapidly (Figures 6-3-3, 6-3-4, 6-3-5, and 6-3-6), patients can present with shortness of breath and tachycardia with hypotension, which are early signs of possible cardiac tamponade.[4] In this situation, the jugular venous pressure is almost always elevated, with preservation of the x descent but absence or attenuation of the y descent due to a blunting of diastolic filling of the ventricle. Pulsus paradoxus, an exaggeration of the normal variation in the pulse during the inspiratory phase of respiration, is commonly found in tamponade and can be quantified by an inspiratory reduction in systolic blood pressure of greater than 10 mm Hg.[4]

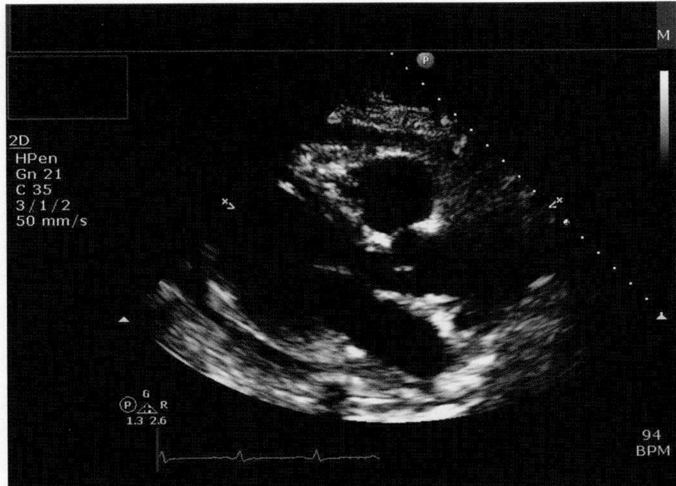

FIGURE 6-3-3 Parasternal long axis image from another patient who presented with chest pain and dyspnea. The echo demonstrates a moderate size pericardial effusion with pericardial thickening ▶ (see Video 6-3-3). She developed worsening dyspnea, tachycardia, and tachypnea. A repeat echo (Figure 6-3-4) demonstrated a much larger effusion.

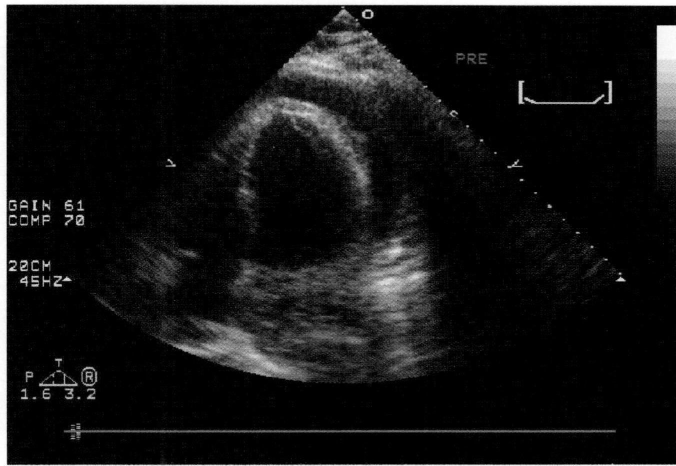

FIGURE 6-3-4 Echo image from the patient in Figure 6-3-3 prior to urgent pericardiocentesis ▶ (see Video 6-3-4).

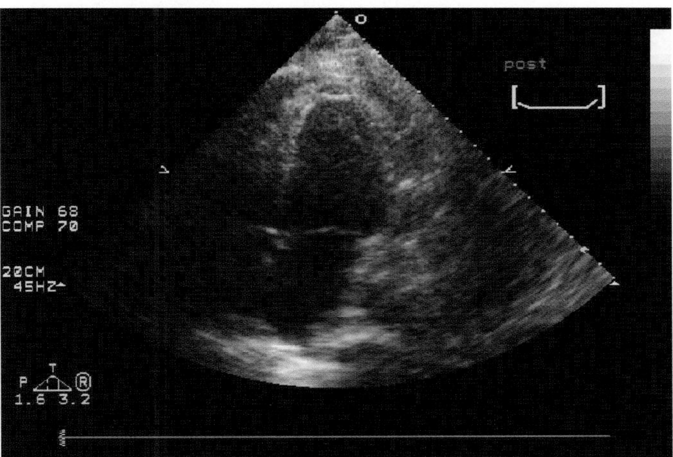

FIGURE 6-3-5 Echo image from the patient in Figure 6-6-3 following urgent pericardiocentesis. There is minimal pericardial fluid ▶(see Video 6-3-5).

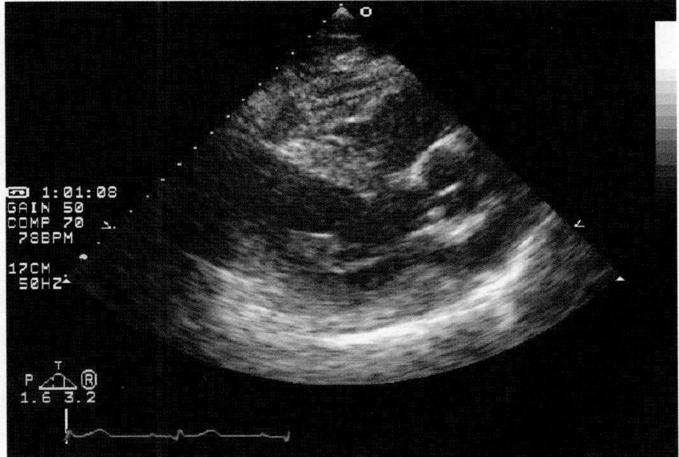

FIGURE 6-3-6 Parasternal long axis view 6 weeks after initial presentation in the patient in Figure 6-3-3. There is minimal pericardial fluid. Pericardial thickening is present. She was asymptomatic and had no clinical or echocardiographic evidence of constriction ▶ (see Video 6-3-6).

LABORATORY STUDIES

- Leukocytosis, raised C-reactive protein concentration, and elevated sedimentation rates are common findings. An elevated thyroid stimulating hormone level may indicate hypothyroidism as the etiology of the pericardial effusion.
- Chronic pericardial effusions may be seen in patients with chronic kidney disease.
- Serological studies might suggest the cause as infectious or autoimmune pericarditis, but are rarely of clinical relevance.
- When studies/laboratory evaluation are inconclusive, the diagnosis of an idiopathic pericardial effusion is made.
- Pericardial fluid measurement should be done of glucose, protein, and lactic dehydrogenase, as well as cell-count, microscopy (including gram and Ziehl-Nielsen stain), bacterial (and occasionally viral) culture, cytological examination, and viral PCR before declaring the effusion idiopathic.[4]

DIFFERENTIAL DIAGNOSIS

Non-idiopathic etiologies of pericardial effusions:[4]

- Infectious
  - Viral (most common: echovirus and coxsackievirus, influenza, Epstein-Barr virus, cytomegalovirus, adenovirus, varicella, rubella, mumps, hepatitis B virus, hepatitis C virus, HIV, parvovirus B19, and human herpesvirus[6]
- Bacterial (most common: tuberculous [4%-5%], other bacterial rare)
- Fungal
- Parasitic (very rare: Echinococcus, Toxoplasma)
- Autoimmune pericarditis
- Neoplastic pericarditis
- Metabolic pericarditis (common: uremia, myxedema)
- Traumatic pericarditis (rare)
- Drug-related pericarditis (rare):
  - Procainamide, hydralazine, isoniazid, and phenytoin (lupus-like syndrome)
  - Penicillins (hypersensitivity pericarditis with eosinophilia)
  - Doxorubicin and daunorubicin (often associated with a cardiomyopathy)

MANAGEMENT

- Pericardial drainage is indicated for tamponade, purulent effusion, or for recurrent or large idiopathic effusions with hemodynamic compromise or suspicion of neoplastic or tuberculous causes.
- If patients have concomitant pericarditis, NSAIDS and colchicine have been shown to improve symptoms, and colchicine may reduce future recurrences.[5]

PATIENT EDUCATION

- Once other conditions have been ruled out, patients need to be instructed to routinely follow-up with a cardiologist and to pay attention to any acute signs of shortness of breath, dyspnea, or confusion as this could suggest impending cardiovascular hemodynamic collapse.

FOLLOW-UP

Small to moderate effusions (<2 cm on echocardiography) should be followed up with repeat imaging studies.[1] If a patient develops symptoms of shortness of breath or confusion, they should seek medical attention. Close follow-up with a cardiologist is essential.

VIDEO LEGENDS

1. Video 6-3-1 A: Transthoracic echo in our patient demonstrating a large effusion in the four chamber view
2. Video 6-3-1 B: Transthoracic echo in our patient demonstrating a large effusion in the short axis view
3. Video 6-3-3: Parasternal long axis image from another patient who presented with chest pain and dyspnea. The echo demonstrates a moderate sized pericardial effusion with pericardial thickening
4. Video 6-3-4: Echo image from the patient in Video 6-3-3 prior to urgent pericardiocentesis. A significant interval increase in the size of the effusion is noted.
5. Video 6-3-5: Echo image from the patient in Video 6-3-3 following urgent pericardiocentesis. There is minimal pericardial fluid.
6. Video 6-3-6: Parasternal long axis view 6 weeks after initial presentation in the patient in figure 3 and Video 6-3-3. There is minimal pericardial fluid. Pericardial thickening is present. She was asymptomatic and had no clinical or echocardiographic evidence of constriction

REFERENCES

1. Troughton RW, Asher CR, Klein AL. Pericarditis. *Lancet.* 2004;363(9410):717-727.
2. Sagristà-Sauleda J, Angel J, Permanyer-Miralda G, Soler-Soler J. Long-term follow-up of idiopathic chronic pericardial effusion. *N Engl J Med.* 1999;341(27):2054-2059.
3. Imazio M. Pericarditis: pathophysiology, diagnosis, and management. *Curr Infect Dis Rep.* 2011;13(4):308-316.
4. Khandaker MH, Espinosa RE, Nishimura RA, et al. Pericardial disease: diagnosis and management. *Mayo Clin Proc.* 2010;85(6):572-593.
5. Imazio M, Bobbio M, Cecchi E, et al. Colchicine in addition to conventional therapy for acute pericarditis: results of the COlchicine for acute PEricarditis (COPE) trial. *Circulation.* 2005;112(13):2012-2016.

SECTION 4

Purulent Pericarditis

Kyle Pfahl, MD

CLINICAL CASE PRESENTATION

A 23-year-old woman with a remote past medical history of intravenous drug abuse presented with a chief complaint of progressive shortness of breath, pleuritic chest pain, and diffuse abdominal pain. Her symptoms initially started after an upper respiratory illness one week prior to presentation and have progressively worsened, especially over the past 48 hours. The patient's chest pain was pleuritic, worse with movement and coughing, and was associated with shortness of breath. She also noted an erythematous, indurated lesion on her left upper extremity that was tender and warm to the touch as well as subjective fevers. She initially presented to an outside hospital, was afebrile with a normal heart rate and blood pressure. A chest CT scan was negative for pulmonary embolism, but did show a small pericardial effusion. She was discharged home with the diagnosis of pleurisy.

She subsequently presented to the Wexner Medical Center at The Ohio State University because of progressive worsening of symptoms. Physical exam revealed a temperature of 102°F (38.8°), tachycardia to 110 beats/min, hypotension with systolic blood pressures in the 80s, normal S_1 and S_2, and no murmurs or rubs. She had reproducible chest pain with movement and palpation, elevated jugular venous distention to 9 cm, clear lungs, no hepatosplenomegaly, and an erythematous, purulent appearing lesion on the left upper extremity. A pulsus paradoxus of 15 mm Hg was present.

The electrocardiogram showed sinus tachycardia with PR depression and diffuse ST- and T-wave changes (Figure 6-4-1). Laboratory evaluation revealed an elevated white blood cell count with a left shift, a minimally elevated troponin, and normal renal function and electrolytes. Blood cultures and cultures from the left upper extremity abscess were positive for methicillin-resistant *Staphylococcus aureus*.

An echocardiogram revealed a large pericardial effusion with evidence of intrapericardial debris and findings suggestive of cardiac tamponade (Figure 6-4-2). She underwent an echo-guided pericardiocentesis. A pericardial drain was placed that revealed purulent pericardial fluid. The pericardial fluid cultures were positive for methicillin-resistant *Staphyloccocus aureus*. The drain was removed after 3 days, when the drain output had slowed to less than 100 cc per day. It was felt that the patient initially developed cellulitis and became

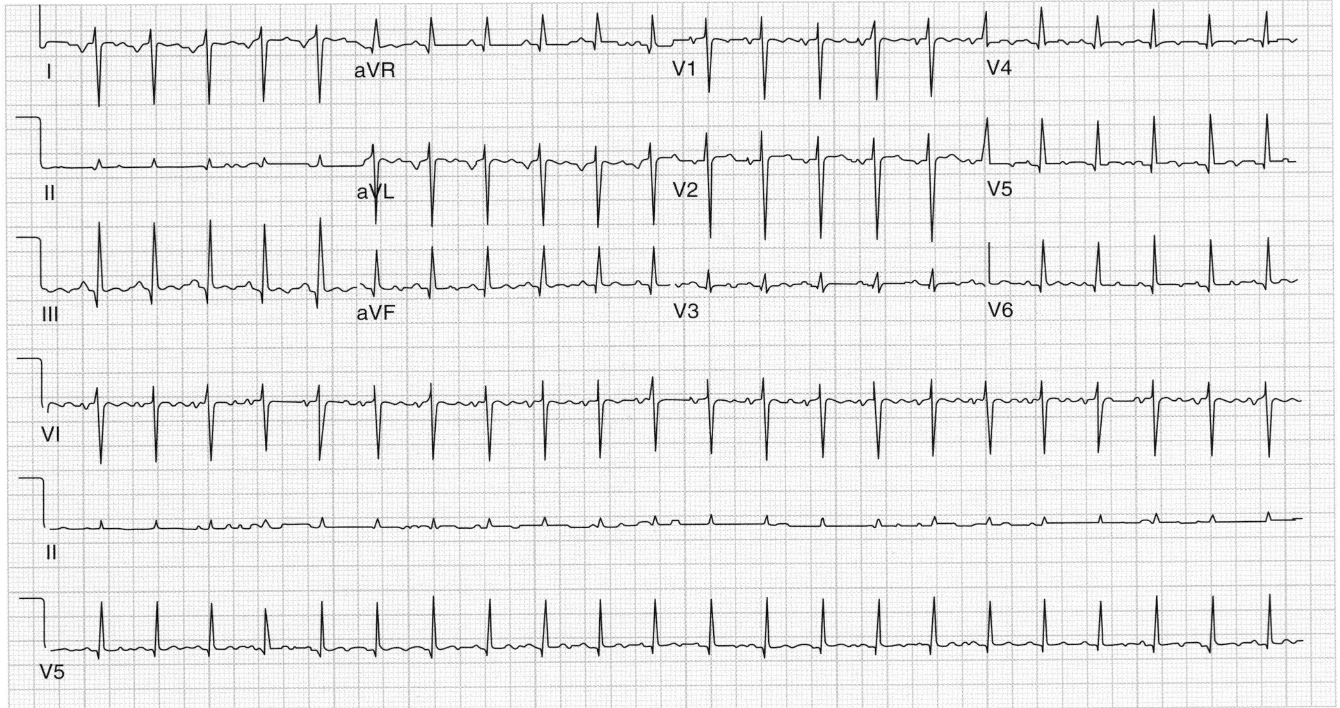

FIGURE 6-4-1 Electrocardiogram in this patient with purulent pericarditis. The electrocardiogram demonstrates sinus tachycardia with PR depression and diffuse ST- and T-wave changes consistent with the patient's diagnosis of pericarditis.

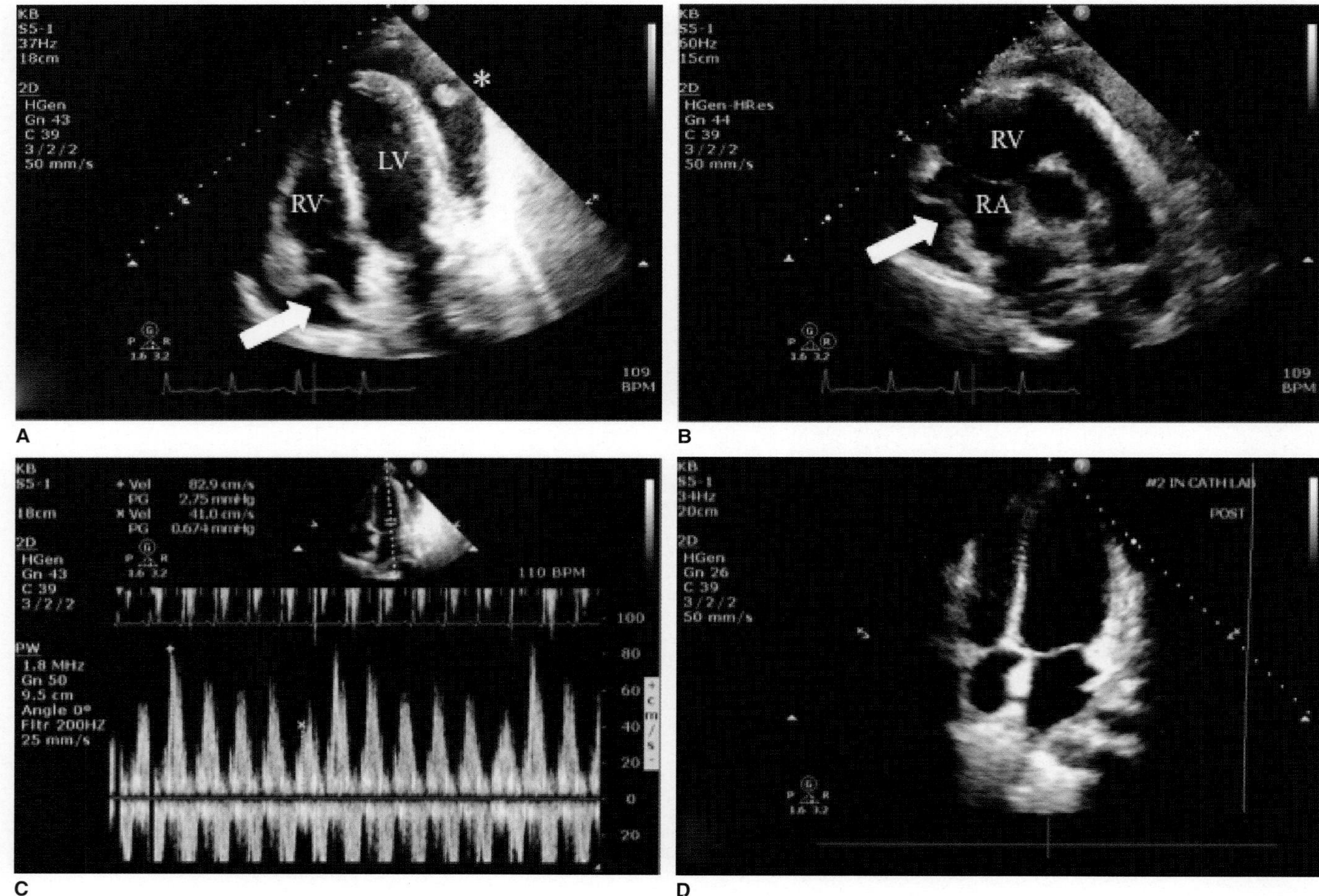

FIGURE 6-4-2 (A) The apical 4 chamber view from the transthoracic echocardiogram demonstrating a large, circumferential pericardial effusion. The star (*) illustrates pericardial debris within the large pericardial effusion. The arrow indicates right atrial collapse suggestive of cardiac tamponade. (B) The parasternal short axis view from the transthoracic echocardiogram demonstrating a large, circumferential pericardial effusion. The arrow illustrates right atrial collapse suggestive of cardiac tamponade. (C) Mitral inflow velocities demonstrating significant respiratory variation suggestive of cardiac tamponade. (D) The 4 chamber view from transthoracic echocardiogram after pericardial drain placement demonstrating resolution of the pericardial effusion ► (see Videos 6-4-2 A-E).

bacteremic, which spread to the pericardium resulting in purulent pericarditis. Clinically, the patient improved with pericardiocentesis and broad-spectrum antibiotics. A repeat echocardiogram revealed resolution of the pericardial effusion (see Video 6-4-5). The patient was placed on 6 weeks of antibiotic therapy with vancomycin with complete resolution of symptoms. A follow-up echocardiogram revealed pericardial thickenening, no effusion, and no evidence of constriction. One year later she remains asymptomatic.

EPIDEMIOLOGY

- In modern practice, purulent pericarditis is rather uncommon. The combined incidence of bacterial pericarditis and tuberculosis-related pericarditis is roughly 4% of all cases of pericarditis.
- Purulent pericarditis is most commonly seen in patients with indwelling venous catheters, immunosuppressed patients, or patients with HIV/AIDS.[1]
- Purulent pericarditis has a high mortality rate (30%-50%), with the majority of deaths resulting from tamponade.[1]

ETIOLOGY AND PATHOPHYSIOLOGY

- There are two major mechanisms involved in the development of purulent pericarditis: hematogenous spread and direct spread from a primary intrathoracic infectious source.
- Virtually any organism can spread from the blood stream to the pericardial sac.
    - The most common pathogens include *Staphyloccocus aureus* and various species of streptococci.
- Direct spread from a primary intrathoracic infectious source, most commonly pneumonia, typically involves *Streptococcus pneumoniae*.
- Other rare causes of purulent pericarditis include extension from another myocardial source (infective endocarditis, myocardial

abscess, perivalvular abscess) (Figures 6-4-3, 6-4-4, and 6-4-5), trauma or post-surgical infections, esophageal rupture with fistula formation, and extension from a retropharyngeal abscess or subdiaphragmatic abscesses.[2,3]

- Overall, *Staphylococcus aureus* accounts for 22% to 31% of all cases, gram negative organisms account for 40% to 45% of all cases, and *Streptococcus pneumoniae* is the most common organism involved in direct spread from an intrathoracic source.[4] Anaerobic infections account for 40% of cases, and mixed infections (aerobic/anaerobic) account for 13% of cases.
- Histoplasma and Candida are the most common fungal causes of purulent pericarditis and almost always occur in patients who are significantly immunosuppressed.
- Tuberculosis results in 2% to 4% of all cases of pericarditis in the United States.[1]

DIAGNOSIS

- A diagnosis of purulent pericarditis is made with pericardiocentesis and pericardial fluid analysis and culture. Pericardial fluid analysis in purulent pericarditis is typically associated with elevated protein level, low glucose (<35 mg/dL), elevated leukocyte counts (>6,000/microliter), and a positive microbiological culture.
- Other diagnostic tools can assist in the diagnosis of purulent pericarditis, including peripheral blood cultures, peripheral leukocytosis, electrocardiogram, chest x-ray, and echocardiography.

CLINICAL FEATURES

- Purulent pericarditis typically presents as an acute febrile illness. Symptoms typically include fever, chest pain (pleurtic and nonpleuritic), and shortness of breath. Unlike other patients with pericardial effusions, patients with purulent pericarditis usually are quite ill systemically and are often quite toxic in appearance.
- Physical exam findings are similar to other causes of pericarditis or tamponade, including tachycardia, hypotension, fevers, elevated jugular venous pressure, reproducible chest pain, hepatosplenomegaly, and lower extremity edema.[4,5] Presentation with fulminate sepsis is common.

LABORATORY STUDIES

- Routine peripheral blood cultures and white blood cell count can be helpful. Inflammatory markers (ESR, CRP) and cardiac biomarkers may be elevated.
- Pericardial fluid analysis should include cell count and differential, bacterial and fungal culture, protein, and glucose. The white blood cell count is typically elevated (>6,000/microliter), protein is typically elevated, and glucose is typically low (<35 mg/dL).[1]

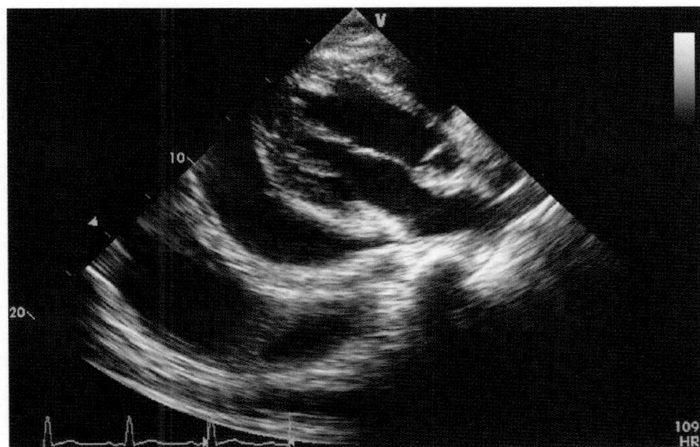

FIGURE 6-4-3 Parasternal long axis image from another patient with purulent pericarditis due to methicillin-resistant staph aureus. He was an IVDA who presented with acute aortic regurgitation due to endocarditis with an aortic root abscess and a purulent pericardial effusion. Note the large left pleural effusion as well ► (see Video 6-4-3).

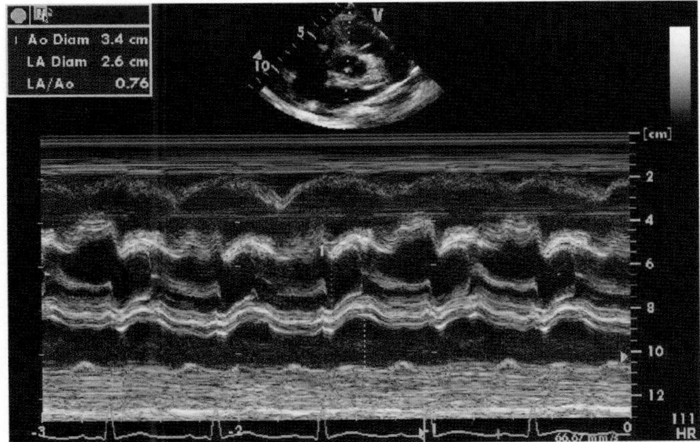

FIGURE 6-4-4 M-mode from the patient in Figure 6-4-3 demonstrating RV diastolic collapse, a finding of cardiac tamponade.

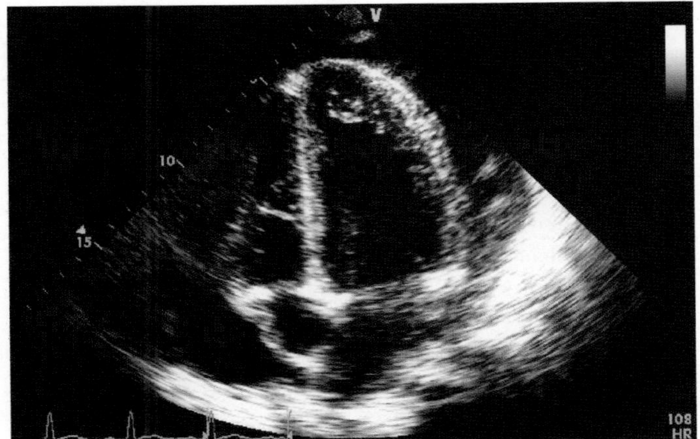

FIGURE 6-4-5 Apical 4 chamber view in this patient again demonstrating a large effusion ► (see Video 6-4-5). He went emergently to the operating room, was found to have purulent pericardial fluid, an aortic root abscess, and multiple AV vegetations. He unfortunately succumbed to multi-organ failure 6 days postoperatively.

DIFFERENTIAL DIAGNOSIS

- Primarily includes other causes of bacteremia/sepsis and pericarditis, which can be ruled out with pericardiocentesis and pericardial fluid analysis.
- It is important to ascertain the source of the infection.

MANAGEMENT

- Treatment typically involves pericardiocentesis and placement of a pericardial drain (until the drainage stops and the patient has responded to antibiotics) or surgical drainage with or without drain placement.
- Initial antibiotic therapy should be broad and then tailored based on the pericardial fluid culture.
- Intravenous antibiotic therapy appropriate for the organism isolated should be given. The duration of antibiotic therapy is not well delineated in the literature, but typically involves 2 to 6 weeks of intravenous therapy.[6]
- Intrapericardial infusion of antibiotics can be considered; however, this method is not sufficient as stand alone therapy. It is unclear which patients, if any, benefit from the use of intrapericardial antibiotics.
- Assessment and management of any remote infection that may have been the source of the bacteremia is also important.
- Pericardiectomy can be considered in patients with persistent pericardial infection, recurrent episodes of tamponade, or the presence of dense intrapericardial adhesions.[6]

PATIENT EDUCATION

- Discussions regarding the avoidance of intravenous drugs is imperative in individuals with such a history
- Education is necessary regarding the signs/symptoms of recurrent infection and instructions to seek immediate medical care if fever or other symptoms return.
- Patients should be informed of the signs/symptoms of pericardial constriction (see Section VI, Constrictive Pericarditis) which can develop after the acute illness resolves.

FOLLOW-UP

- Follow-up care with specialists (infectious disease and cardiology) should be arranged on an individualized basis. No specific follow-up regimen is indicated. A repeat echocardiogram following completion of therapy is reasonable to determine if there is any residual pericardial fluid present and to assess for any evidence of pericardial constriction.

VIDEO LEGENDS

1. Video 6-4-2 A: Parasternal long axis view from the transthoracic echocardiogram demonstrating a large, circumferential pericardial effusion.
2. Video 6-4-2 B: RV inflow view from the transthoracic echocardiogram of the right ventricle and right atrium demonstrating a large pericardial effusion and right atrial collapse, suggestive of cardiac tamponade.
3. Video 6-4-2 C: Parasternal short axis view from transthoracic echocardiogram demonstrating a large, circumferential pericardial effusion as well as right atrial and right ventricular collapse suggestive of cardiac tamponade.
4. Video 6-4-2 D: Four chamber view from transthoracic echocardiogram demonstrating a large pericardial effusion as well as pericardial debris.
5. Video 6-4-2 E: Four chamber view from transthoracic echocardiogram after pericardial drain placement demonstrating resolution of the previous large pericardial effusion.
6. Video 6-4-3: Parasternal long axis image from another patient with purulent pericarditis due to methicillin resistant staph aureus. He was an IVDA who presented with acute aortic regurgitation due to endocarditis with an aortic root abscess and a purulent pericardial effusion. Note the large left pleural effusion as well
7. Video 6-4-5: Apical 4 chamber view in this patient again demonstrating a large effusion. He went emergently to the operating room, was found to have purulent pericardial fluid, an aortic root abscess and multiple AV vegetations.

REFERENCES

1. Shiber JR. Purulent pericarditis: acute infections and chronic complications. *Hosp Physician*. 2008;44:9-18.
2. Boyle JD, Pearce ML, Guze LB. Purulent pericarditis. Review of the literature and report of eleven cases. *Medicine*. 1961;40:119-144.
3. Kauffman CA, Watanakunakorn C, Phair JP. Purulent pneumococcal pericarditis. A continuing problem in the antibiotic era. *Am J Med.* 1973;54:753
4. Ruben RH, Moellering RC Jr. Clinical, microbiological, and therapeutic aspects of purulent pericarditis. *Am J Med.* 1975; 59:68.
5. Sagristá-Sauleda J, Barrabés JA, Permanyer-Miralda G, Soler-Soler J. Purulent pericarditis: review of a 20-year experience in a general hospital. *J Am Coll Cardiol.* 1993;22:1661.
6. Maisch B, Seferović PM, Ristić AD, et al. Guidelines on the diagnosis and management of pericardial disease executive summary; the task force on the diagnosis and management of pericardial disease of the European Society of Cardiology. *Eur Heart J.* 2004;25:587.
7. Roy CL, Minor MA, Brookhart A, Choudhry NK. Does this patient with a pericardial effusion have cardiac tamponade? *JAMA.* 2007;297(16):1810.

SECTION 5

Acute Pericardial Effusion Due to Lead Perforation and the Role of Echocardiography

Sakima A. Smith, MD

CLINICAL CASE PRESENTATION

A 55-year-old man with history of ischemic cardiomyopathy had a recent implantation of a dual-chamber implantable cardioverter-defibrillator (ICD). He was discharged in stable condition. He was readmitted to the hospital due to ongoing chest pain and subsequently had an ICD shock for atrial fibrillation with rapid ventricular rates. Device interrogation revealed noncapture and very poor sensing of the right ventricular (RV) ICD lead, significantly different from his immediate post-implant evaluation. A chest x-ray was concerning for RV perforation (Figure 6-5-1). An echocardiogram in the emergency department demonstrated that the RV lead had perforated the RV apex resulting in a pericardial effusion (Figure 6-5-2). He was referred to the electrophysiology (EP) lab for RV lead revision. A transthoracic echocardiogram in the EP lab showed a moderate-sized pericardial effusion with evidence of RV lead perforation. A pericardial drain was placed with removal approximately 400 cc of blood. With the pericardial drain in place, the RV ICD lead was removed, and a new RV ICD lead was placed along the RV septum. During the procedure, the patient remained hemodynamically stable. There was good sensing capture threshold impedance with the new RV ICD lead. Once the new lead was in place, the postprocedural chest x-ray (Figure 6-5-3) confirmed that the lead was in a good position.

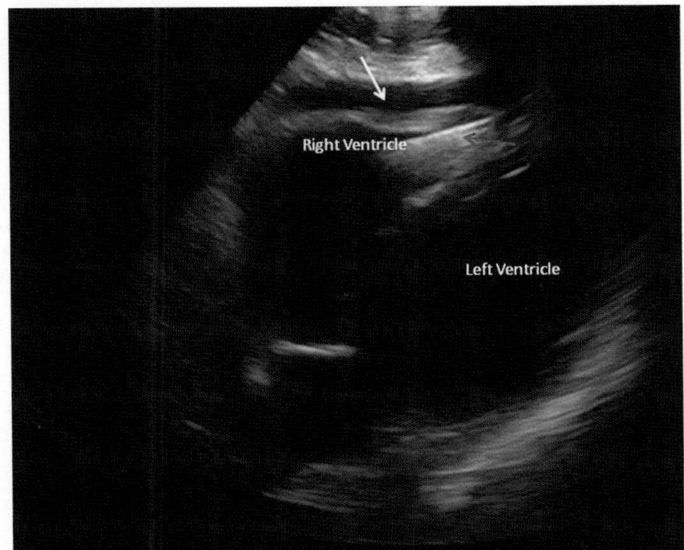

FIGURE 6-5-2 Subcostal view demonstrating a small pericardial effusion (white arrow) and evidence of perforation of the RV lead (red arrow) through the RV myocardium.

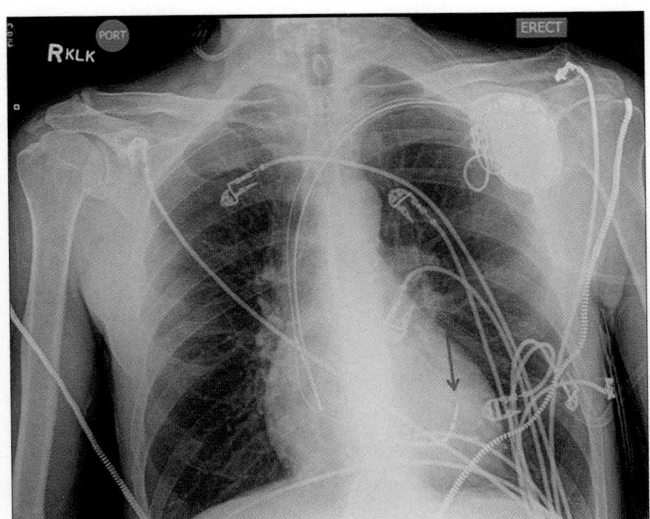

FIGURE 6-5-1 Chest x-ray demonstrating an abnormal position of the right ventricular lead which had migrated since the initial postprocedure x-ray.

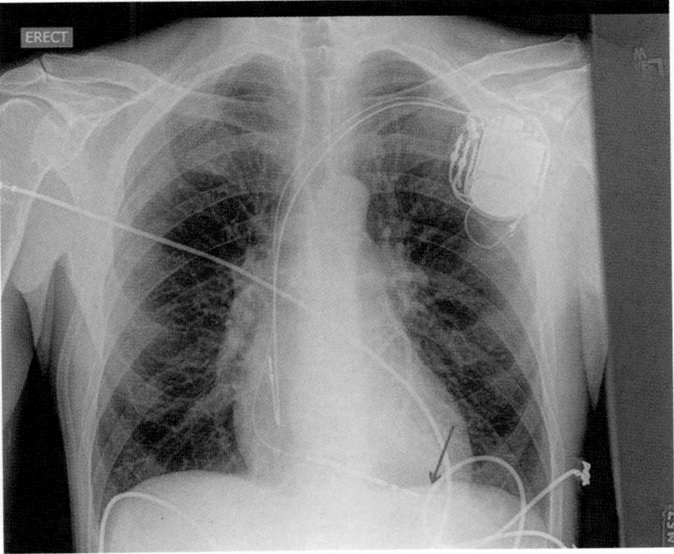

FIGURE 6-5-3 Chest x-ray post-lead revision demonstrating the RV lead in the RV apex.

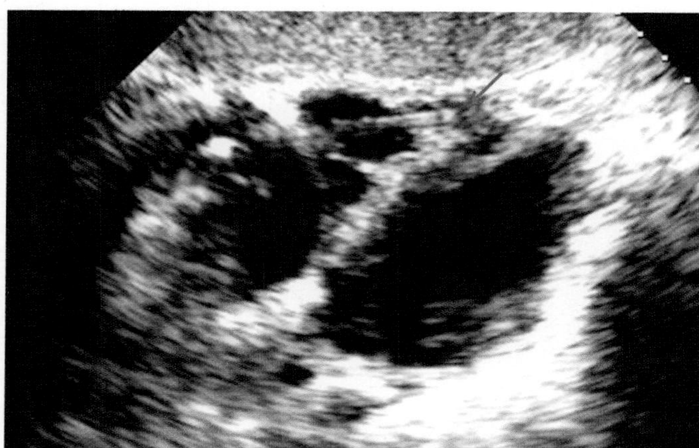

FIGURE 6-5-4 Post pericardial drain removal subcostal view demonstrating resolution of the pericardial effusion.

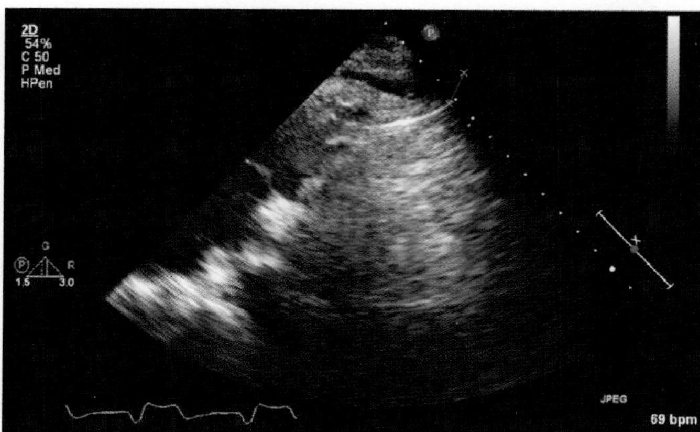

FIGURE 6-5-5 Subcostal image from a different patient with a more impressive perforation which was seen immediately post-pacer implantation. This patient developed acute tamponade, was treated with lead removal and pericardial drainage. She did not require surgical repair.

There was no further drainage from the pericardial drain, which was then removed. A follow-up echocardiogram revealed resolution of the effusion (Figure 6-5-4). The patient was discharged without any further events and continues to do well.

EPIDEMIOLOGY

Lead perforation:

- Permanent pacemakers and implantable cardiac defibrillators (ICDs) are implanted in over 250,000 patients a year in the United States.[1]
- Lead perforation via the right atrium or ventricle is rare, with an incidence of 0.6% to 5%.[2]

PATHOPHYSIOLOGY

A higher rate of right ventricular perforations may be seen in patients who had ICDs compared with pacemakers. This is probably due to the larger diameter of the ICD lead and more complex nature of an ICD lead compared to a pacemaker lead.[1]

DIAGNOSIS

- Cardiac echocardiography provides a rapid, accurate, noninvasive assessment of pericardial and cardiac morphology, the physiological importance of complications, and an overall assessment of the relative amount of pericardial fluid.
- Occasionally the perforated lead can be visualized (Figure 6-5-2), which usually leads to an acute or subacute accumulation of pericardial fluid. If the fluid accumulates rapidly or a large effusion develops over time, cardiac tamponade can result in some instances (Figures 6-5-5 and 6-5-6).
- Chest radiography and computed tomography (CT) are also helpful and can identify abnormal lead placement. In one series of asymptomatic patients, late lead perforation on CT was found in 15% of cases.[1]

CLINICAL FEATURES

- The clinical presentation can be quite varied. Patients can range from being totally asymptomatic to presenting in extremis with cardiac tamponade.
- Due to abnormal sensing and capturing from the perforated lead, atrial and ventricular arrhythmias may occur. The patient may also lose pacing function.
- Nonspecific chest pain may also be present.
- If a large effusion develops rapidly, hemodynamic compromise (tamponade) may develop.

LABORATORY STUDIES

Laboratory studies are not helpful in this clinical situation

DIFFERENTIAL DIAGNOSIS

If a pericardial effusion is present in the absence of lead perforation, then other causes of pericardial effusion need to be considered[3]:

- Infectious
  - Viral (most common: echovirus and coxsackievirus, influenza, Epstein-Barr virus, cytomegalovirus, adenovirus, varicella, rubella, mumps, hepatitis B virus, hepatitis C virus, HIV, parvovirus B19, and human herpesvirus.[6]

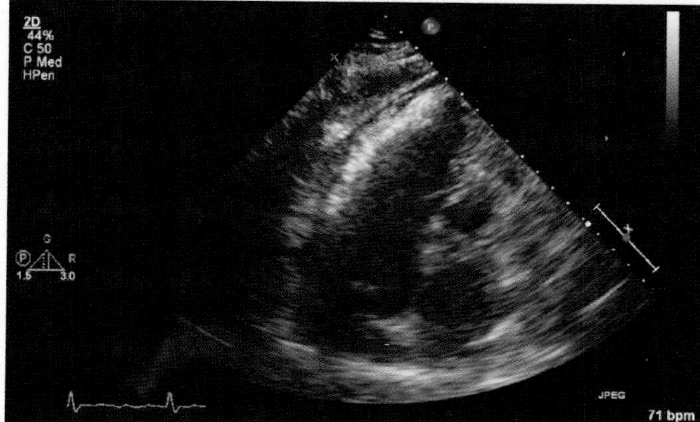

FIGURE 6-5-6 Subcostal image from another patient with a lead perforation. There is evidence of a subepicardial hematoma (arrow) along the RV free wall ► (see Video 6-5-6).

- Bacterial (most common: tuberculous [4%-5%], other bacterial rare)
- Fungal
- Parasitic (very rare: Echinococcus, Toxoplasma)
- Autoimmune pericarditis
- Neoplastic pericarditis
- Metabolic pericarditis (common: uremia, myxedema)
- Traumatic pericarditis (rare)
- Drug-related pericarditis (rare)
    - Procainamide, hydralazine, isoniazid, and phenytoin (lupus-like syndrome)
    - Penicillins (hypersensitivity pericarditis with eosinophilia)
    - Doxorubicin and daunorubicin (often associated with a cardiomyopathy)

MANAGEMENT

- Management of acute hemodynamic issues, if present, are employed (fluid resuscitation, transfusion, urgent pericardiocentesis).
- If there is a large effusion or evidence of tamponade, pericardiocentesis is warranted.
- Lead extraction/replacement or lead repositioning is the preferred method of managing lead perforations. Operator experience is vital in determining success of lead extraction as familiarity of a wide array of techniques will increase the likelihood of uncomplicated extraction.
    - Long implantation time, lack of operator experience, ICD lead type and female gender are risk factors for life-threatening complications.[4]
    - Lead extraction should, therefore, ideally be performed in high volume centers with experienced staff and on-site support from a cardiothoracic surgical team able to deal with bleeding complications from cardiovascular perforation.[4]

PATIENT EDUCATION

- Once other conditions have been ruled out, patients need to be instructed to routinely follow-up with a cardiologist and to pay attention to any acute signs of shortness of breath, dyspnea, or confusion as this could suggest impending cardiovascular hemodynamic collapse.

FOLLOW-UP

- After lead replacement and pericardiocentesis (if a significant effusion developed) to drain the related effusion, a follow-up echocardiogram is often performed to confirm that there is resolution of the pericardial effusion.
- A chest x-ray is also obtained prior to discharge to confirm correct lead placement.
- If a patient develops symptoms of shortness of breath or confusion they should seek medical attention. Close follow-up with a cardiologist is essential.

VIDEO LEGEND

1. Video 6-5-6: Subcostal image from a patient with a lead perforation. There is evidence of a subepicardial hematoma along the RV free wall

REFERENCES

1. Hirschl DA, Jain VR, Spindola-Franco H, Gross JN, Haramati LB. Prevalence and characterization of asymptomatic pacemaker and ICD lead perforation on CT. *Pacing Clin Electrophysiol.* 2007;30(1):28-32.
2. Khan MN, Joseph G, Khaykin Y, Ziada KM, Wilkoff BL. Delayed lead perforation: a disturbing trend. *Pacing Clin Electrophysiol.* 2005;28(3):251-253.
3. Imazio M. Pericarditis: pathophysiology, diagnosis, and management. *Curr Infect Dis Rep.* 2011;13(4):308-316.
4. Farooqi FM, Talsania S, Hamid S, Rinaldi CA. Extraction of cardiac rhythm devices: indications, techniques and outcomes for the removal of pacemaker and defibrillator leads. *Int J Clin Pract.* 2010;64(8):1140-1147.

SECTION 6

Constrictive Pericarditis

Sakima A. Smith, MD, and
David A. Orsinelli, MD, FACC, FASE

CLINICAL CASE PRESENTATION

A 56-year-old man with history of hepatitis B and C, COPD, and cirrhosis presented to The Ohio State Medical Center with a chief complaint of "increased swelling of my body from the chest down." These complaints began 3 months ago, and he now has had a 40 lb weight gain with swelling in his abdomen and legs. There were no recent dietary or medication changes. His examination revealed jugular venous distension, a normal S_1 and with a loud P_2, a 2/6 systolic murmur at the right upper sternal border, a right ventricular heave, clear lungs, and a distended abdomen with bilateral 3+ pitting edema above the knees. His chest radiograph (Figure 6-6-1) and CT scan revealed pericardial calcification. The ECG demonstrated nonspecific

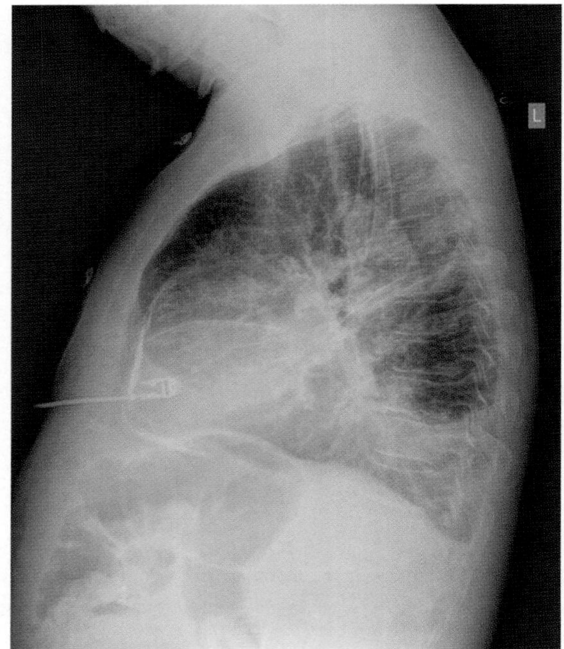

FIGURE 6-6-1 Chest x-ray demonstrating pericardial calcification.

T-wave changes. Echocardiography revealed a “septal bounce,” inferior vena cava distension, and hepatic vein diastolic flow reversal (Figures 6-6-2 to 6-6-4). During his hospitalization, he underwent cardiac catheterization which confirmed the diagnosis of pericardial constriction (Figure 6-6-5). He subsequently underwent a successful pericardiectomy. Pathology was not able to elucidate a specific etiology other than demonstrating chronic inflammation, which may have played a role (Figure 6-6-6).

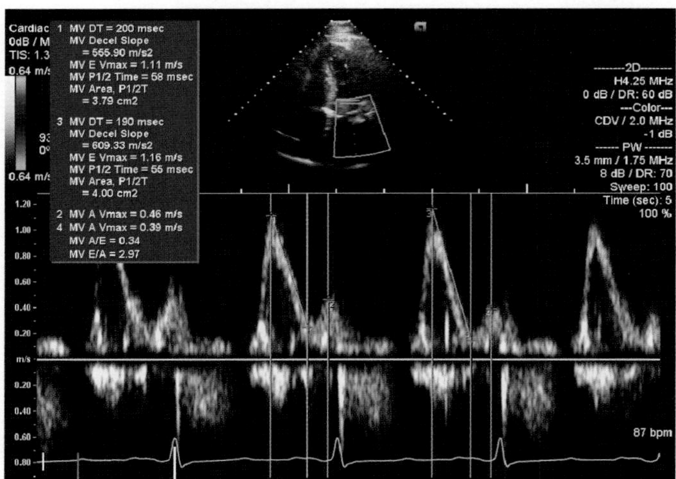

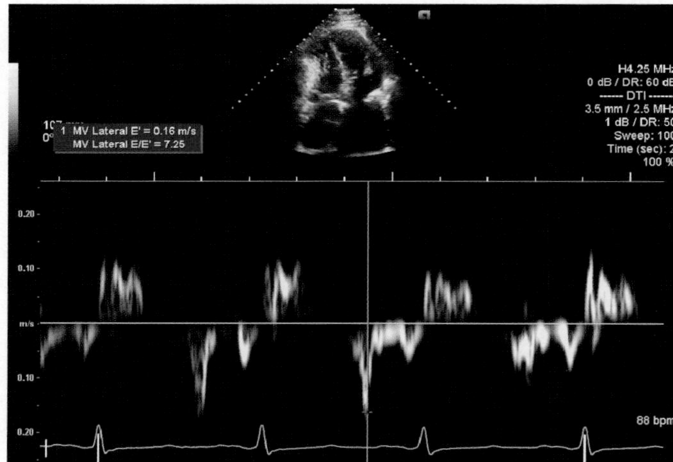

FIGURE 6-6-3 Transmitral flow (top panel) and tissue Doppler imaging (bottom panel) demonstrate “E” wave predominance and increased tissue Doppler e′ velocity.

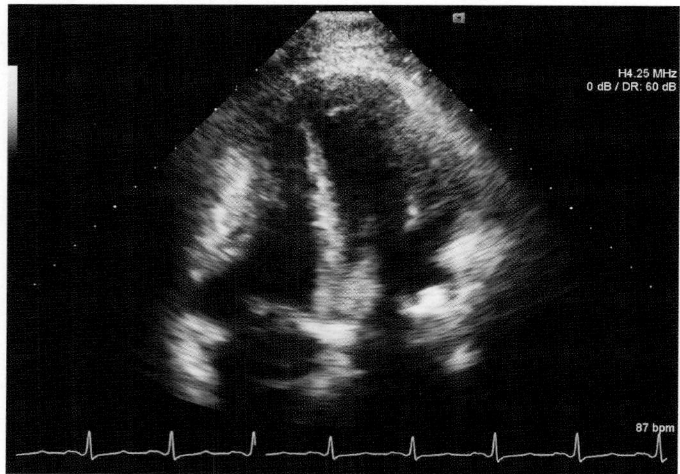

FIGURE 6-6-2 Apical 4 chamber view demonstrating abnormal septal motion (“septal bounce”) ▶ (see Video 6-6-2).

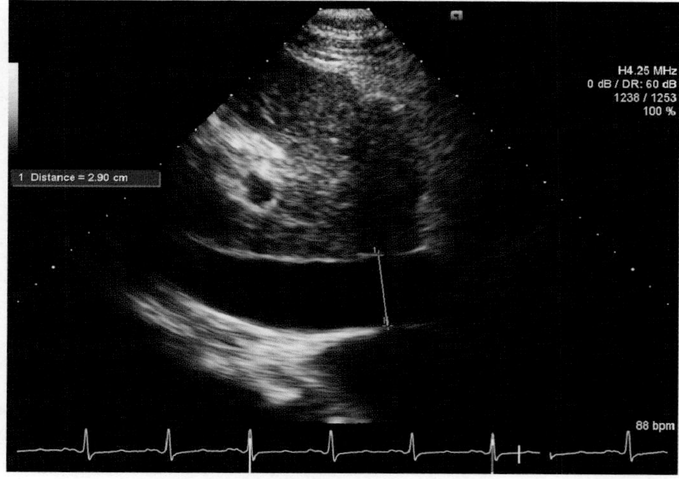

FIGURE 6-6-4 Subcostal view demonstrating IVC plethora ▶ (see Video 6-6-4).

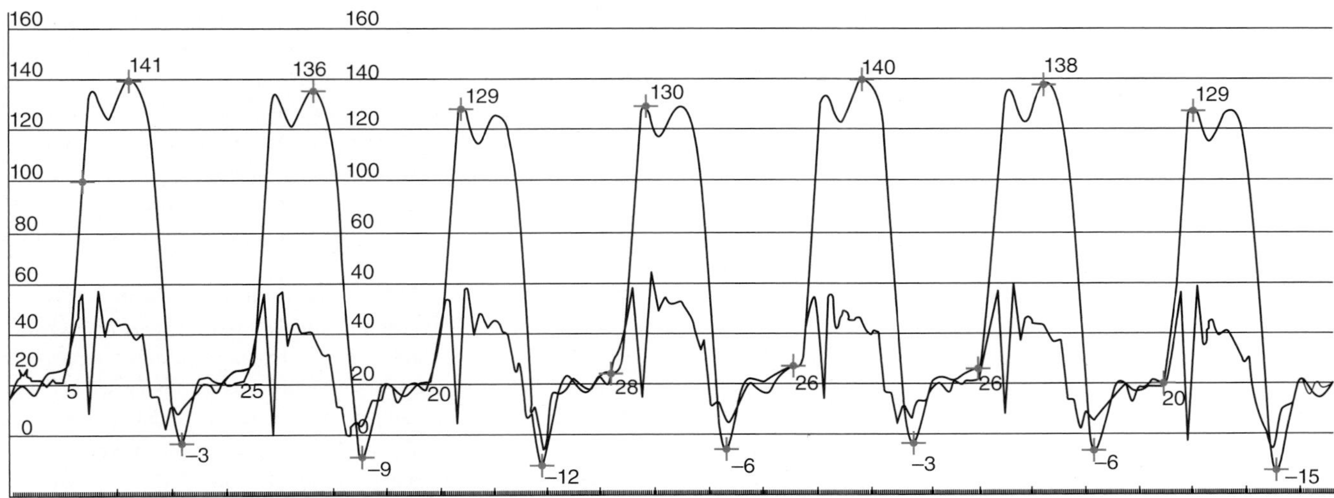

FIGURE 6-6-5 Cardiac catheterization showing left and right ventricular pressure waveforms demonstrating diastolic equilibration of pressures and the dip and plateau ("square root sign").

CLINICAL FEATURES

- Most patients present with signs and symptoms of heart failure such as peripheral edema, increasing abdominal girth, dyspnea, and fatigue. On physical examination, marked pitting edema or even anasarca may be present; ascites may be detected. The lung fields are typically clear.
- Cardiovascular examination findings include jugular venous distention with prominent "y" descents and preserved "x" descents. Kussmaul's sign is frequently present (Kussmaul's sign is the observation of a jugular venous pressure that rises with inspiration and suggests impaired filling of the right ventricle). Murmurs are uncommon. A pericardial "knock" may be heard (a low-frequency sound that is heard 80 to 100 msec after the second heart sound that is usually audible over the precordium).

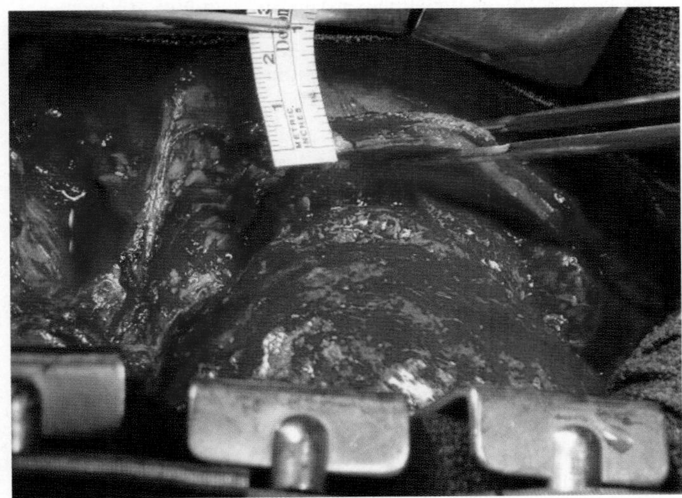

FIGURE 6-6-6 Thickened, inflamed pericardium found at pericardiectomy.

EPIDEMIOLOGY

- The overall incidence and prevalence of constrictive pericarditis is difficult to define due to the diagnostic challenges inherent to the disease process, but if one were to make an estimate based on the current level of 725,000 pericardiectomies performed annually in the United States, a conservative 0.3% incidence could yield up to 2200 new cases annually.[1]

PATHOPHYSIOLOGY AND ETIOLOGY

- Constrictive pericarditis is caused by fibrosis and/or calcification of the pericardium.
- The hemodynamic features are due to the fixed end-diastolic volume (the heart is constrained by the rigid pericardium and cannot fill further) as well as the isolation of the cardiac chambers from changes in intrathoracic pressure related to respiration.[2] Ventricular filling is impeded after the initial increase in volume early in diastole.[2,3] The high driving pressure across the valves at the time of MV valve opening results in early rapid diastolic filling, an abrupt increase in ventricular pressure, and the termination of flow in early diastole, with the end result being a significant increase of diastolic pressures in all four chambers.[2,3]
- Ventricular interdependence is exaggerated due to pericardial constraint.[2] Thus filling of the right ventricle comes at the expense of left ventricular filling and vice-versa. These hemodynamic changes result in the signs/symptoms of right-sided congestion and may also account for the symptoms of fatigue and dyspnea.
- The etiology of pericardial constriction has changed over time, and the underlying causes vary depending on the population studied. Historically, tuberculous pericardial disease was the most common cause of constrictive pericardial disease.[1,4] This would result in severe calcification of the entire pericardium.[1] In the modern era, chest radiation for malignancies and cardiac surgical procedures are often the underlying cause, though most current cases are sequelae of idiopathic or viral pericarditis.[1,4] Other causes include

malignant pericardial disease, post trauma, drug-related, asbestosis, sarcoidosis, other connective tissue diseases, uremia and bacterial pericarditis.[1,4]

ECHOCARDIOGRAPHY

- Patients presenting with signs/symptoms of congestive heart failure such as dyspnea and edema often undergo echocardiography early in their diagnostic evaluation. Pericardial disease, and in particular, constrictive pericarditis is in the differential diagnosis.
- There are many echocardiographic findings that may lead to the diagnosis of constriction. Unless there are concomitant abnormalities, left and right ventricular chamber size and function are normal.
  - M-mode and two-dimensional echo may demonstrate a "septal bounce." This finding is a consequence of prominent early diastolic filling of the ventricles with abrupt cessation of inflow resulting in displacement of the septum and reflects the exaggerated ventricular interdependence.[2,5]
  - The abrupt cessation of diastolic filling may be reflected in "flattening" of the posterior wall in mid- and late-diastole demonstrated on M-mode.[2]
  - The inferior vena cava is usually dilated, reflecting increased right atrial pressure.
  - While not very sensitive, the pericardium may appear thickened. Transeophageal echocardiography may be more sensitive to detect pericardial thickening.[2]
  - Other M-mode and 2-D findings suggestive of constriction include a steep mitral E-F slope, premature opening of the pulmonary valve, sharp early diastolic posterior displacement of the posterior aortic root, blunting of the angle between the posterior LA and LV walls, and bowing of the inter-atrial septum to the left with inspiration.[2]
  - Spectral Doppler interrogation of mitral and tricuspid valve inflow patterns as well as hepatic vein and pulmonary vein flow aids in making the diagnosis of constriction and differentiating constriction from restriction. The normal respirophasic changes in inflow patterns are exaggerated due to the underlying pathophysiology. Early mitral filling velocity is increased with a short deceleration time.[2] With inspiration, the mitral valve "E" wave decreases and the tricuspid valve "E" wave increases. With expiration, as intrathoracic pressure increases and the driving pressure for the LA to the LV increases, the mitral "E" wave increases. These dynamic respirophasic changes are not seen with restrictive cardiomyopathy.
  - Other conditions (for example severe COPD or asthma that result in marked changes in intrathoracic pressure) as well as right ventricular failure may lead to similar findings.[2]
  - Assessment of hepatic vein flow on Doppler echo may demonstrate increased diastolic flow reversal which is due to decreased right ventricular filling with decreased hepatic vein forward diastolic flow.[5] This flow reversal is exaggerated with inspiration.[2] In addition, interrogation of the pulmonary veins also demonstrates marked respirophasic changes, with increases in the antegrade systolic and early diastolic velocities (reflected in increases in the mitral "E" wave) and decreases in the velocities with inspiration.[2]
  - Tissue Doppler interrogation may also help to differentiate constriction form restriction. Since left ventricular diastolic function and relaxation are normal (unless there is concomitant myocardial disease such as ischemia), tissue Doppler demonstrates normal e' velocities reflecting normal relaxation. In fact, with constrictive physiology, e' velocities may be increased.[2] This may help to differentiate constriction from a restrictive myocardial process (in which tissue e' velocities are often reduced).
  - Newer techniques to evaluate myocardial mechanics such as strain imaging (either with tissue Doppler or speckle tracking techniques), twist and torsion, while not routinely employed in most clinical echocardiography labs, may in the future become routinely incorporated into the echocardiographic assessment of pericardial disease. Preliminary data suggests that while longitudinal strain is normal, circumferential strain, twist angle and untwisting velocity are decreased in constriction. Conversely, in restrictive myopathic processes, strain is decreased while twist angle and untwisting velocity are normal.[2]
  - The interested reader is referred to an excellent review[2] of echocardiography in the diagnosis of constriction. This well-referenced article contains detailed descriptions of the echocardiographic features and sensitivities/specificities of these findings gleaned from the literature.

OTHER DIAGNOSTIC TESTING AND PROCEDURES

- The clinical evaluation of a patient with suspected pericardial constriction should include a careful history and physical examination to elicit the historical features and examination findings noted above.
- Laboratory studies are not very specific for the diagnosis, though it may be useful to check studies for evidence of chronic inflammation (CRP, ESR), serum markers suggesting a connective tissue disease, and a tuberculin skin test to assess for evidence of tuberculosis.
- A chest x-ray should be obtained. While often unremarkable, the chest x-ray findings may include clear lung fields and evidence of pericardial calcification as was found in the current patient.
- The electrocardiogram findings are nonspecific. Low voltage may be present.[5]
- Cardiac computed tomography (CT) and magnetic resonance imaging (MRI) may be useful. CT may demonstrate small areas of calcification, a finding suggestive of pericardial constriction. Additional CT findings include pericardial thickening (>4 mm), deformation of the right ventricle, small left ventricular cavity size and findings suggestive of elevated right-sided pressures similar to those described with echocardiography.[6] MRI may also demonstrate pericardial thickening and other findings as described above with CT. In addition, MRI may demonstrate abnormal septal motion in diastole.[6]
- Cardiac catheterization demonstrates elevated filling pressures. The "square root sign" (an early diastolic dip followed by a plateau of diastasis, the last stage of diastole just before contraction) and diastolic equalization are seen about 77% and 81% of the time, respectively.[7] The diagnosis by cardiac catheterization alone can be made about 60% of the time.[7]

DIFFERENTIAL DIAGNOSIS

- The clinical presentation of right-sided heart failure can mimic many cardiac and noncardiac diseases such as biventricular congestive heart failure, valvular heart disease, hepatic or renal failure, and nephrotic syndrome. An important point to remember is that hepatic cirrhosis can sometimes prompt a GI work-up, but in reality it may be due to right-sided heart failure from constriction.
- A careful history to elicit potential underlying etiologies of constrictive pericardial disease (eg, prior chest radiation, cardiac surgical procedures, pericarditis etc.) is important.
- One diagnostic challenge is to differentiate constrictive pericarditis from restrictive cardiomyopathy.[5] A history of radiation exposure or a previous open heart surgical procedure will point towards constrictive pericarditis. Restrictive cardiomyopathy is a heart-muscle disease that results in impaired ventricular filling with normal or decreased diastolic volume. The increased stiffness of the myocardium causes pressure within the ventricle to rise precipitously with only small increases in volume. Murmurs are more common with restriction, but the pericardial knock is absent.
- Cardiac catheterization is very helpful to differentiate restriction from constriction. Also, chest x-ray and CT will not reveal pericardial calcifications in restriction.
- Several echocardiographic features (as previously discussed) may help to differentiate constriction from restriction.

DIAGNOSIS

- The diagnosis is usually made by a combination of clinical features, echocardiographic findings, cardiac catheterization features, and pericardial calcification that is seen on CT or chest x-ray. Cardiac MRI may also be helpful.

MANAGEMENT

- The definitive therapy for constrictive pericarditis is a pericardiectomy. Recent data suggests that the perioperative mortality is approximately 6%.[8] The mortality also depends on the underlying etiology, with a mortality rate of 2.7% in idiopathic constriction, 8.3% in postsurgical constriction, and 21.4% in post-radiation constriction.[8] Although when compared to an age- and sex-matched cohort long-term mortality may be decreased after a pericardiectomy, patients experience marked symptomatic improvement after pericardiectomy, with up to 83% being either asymptomatic or mildly symptomatic.[1]

FOLLOW-UP

- It is imperative that a patient with a diagnosis of constrictive pericarditis be evaluated and follow-up with a cardiologist, who may then refer the patient to a cardiothoracic surgeon for definitive treatment (pericardiectomy). Surgical treatment may not only be diagnostic but therapeutic for symptomatic patients.

VIDEO LEGENDS

1. Video 6-6-2: Apical 4 chamber view demonstrating abnormal septal motion ("septal bounce") in a patient with constrictive pericarditis.
2. Video 6-6-4: Subcostal view demonstrating IVC plethora in a patient with constrictive pericarditis.

REFERENCES

1. Ling LH, Oh JK, Schaff HV, et al. Constrictive pericarditis in the modern era: evolving clinical spectrum and impact on outcome after pericardiectomy. *Circulation.* 1999;100(13):1380-1386.
2. Dal-Bianco JP, Sengupta PP, Mookadam F, Chandrasekaran K, Tajik AJ, Khanderia BK. Role of echocardiography in the diagnosis of constricive pericarditis. *J Am Soc Echocardiogr.* 2009;22:24-33.
3. Nishimura RA. Constrictive pericarditis in the modern era: a diagnostic dilemma. *Heart.* 2001;86(6):619-623.
4. Imazio M, Brucato A, Maestroni S, et al. Risk of constrictive pericarditis after acute pericarditis. *Circulation.* 2011;124: 1270-1275.
5. Kushwaha SS, Fallon JT, Fuster V. Restrictive cardiomyopathy. *N Engl J Med.* 1997;336(4):267-276.
6. Yared K, Baggish AL, Picard MH, Hoffmann U, Hung J. Multimodality imaging of pericardial diseases. *JACC Cardiovasc Imaging.* 2010;3:650-660.
7. Talreja DR, Edwards WD, Danielson GK, et al. Constrictive pericarditis in 26 patients with histologically normal pericardial thickness. *Circulation.* 2003;108(15):1852-1857.
8. Bertog SC, Thambidorai SK, Parakh K, et al. Constrictive pericarditis: etiology and cause-specific survival after pericardiectomy. *J Am Coll Cardiol.* 2004;43(8):1445-1452.

7 ECHOCARDIOGRAPHIC EVALUATION OF AORTIC PATHOLOGY

Gbemiga Sofowora, MBChB, FACC and
Nkechinyere N. Ijioma, MBBS

INTRODUCTION

Aortic pathology can present in many ways, including acute aortic syndromes, such as an aortic dissection, or chronically, as in cases with aortic aneurysmal disease or atherosclerotic disease. Echocardiography is especially valuable in the acute setting due to its rapid availability and portability, enabling its use in the emergency department (ED) and the operating room. While transthoracic echocardiography (TTE) is useful to evaluate the proximal aorta, the aortic valve, left ventricular function, and the presence of pericardial effusion, it is relatively insensitive for the diagnosis of acute pathology such as dissection. Transesophageal echocardiography is a more sensitive and specific modality to evaluate the aorta and is often used in the emergent setting or in the operating room. Computed tomographic angiography (CT angiography) is often even more readily available in the ED and in many institutions, including our own, has supplanted the use of TEE in the acute setting unless there are contraindications to its use. Magnetic resonance angiography (MRA) is an ideal imaging modality for the evaluation and follow-up of patients with aortic pathology; however, its role in the emergent situation, especially in hemodynamically unstable patients, is limited.

In this chapter, Drs. Sofowora and Ijioma will explore the use of echocardiography in a variety of clinical settings in patients with suspected or known aortic pathology, including patients with suspected acute aortic syndromes (aortic dissection, acute intramural hematoma), atheroembolic events due to aortic atherosclerosis, and chronic aortopathies in patients with connective tissue disease such as Marfan syndrome and bicuspid aortic valves.

SECTION 1

Acute Aortic Dissection

CLINICAL CASE PRESENTATION

The patient is a 79-year-old woman with a longstanding history of hypertension and a 40 pack-year cigarette smoking history presented to the emergency department with severe chest pain that was described as tearing in nature and was followed by fainting. Her daughter-in-law saw her at the house and called emergency services. On arrival in the emergency department, she was diaphoretic and moaning in pain. An ECG demonstrated normal sinus rhythm with evidence of left ventricular hypertrophy and nonspecific ST-segment changes. On physical examination, her pulses were thready, her blood pressure was 90/30 mm Hg, her apex beat was thrusting, and she had a fourth heart sound with a loud A_2. She had a mid-diastolic murmur that was best heard along the sternal border with her leaning forward in expiration. Her lungs were clear and she had no edema. She had a dialysis fistula in her left arm. A transthoracic echocardiogram showed a linear opacity in her ascending aorta and at least moderate aortic regurgitation (Figures 7-1-1 and 7-1-2). After an emergent CT scan confirmed a type A dissection, she was taken to the operating room (OR). Representative intraoperative TEE images are shown in Figures 7-1-3 to 7-1-8. Her dissection was repaired, and the ascending aorta was replaced with a prosthetic graft. She was initially stable following her surgery, but 10 days later she died from surgical complications.

CLINICAL FEATURES AND NATURAL HISTORY

- Patients may present with chest pain. This pain is usually acute, of sudden onset, and severe intensity. However, painless dissection may occur with Marfan syndrome or in patients with neurologic complications.
- The pain may be described as tearing/ripping and radiates to the back or abdomen.
- The site of dissection may be inferred from the location of the pain. Anterior chest pain usually involves the anterior arch or aortic root, interscapular pain usually involves the descending aorta, while neck/jaw pain suggests aortic arch and great vessel involvement.
- Radiation to the neck suggests a type A dissection, while interscapula radiation suggests type B dissection (refer to text below for classification scheme).
- Loss of consciousness may occur.
- There may be a painless interval after the initial episode of pain lasting anywhere from 1 hour to 5 days followed by a return of pain and death.
- Neurologic deficits including symptoms of cerebrovascular accident (CVA), syncope, or altered mental state can occur. Horner's syndrome can result from interruption of the cervical sympathetic ganglia.

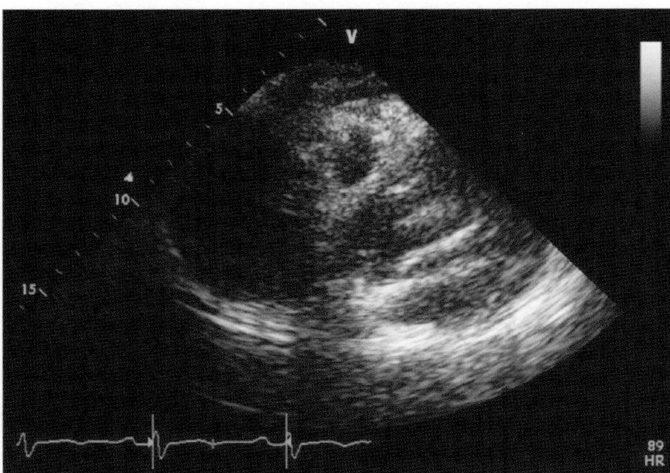

FIGURE 7-1-1 Focused parasternal long axis view. There is a type A dissection with a dissection flap visualized on this TTE ► (see Video 7-1-1).

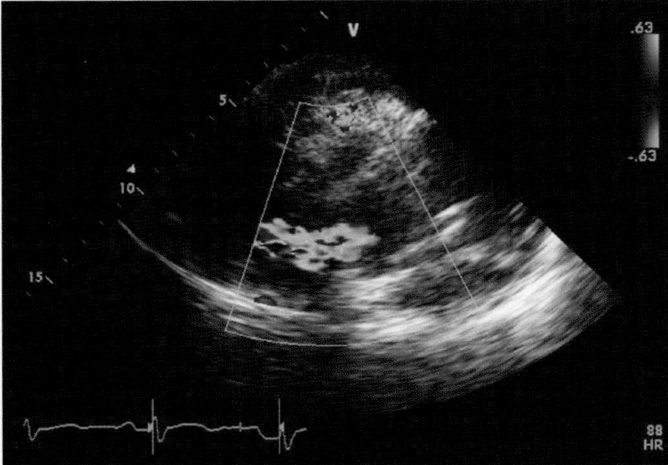

FIGURE 7-1-2 Parasternal long axis view with color Doppler demonstrating the dissection flap with significant AR due to the aortic dissection ► (see Video 7-1-2).

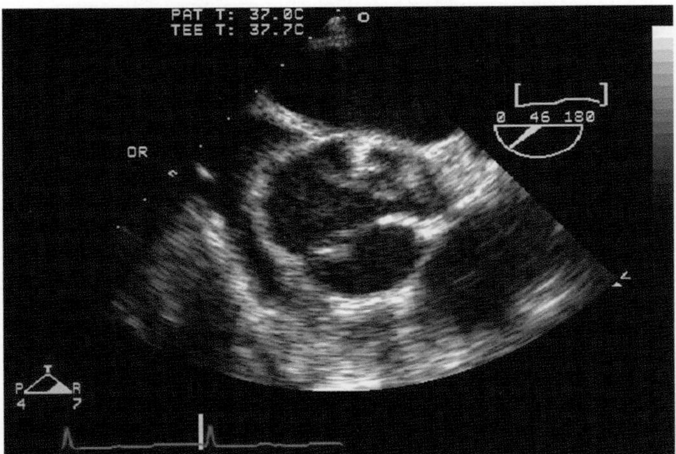

FIGURE 7-1-3 Intraoperative TEE short axis view of the aorta. There is a type A dissection with a large mobile dissection flap. Note the dissection flap prolapsing across the AV, which contributes to the AR ► (see Video 7-1-3).

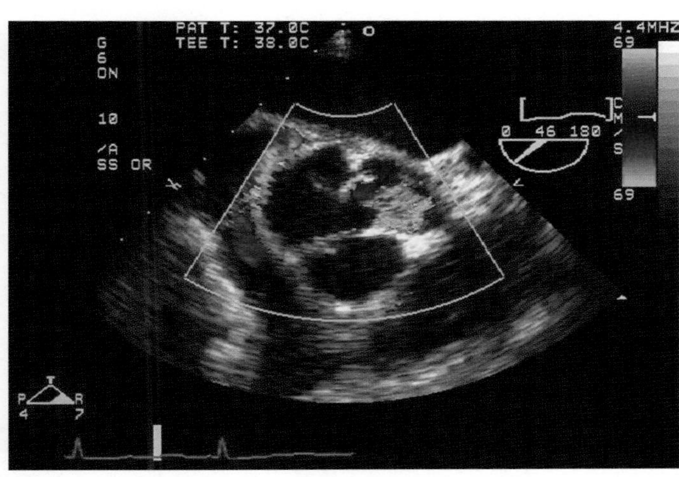

FIGURE 7-1-4 Intraoperative TEE short axis view of the aortic root and aortic valve with color Doppler. There is significant AR caused in part by the dissection flap prolapsing across the AV ► (see Video 7-1-4).

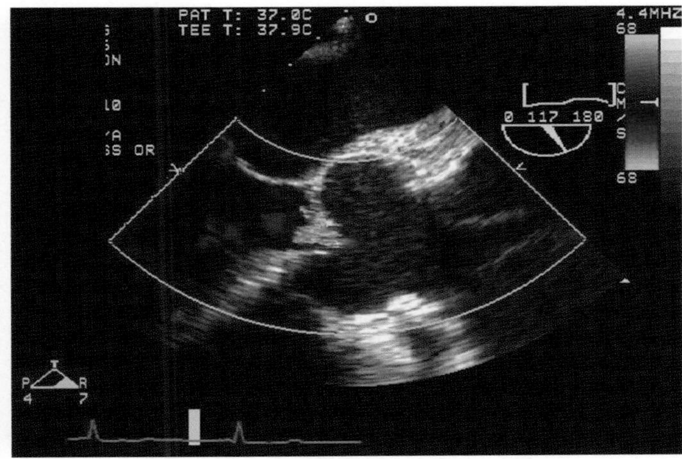

FIGURE 7-1-5 Intraoperative TEE long axis view with color Doppler again demonstrating the dissection flap and associated AR ► (see Video 7-1-5).

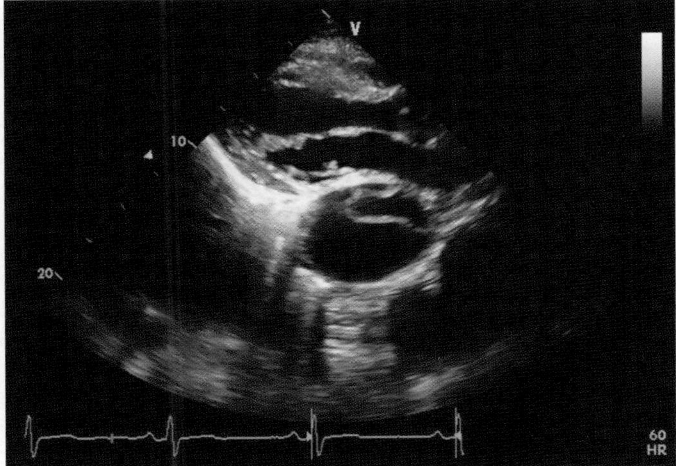

FIGURE 7-1-6 Parasternal long axis view demonstrating a dilated descending aorta with a dissection flap in a different patient with a known chronic type B dissection.

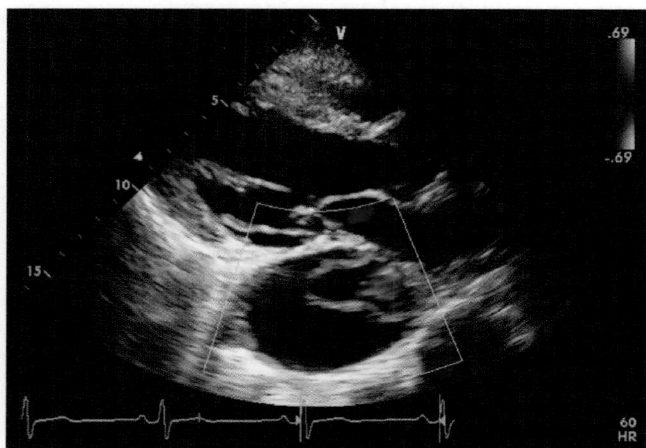

FIGURE 7-1-7 Parasternal long axis view from the same patient in Figure 7-1-6 with color flow Doppler demonstrating flow in the true lumen.

- Dissection into the pleura can manifest with dyspnea and hemoptysis.
- Damage to the kidneys and intestines may occur as a complication of type B dissection and may manifest with hematuria and bowel ischemia.
- Patients may be hypotensive (due to excessive vagal tone, cardiac tamponade, or hypovolemia from aortic rupture) or hypertensive (from catecholamine surge or essential hypertension).
- With type A dissections, clinical signs of aortic regurgitation may be present (bounding pulses, diastolic murmur, increased pulse pressure). Severe aortic regurgitation may present with acute dyspnea.
- Asymmetric pulses and inter-arm systolic blood pressure difference >20 mm Hg may be present.
- Mortality is high.[1]

EPIDEMIOLOGY

- The incidence of aortic dissection is approximately 2.9 to 3.5 per 100,000 person years.[2]
- Usually affects persons in their sixth decade of life.

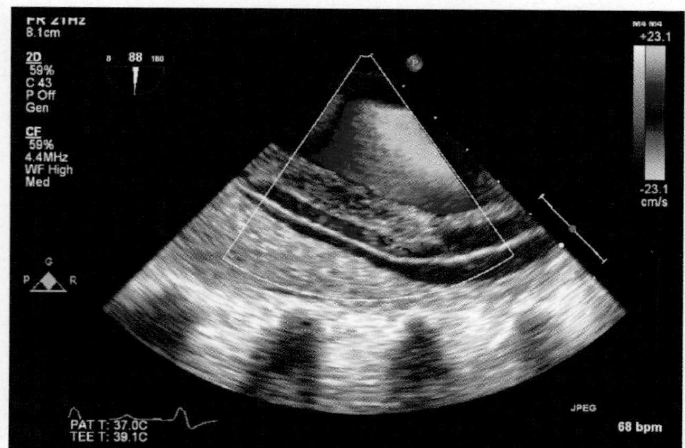

FIGURE 7-1-8 Intraoperative TEE image of another patient with a type A dissection that extended into the descending aorta. There is evidence (color Doppler) of flow in both lumens ▶ (see Video 7-1-8).

- The most common predisposing features include: hypertension, genetic conditions (Marfan syndrome, Ehlers-Danlos syndrome, bicuspid aortic valve, Turner syndrome, Loeys-Dietz syndrome), aortic aneurysm, inflammatory vasculitis (giant cell arteritis, Takayasu arteritis), pregnancy, cocaine abuse, iatrogenic (interventional procedures such as cardiac catherization).

PATHOPHYSIOLOGY AND ETIOLOGY

- The initial lesion is usually a tear in the intima. The resulting column of blood results in dissection of the intimal and medial layers both proximally and distally from the site of the initial tear. Often, several intimal tears are present.
- An intramural hematoma is caused by rupture of the vasa vasorum in the intima and is defined by the absence of an entry point and lack of free flow within the aortic wall. It may, however, progress to a typical dissection if the intima tears.
- Dissections affecting the thoracic aorta may be classified based on the location of the intimal tear or "entry point." There are two classification schemes (Stanford and Debakey).
  - Stanford type A includes all dissections involving the ascending aorta, while Stanford type B includes all dissections not involving the ascending aorta.
  - Debakey type I includes all dissections which involve the ascending aorta and extend into the arch; they may extend distally in to the descending aorta. Debakey type II includes all dissections involving and limited to the ascending aorta. Debakey type III includes dissections limited to the descending aorta.

ECHOCARDIOGRAPHY

- Transthoracic echocardiography (TTE) may be useful for detecting ascending aortic dissections, but it has limited ability to visualize the distal ascending aorta and is relatively insensitive compared to other imaging modalities. Complications of a type A dissection (eg, aortic valve incompetence, pericardial effusion, LV dysfunction due to compromise of blood coronary flow) are readily detected by TTE.
- TTE may also demonstrate baseline abnormalities of the aortic valve or root such as aortic stenosis, a bicuspid aortic valve, or dilation of the aortic root, which are predisposing factors for dissection.
- A dissection of the ascending aorta may lead to aortic incompetence in one of 4 ways.
  - Primary aortic valve abnormality such as a bicuspid aortic valve or preexisting aortic dilation with resultant malcoaptation of the aortic cusps
  - Extension of the dissection flap into the sino-tubular junction leading to malcoaptation of an aortic valve cusp
  - Extension of the dissection flap into the base of an aortic valve cusp leading to malcoaptation
  - Extension of the dissection flap in between the aortic valve cusps
- A dissection flap may be visualized in the proximal ascending aorta.
- The absence of aortic regurgitation and a normal proximal ascending aorta and arch make the presence of an ascending aortic dissection unlikely.

- Transesophageal echocardiography (TEE) is more sensitive than TTE to detect aortic dissection, it can demonstrate the presence and location of an entry point and the extent of the dissection, and it may distinguish both the true and false lumens. Clues to help distinguish between the true and false lumen include:
  - The lumen into which the aortic valve opens is, by definition, the true lumen.
  - The true lumen wall is usually round or oval in cross-section.
  - The true lumen in the descending aorta is usually smaller.
  - The wall of the true lumen is usually pulsatile.
  - The presence of swirling echoes or thrombus usually suggests a false lumen.
  - There may be collagenous strands seen in the false lumen.
- TEE may also demonstrate the presence of other complications:
  - Cardiac tamponade due to dissection into the pericardial space
  - LV wall motion abnormalities due to extension of the dissection usually into the ostium of the right coronary artery
  - Extension of the dissection into one of the great vessels of the aortic arch
- Several structures may be confused with a dissection on TEE, including:
  - The brachiocephalic vein. This may be distinguished from a dissection flap by demonstrating venous flow within the vessel or by injecting agitated saline in to the left arm and demonstrating saline opacification in the vessel.
  - Side lobe artifacts. These may be distinguished from a dissection flap by their relative immobility.

OTHER DIAGNOSIS TESTING AND PROCEDURES

- ECG is recommended for all patients to evaluate for myocardial infarction.[3]
  - The absence of ECG abnormalities in a patient with severe chest pain may suggest an aortic dissection.
  - Since a dissection may extend into a coronary sinus (usually the right) and dissect in to a coronary artery ostium, it may cause an acute myocardial infarction, which can be detected on ECG.
- D-dimer may be helpful to exclude a pulmonary embolism.
- The Chest x-ray may demonstrate a widened mediastinum, cardiomegaly (due to a pericardial effusion) or pleural fluid.
- Definitive diagnosis of a thoracic aortic aneurysm/dissection is by transesophageal echocardiography (TEE), CT scan, or MRI.
- TEE has a sensitivity of 100% for detection of a thoracic aortic dissection and 60% for aortic arch vessel involvement, while its specificities were 94% and 85% respectively.[4] Its advantages are that it can be deployed quickly in an acute situation and interpreted virtually instantaneously. No radiation or contrast is involved. It can be used irrespective of renal dysfunction, is relatively portable, and may be able to demonstrate the presence of complications.
- Disadvantages of TEE include:
  - Dependence on superior technical/operator skill.
  - Need for conscious sedation and a secure airway.
  - Blind spot that corresponds to the crossing of the bronchus across the distal ascending aorta and proximal arch. However, a dissection that is strictly limited to this area is extremely unlikely.
  - Obesity, pulmonary emphysema, and mechanical ventilation can reduce the accuracy of TEE.
- CT scan has a sensitivity of 100% for detection of a thoracic aortic dissection and 93% for an arch vessel involvement with specificities of 100% and 97% respectively.[4] Its positive and negative predictive values were 100% and 89% respectively.[5] It may help delineate the extent of the dissection all the way to the mesenteric, renal, and iliac arteries. It is also more accurate than TEE or MRI in detecting arch vessel involvement. A significant disadvantage is its inability to show the presence of aortic incompetence and the need for iodinated contrast.
- MRI has a sensitivity of 100% and specificity of 94% for a thoracic aortic dissection and sensitivity of 67% with a specificity of 88% for arch vessel involvement.[4] MRI may not be used in patients with metal devices or pacemakers and its use is limited in patients who are claustrophobic. Reports of nephrogenic systemic fibrosis following use of gadolinium in patients with moderate to severe renal insufficiency may limit its use as well. MRI is also limited by its lack of portability.
- The recently published guidelines on management of thoracic aortic disease,[3] encourage the use of clinical pretest probability to guide the imaging algorithm for diagnosis.
  - Three categories of patients are identified based on the aortic dissection diagnosis (ADD) score. Scoring is based on presence or absence of three features:
- High-risk conditions (Marfan syndrome, family history of aortic disease, known aortic valve disease, known thoracic aortic aneurysm, recent aortic manipulation)
- High-risk pain features (abrupt onset, severe, tearing/ripping chest, back or abdominal pain)
- High-risk exam features (pulse deficits, difference in systolic blood pressure, hypotension or shock, new aortic regurgitation murmur, focal neurologic deficit).
  - Each feature is assigned a score of one (1). This diagnostic algorithm has been shown to be highly sensitive (95% sensitivity) for the diagnosis of acute aortic dissection.[6] The specificity is unknown.
  - The expedited aortic imaging modalities are identified as computed tomography imaging (CT) with angiography, magnetic resonance (MR) imaging with MR angiography (MRA), or TEE with color Doppler flow. In unstable patients, TEE or CT are the imaging modalities of choice.
- A chest x-ray is recommended for all patients with low and intermediate risk pretest probability.[3] This may demonstrate widening of the mediastinum and unfolding of the aorta. The absence of these features, however, does not rule out a dissection.
- For patients with high pretest probability (ADD score 2-3), immediate surgical consultation and expedited aortic imaging is recommended.[3]
  - For patients with intermediate pretest probability (ADD score 1), expedited aortic imaging is recommended if the ECG is not consistent with an ST-elevation myocardial infarction (STEMI) and if

no alternate diagnosis are suggested by history, physical exam, or chest x-ray.[3]

- For a low pretest probability (ADD score 0), recommendation is to proceed with diagnostic evaluation as indicated by the clinical presentation. If no alternate diagnosis is identified and there is widened mediastinum on CXR or unexplained hypotension, the recommendation is to proceed with expedited aortic imaging.[3]

DIFFERENTIAL DIAGNOSIS

- Acute myocardial infarction
- Pulmonary embolism
- Spontaneous pneumothorax
- Acute pericarditis
- Mesenteric ischemia

DIAGNOSIS

- The diagnosis of an aortic dissection is made by demonstrating an intimal flap with any of the above imaging modalities, which can also demonstrate complications of the dissection and help to guide management.

MANAGEMENT

- Definitive treatment of a type A aortic dissection is surgical. Dissections involving the descending aorta (type B) are treated medically unless there is intractable pain, uncontrolled hypertension, extension of the dissection, or end organ damage (limb or visceral ischemia).
- Medical management (acutely prior to surgery for a type A dissection and for all type B dissections) includes:
  - Pain control with opiates may help with blood pressure management.
  - β-Blockers can reduce the heart rate and blood pressure and therefore minimize hemodynamic shear stress on the aorta. Target blood pressure is <120 mm Hg systolic, and a target heart rate is <60 beats per minute. Calcium channel blockers may be used for persons intolerant of β-blockers.
  - If the blood pressure remains elevated, then a vasodilator such as nitroprusside may be added in addition to a β-blocker.

FOLLOW-UP

- Lifelong blood pressure (BP) control is required post discharge. Goal BP is <120/80 mm Hg.
- Regular imaging is also required at 1, 3, 6 and 12 months after the initial event, looking for signs of aortic expansion, aneurysm formation, malperfusion and leakage at anastomotic sites. Thereafter, yearly imaging is recommended. CT or MRI is usually employed for follow-up imaging.
- Patient education regarding the signs and symptoms of recurrent dissection or potential postdissection complications is also recommended.

VIDEO LEGENDS

1. Video 7-1-1: Focused parasternal long axis view. There is a Type A dissection with a dissection flap visualized on this TTE.
2. Video 7-1-2: Parasternal long axis view with color Doppler demonstrating the dissection flap with significant AR due to the aortic dissection.
3. Video 7-1-3: Intraoperative TEE short axis view of the aorta. There is a type A dissection with a large mobile dissection flap. Note the dissection flap prolapsing across the AV.
4. Video 7-1-4: Intraoperative TEE short axis view of the aortic root and aortic valve with color Doppler. There is significant AR caused in part by the dissection flap prolapsing across the AV.
5. Video 7-1-5: Intraoperative TEE long axis view with color Doppler again demonstrating the dissection flap and associated AR.
6. Video 7-1-8: Intra-operative TEE image of another patient with a Type A dissection that extended in to the descending aorta. There is evidence (color Doppler) of flow in both lumens.

REFERENCES

1. Miller DC, Mitchell RS, Oyer PE, Stinson EB, Jamieson SW, Shumway NE. Independent determinants of operative mortality for patients with aortic dissections. *Circulation.* 1984;70(3 Pt 2): I153-164.
2. Clouse WD, Hallett JW Jr, Schaff HV, et al. Acute aortic dissection: population-based incidence compared with degenerative aortic aneurysm rupture. *Mayo Clin Proc.* Feb 2004;79(2):176-180.
3. Hiratzka LF, Bakris GL, Beckman JA, et al. 2010 ACCF/AHA/AATS/ACR/ASA/SCA/SCAI/SIR/STS/SVM guidelines for the diagnosis and management of patients with thoracic aortic disease. A report of the American College of Cardiology Foundation/American Heart Association Task Force on Practice Guidelines, American Association for Thoracic Surgery, American College of Radiology, American Stroke Association, Society of Cardiovascular Anesthesiologists, Society for Cardiovascular Angiography and Interventions, Society of Interventional Radiology, Society of Thoracic Surgeons, and Society for Vascular Medicine. *J Am Coll Cardiol.* 2010;55(14):e27-e129.
4. Sommer T, Fehske W, Holzknecht N, et al. Aortic dissection: a comparative study of diagnosis with spiral CT, multiplanar transesophageal echocardiography, and MR imaging. *Radiology.* 1996;199(2):347-352.
5. Erbel R, Engberding R, Daniel W, Roelandt J, Visser C, Rennollet H. Echocardiography in diagnosis of aortic dissection. *Lancet.* 1989;1(8636):457-461.
6. Rogers AM, Hermann LK, Booher AM, et al. Sensitivity of the aortic dissection detection risk score, a novel guideline-based tool for identification of acute aortic dissection at initial presentation: results from the international registry of acute aortic dissection. *Circulation.* 2011;123(20):2213-2218.

SECTION 2

Aortic Intramural Hematoma

CLINICAL CASE PRESENTATION

The patient is a 36-year-old woman who was driving home from a Thanksgiving party. She drove her car into a lamppost, and the steering wheel drove into her chest. When emergency services arrived, she was unconscious and had to be transferred to a nearby tertiary care hospital. She had several lacerations over her face and chest wall. A toxicology screen revealed a blood alcohol level over 3 times the legal limit. CT scan showed an unusual thickening of the lumen of her aortic arch and descending aorta. She was immediately taken to the operating room where the thickening was found to be an intramural hematoma in the arch of her aorta and extending down the proximal descending aorta. Intraoperative images are shown in Figures 7-2-1 to 7-2-3. She subsequently received a graft to the affected parts of her aorta and had a benign postoperative course. She was counseled extensively on the perils of driving while intoxicated.

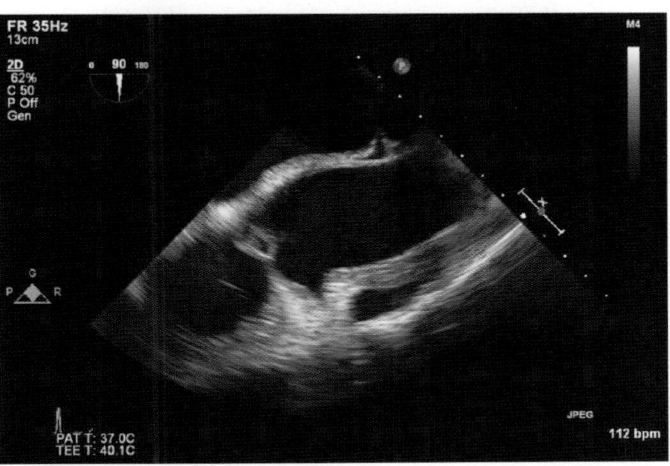

FIGURE 7-2-1 Intraoperative TEE. Long axis view of the proximal aorta demonstrating the intramural hematoma ► (see Video 7-2-1).

PATHOGENESIS

- A variant of an aortic dissection, an intramural hematoma may be present in the ascending aorta, arch, or descending aorta. It is usually characterized by the absence of an entry point and lack of flow within the tear. It usually measures at least 7 mm in width and extends longitudinally from 3 to 20 cm. It may be due to trauma (as in this case) or occur spontaneously.
- Rupture of the vasa vasorum within the aortic wall leads to an intramural hematoma.
- It can occur either spontaneously or due to trauma.

EPIDEMIOLOGY

- Constitutes 4% to 27% of cases originally diagnosed as a dissection.[1]
- In a meta-analysis, 61% were male.[2]

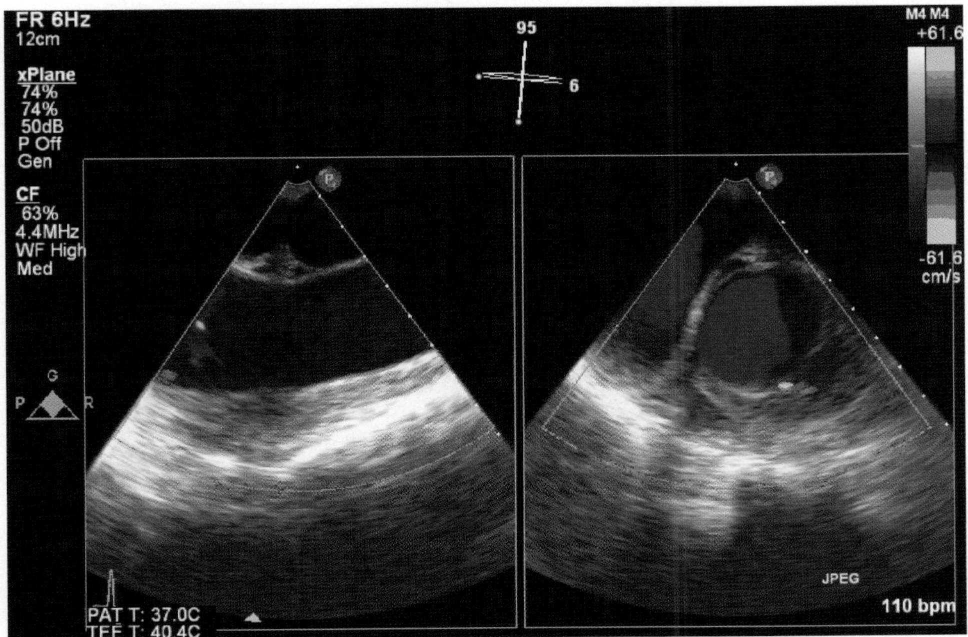

FIGURE 7-2-2 Intraoperative TEE Biplane view of the patient with an intramural hematoma on intraoperative TEE with color Doppler ► (see Video 7-2-2).

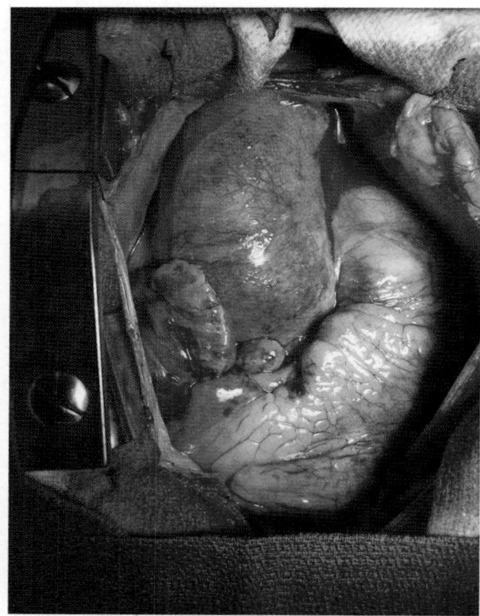

FIGURE 7-2-3 Intraoperative photo of the intramural hematoma taken by the surgeon at the time of surgical repair.

- The most common predisposing factor was hypertension.[3]
- Most cases occur in the descending aorta.[3]
- For traumatic intramural hematomas, the most common cause was a motor vehicle accident. The second leading cause was an intra-aortic balloon pump.[2]

NATURAL HISTORY

- May progress to dissection, aortic rupture, or aneurysm.[4,5]
- May regress or be resorbed.
- The most important factor favoring early progression (<30 days) was ascending aorta location.
- Factors favoring late progression were younger age and absence of β-blocker use during follow up.[5]

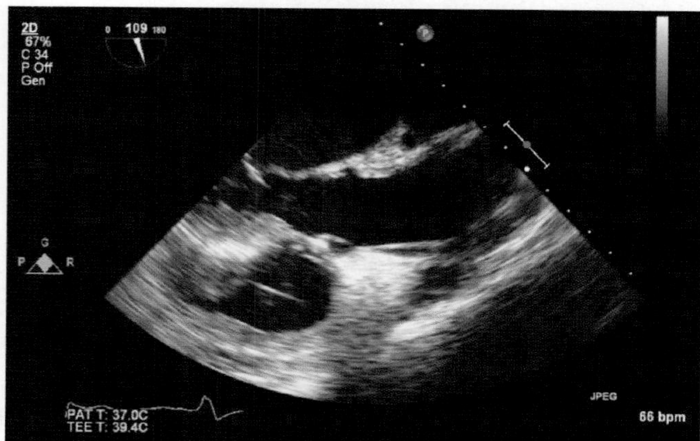

FIGURE 7-2-4 Intraoperative TEE demonstrating a spontaneous intramural hematoma (type A) in a different patient presenting with severe chest pain and a BP of 190/120 mm Hg. No dissection flap was seen. The patient underwent successful ascending aorta repair ▶ (see Video 7-2-4).

ECHOCARDIOGRAPHY

- The presence of focal crescentic thickening within the aortic wall, an eccentric aortic lumen, displaced intimal calcium and echolucent areas, and the absence of an intimal flap or an entry point all suggest the diagnosis of an intramural hematoma.[6] A traumatic intramural hematoma may be concentric rather than eccentric.
- Differential diagnosis includes aortic atherosclerosis, aortic aneurysm with thrombosis, and aortic dissection.
- The presence of a smooth rather than irregular surface and homogeneity rather than heterogeneity suggest intramural hematoma over atherosclerosis. Extension of the thickening for >5 cm suggests hematoma rather than atherosclerosis.[2]
- Thickening beneath the bright echodense intima suggests an intramural hematoma, while thickening above it suggests thrombosis within the aorta.

MANAGEMENT

- Intramural hematoma without intimal rupture should be managed similar to aortic dissection of the corresponding aortic segment.[7] Surgery is recommended for type A intramural hematoma. Aggressive medical therapy (pain control and optimization of blood pressure) is recommended for initial management of type B intramural hematoma.

FOLLOW-UP

- Careful attention to blood pressure control and the management of concomitant risk factors, especially the treatment of dyslipidemia, is warranted.
- See Section I, Acute Aortic Dissection, for further recommendations.

VIDEO LEGENDS

1. Video 7-2-1: Intraoperative TEE. Long axis view of the proximal aorta demonstrating the intramural hematoma.
2. Video 7-2-2: Intraoperative TEE Biplane view of the patient with an intramural hematoma on intraoperative TEE with color Doppler.
3. Video 7-2-4: Intra-operative TEE demonstrating a spontaneous intramural hematoma (Type A) in a different patient presenting with severe chest pain and a BP = 190/120. No dissection flap was seen. The patient underwent successful ascending aorta repair.

REFERENCES

1. Sawhney NS, DeMaria AN, Blanchard DG. Aortic intramural hematoma: an increasingly recognized and potentially fatal entity. *Chest.* 2001;120(4):1340-1346.
2. Maraj R, Rerkpattanapipat P, Jacobs LE, Makornwattana P, Kotler MN. Meta-analysis of 143 reported cases of aortic intramural hematoma. *Am J Cardiol.* 2000;86(6):664-668.
3. Ganaha F, Miller DC, Sugimoto K, et al. Prognosis of aortic intramural hematoma with and without penetrating atherosclerotic ulcer: a clinical and radiological analysis. *Circulation.* 2002;106(3):342-348.

4. Evangelista A, Mukherjee D, Mehta RH, et al. Acute intramural hematoma of the aorta: a mystery in evolution. *Circulation.* 2005;111(8):1063-1070.
5. von Kodolitsch Y, Csosz SK, Koschyk DH, et al. Intramural hematoma of the aorta: predictors of progression to dissection and rupture. *Circulation.* 2003;107(8):1158-1163.
6. Harris KM, Braverman AC, Gutierrez FR, Barzilai B, Davila-Roman VG. Transesophageal echocardiographic and clinical features of aortic intramural hematoma. *Journal Thorac Cardiovasc Surg.* 1997;114(4):619-626.
7. Hiratzka LF, Bakris GL, Beckman JA, et al. 2010 ACCF/AHA/AATS/ACR/ASA/SCA/SCAI/SIR/STS/SVM guidelines for the diagnosis and management of patients with thoracic aortic disease. A report of the American College of Cardiology Foundation/American Heart Association Task Force on Practice Guidelines, American Association for Thoracic Surgery, American College of Radiology, American Stroke Association, Society of Cardiovascular Anesthesiologists, Society for Cardiovascular Angiography and Interventions, Society of Interventional Radiology, Society of Thoracic Surgeons, and Society for Vascular Medicine. *J Am Coll Cardiol.* 2010;55(14):e27-e129.

SECTION 3

Aortic Atherosclerosisand Atherosclerotic Debris

CLINICAL CASE PRESENTATION

The patient is a 60-year-old man with a past history of hypertension who had had several episodes of transient blindness affecting his left eye. Each episode of blindness lasted anywhere from 20 minutes to an hour. Concerned, he mentioned this to his family physician who immediately referred him to a Neurologist. A CT of the brain was obtained and was unremarkable, as was a carotid duplex scan. A TEE was ordered to assess for a potential cardiac source of embolism. There was evidence of mild left ventricular hypertrophy. There was no evidence of intracardiac thrombus, spontaneous contrast, or shunting. There was, however, extensive atherosclerotic disease of the aorta with plaque extending more than 5 mm into the lumen of the descending aorta. The ascending aorta and arch also had extensive plaque with a mobile component to one plaque seen in the arch, most likely representing superimposed thrombus on an ulcerated plaque (Figures 7-3-1 and 7-3-2). The patient was treated with a combination of statin therapy and aspirin. He has had no clinically evident recurrent events.

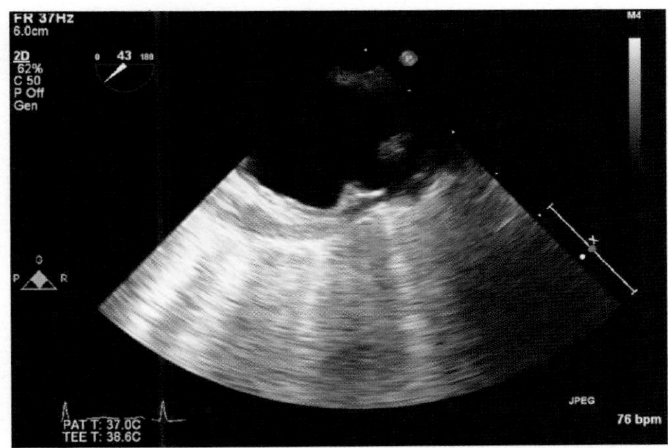

FIGURE 7-3-1 TEE image of the aortic arch in our patient demonstrating complex plaque in the aortic arch with mobile debris ► (see Video 7-3-1).

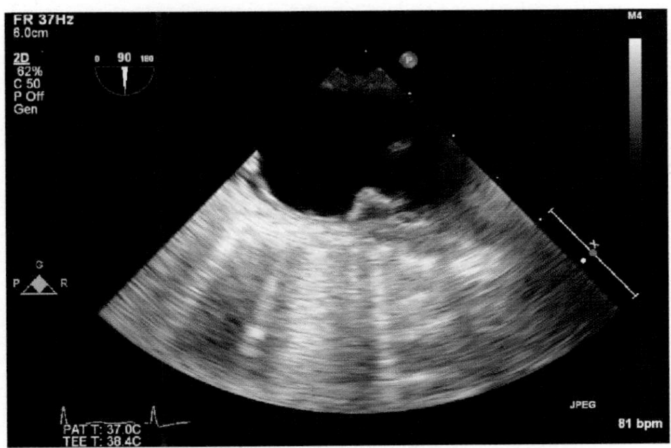

FIGURE 7-3-2 Another TEE image from this patient demonstrating mobile debris in the arch, the most likely cause of this patient's neurologic event ► (see Video 7-3-2).

CLINICAL FEATURES AND NATURAL HISTORY

- Most patients are asymptomatic. They may be symptomatic from concomitant coronary, cerebral, or peripheral vascular disease.
- Atherosclerotic disease of the aorta may be an incidental finding during imaging of the aorta or during work-up for a cardiac source of embolus.
- The natural history of atherosclerosis is one of slowly progressive inflammation with gradual formation of plaque occurring over several decades. Atherosclerotic plaque may be classified in the following ways:
  - Complex plaque is defined as plaque extending ≥4 mm into the aortic lumen, or which has a thrombotic component, or has a mobile component. Simple plaque is the absence of any of these features.

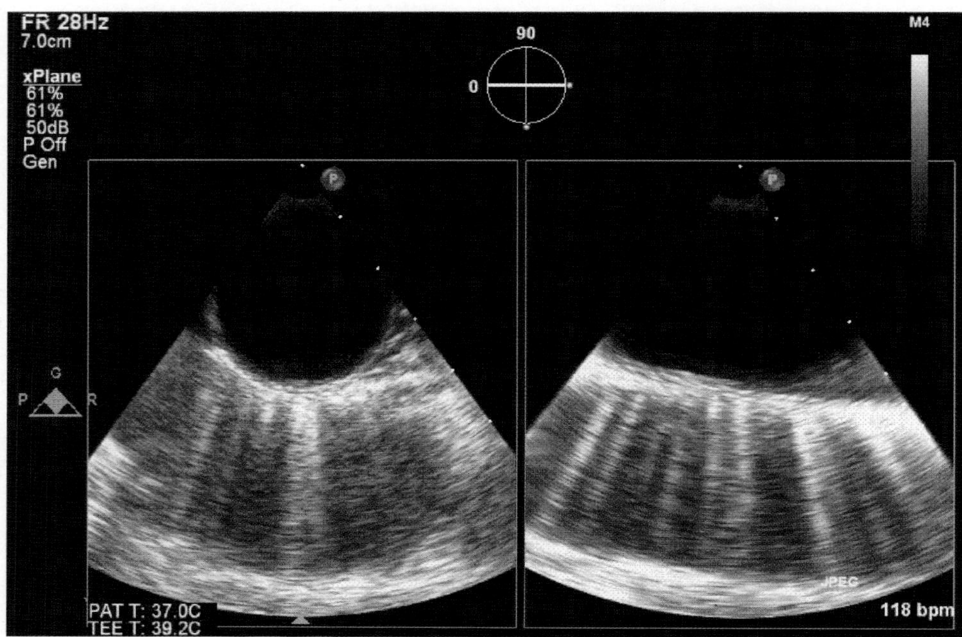

FIGURE 7-3-3 Aortic atheroma grade 1 (normal aortic intima).

- Ribakov's classification (Figures 7-3-3 to 7-3-7)
  - Grade 1: No disease or intimal thickening
  - Grade 2: Intimal thickening
  - Grade 3: Atheroma <5 mm
  - Grade 4: Atheroma >5 mm
  - Grade 5: Mobile atheroma
  - In a transesophageal study of the natural history of atheromatous disease of the thoracic aorta, 67% of lesions remained stable by atheroma grade; however, dynamic changes in individual lesions were noted. Of patients with grade 5 disease in this study, while 57% no longer had the initial mobile component present on follow-up, all had evidence of new mobile lesions.[1]

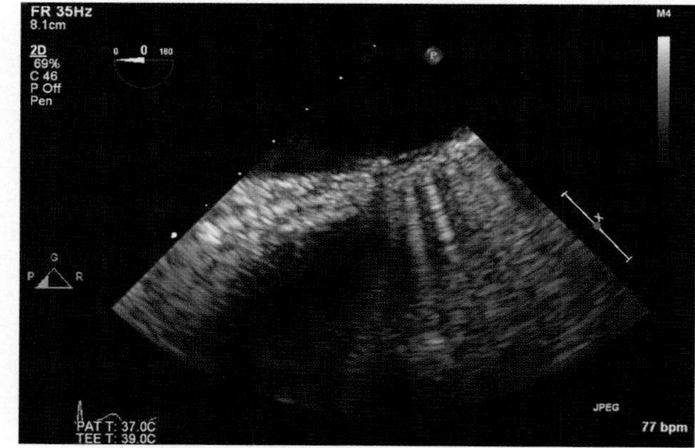

FIGURE 7-3-4 Aortic atheroma grade 2 ► (see Video 7-3-4).

EPIDEMIOLOGY

- In one study of 588 randomly sampled subjects aged ≥45 years, the incidence of simple and complex plaque were 43.7% and 7.6% respectively.[2]
- The incidence and severity of aortic atheroma increases with age with severe atheroma seen in >20% of patients older than 74 years.[2,3]
- Ulcerated plaque was noted in 28% of patients who died of cerebrovascular disease compared with 5% of patients dying of other neurological disease.[3]
- Identification of plaque ≥4 mm is associated with a nine-fold increase in risk for ischemic stroke.[4] The odds ratio for stroke or peripheral embolism in patients with aortic atheroma is 4.0. This increases in patients with mobile plaque to 12.[3]
- Other risk factors for stroke are: noncalcified plaque (odds ratio: 10.3)[4,5] and ascending aorta location.

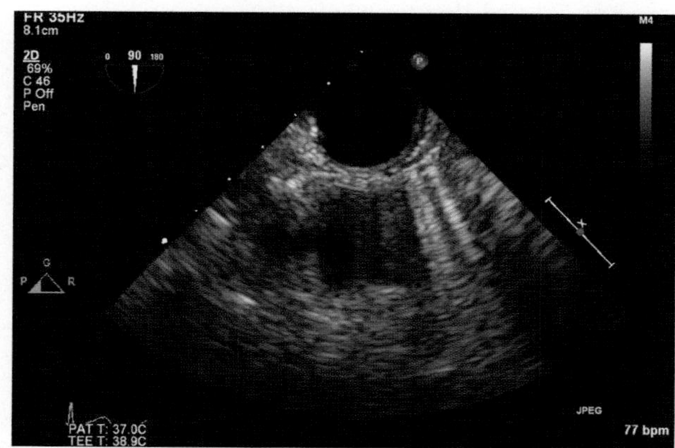

FIGURE 7-3-5 Aortic atheroma grade 3 ► (see Video 7-3-5).

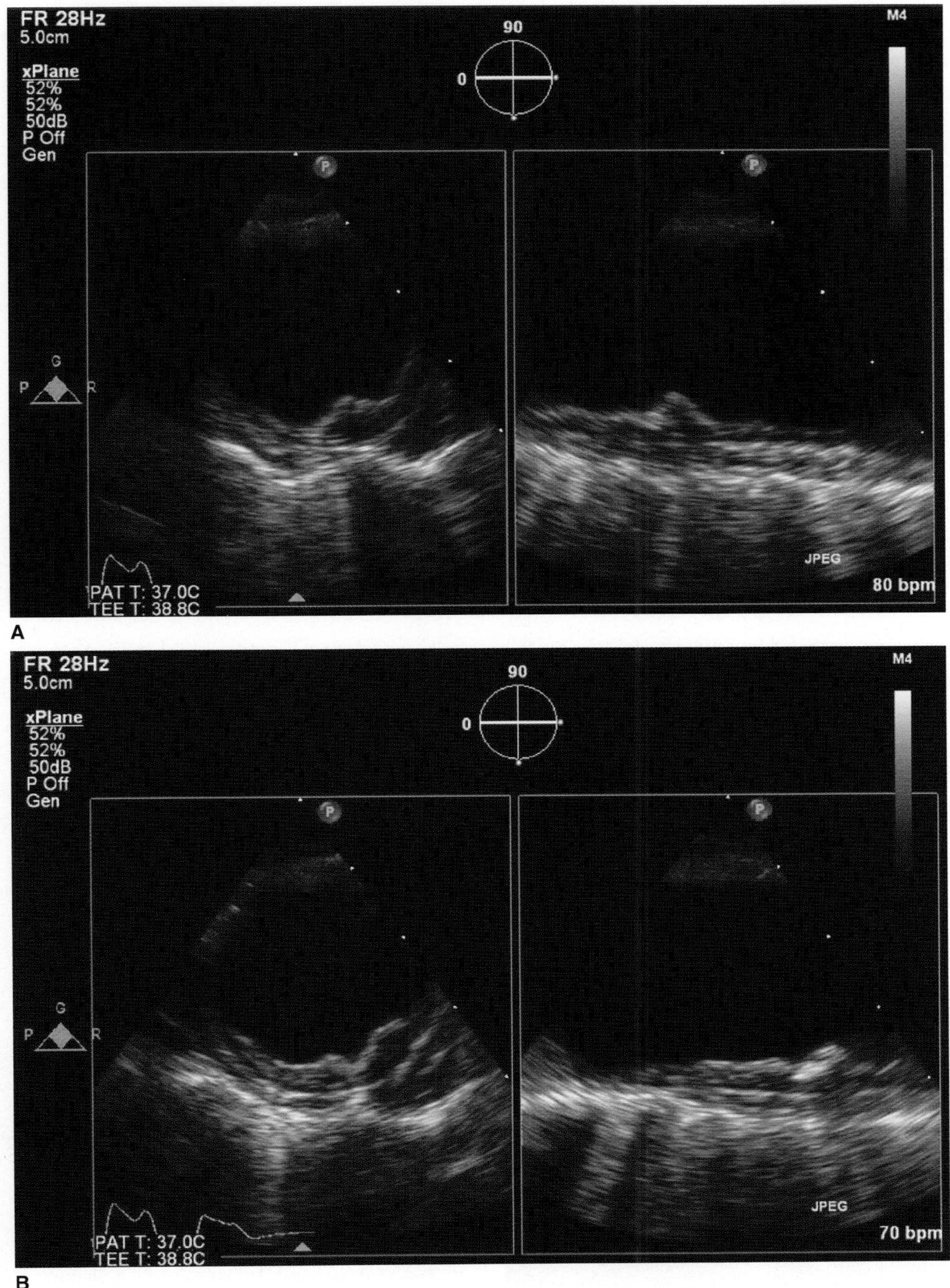

FIGURE 7-3-6 (A/B) Aortic atheroma grade 4. Note the raised, somewhat ulcerated plaque in these 2 examples of grade 4 atheroma ▶ (see Videos 7-3-6 A and B).

ECHOCARDIOGRAPHY

- Transthoracic echo is rather insensitive for the detection of atherosclerotic aortic disease.
- Aortic plaque is usually seen as an area of intimal thickening and in complex plaque may protrude into the aortic lumen. Thrombus, ulceration, or calcification may also be seen.
- TEE provides excellent visualization of most of the thoracic aorta. Compared to other imaging modalities, it has the advantage of ease of use and portability, is not limited in patients with renal insufficiency, and can be used in patients with pacemakers. It also has the advantage of being able to visualize the mobile components of a plaque.
- Transesophageal echocardiography has a “blind spot” at the junction of the ascending aorta and the arch corresponding to the crossover of the trachea.
- Epiaortic ultrasonography is often used intraoperatively. It can influence the decision to perform surgery with or without cardiopulmonary bypass (off-pump or on-pump) and in guiding the placement of aortic cannulas prior to surgery.

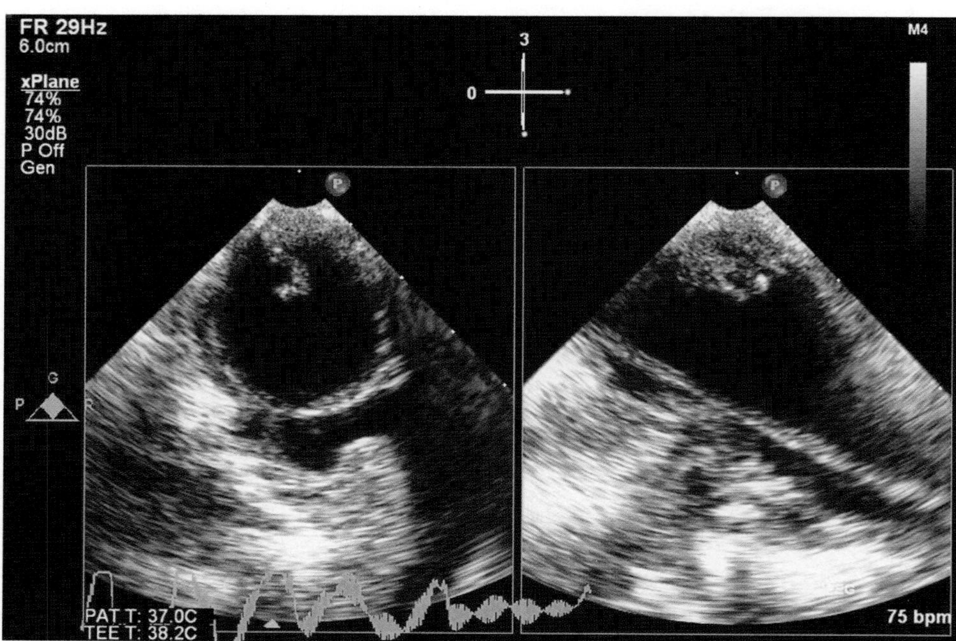

FIGURE 7-3-7 Aortic atheroma grade 5. Note the mobile debris in this x-plane view of the descending aorta ▶ (see Video 7-3-7).

- The use of epiaortic ultrasound guided on-pump coronary artery bypass grafting has been associated with a significant reduction in stroke.

DIAGNOSIS

- The diagnosis of aortic atherosclerosis is made by demonstrating the presence of plaque with imaging. Ulceration and superimposed thrombus can also be detected.

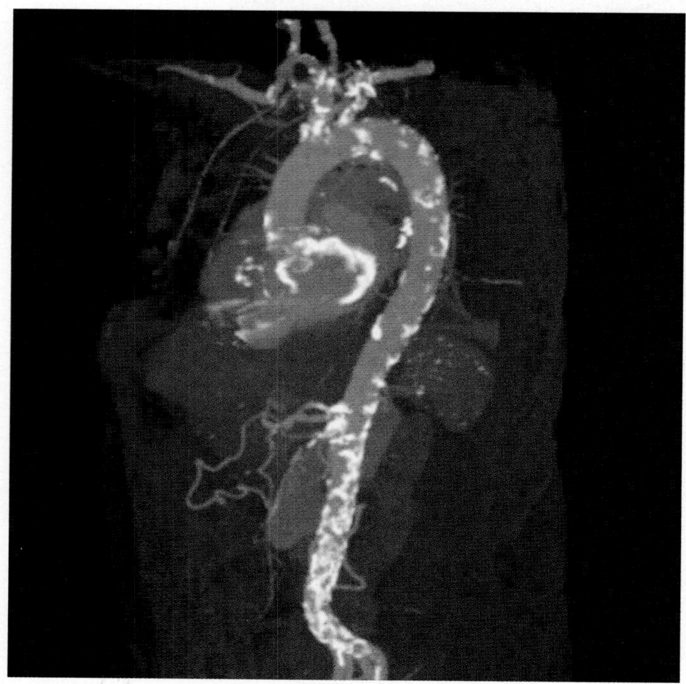

FIGURE 7-3-8 Three-dimensional CT angiogram demonstrating extensive aortic calcification.

OTHER DIAGNOSTIC IMAGING MODALITIES

- Both MR angiography and CT scanning can detect aortic atherosclerosis and can define the entire aorta and the peripheral vasculature.
- Intraoperative imaging with epiaortic ultrasonography is employed as previously discussed.

MANAGEMENT

- Management of the results of the atheroembolic process (stroke/TIA/peripheral embolism) depends on the organ system involved.
- There are no randomized trials demonstrating the benefit of any one therapy.
- Nonrandomized trials have demonstrated favorable results with the use of both oral anticoagulants and antiplatelet agents.[6]
- Statins have been shown to reduce plaque volume following 6 months of therapy.[7]
- At our institution, most patients are treated with antiplatelet therapy and statins, as well as control of other risk factors such as hypertension and diabetes. Smoking cessation is also critical.

FOLLOW-UP

- Patients should be educated as to the signs and symptoms of embolic events.
- Treatment of underlying risk factors should be emphasized, including the critical role of smoking cessation.
- Serial imaging is rarely indicated.

VIDEO LEGENDS

1. Video 7-3-1: TEE image of the aortic arch in our patient demonstrating complex plaque in the aortic arch with mobile debris.
2. Video 7-3-2: Another TEE image from this patient again demonstrating mobile debris in the arch, the most likely cause of this patient's neurologic event
3. Video 7-3-4: Aortic atheroma Grade 2
4. Video 7-3-5: Aortic atheroma Grade 3
5. Video 7-3-6 A: Aortic atheroma Grade 4. Note the raised, somewhat ulcerated plaque in this example of Grade 4 atheroma
6. Video 7-3-6 B: Aortic atheroma Grade 4. Note the raised, somewhat ulcerated plaque in this example of Grade 4 atheroma
7. Video 7-3-7: Aortic atheroma Grade 5. Note the mobile debris in this X-plane view of the descending aorta.

REFERENCES

1. Montgomery DH, Ververis JJ, McGorisk G, Frohwein S, Martin RP, Taylor WR. Natural history of severe atheromatous disease of the thoracic aorta: a transesophageal echocardiographic study. *J Am Coll Cardiol.* 1996;27(1):95-101.
2. Meissner I, Khandheria BK, Sheps SG, et al. Atherosclerosis of the aorta: risk factor, risk marker, or innocent bystander? A prospective population-based transesophageal echocardiography study. *J Am Coll Cardiol.* 2004;44(5):1018-1024.
3. Macleod MR, Amarenco P, Davis SM, Donnan GA. Atheroma of the aortic arch: an important and poorly recognised factor in the aetiology of stroke. *Lancet Neurol.* 2004;3(7):408-414.
4. Amarenco P, Cohen A, Tzourio C, et al. Atherosclerotic disease of the aortic arch and the risk of ischemic stroke. *New Engl J Med.* Dec 1 1994;331(22):1474-1479.
5. Gottsegen JM, Coplan NL. The atherosclerotic aortic arch: considerations in diagnostic imaging. *Prev Cardiol.* 2008;11(3):162-167.
6. Dressler FA, Craig WR, Castello R, Labovitz AJ. Mobile aortic atheroma and systemic emboli: efficacy of anticoagulation and influence of plaque morphology on recurrent stroke. *J Am Coll Cardiol.* 1998;31(1):134-138.
7. Lima JA, Desai MY, Steen H, Warren WP, Gautam S, Lai S. Statin-induced cholesterol lowering and plaque regression after 6 months of magnetic resonance imaging-monitored therapy. *Circulation.* 2004;110(16):2336-2341.

SECTION 4

Marfan Syndrome

CLINICAL CASE PRESENTATION

A 20-year-old man was brought to the ED with sudden onset tearing chest pain, which caused him to lose consciousness briefly. His mother found him and called 911. On arrival, he was a 6'4" tall, thin young man in obvious pain. His blood pressure was 82/31 mm Hg, and his pulse was thready. His father had had a similar presentation at about the same age that resulted in surgery. On examination, he wore glasses, had retrognathia, and an unusually prominent chest wall. Auscultation revealed a high-pitched diastolic murmur best heard along the left sternal border leaning forward in expiration. He had scars over his lower abdominal wall due to two previous hernia repairs. An ECG showed no ST segment changes and troponin levels were minimally elevated. An emergent echocardiogram was obtained. The images were suboptimal due to his chest wall deformity, but demonstrated normal LV function. An ill-defined linear echo density adjacent to the aortic wall was noted (Figure 7-4-1). Given the patient's hemodynamic instability and the clinical suspicion for an acute aortic dissection, the patient was taken directly to the operating room, where a TEE confirmed the diagnosis. He underwent a Bentall operation with a mechanical valve/conduit. Postoperatively, he made an uneventful recovery and was discharged on a β-blocker and warfarin. A diagnosis of Marfan syndrome was made. His other first-degree relatives were evaluated; none were diagnosed with Marfan syndrome.

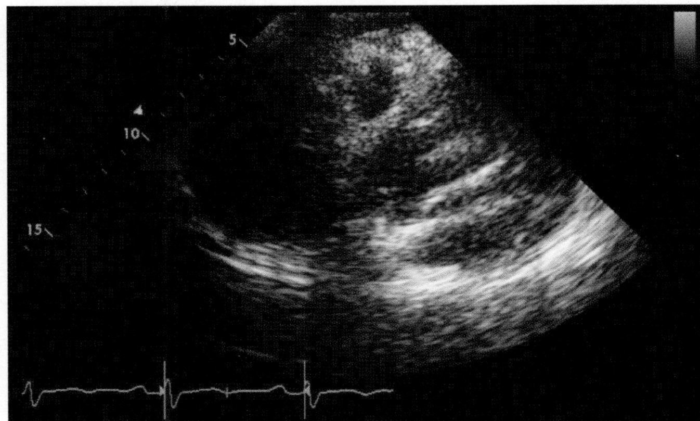

FIGURE 7-4-1 Limited TTE view of the patient with findings suspicious for a dissection.

NATURAL HISTORY OF AORTOPATHY IN MARFAN SYNDROME

- Death is usually due to aortic dissection. Factors favoring dissection include:
  - Aortic diameter >5.0 cm
  - Increase in diameter of >5% per year or 2 mm/year in the adult
  - Dilation beyond the sinuses
  - Family history of dissection

EPIDEMIOLOGY

- The prevalence of Marfan syndrome is estimated to be between 4.6/100,000[1,2] to 1-2/10,000 people.[3]
- Risk of dissection and death is 0.17% per year and increases with increasing aortic diameter from 0.09% per year with an aortic diameter of <40 mm to 0.3% per year with aortic diameters of 45 to 49 mm to 1.33% per year with diameters of 50 to 54 mm.[4]

PATHOPHYSIOLOGY AND ETIOLOGY

- Marfan syndrome is inherited as an autosomal dominant disorder. Up to 25% of cases may be due to sporadic mutation.
- There is usually a mutation in the fibrillin-1 gene. This can lead to alterations in the extracellular matrix of the microfibrillar apparatus with stiffening of the aorta. Multiple possible mutations exist, and there is no correlation between mutations and phenotypic expression. The disease is highly penetrant but has highly variable phenotypic expression.

ECHOCARDIOGRAPHY

- Both transthoracic and transesophageal echocardiography are useful in the evaluation and management of the patient with known or suspected Marfan syndrome (Figures 7-4-2 to 7-4-7).
    - TTE can detect proximal aortic involvement and abnormalities of the mitral valve/annulus.
    - TEE is better suited to visualize more of the aorta and is more sensitive for the diagnosis of an aortic dissection.
- Dilation of the ascending aorta up to the sinuses is suggestive of Marfan syndrome as is a type A dissection in a young person.
- Other features detected with echocardiography include:
    - Dilation of the pulmonary artery in the absence of valvular or peripheral pulmonic stenosis in a patient less than age 40.
    - Mitral valve prolapse with or without regurgitation
    - Mitral annular calcification in a patient less than age 40.
    - Aneurysm and/or dissection of the descending thoracic or abdominal aorta in a patient less than age 50.

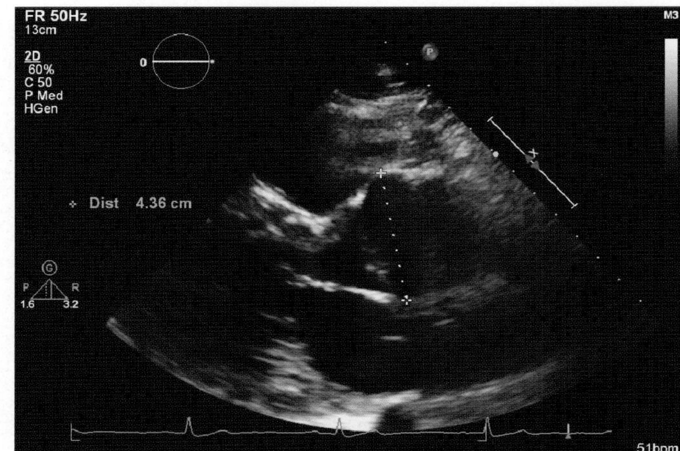

FIGURE 7-4-3 TTE image of the aorta in a patient with Marfan syndrome showing moderate aortic dilation.

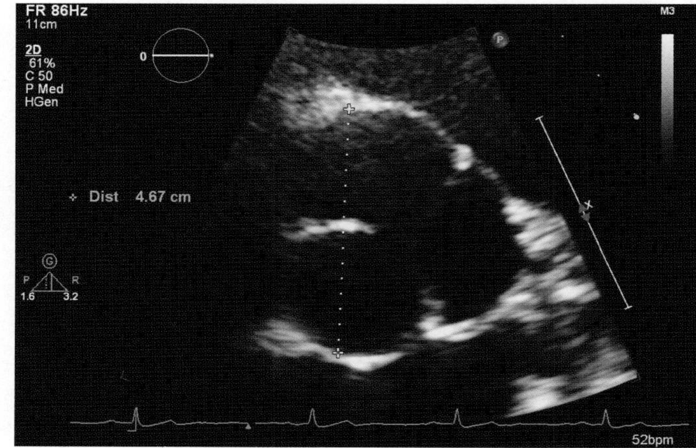

FIGURE 7-4-4 TEE image of the aortic root (short axis) in a patient with Marfan syndrome demonstrating aortic dilation.

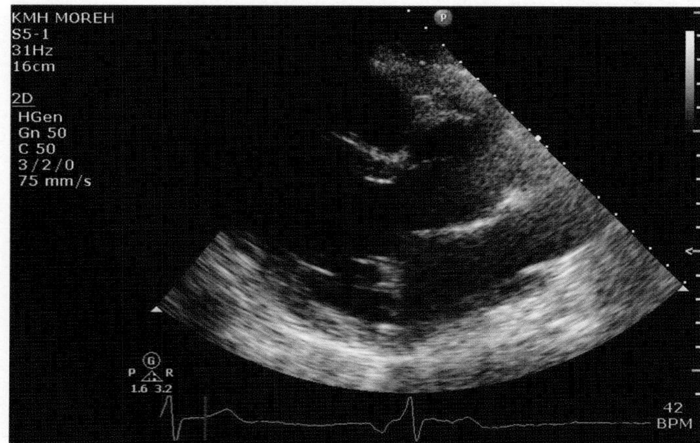

FIGURE 7-4-2 TTE parasternal long axis view of a patient with Marfan syndrome demonstrating mild mitral valve prolapse involving the posterior leaflet. The aortic root is also dilated. ► (see Video 7-4-2).

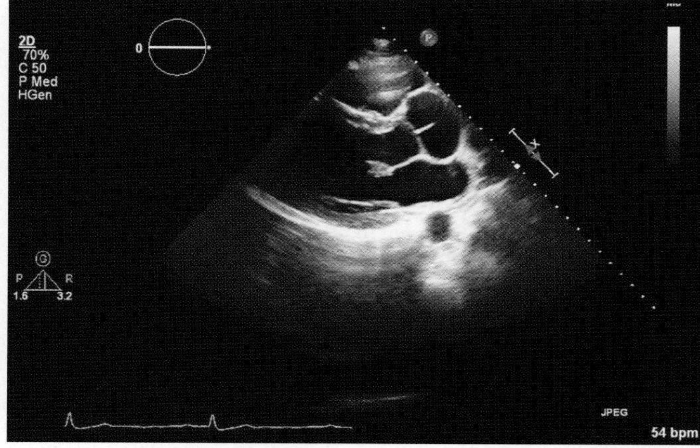

FIGURE 7-4-5 Parasternal long axis view (TTE) demonstrating a "teardrop" shaped, dilated aortic root as well as a thickened MV that prolapses ► (see Video 7-4-5).

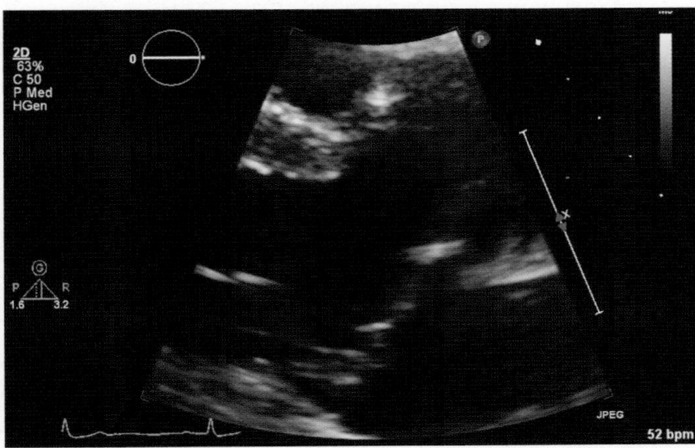

FIGURE 7-4-6 Bi-leaflet MVP in another patient with Marfan syndrome. In contrast to the other patients, this individual has a normal aorta ▶ (see Video 7-4-6).

OTHER IMAGING MODALITIES

- As is the case with other aortopathies, CT angiography and MRA of the aorta can be used to evaluate the aorta in order to detect aortic involvement in a patient with suspected Marfan syndrome.

DIAGNOSIS

- The diagnosis of Marfan syndrome requires examination by an orthopedic surgeon, cardiologist, and ophthalmologist with possible input from a geneticist.
- The Ghent diagnostic criteria are used to diagnose Marfan syndrome clinically.
- It includes major and/or minor criteria in:
  - The cardiovascular system
  - The skeletal system
  - The eyes
  - The lungs
  - The skin
  - The dura mater
  - Family history
- The clinical diagnosis of Marfan syndrome requires the presence of major criteria in two organ systems and involvement of a third organ system.
- In a patient with a family history of Marfan syndrome in a first-degree relative, a major criterion in one organ system with involvement of a second organ system is all that is required for diagnosis.

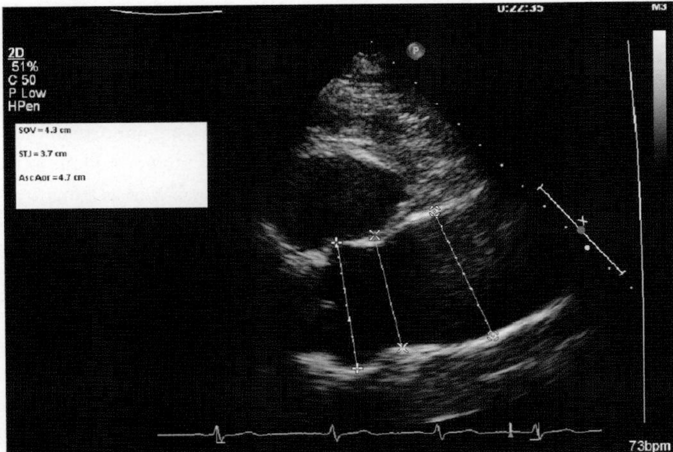

FIGURE 7-4-7 Marfan patient with aortic dilation. In this case, the ascending aorta is larger than the sinuses of Valsalva.

MANAGEMENT

- Medical management is a multi-specialty approach involving the cardiologist, ophthalmologist, orthopedist, and geneticist.
- Medical management includes the use of β-blockade to reduce the risk of aortic dilation.
- TTE can be used to assess the mitral valve, aortic valve, aortic root, and proximal ascending aorta.
- The entire aorta should be imaged. CT angiography or MRA can be used for long-term serial assessment of the aorta. In cases where there are contraindications to these tests (eg, contrast allergy, renal insufficiency, pacemakers), TEE can be employed.
- Patients are advised not to smoke, to control their blood pressure, and not to participate in full-contact sports.
- When the aortic root reaches a diameter of ≥5.0 cm, surgery is recommended.
- Surgery involves replacement of the aortic root/arch with or without sparing of the valve, depending on the presence and severity of aortic regurgitation.
- Screening of first-degree relatives of an index patient is recommended.

PATIENT EDUCATION AND FOLLOW-UP

- Patients should be informed of the genetic nature of their condition.
- Education regarding the signs/symptoms of aortic dissection is imperative.
- The importance of periodic assessment of their cardiovascular status should be stressed.

VIDEO LEGENDS

1. Video 7-4-2: TTE parasternal long axis view of a patient with Marfan syndrome demonstrating mild mitral valve prolapse involving the posterior leaflet. The aortic root is also dilated
2. Video 7-4-5: Parasternal long axis view (TTE) demonstrating a "tear-drop" shaped, dilated aortic root as well as a thickened MV which prolapses
3. Video 7-4-6: Bi-leaflet MVP in another patient with Marfan syndrome. In contrast to the other patients, this individual has a normal aorta

REFERENCES

1. Fuchs J. Marfan syndrome and other systemic disorders with congenital ectopia lentis. A Danish national survey. *Acta Paediatr.* 1997;86(9):947-952.
2. Gray JR, Bridges AB, Faed MJ, et al. Ascertainment and severity of Marfan syndrome in a Scottish population. *J Med Genet.* 1994;31(1):51-54.
3. Pyeritz RE. The Marfan syndrome. *Annu Rev Med.* 2000;51:481-510.
4. Jondeau G, Detaint D, Tubach F, et al. Aortic event rate in the Marfan population: a cohort study. *Circulation.* 2012;125(2):226-232.

SECTION 5

Aortopathy in Bicuspid Aortic Valve Disease

CLINICAL CASE PRESENTATION

The patient is a 50-year-old cardiologist. During physical examination classes in his medical school he noticed he had an unusual high-pitched diastolic murmur best heard over the aortic area that radiated down the left side of his sternum. Intrigued, he obtained an M-mode echocardiogram of his heart once the technology was available and noticed a mildly dilated aortic root and eccentric coaptation of his aortic leaflets. Once 2-D echocardiography became available, he underwent an echocardiogram which demonstrated systolic doming of the aortic valve leaflets. The valve was bicuspid with fusion of the right and left coronary cusps with a midline raphe. There was mild to moderate aortic regurgitation. He has remained asymptomatic but has yearly echocardiograms to monitor the size of his aortic root.

NATURAL HISTORY

- The size of the aorta in children with a bicuspid aortic valve is greater than in children without.
- The rate of dilation of the aorta is greater the larger the size at baseline.
- The median increase in aortic sinus dimension was found to be 0.2 mm/year in patients with a bicuspid aortic valve.[1]
- Risk factors for dilation include: age, male sex, systolic blood pressure, and significant valve disease.[1]
- The rate of dissection is 0.1% per patient year of follow-up[1] and usually involves the ascending aorta.

EPIDEMIOLOGY

- Bicuspid aortic valve is the most common congenital heart defect and has an overall prevalence of 1% to 2%
- Fusion of the right and left cusps occurs in 80% of bicuspid aortic valves, and fusion of the right and noncoronary occurs in 20%. Fusion of the left and noncoronary is exceedingly rare.
- There is a 9- to 18-fold higher incidence of aortic aneurysms in individuals with bicuspid aortic valve.[2]
- The high incidence of familial clustering is compatible with autosomal dominant inheritance with reduced penetrance.[3]

PATHOGENESIS

- Bicuspid aortic valve is associated with several complications, including valvular stenosis and regurgitation (see Chapter 3, Echocardiographic Assessment of Valvular Heart Disease), as well as aortic pathology including aortic dilation, aortic aneurysm and aortic dissection, and coarctation of the aorta.
- The condition is associated with Erdheims cystic medial necrosis, which consists of the triad of:
  - Noninflammatory loss of smooth muscle cells
  - Fragmentation of elastic fibers
  - Accumulation of basophilic ground substance within the medial wall
- There is loss of smooth muscle cells in the aortic media and matrix disruption leading to accelerated degeneration of the media.
- Familial studies suggest a genetic predisposition, and bicuspid aortic valve may be due to more than one genetic mutation with different patterns of inheritance.
- Aortic dilation may manifest in patients with bicuspid aortic valve without evidence of stenosis or regurgitation, and up to 50% of patients with normally functioning bicuspid aortic valves have echocardiographic evidence of aortic dilation.[4]

DIAGNOSIS OF AORTOPATHY AND ASSOCIATED CONDITIONS

- This involves identification of some of the associated abnormalities associated with a bicuspid aortic valve. This includes dilation/aneurysm of the aortic root and ascending aorta as well as aortic coarctation.
- On physical examination, patients with aortic regurgitation may have a wide pulse pressure. A high-pitched diastolic murmur best heard over the left sternal border leaning forward in expiration may be appreciated. With aortic stenosis, a systolic ejection murmur radiating to the carotids with a fourth heart sound, split second heart sound, and soft aortic component of the second heart sounds may be heard. The pulse is usually described as slow rising (pulsus parvus et retardus) with severe AS. An ejection click may be appreciated.

ECHOCARDIOGRAPHY

- Transthoracic echo and Doppler echocardiography are well suited to evaluate the aortic valve, proximal ascending aorta, and in some individuals, the aortic arch and descending aorta.
  - M-mode echocardiography may demonstrate a dilated aortic root and asymmetric coaptation point of the AV closure line, suggesting a bicuspid aortic valve.
  - Two-dimensional echocardiogram in the parasternal long axis view may show systolic doming of the aortic valve or prolapse of one of the cusps.
  - Diagnosis rests upon viewing the valve cusps in systole in the parasternal short axis view. This helps differentiate a bicuspid aortic valve with a raphe from a normal tricuspid valve or a unicuspid valve.
  - Doppler echocardiography is employed to assess aortic valve hemodynamics (stenosis and regurgitation) and can be used to detect a systolic gradient in the descending aorta, indicative of coarctation.
- Transesophageal echocardiography may better visualize the aortic valve morphology.
  - TEE is often better suited to assess the aorta in terms of the presence and extent of dilation, aneurysm, dissection, or coarctation.

ALTERNATE IMAGING MODALITIES

- Similar to the evaluation of other aortopathies, MRA and CT angiography may be employed.
- A chest x-ray may demonstrate a widened mediastinum with dilation of the ascending aorta and arch.

MANAGEMENT

- Serial assessment of the aortic valve by echocardiography is essential. The frequency of serial assessment depends on the degree of insufficiency or stenosis and the left ventricular chamber size/function (see Chapter 3, Echocardiographic Assessment of Valvular Heart Disease).
- Indications for aortic valve replacement are discussed in Chapter 3, Echocardiographic Assessment of Valvular Heart Disease.
- Aortic root dilation should be carefully monitored by echocardiography, CT angiography, or MRA.
- Aortic root replacement is recommended earlier (4-5 cm) than for patients with a tricuspid valve (5-6 cm).[5]
- The benefit of β-blockers to prevent aortic dilation in bicuspid aortopathy is not clear, but hypertension should be treated.[6]

PATIENT EDUCATION AND FOLLOW-UP

- Patients should be educated concerning the signs and symptoms of acute aortic syndromes such as dissection and should be promptly evaluated in an emergency department if such symptoms develop.
- Since symptoms may mimic a myocardial infarction, patients should inform emergency department staff of their diagnosis, as conventional treatment for a myocardial infarction can be devastating for patients with a dissection.

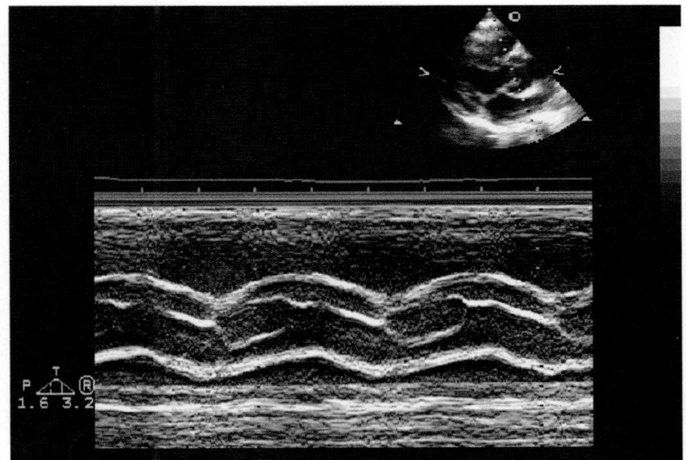

FIGURE 7-5-1 M-mode of the patient demonstrating a minimally dilated aortic root and eccentric closure of the AV.

- Patients must understand the need for serial clinical evaluations and imaging.
- Serial assessment of the aorta is usually performed with MRA or CT angiography (unless contraindicated). In those cases, TEE may be employed.

VIDEO LEGENDS

1. Video 7-5-2: Bicuspid aortic valve in the parasternal short axis view
2. Video 7-5-5: Associated coarctation of the aorta in a different patient with a bicuspid aortic valve: Suprasternal notch view of the arch and upper descending aorta with color Doppler
3. Video 7-5-9: Parasternal long axis view of a different patient with a severely dilated aortic root (7 cm) who presented with congestive heart failure from chronic AR. Note the dilated, hypokinetic LV.

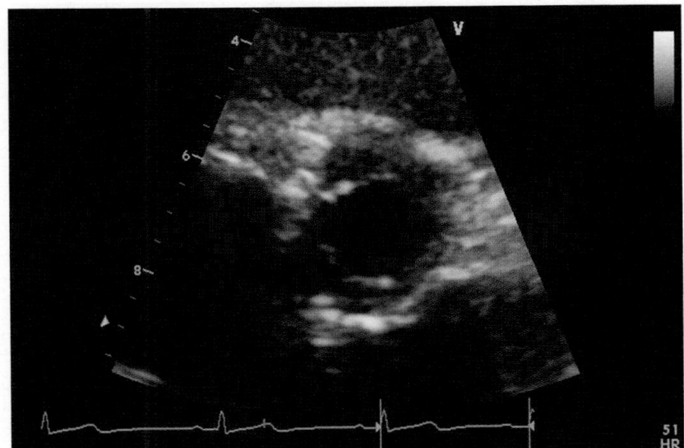

FIGURE 7-5-2 Bicuspid aortic valve in a parasternal short axis view ► (see Video 7-5-2).

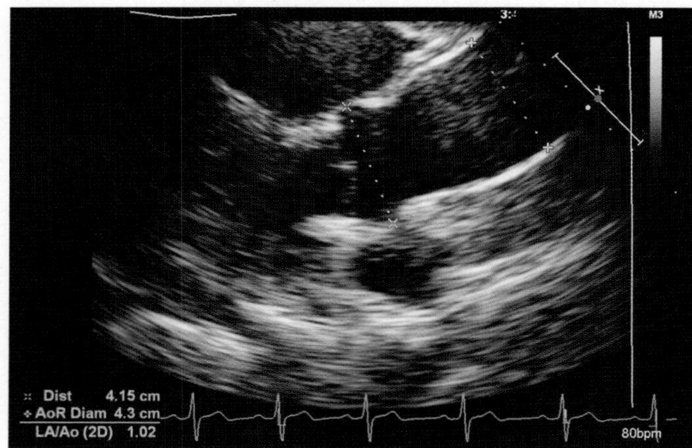

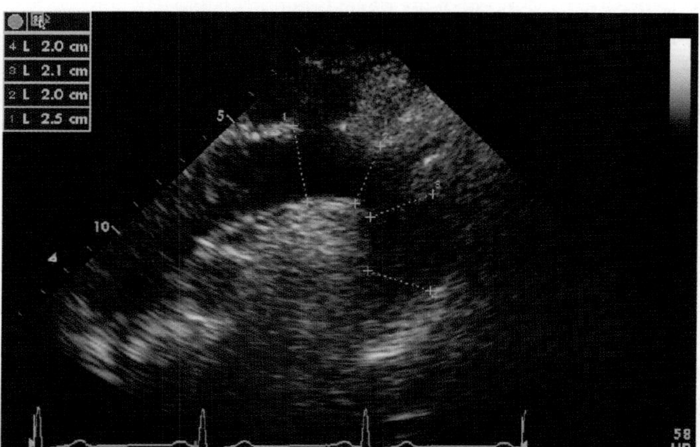

FIGURE 7-5-3 Recent TTE images from our patient. The dilated aortic root and ascending aorta are noted, and dimensions have been stable (top panel). The arch and descending aorta are normal (bottom panel).

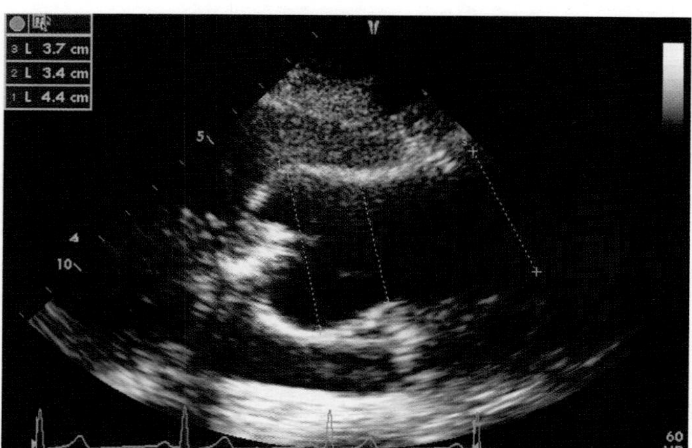

FIGURE 7-5-4 TTE image from another patient demonstrating more significant aortic enlargement.

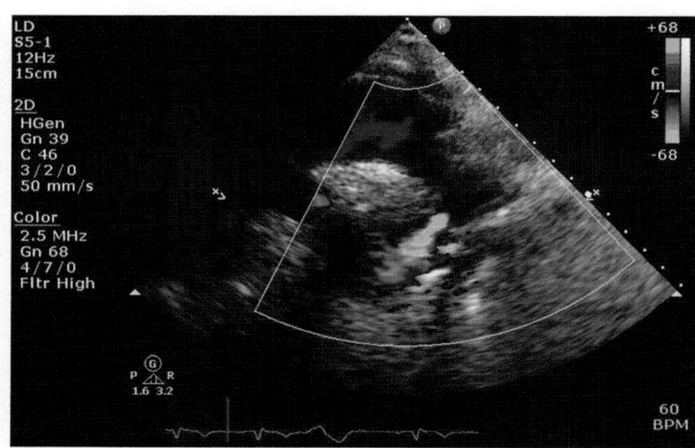

FIGURE 7-5-5 Associated coarctation of the aorta in a different patient with a bicuspid aortic valve. Suprasternal notch view of the arch and upper descending aorta with color Doppler ► (see Video 7-5-5).

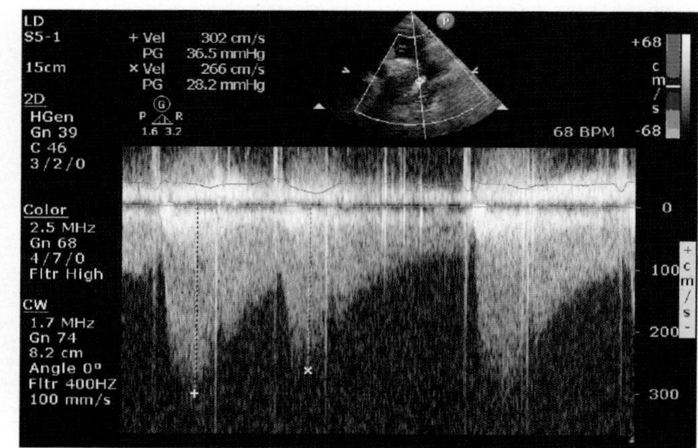

FIGURE 7-5-6 Estimated gradients across the coarctation. Note that gradients may be underestimated in this case because of the angle between the Doppler beam and jet direction.

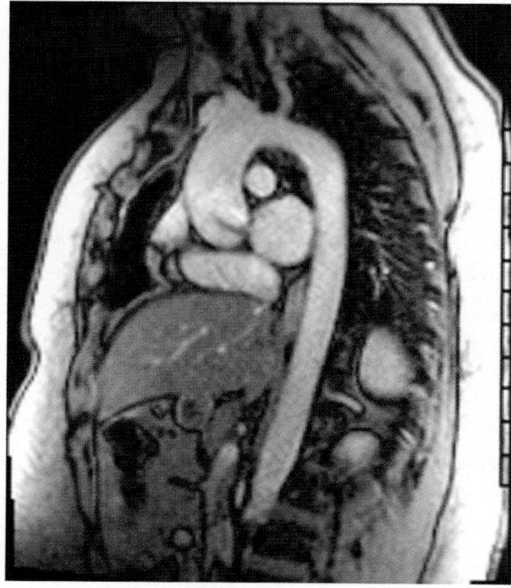

FIGURE 7-5-7 MRA demonstrating ascending aorta dilation in a patient with a bicuspid AV. The remainder of the aorta is normal in this patient.

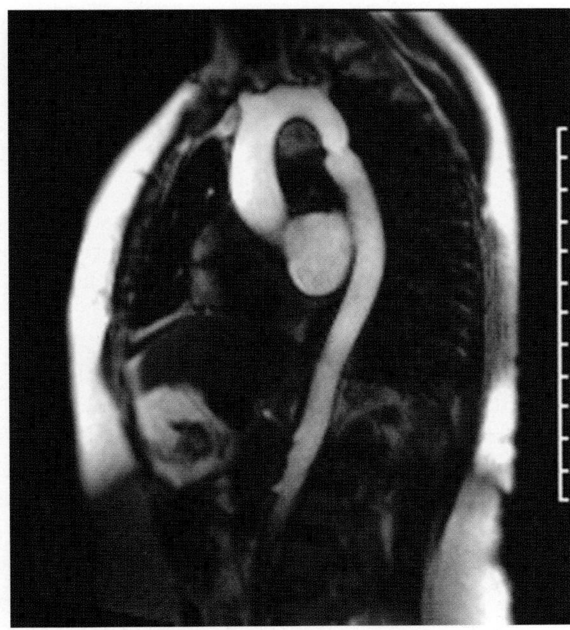

FIGURE 7-5-8 MRA demonstrating coarctation and a dilated ascending aorta from a patient with a bicuspid aortic valve.

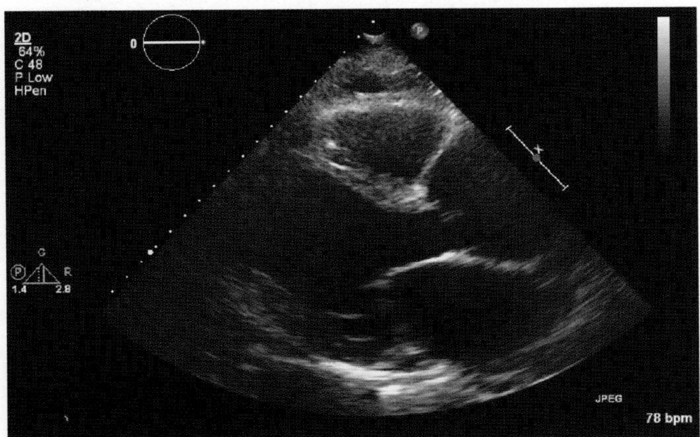

FIGURE 7-5-9 Parasternal long axis view of a different patient with a severely dilated aortic root (7 cm) who presented with congestive heart failure from chronic AR. Note the dilated, hypokinetic LV ▶ (see Video 7-5-9). His brother had a bicuspid valve with a normal aorta. This patient never underwent screening for aortopathy.

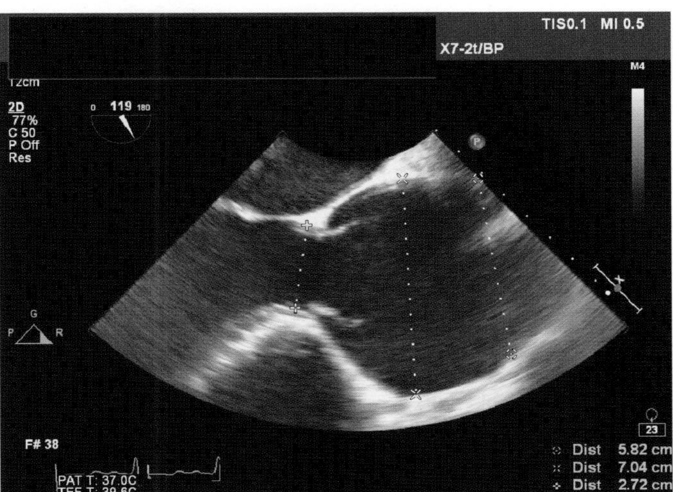

FIGURE 7-5-10 Intraoperative TEE of the patient in Figure 7-5-9 at the time of his Bentall procedure. He did well postoperatively with improvement in his LVEF and symptoms.

REFERENCES

1. Tzemos N, Therrien J, Yip J, et al. Outcomes in adults with bicuspid aortic valves. *JAMA*. 2008;300(11):1317-1325.
2. Bonderman D, Gharehbaghi-Schnell E, Wollenek G, Maurer G, Baumgartner H, Lang IM. Mechanisms underlying aortic dilatation in congenital aortic valve malformation. *Circulation*. 1999;99(16):2138-2143.
3. Huntington K, Hunter AG, Chan KL. A prospective study to assess the frequency of familial clustering of congenital bicuspid aortic valve. *J Am Coll Cardiol*. 1997;30(7):1809-1812.
4. Nistri S, Sorbo MD, Marin M, Palisi M, Scognamiglio R, Thiene G. Aortic root dilatation in young men with normally functioning bicuspid aortic valves. *Heart*. 1999;82(1):19-22.
5. Ergin MA, Spielvogel D, Apaydin A, et al. Surgical treatment of the dilated ascending aorta: when and how? *Ann Thorac Surg*. 1999;67(6):1834-1839; discussion 1853-1836.
6. Fedak PW, Verma S, David TE, Leask RL, Weisel RD, Butany J. Clinical and pathophysiological implications of a bicuspid aortic valve. *Circulation*. 2002;106(8):900-904.

8 ECHOCARDIOGRAPHIC ASSESSMENT OF THE PATIENT WITH STROKE OR TIA: A NEUROLOGIST'S PERSPECTIVE

Chad M. Miller, MD, and Andrew Slivka, MD

INTRODUCTION

Stroke affects more than 700,000 Americans each year, with approximately 85% of these being ischemic in nature.[1] A substantial portion of these individuals suffered a prior stroke or TIA (200,000), thus creating the opportunity for secondary prevention and risk factor modification. Among ischemic strokes, 15% to 33% are thought to be embolic in origin with the highest rates of embolization seen among younger individuals (<45 years old).[2] Embolic strokes are characteristically associated with increased rates of disability and mortality compared to other stroke mechanisms.[3]

Strokes from an embolic source often have sudden onset of the worst neurological symptoms, multifocal presentation, aphasia without hemiparesis, or co-occurrence of systemic emboli. Embolism should be suspected in individuals who demonstrate ischemic involvement in multiple vascular territories or lack a clearly identifiable etiology for stroke on brain and vascular imaging. The most common sources of cerebral emboli are nonvalvular atrial fibrillation, valvular heart disease, and left ventricular thrombi. The similarity of cardiovascular and cerebrovascular risk factors makes determination of a embolic etiology particularly challenging. Despite this, identification of the etiology of stroke as embolic has critical importance in selection of the most appropriate treatment.

The correlation of potential cardiac sources of emboli to stroke occurrence is variable. As a result, adequate evaluation of TIA and stroke patients should also include exploration of noncardiac causes. Vascular imaging with carotid duplex, transcranial Doppler, magnetic resonance (MR) or computed tomography (CT) arteriography are helpful in evaluating potential arterial sources of stroke. Small subcortical infarcts (lacunar strokes) are often associated with small vessel disease, particularly in patients with hypertension and diabetes mellitus. Younger patients may have vascular pathology other than atherosclerosis such as arterial dissection, fibromuscular dysplasia, dolichoectatic arteries, fusiform aneurysms, and primary central nervous system or systemic vasculitides. Brain imaging with MR or CT is valuable in identifying structural abnormalities that may present as stroke mimics.

Considering the importance of the heart and great vessels as sources of emboli, echocardiography has a fundamental role in the evaluation of the patient with suspected embolic infarction, particularly those with multiple vascular distribution stroke or those without a clear vascular etiology for the stroke. Both the Clinical Guidelines for the Use of Echocardiography[4] and the Appropriate Use Criteria for Echocardiography[5] support the role of echocardiography in the evaluation of selected patients with a suspected cardio-embolic event, especially younger patients and those with no obvious other etiology of their neurologic event. The use of echocardiography is a Class III indication[4] and felt to be an inappropriate use of echo[5] in patients in whom management decisions will not be altered by the echocardiographic findings.

While transesophageal echocardiography (TEE) is superior to transthoracic echocardiography (TTE) in detecting many potential cardio-embolic sources, evidence for the superiority of warfarin over antiplatelet therapy in treating most of these sources is lacking, as will be discussed.

This chapter will evaluate the role of echocardiography in evaluating and managing the stroke patient with a patent foramen ovale, valvular strands, noninfectious vegetations, aortic pathology, and/or intracardiac thrombus—all potential embolic sources of cerebral infarction.

SECTION 1

Patent Foramen Ovale

CLINICAL CASE PRESENTATION

The patient is a 51-year-old man with a past history of hyperlipidemia and hypertension who presented with a right-sided headache, nausea, diaphoresis, and vertigo. He had a similar episode of vertigo for 30 minutes 6 weeks prior to his presentation.

General physical examination including cardiac exam was normal. Neurological examination was normal except for slight fine horizontal nystagmus to right gaze and rotatory nystagmus to left gaze. MR scan of the brain demonstrated a right inferior cerebellar infarct. MR angiogram of the head and neck was normal except the right posterior inferior cerebellar artery was not visualized. Transthoracic echocardiography revealed normal left ventricular size and function, no

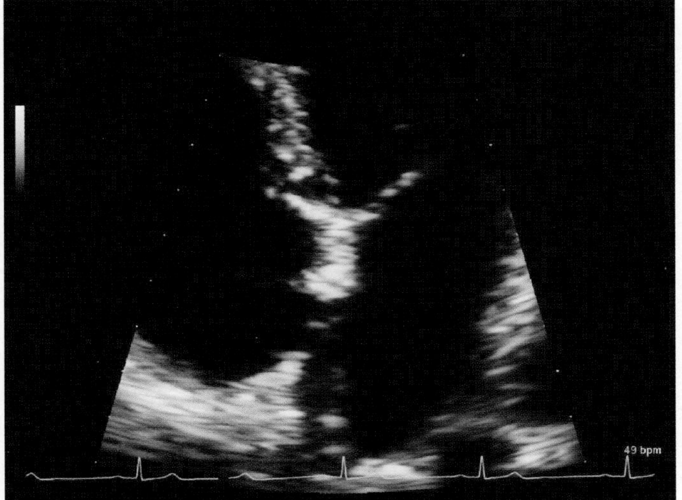

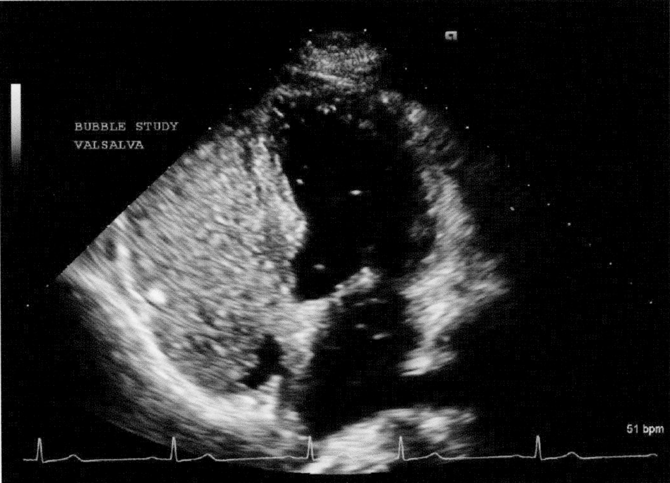

FIGURE 8-1-1 Transthoracic echo demonstrating a hypermobile atrial septum (top panel) and an atrial level right-to-left shunt with Valsalva (bottom panel) ► (see Videos 8-1-1 L and R).

valvular disease. With saline contrast, a right-to-left shunt was seen consistent with a patent foramen ovale (Figure 8-1-1). Lower extremity duplex was normal. No venous thrombosis was identified. ECG and telemetry during his hospitalization revealed normal sinus rhythm. He was begun on aspirin 81 mg daily. His vertiginous symptoms resolved in 1 to 2 weeks.

CLINICAL FEATURES

- A patent foramen ovale (PFO) is a functional anatomical opening in the interatrial septum that allows fetal shunting of oxygenated blood from systemic venous return to the left side of the heart in utero.
- When this anatomical remnant persists into childhood and adult life, it rarely results in pathology.
- In the setting of right-to-left heart shunting, PFOs have been implicated in contributing to postural desaturation syndromes, migraine headaches, decompression illness after deep-water scuba diving, and ischemic stroke related to paradoxical embolization.

EPIDEMIOLOGY

- PFOs are found in up to 27% of adults. Their incidence continues to decline with aging.[1]
- The relationship between PFO and embolic stroke related to paradoxical embolization is controversial. Some studies suggest that PFOs are more common in patients suffering a cryptogenic stroke, though ultimate causality has not been established.[1]
- Shunting may occur across a PFO during Valsalva or other causes of elevated right atrial pressures. The presence of a PFO with persistent/continuous right-to-left shunt may confer a higher stroke risk than intermittent shunting.
- An atrial septal aneurysm (ASA) is a hypermobile septum primum that demonstrates >10 mm of excursion into the alternating atria during the cardiac cycle (Figure 8-1-2). It is found in 2% of adults and may further increase the risk of stroke when associated with a PFO and right-to-left atrial shunting.[6]

PATHOPHYSIOLOGY AND ETIOLOGY

- Right-to-left shunting across a PFO occurs most commonly in early systole, when the right atrial pressure is highest.
- Stroke caused by paradoxical embolization requires introduction of thrombus, air, bone, fat, or other substances capable of entering the venous system and shunting through the PFO to avoid filtration within the lung.

ECHOCARDIOGRAPHY

- Multiplane transesophageal echocardiography (TEE) using Doppler imaging and contrast injection with the Valsalva maneuver is the gold standard for detection of PFO and associated septal pathology.[7]
- For contrast studies, 9 cc of saline is mixed with a small amount of air (eg, 0.5-1 cc) with or without the addition of a small amount of the patient's blood (0.5-1 cc). This solution is then agitated

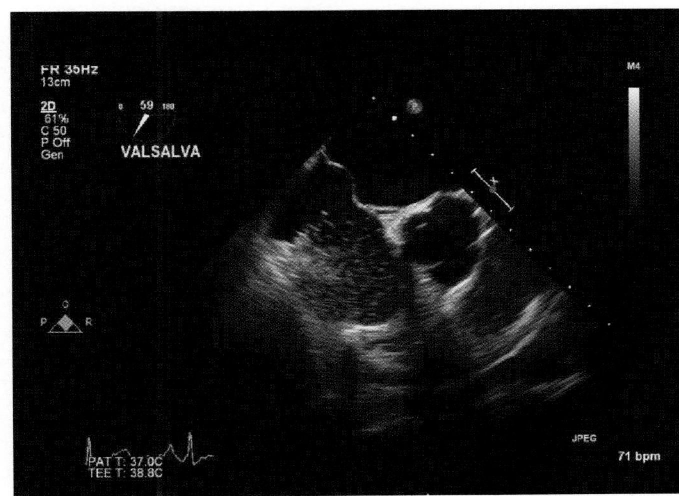

FIGURE 8-1-2 Transesophageal echo demonstrating an atrial septal aneurysm with a right-to-left shunt via a patent foramen ovale (PFO) ► (see Video 8-1-2).

between two 10-cc syringes attached to an antecubital IV through a triple port stopcock apparatus. After the solution has become opaque due to vigorous agitation, the contents are injected intravenously during a Valsalva maneuver. Contrast seen by echocardiography in the left atria during the first 3 to 5 cardiac cycles are suggestive of right-to-left shunting at the atrial level. Less than 20 bubbles are seen with small PFOs. Twenty to fifty bubbles are seen with moderate sized PFOs. Greater than 50 bubbles are noted with large PFOs.[7]

- Three-dimensional TEE allows for improved determination of PFO size and structure. Additionally, color flow Doppler can demonstrate flow through the PFO, which may be bidirectional.
- Some evidence exists favoring femoral, rather than antecubital, injection of echo contrast, since the trajectory of blood flow from the inferior vena cava may more readily reveal shunting.[7]

OTHER DIAGNOSTIC TESTING AND PROCEDURES

- Cardiac MRI has been used to identifying atrial septal pathology, though data regarding its sensitivity is mixed. Even less data is available for cardiac CT in the evaluation of PFO.
- Transcranial Doppler (TCD) is an ultrasonic technique that can identify emboli passing through the proximal intracranial vessels. Systemic shunting can be exhibited by peripheral agitated saline/contrast administration. TCD identifies emboli resulting from TEE-demonstrated PFOs with a high degree of sensitivity (94%) and has been shown to discover additional shunts not seen via TEE techniques.[7] TCD detects emboli from pulmonary and systemic arterial venous malformations (AVMs) as well as other sources of shunting and arterial embolism. TCD and TEE are complimentary tools in the detection of cardioembolic disease.
- For patients with pathology allowing paradoxical embolism, lower extremity duplex or CT venogram of the pelvis and lower extremity can be used to identify deep vein thrombus at risk for paradoxical embolization.

DIFFERENTIAL DIAGNOSIS

- Atrial septal defects, including sinus venosus defects, and intrapulmonary AVMs may cause right-to-left shunting thought to be caused by PFOs. Pulmonary AVMs produce left atrial bubbles typically delayed greater than 3 to 5 cardiac cycles after intravenous injection.

DIAGNOSIS

- Echocardiography with a contrast bubble study is recommended for identification of PFO. TEE studies have greater sensitivity, though many institutions prefer to screen patients utilizing a transthoracic echocardiogram (TTE). Given the uncertain relationship between PFO and stroke, the aggressiveness of diagnostic testing should take into account the impact that this diagnosis may or may not have on subsequent stroke therapy.

MANAGEMENT

- In the PICSS study, a subset of patients having PFO were randomized to warfarin or aspirin and followed for 2 years for evidence of cerebral infarction. No difference in the stroke rate was seen between these two therapies.[8] As a result, patients with PFO and stroke should be treated with antiplatelet agents for secondary stroke prevention.
- In a recently released randomized study evaluating the impact of PFO closure on recurrent stroke, rates of stroke were not reduced with PFO closure. Additionally, identification of recurrent stroke was associated with factors unrelated to the PFO, namely paroxysmal atrial fibrillation.[9] The PRECISE study failed to show conclusive evidence that interventional PFO closure reduces cryptogenic stroke rate.[10] Only 70% to 71% of patients had complete closure of their PFO on repeat TEE in each of these studies. While PFO closure may not reduce the risk of stroke, there is some evidence that postprocedure rates of atrial fibrillation are increased.
- Despite the possible increased risk of stroke with PFO with an ASA, there is no proven benefit in therapeutic anticoagulation for these patients.[1]
- Regardless of the suspicion of paradoxical embolization, noninfectious deep venous thrombosis should be treated with unfractionated or low molecular weight heparin followed by warfarin with a goal INR of 2.0 to 3.0. Inferior vena cava filters may be indicated for patients with contraindications to anticoagulant therapy.

FOLLOW-UP

- Given the lack of causality between PFO and embolic stroke, routine follow-up with echocardiography is not recommended. Recurrent stroke should prompt a reevaluation of the patient's modifiable risks and perhaps exploration of other cardioembolic risks that would prompt changes in preventive strategy. Patients with recurrent events may be considered for enrollment in ongoing clinical trials exploring the role of PFO closure.

VIDEO LEGENDS

1. Video 8-1-1 L: Transthoracic echo demonstrating a hypermobile atrial septum
2. Video 8-1-1 R: Transthoracic echo demonstrating an atrial level right to left shunt with Valsalva. Note the saline contrast bubbles in the left heart.
3. Video 8-1-2: Transesophageal echo demonstrating an atrial septal aneurysm with a right to left shunt via a patent foramen ovale (PFO).

REFERENCES

1. Furie KL, Kasner SE, Adams RJ, et al. Guidelines for prevention of stroke in patients with ischemic stroke or transient ischemic attack. A guideline for healthcare professionals from the American Heart Association/American Stroke Association. *Stroke.* 2011;42:227-276.
2. Dafer RM, Pasnoor M, Gorton ME, and Gollub S. Chordae tendinae tumor as the cause of cardioembolic stroke. *J Stroke Cerebrovasc Dis.* 2006;15(2):72-73.
3. Arboix A, and Alio J. Cardioembolic stroke: clinical features, specific cardiac disorders and prognosis. *Curr Cardiol Rev.* 2010;6:150-161.

4. Cheitlin MD, Armstrong WF, Aurigemma GP, et al. ACC/AHA/ASE 2003 guideline update for the clinical application of echocardiography - summary article. A report of the American College of Cardiology/American Heart Association Task Force on practice guidelines. (ACC/AHA/ASE 2003 Committee to Update the 1997 Guidelines for the Clinical Application of Echocardiography). *J Am Coll Cardiol.* 2003;42:954-970.

5. Douglas PS, Garcia MJ, Haines DE, et al. ACCF/ASE/AHA/ASNC/HFSA/HRS/SCAI/SCCM/SCCT/SCMR 2011 appropriate use criteria for echocardiography: a report of the American College of Cardiology Foundation Appropriate Use Criteria Task Force, American Society of Echocardiography, American Heart Association, American Society of Nuclear Cardiology, Heart Failure Society of America, Heart Rhythm Society, Society of Cardiovascular Angiography and Interventions, Society of Critical Care Medicine, Society of Cardiovascular Computed Tomography, and Society of Cardiovascular Magnetic Resonance. *J Am Coll Cardiol.* 2011;57(9):1126-1166. doi: 10.1016/j.jacc.2010.11.002.

6. Mas JL, Arquizan C, Lamy C, et al; Patent Foramen Ovale and Atrial Septal Aneurysm Study Group. Recurrent cerebrovascular events associated with patent foramen ovale, atrial septal aneurysm, or both. *New Engl J Med.* 2001;345:1740-1746.

7. Buchholz S, Shakil A, Figtree GA, Hansen PS, Bhindi R. Diagnosis and management of patent foramen ovale. *Postgrad Med J.* 2012;88:217-225.

8. Homma S, Sacco RL, DiTullio MR, Sciacca RR, Mohr JP; PFO in Cryptogenic Stroke Study (PICSS) Investigators. Effect of medical treatment in stroke patients with patent foramen ovale: patent foramen ovale in Cryptogenic Stroke Study. *Circulation.* 2002;105:2625-1631.

9. Furlan AJ, Reisman M, Massaro J, et al. Closure or medical therapy for cryptogenic stroke with patent foramen ovale. *N Engl J Med.* 2012;366:991-999.

10. Wohrle J, Bertrand B, Sondergaard L, et al. PFO closuRE and CryptogenIc StrokE (PRECISE) registry: a multi-center, international registry. *Clin Res Cardiol.* 2012;101(10):787-793. Epub 2012 Apr 10.

SECTION 2

Valvular Strands

CLINICAL CASE PRESENTATION

The patient is a 28-year-old woman with a past history of migraine headaches, and meningitis as a child who presented with aphasia and right-sided weakness. General physical examination including cardiac exam was normal. Neurological examination was normal except for decreased fluency but normal naming, repetition, comprehension, reading, and writing and mild right upper and lower extremity weakness. MR scan of the brain demonstrated a left medial frontal, parietal infarct. MR angiogram of the head and neck revealed a proximal left anterior cerebral artery occlusion. Transthoracic and transesophageal echocardiography revealed normal left ventricular size and function and no hemodynamically significant valvular disease or shunts. Valvular strands were seen on the aortic valve on transthoracic echocardiography (Figure 8-2-1) and on both the mitral and aortic valves on TEE (Figure 8-2-2). ECG and telemetry during her hospitalization revealed normal sinus rhythm.

She was begun on aspirin 81 mg daily. Her symptoms improved over days and resolved within weeks.

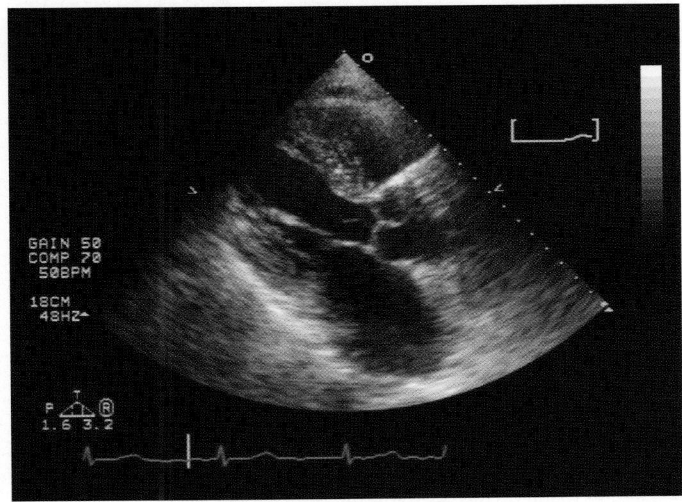

FIGURE 8-2-1 Transthoracic echo demonstrating a large strand on the aortic valve ► (see Video 8-2-1).

CLINICAL FEATURES

- Valvular strands are also called Lambl's excresences. They are filiform structures that can be found on native or prosthetic valves. They commonly occur on the ventricular side of the aortic valve, or the atrial side of the mitral valve.[1]
- Valvular strands are usually clinically asymptomatic.

EPIDEMIOLOGY

- Valvular strands can be found in 5.5% of the general population and tend to occur in younger individuals.[2,3]
- Strands are comprised of a fibroelastic avascular core covered by a single layer of endothelial cells.[3] This single layer differentiates them from papillary fibroelastomas. The pathogenesis of Lambl's excresences is unclear, but they may arise from valvular denuding that occurs under high shear stress that is subsequently covered by fibrin.

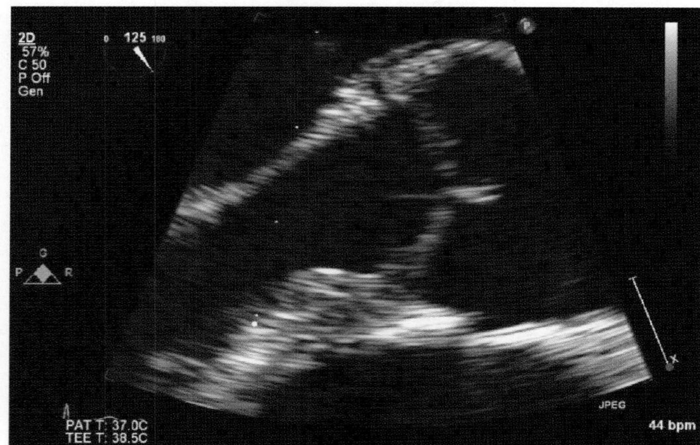

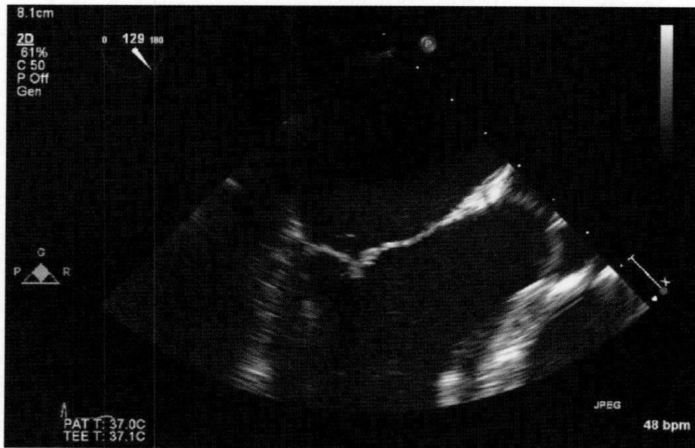

FIGURE 8-2-2 Transesophageal echo demonstrating valve strands on the aortic valve (top panel) and mitral valve (bottom panel) ► (see Videos 8-2-2 L and R).

- Valvular strands are a potential embolic source, though their occurrence has not been consistently shown to increase stroke risk.[4]

PATHOPHYSIOLOGY AND ETIOLOGY

- Valvular strands, seen on both native and prosthetic valves, have been hypothesized to cause stroke or TIA from embolization. It is unclear if the strands embolize or if thrombus forms on the strands and subsequently embolizes.

ECHOCARDIOGRAPHY

- Excrescences are typically less than 2 mm in diameter and are elongated in shape.[4] They are typically positioned near the leaflet closure lines, differentiating them from other valvular pathology.
- Strands are twice as common on the mitral valve and on valves that are thickened or redundant.[5]
- Mitral and aortic valves and other left heart structures are better seen on TEE than TTE.[6]

OTHER DIAGNOSTIC TESTING AND PROCEDURES

- Echocardiography is the primary modality for identification of valvular strands. Given the benign nature of this finding, diagnostic testing after stroke should be targeted toward tests capable of identifying more likely sources of emboli.

DIFFERENTIAL DIAGNOSIS

- Valvular strands must be differentiated from myxomas, valvular thrombi and vegetations, cardiac metastases, primary cardiac neoplasms, and fibroelastomas.[3] Papillary fibroelastomas are the most common valvular tumor and are histopathologically distinct from strands in their multiple endothelial layers.[7]

DIAGNOSIS

- Diagnosis of valvular strands is made by echocardiography. Identification of strands after ischemic stroke does not alter the recommended treatment of antiplatelet therapy. Diagnostic rigor should follow the clinical concern for other valvular pathology.

MANAGEMENT

- In patients with valvular strands, no difference in recurrent stroke risk has been noted when comparing antiplatelet and anticoagulant therapy.[8] Therefore, antiplatelet therapy is recommended for secondary stroke prevention.[4]
- These strands may be considered a potential embolic source or as a marker of potential embolic risk, especially when detected on prosthetic valves.[9]
- When valvular strands arise from mechanical prosthetic valves, warfarin anticoagulation with a goal INR between 2.5 and 3.5 is recommended. If stroke recurs despite this regimen, low-dose aspirin (75-100 mg) should be added to warfarin, if the patient has previously not been on aspirin therapy.[4,9]

FOLLOW-UP

- No specific echocardiographic follow-up is required for asymptomatic patients with valvular strands.
- No specific therapy is recommended for asymptomatic patients with native valve strands.
- For patients with prosthetic valve strands, meticulous attention to anticoagulation status is recommended.[9]

VIDEO LEGENDS

1. Video 8-2-1: Transthoracic echo demonstrating a large strand on the aortic valve.
2. Video 8-2-2 L: Transesophageal echo demonstrating valve strands on the aortic valve.
3. Video 8-2-2 R: Transesophageal echo demonstrating valve strands on the mitral valve.

REFERENCES

1. Rhee HY, Choi H, Kim S, Shin W, Kim SH. Acute ischemic stroke in a patient with a native valvular strand. *Case Rep Neurol.* 2010;2:91-95.
2. Freedberg RS, Goodkin GM, Perez JL, Tunick PA, Kronzon I. Valve strands are strongly associated with systemic embolization: a transesophageal echocardiographic study. *J Am Coll Cardiol.* 1995;26:1709-1712.

3. Ker, J. The serpentine mitral valve and cerebral embolism. *Cardiovasc Ultrasound.* 2011;9:7-9.

4. Whitlock RP, Sun JC, Fremes SE, Rubens FD, Teoh KH. Antithrombotic and thrombolytic therapy for valvular disease: antithrombotic therapy and prevention of thrombosis, 9th ed: American College of Chest Physicians Evidence-Based Clinical Practice Guidelines. *Chest.* 2012;141:e576S-e600S.

5. Nighoghossian N, Derex L, Perinetti M, et al. Course of valvular strands in patients with stroke: cooperative study with transesophageal echocardiography. *Am Heart J.* 1998;136:1065-1069.

6. Weir NU. An update on cardioembolic stroke. *Postgrad Med J.* 2008;84:133-142.

7. Dafer RM, Pasnoor M, Gorton ME, Gollub S. Chordae tendinae tumor as the cause of cardioembolic stroke. *J Stroke Cerebrovasc Dis.* 2006;15(2):72-73.

8. Homma S, Di Tullio MR, Sciacca RR, Sacco RL, Mohr JP. Effect of aspirin and warfarin therapy in stroke patients with valvular strands. *Stroke.* 2004;35:1436-1442.

9. Orsinelli DA. Prosthetic valve strands: clinically significant or irrelevant to management? *J Am Soc Echocardiogr.* 2009;22:895-898.

SECTION 3

Noninfective Vegetations

CLINICAL CASE PRESENTATION

The patient is a 38-year-old man with a past history of hypertension, Wolff-Parkinson-White syndrome, status post ablation, traumatic brain injury following an automobile accident, obstructive sleep apnea, renal calculi who presented with headache, right visual field deficit, and right sided numbness.

General physical examination including cardiac exam was normal. Neurological examination revealed a right homonymous hemianopia, and decreased pin and touch sensation over the right face, arm, and leg. MR scan of the brain demonstrated a left occipital, medial temporal, and thalamic infarct in the distribution of the left posterior cerebral artery. MR angiogram of the head and neck was normal except for a small irregular distal left posterior cerebral artery with poor distal flow. Transthoracic echocardiography revealed normal left ventricular size and function and no valvular disease. Transesophageal echocardiography showed small vegetations on the tip of the anterior and posterior mitral valve, the largest being 4.3 × 3.8 mm at the tip of the mitral valve (Figures 8-3-1 and 8-3-2). Blood cultures were negative. ECG and telemetry during his hospitalization revealed normal sinus rhythm.

He was discharged on warfarin. His symptoms improved over 2 months. When seen in follow-up, he had decided not to take the warfarin and was not on any antithrombotic medication. Warfarin was again prescribed. Follow-up transesophageal echocardiography done 4 months later (6 months after the stroke) showed only a modest decrease in the size of the mitral valve vegetation (Figure 8-3-3 top panel). He had still not begun on warfarin. At this point he did begin taking warfarin. Follow-up transesophageal echocardiography done 7 months later (13 months after the stroke) showed a minimal decrease in the size of the mitral valve vegetation. His exam was normal by this time. He remained on warfarin. Follow-up transesophageal echocardiography done 5.5 months later (18.5 months after the stroke) showed a further decrease in the size of the mitral valve

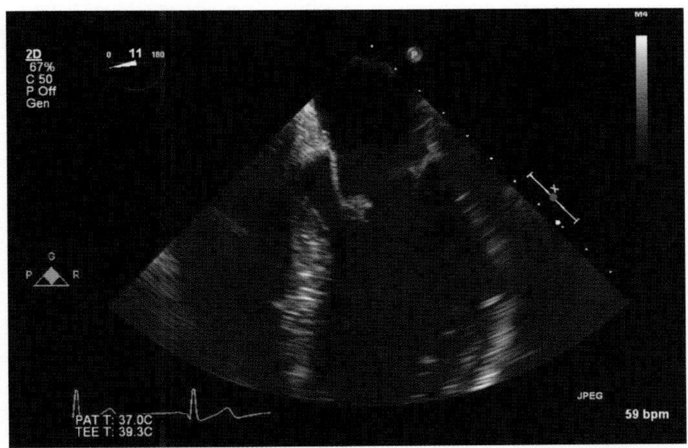

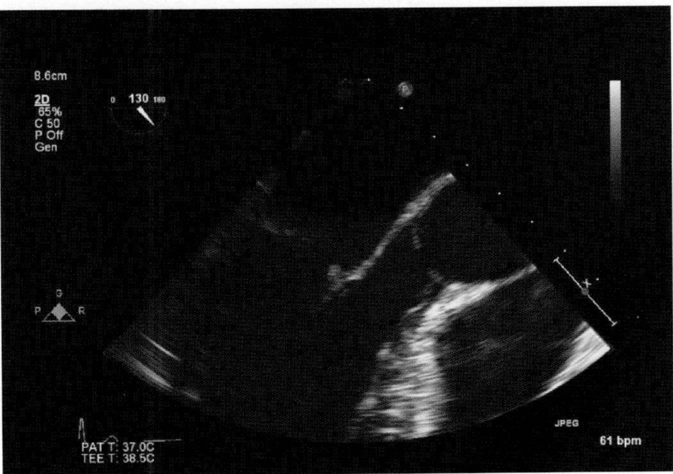

FIGURE 8-3-1 Transesophageal echo demonstrating a large vegetation on the anterior mitral valve leaflet in a 4 chamber view (top panel) and 3 chamber view (bottom panel) ▶ (see Videos 8-3-1 L and R).

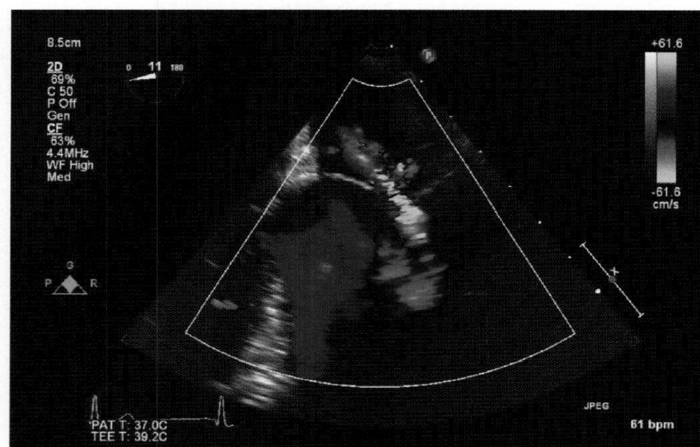

FIGURE 8-3-2 Color flow Doppler demonstrating mitral insufficiency due to NBTE ► (see Video 8-3-2).

vegetation, measuring 0.2 × 0.3 mm (Figure 8-3-3 bottom panel). His prescription for warfarin had run out 1 month prior to that clinic visit, and he did not wish to resume the warfarin or any other antithrombotic. He had no recurrent ischemic events during follow-up.

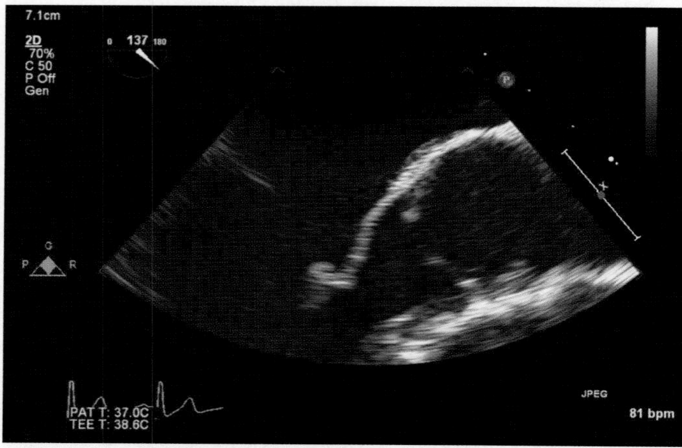

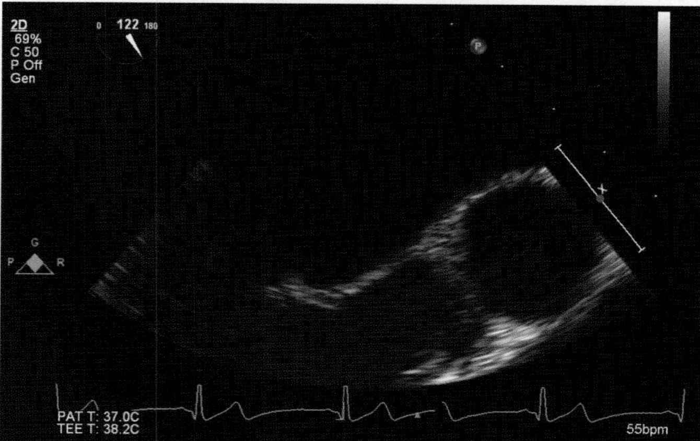

FIGURE 8-3-3 Follow-up TEE demonstrating minimal change in the size of the vegetation at initial follow-up (top panel) and further decrease in size at last follow-up (bottom panel) ► (see Videos 8-3-3 L and R).

CLINICAL FEATURES

- Nonbacterial thrombotic endocarditis (NBTE) is a noninfectious endocarditis primarily affecting the atrial surfaces of the atrioventricular valves and the ventricular surfaces of the semilunar valves. Compared to excresences, noninfective vegetations tend to be more round, sessile, and heterogenous in shape.[1]
- Libman-Sacks endocarditis is a sterile verrucous valvular lesion commonly associated with systemic lupus erythematosis (SLE) and the antiphospholipid antibody syndrome.[2] While most valvular lesions are asymptomatic, the disease can be severe in some individuals.
- Most noninfective vegetations are associated with an underlying coagulopathy.

EPIDEMIOLOGY

- NBTE most commonly affects individuals in the 4th to 8th decades of life.[1] The condition may be related to sepsis or an underlying systemic malignancy.
- The antiphospholipid antibody syndrome (AAS) has a prevalence of 1% to 6.5% and predisposes patients to noninfective vegetations.[3] AAS may be associated with SLE, which is related to a high occurrence of valvular echocardiographic findings. Thickening of valves is noted in 51% of SLE patients, while vegetations are found in 43%.[4] On serial echocardiograms, it is common for the valvular lesions to undergo morphological changes.

PATHOPHYSIOLOGY AND ETIOLOGY

- Libman-Sacks (LS) endocarditis results from deposition of fibrin and platelet thrombi upon the valve surface.[2] While valve necrosis and mononuclear infiltration is common, the presence of polymorphonuclear leukocytes should prompt concern of secondary bacterial infection.
- Libman-Sacks endocarditis may be distinguished pathologically from nonbacterial thrombotic endocarditis. The vegetations from LS endocarditis are densely adherent to the endocardium, occur frequently on the valve rings and commissures, and may involve the mural endocardium, chordae tendinae, and papillary musculature. Microscopically, fibrin, fibrous tissue, and mild inflammation with plasma cells or mononuclear cells may be present. Vegetations with nonbacterial endocarditis are typically found on contact surfaces of the valve leaflets, atrial surfaces of the atrioventricular valves, or the ventricular surface of the semilunar valves. Acellular thrombi are seen microscopically.[5]

ECHOCARDIOGRAPHY

- LS lesions are most commonly found on the posterior mitral leaflet, but they can also be located on the endocardial surface, chordae tendonae, or papillary muscles.[2] In addition to embolization, these lesions may result in valvular insufficiency or stenosis.
- NBTE lesions are often rounded, sessile, and greater than 3 mm in diameter. They demonstrate a heterogenous echoreflectance.[1]
- Noninfective vegetations tend to be smaller than their infective counterparts, and, therefore, may be more challenging to identify on echocardiography.[2]

- TEE is more sensitive in identifying LS endocarditis than TTE.[2,6] In one cohort of SLE patients, TTE was able to identify only 63% of lesions apparent on TEE.[7]

OTHER DIAGNOSTIC TESTING AND PROCEDURES

- While MRI and CT imaging techniques may incidentally identify some valvular abnormalities, TEE remains the diagnostic test of choice for evaluating valvular lesions.
- Blood cultures should be drawn in any patient who may be suspected of harboring primary or secondarily infected valve lesions.

DIFFERENTIAL DIAGNOSIS

- Bacterial endocarditis, fibroelastomas, valvular myxomas, and valvular stranding or thickening comprise the differential diagnosis for noninfected vegetations. Atrial myxomas make up more than 50% of all primary cardiac tumors and may present with embolization.

DIAGNOSIS

- Noninfected valvular vegetations may persist unnoticed prior to embolization and stroke. While more common with infected vegetations, fever, arthritis, cardiac murmurs, and splinter hemorrhages have been described with noninfectious lesions.
- Suspicion of a valvular lesion should be pursued with serial blood cultures and TEE.

MANAGEMENT

- Since noninfectious vegetations may be the result of a systemic malignancy, coagulopathy, or connective tissue diseases, primary treatment of the underlying disorder is the mainstay of therapy.
- Appropriate management of incidentally discovered noninfected valvular lesions is unclear.
- For patients suffering embolic complications of NBTE, treatment with full dose intravenous unfractionated heparin or low molecular weight heparin[8] is recommended, based on the experience in patients with cancer. In patients without underlying malignancies, warfarin seems a reasonable alternative though the duration of treatment is unclear.

FOLLOW-UP

- Nonembolized valvular lesions do not require echocardiographic follow-up. Appropriate treatment for disease progression in the setting of full anticoagulation is unclear.
- Echocardiography may be useful in determining the duration of anticoagulation in patients suffering embolic complications. Resolution of the vegetation may allow consideration of transition to antiplatelet therapy.

VIDEO LEGENDS

1. Video 8-3-1 L: Transesophageal echo demonstrating a large vegetation on the anterior mitral valve leaflet in a four chamber view.
2. Video 8-3-1 R: Transesophageal echo demonstrating a large vegetation on the anterior mitral valve leaflet in a 3 chamber view.
3. Video 8-3-2: Color flow Doppler demonstrating mitral insufficiency due to NBTE
4. Video 8-3-3 L: Follow-up TEE demonstrating minimal change in the size of the vegetation at initial follow up.
5. Video 8-3-3 R: Follow-up TEE demonstrating a further decrease in size of the vegetation at last follow up.

REFERENCES

1. Salem DN, O'Gara PT, Madias C, Pauker SG. Valvular and structural heart disease: American College of Chest Physicians Evidence-Based Clinical Practice Guidelines, 8th ed. *Chest.* 2008;133:593S-629S.
2. Lee JL, Naguwa SM, Cheema GS, Gershwin E. Revisiting Libman-Sacks endocarditis: a historical review and update. *Clinic Rev Allerg Immunol.* 2009;36:126-130.
3. Vila P, Hernandez MC, Lopez-Fernandez MF, Battle J. Prevalence, follow-up, and clinical significance of the anticardiolipin antibodies in normal subjects. *Thromb Haemost.* 1994;72:1311-1315.
4. Roldan CA, Shively BK, Crawford MH. An echocardiographic study of valvular heart disease associated with systemic lupus erythematosus. *New Engl J Med.* 1996;335:1424-1430.
5. Joffe II, Jacobs LE, Owen AN, Ioli A, Kotler MN. Noninfective valvular masses: review of the literature with emphasis on imaging techniques and management. *Am Heart J.* 1996;131:1175-1183.
6. Walz ET, Slivka AP, Tice FD, Gray PC, Orsinelli DA, Pearson AC. Noninfective mitral valve vegetations identified by transesophageal echocardiography as a cause of stroke. *J Stroke Cerebrovasc Dis.* 1998;7(5):310-314.
7. Roldan CA, Qualls CR, Sopko KS, Sibbit WL Jr. Transthoracic versus transesophageal echocardiography for detection of Libman-Sacks endocarditis: a randomized controlled study. *J Rheumatol.* 2008;35:224-229.
8. Whitlock RP, Sun JC, Fremes SE, Rubens FD, Teoh KH. Antithrombotic and thrombolytic therapy for valvular disease: Antithrombotic Therapy and Prevention of Thrombosis, 9th ed: American College of Chest Physicians Evidence-Based Clinical Practice Guidelines. *Chest.* 2012;141:e576S-e600S.

SECTION 4

Aortic Pathology

CLINICAL CASE PRESENTATION

The patient is a 69-year-old man with a past history of chronic obstructive pulmonary disease, status post right-lung transplant, coronary artery disease, status postcoronary bypass surgery, gastroesophageal reflux, and hypothyroidism who presented with loss of vision in the lower half of his left eye. He was seen by ophthalmology, who diagnosed a retinal branch occlusion, and was treated with laser embolectomy. His vision gradually improved over several days. By the time he was seen, he had slight blurring of vision in the left eye.

General physical examination including cardiac exam was normal. Neurological examination was normal. Carotid duplex showed 50% to 69% stenosis of the right internal carotid and 20% to 49% stenosis of the left internal carotid. Transesophageal echocardiography revealed normal left ventricular size and function and no valvular disease. Severe, complex atherosclerosis was seen in the aortic arch (Figure 8-4-1).

He was discharged on warfarin. He had been on clopidogrel previously. Follow-up transesophageal echocardiography done 4 months later showed severe atherosclerosis of the aortic arch but resolution of the mobile plaque. Warfarin was discontinued, and he was restarted on clopidogrel. He had no recurrent ischemic events during follow-up.

CLINICAL FEATURES

- Aortic disease results in cerebral infarction through embolization of clot or atherosclerotic materials to the cerebral vasculature. Less commonly, extensive atherosclerotic disease can narrow the ostia of the left carotid artery in a flow limiting fashion. A full review of aortic dissection, intramural hematoma, and other aortic disease may be found in Chapter 7, Echocardiographic Evaluation of Aortic Pathology. This section will focus upon embolic disease of the aorta emanating from atherosclerotic plaque.
- Stroke originating from aortic debris should be suspected in patients with evidence of systemic embolization. Signs include renal failure with evidence of eosinophils on urinalysis, Hollenhorst plaques, and digit discoloration related to appendicular infarction. Radiographically, splenic and solid organ infarctions may be appreciated.
- Asymmetry in upper extremity pulses or blood pressure readings can be indicative of severe aortic disease.
- Inflammatory conditions with propensity toward the great vessels (Takayasu's arteritis) and congenital valvular disease with aortic manifestations may demonstrate rare and unique findings on clinical exam.

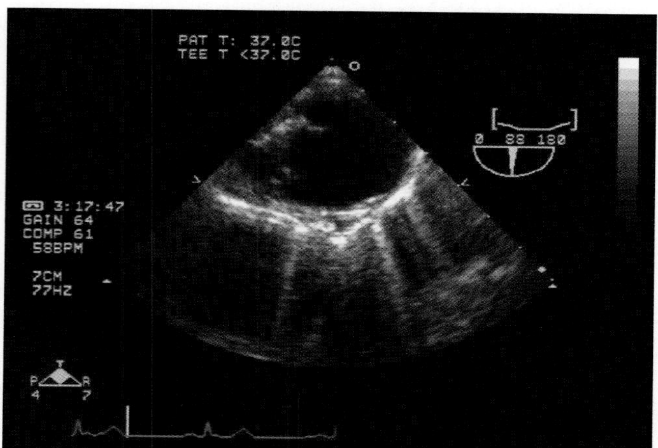

FIGURE 8-4-1 TEE of the aortic arch demonstrating a large plaque in the distal aortic arch with mobile debris ▶ (see Video 8-4-1).

EPIDEMIOLOGY

- Both atheroemboli and thromboemboli may originate from the aorta (Figure 8-4-2). The presence of aortic plaque is more common in individuals with cryptogenic stroke and has been associated with a greater overall risk.[1] Those patients with ulcerated plaque appear to be at greatest risk of embolic stroke, particularly if plaque thickness exceeds 4 mm.[1,2] A lack of calcification within the aortic plaque confers a greater risk of embolization.[1]
- In the SPAF trial, those individuals with aortic disease had a substantially higher annual rate of stroke (12%-20% versus 1.2%).[1]
- High-intensity transient signals (HITS) on transcranial ultrasound are more common in patients with aortic disease.[3]

PATHOPHYSIOLOGY AND ETIOLOGY

- Aortic atherosclerosis shares common risk factors with systemic atherosclerosis, including hypercholesterolemia, hypertension, and smoking history.
- Newly formed thrombi on the surface of atherosclerotic lesions are more likely to embolize than the plaque elements themselves.

ECHOCARDIOGRAPHY

- Given its location within the chest, the aortic arch is better seen with TEE than TTE. This discrepancy is magnified in patients with pulmonary disease or unusually large body habitus.

OTHER DIAGNOSTIC TESTING AND PROCEDURES

- Transcranial Doppler can identify HITS resulting from aortic emboli.
- Intraoperatively, aortic disease can be identified by epiaortic ultrasound.[2]
- Magnetic resonance arteriography can be used to assess aortic plaque, but suffers from decreased sensitivity in identifying

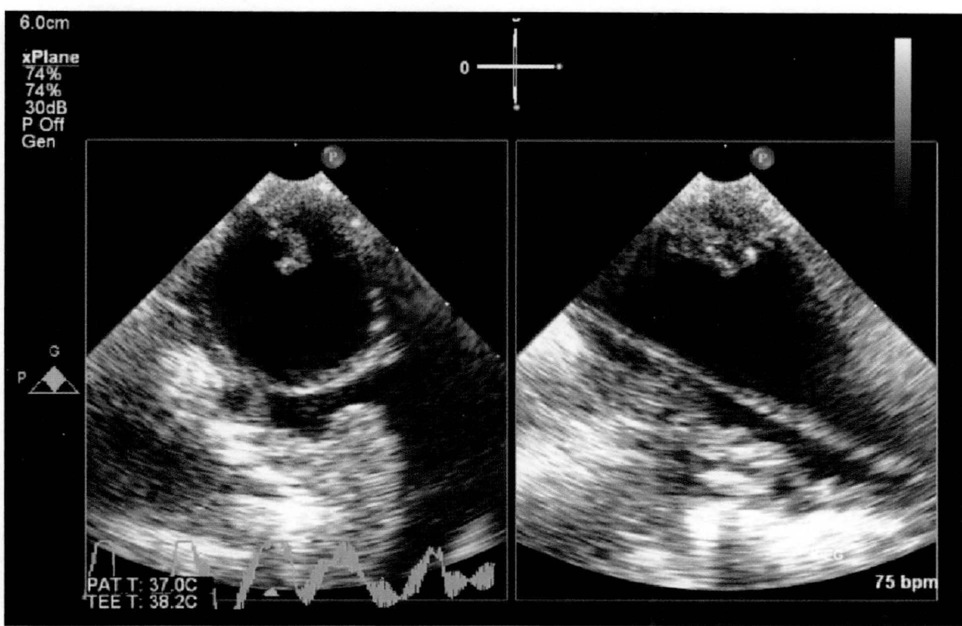

FIGURE 8-4-2 Mobile debris in the descending aorta of another patient with a stroke and lower extremity embolization after an interventional procedure ► (see Video 8-4-2).

high risk lesions and accurately assessing plaque thickness.[2] Electrocardiogram-gated multidetector row computed tomography (MDCT) has shown some efficacy in diagnosis of aortic lesions.[5]

DIFFERENTIAL DIAGNOSIS

- Aortic atherosclerosis must be differentiated from other sources of emboli, such as dissection, intramural hematoma, and vasculitis.
- Inflammatory vasculitides present with fever, malaise, decreased upper extremity pulses, and blood pressure asymmetry. Takayasu's arteritis results in TIA or stroke in 10% to 20% of patients.[6]

DIAGNOSIS

- Transthoracic imaging of the aorta is relatively insensitive. Optimal evaluation of the aortic arch by echocardiography is achieved with TEE.

MANAGEMENT

- Because of the atherosclerotic nature of the lesions, aggressive cholesterol management is important in controlling aortic embolic risk.
- Comparisons of warfarin and antiplatelets for prevention of stroke from aortic emboli have had mixed results. Aortic atherosclerotic lesions should be treated with low dose aspirin therapy (50-100 mg/day).[8] For mobile aortic arch thrombi, anticoagulation with a goal INR of 2 to 3 or low dose aspirin can be considered.

FOLLOW-UP

- It is unclear if echocardiographic follow-up of aortic atherosclerosis provides useful therapeutic information regarding response to therapy.
- For patients who are anticoagulated due to aortic arch thrombi, repeat echocardiography may guide transition to antiplatelet therapy upon resolution of the embolic source.

VIDEO LEGENDS

1. Video 8-4-1: TEE of the aortic arch demonstrating a large plaque in the distal aortic arch with mobile debris.
2. Video 8-4-2: Mobile debris in the descending aorta of another patient with a stroke and lower extremity embolization after an interventional procedure.

REFERENCES

1. Whitlock RP, Sun JC, Fremes SE, Rubens FD, Teoh KH. Antithrombotic and thrombolytic therapy for valvular disease: Antithrombotic Therapy and Prevention of Thrombosis, 9th ed: American College of Chest Physicians Evidence-Based Clinical Practice Guidelines. *Chest.* 2012;141:e576S-e600S.
2. Tunick PA, Kronzon I. Atheromas of the thoracic aorta: clinical and therapeutic update. *J Am Coll Cardiol.* 2000;35:545-554.
3. Tundek T, DiTullio MR, Sciacca RR, et al. Association between large aortic arch atheromas and high-intensity transient signals in elderly stroke patients. *Stroke.* 1999;30:2683-2686.
4. Ko Y, Park J, Yang MH, et al. Significance of aortic atherosclerotic disease in possibly embolic stroke: 64-multidetector row computed tomography study. *J Neurol.* 2010;257:699-705.
5. Zhou L, Ni J, Gao S, Peng B, Cui L. Neurological manifestations of takayasu arteritis. *Chin Med Sci J* 2011;26(4):227-230.
6. Weir NU. An update on cardioembolic stroke. *Postgrad Med J.* 2008;84:133-142.
7. Salem DN, O'Gara PT, Madias C, Pauker SG. Valvular and structural heart disease: American College of Chest Physicians Evidence-Based Clinical Practice Guidelines, 8th ed. *Chest.* 2008;133:593S-629S.

SECTION 5

Intracardiac Thrombus

CLINICAL CASE PRESENTATION

The patient is a 50-year-old man with a past history of bipolar disorder and hyperlipidemia who presented with dysarthria, left-sided weakness, and numbness. He had elevated troponin of 17 ng/mL.

General physical examination including cardiac exam was normal. Neurological examination showed a left homonymous hemianopia, left lower facial weakness, left upper, and lower extremity weakness in the 0 to 1 range, decreased pin, touch left face upper, lower extremity, left sided neglect, hyperrelexia on the left, and left Babinski sign. MR demonstrated a large right frontal, temporal, parietal infarct. Carotid duplex showed less than 50% stenosis of both proximal internal carotid arteries. MR angiogram of the brain revealed a proximal right middle cerebral artery occlusion. Transesophageal echocardiography demonstrated no valvular disease. There was severe segmental left ventricular dysfunction with an ejection fraction of 25% to 30% and thrombus in the apex of the left ventricle and a large left atrial appendage thrombus (Figure 8-5-1).

His hospital course was complicated by aspiration pneumonia and a urinary tract infection. He had a gastrostomy tube placed. Repeat CT scan 9 days after presentation did not demonstrate hemorrhagic conversion of the infarction. He was begun on warfarin with bridging enoxaparin.

CLINICAL FEATURES

- Atrial fibrillation, left ventricular systolic dysfunction, mechanical valve replacement and congestive heart failure increase the risk for the formation of intracardiac thrombus. It is rare for intracardiac thrombus to produce identifying signs or symptoms independent from the underlying cardiac disease or the symptoms that result from embolization.

EPIDEMIOLOGY

- Atrial fibrillation commonly results in thrombus within the left atrial appendage, which may embolize and result in ischemic stroke. Atrial fibrillation affects over 2 million Americans, and 75,000 strokes are caused by atrial fibrillation each year.[1]
- Concomitant risk factors greatly impact the risk of stroke resulting from atrial fibrillation. Congestive heart failure, age, hypertension, diabetes, and prior stroke result in the greatest risk.
- Patients with valvular disease and atrial fibrillation have a risk of stroke 17 times greater than age-matched controls.[2]
- Intraventricular thrombus may develop in patients with recent myocardial infarction, particularly those with apical and anterior hypokinesis. Stroke occurs in 12% of patients with acute myocardial infarction complicated by left ventricular thrombus. The rate of embolization is greatest in the first to third month, and the thrombus may remain for greater than a year in over one-third of patients.[1]
- Similarly, intraventricular thrombus may result from congestive heart failure due to cardiomyopathy. The mean ejection fraction for those harboring a thrombus is 18%.[3] The risk of embolization is related to the degree of systolic dysfunction and increases 18% for every 5% decrement in ejection fraction.[1]

PATHOPHYSIOLOGY AND ETIOLOGY

- Atrial fibrillation causes stasis of blood within the atrial chamber that results in thrombus formation (Figures 8-5-2 to 8-5-4). The duration of atrial fibrillation and the size of the atria correlate with the likelihood of thrombus formation.
- In patients with left ventricular dysfunction, thrombus may develop in the ventricle due to stasis of blood, especially in the apex, in patients with myocardial infarction.

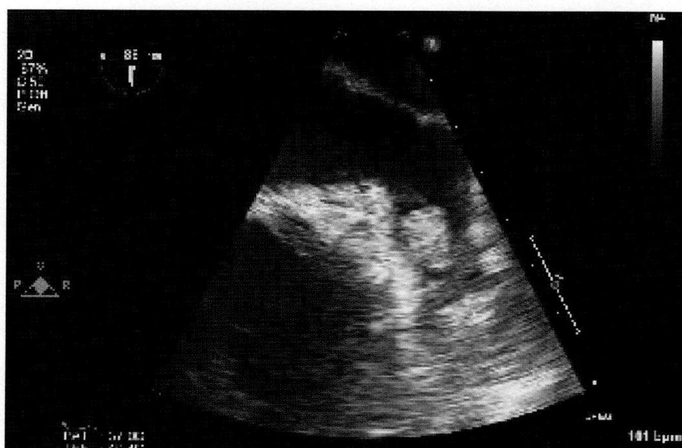

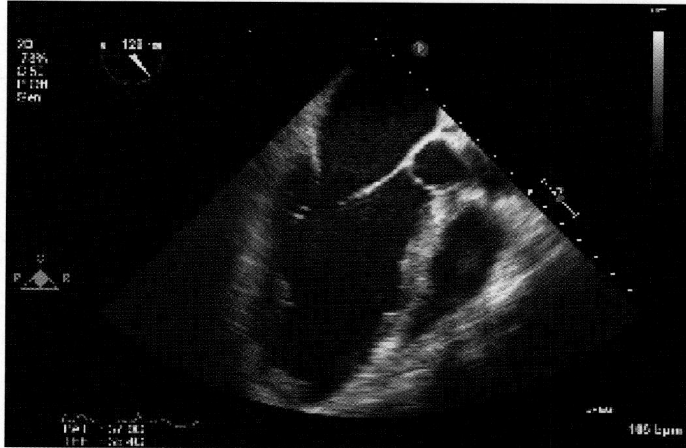

FIGURE 8-5-1 TEE demonstrating both a left atrial appendage (top panel) and left ventricular apical (bottom panel) thrombus ► (see Videos 8-5-1 L and R).

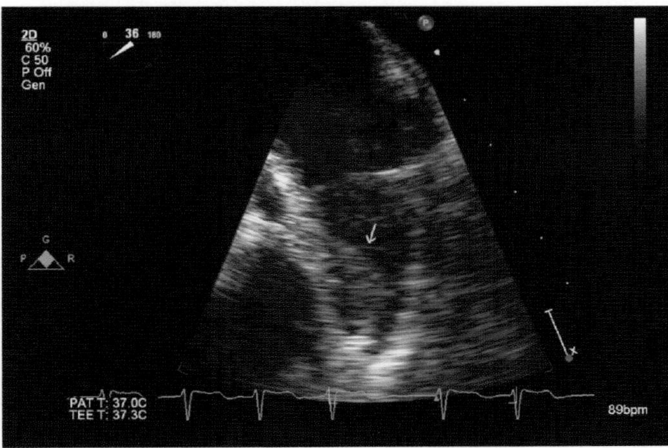

FIGURE 8-5-2 TEE of the left atrial appendage in another patient who presented with a TIA, which demonstrates spontaneous contrast and a large thrombus in the left atrial appendage ▶ (see Video 8-5-2).

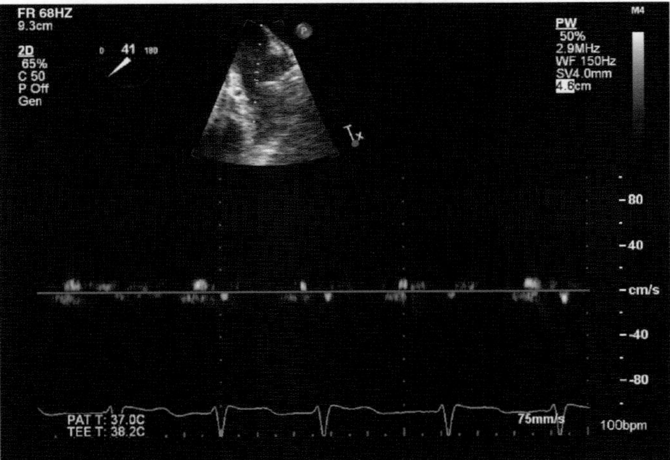

FIGURE 8-5-3 Pulsed wave Doppler of the left atrial appendage demonstrating severely impaired emptying velocities, which are associated with an increased risk of stroke.

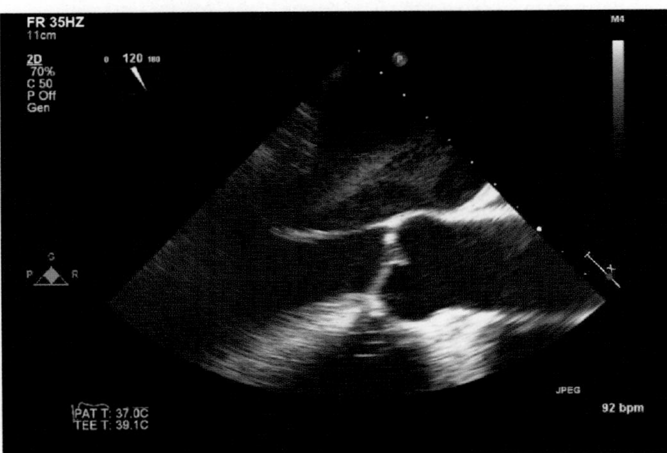

FIGURE 8-5-4 TEE demonstrating severe spontaneous contrast in an enlarged left atrium, which is associated with an increased risk of thromboembolism ▶ (see Video 8-5-4).

ECHOCARDIOGRAPHY

- Echocardiographic features may predict the likelihood of embolic stroke due to atrial fibrillation. Left atrial enlargement, left ventricular dysfunction, mitral annular calcification, visible left atrial thrombus, and spontaneous echo contrast all increase risk of embolization.[1]
- In addition to increased risk of thrombus formation, left atrial size correlates adversely with success of cardioversion. Peak Doppler flow filling velocities >25 cm/sec are associated with low probability of stroke. Similarly, spontaneous echo contrast increases risk of stroke from 3% to 12% per year.[4]
- Most atrial thrombi are found in the left atrial appendage which is best visualized with TEE.[2] In a study of over 200 patients with cryptogenic stroke, 55% were discovered to have a source of embolism. Among the cohort with normal TTE studies, 40% had findings on TEE, 13% of which prompted anticoagulation.

OTHER DIAGNOSTIC TESTING AND PROCEDURES

- Cardiac CT may be helpful in identifying atrial thrombi. In one series of 101 patients, 64-slice cardiac CT identified all clots seen on TEE and identified undiscovered thrombus in a small subset of patients.[5]
- Contrast enhanced MRI has utility in discovering atrial thrombus and demonstrated the highest sensitivity for surgically confirmed thrombi in one series of 160 patients.[6]

DIFFERENTIAL DIAGNOSIS

- Primary and metastatic cardiac tumors, valvular abnormalities, and thickened chordae tendonae and papillary muscles must be differentiated from intracardiac thrombus.

DIAGNOSIS

- Echocardiography is the main method of identification of intracardiac thrombi. Use of TTE prior to TEE evaluation should depend upon the clinical setting, TEE availability, individual patient features, and institution-specific data regarding study quality.
- Holter and telemetry monitoring is useful in identify paroxysmal atrial fibrillation. Unrecognized atrial fibrillation is an underappreciated source of cryptogenic stroke.

MANAGEMENT

- Guidelines recommend anticoagulation for patients aged 60 and older with atrial fibrillation and concomitant hypertension, diabetes mellitus, coronary artery disease, prior thromboembolism, systolic heart dysfunction or heart failure. Anticoagulation is recommended for all atrial fibrillation patients aged 75 and older who do not have a contraindication to anticoagulation.[7] These risks are consistent with a CHADS2 score of 2 or greater, which correlates with an annual stroke risk greater than 2.5%.[4] Goal INR for anticoagulation is 2 to 3 and should be started within the first 2 weeks after infarction. Warfarin has been shown to reduce the relative risk of stroke by 68%.[1] It is unclear if bridging with unfractionated or low molecular weight heparin is valuable in all patients, but it should be considered in those with Protein C or S deficiency or in those with intracardiac thrombus and early recurrent systemic embolization despite antiplatelet therapy.[8] The annual risk of hemorrhage on warfarin is 1.3%. Patients not able to tolerate warfarin may be treated with 325 mg of daily aspirin, which provides a 21% relative risk-reduction of stroke.[1] Patients experiencing a stroke while adequately anticoagulated are not likely to benefit from a higher goal INR or addition of antiplatelet medications.

- The role of atrial appendage closure and resection for stroke prevention is unclear.[10]
- Many new anticoagulant agents have been developed for the purpose of reducing stroke risk while providing an improved safety profile, freedom from INR monitoring, and fewer drug and food interactions. Dabigatran is an antifactor Xa agent recently evaluated in an open label trial. The medication demonstrated superior efficacy in preventing stroke and systemic embolization while limiting hemorrhage.[11] It remains to be seen if this performance is maintained with greater volume of use. The ROCKET AF study demonstrated that rivaroxaban, a factor Xa inhibitor, was comparable to warfarin in regards to preventing stroke while resulting in fewer complications of intracranial hemorrhage. While the promise of the new agents (dabigatran, rivaroxaban and apixaban) to decrease the risk of stroke in patients with non valvular AF is exciting, their safety and efficacy will ultimately be realized over time with routine use outside of clinical trials. In the event of serious bleeding, strategies for effective reversal of each of these agents have been ineffective.
- Patients with cardiomyopathy, low ejection fraction, and stroke are often anticoagulated, but there are no randomized trials to support this practice. Anti-platelet use is a reasonable alternative option. WARCEF found no benefit of warfarin over aspirin in patients with cardiomyopathy, EF <35%, though only 12% to 13% of patients in the study had prior TIA, stroke, and incidence of intracardiac thrombus not mentioned.[12]
- Patients with intraventricular thrombus after myocardial infarction are commonly anticoagulated for 3 months to one year.[1] Late embolization is uncommon in this cohort.

FOLLOW-UP

- Persistent or paroxysmal atrial fibrillation requires lifetime anticoagulation in a patient with a stroke or TIA.
- Serial TEE to follow the course of a documented left atrial thrombus in not indicated, unless restoration of sinus rhythm is planned.
- Given the questioned value of anticoagulation with cardiomyopathy-associated thrombus, and the decreased risk of late embolization in myocardial infarction patients, the value of routine echocardiographic follow-up is uncertain.

VIDEO LEGENDS

1. Video 8-5-1 L: TEE demonstrating a left atrial appendage thrombus.
2. Video 8-5-1 R: TEE demonstrating a left ventricular apical thrombus.
3. Video 8-5-2: TEE of the left atrial appendage in another patient who presented with a TIA which demonstrates spontaneous contrast and a large thrombus in the left atrial appendage
4. Video 8-5-4: TEE demonstrating severe spontaneous contrast in an enlarged left atrium which is associated with an increased risk of thromboembolism.

REFERENCES

1. Furie KL, Kasner SE, Adams RJ, et al. Guidelines for prevention of stroke in patients with ischemic stroke or transient ischemic attack. A guideline for healthcare professionals from the American Heart Association/American Stroke Association. *Stroke.* 2011;42:227-276.
2. Weir NU. An update on cardioembolic stroke. *Postgrad Med J.* 2008;84:133-142.
3. Sharma ND, McCullough PA, Philbin EF, Weaver WD. Left ventricular thrombus and subsequent thromboembolism in patients with severe systolic dysfunction. *Chest.* 2000;117:314-320.
4. Babarro EG, Rego AR, Gonzalez-Juanatey JR. Cardioembolic stroke: call for a multidisciplinary approach. *Cerebrovasc Dis.* 2009;27(suppl 1):82-87.
5. Hur J, Kim YJ, Nam JE, et al. Thrombus in the left atrial appendage in stroke patients: detection with cardiac CT angiography—a preliminary report. *Radiology.* 2008;249:81-87.
6. Srichai MB, Junor C, Rodriquez IL, et al. Clinical, imaging, and pathological characteristics of left ventricular thrombus: a comparison of contrast-enhanced magnetic resonance imaging, transthoracic echocardiography, and transesophageal echocardiography with surgical or pathological validation. *Am Heart J.* 2006;152:75-84.
7. Fuster V, Ryden LE, Asinger RW, et al. Guidelines for the management of patients with atrial fibrillation: executive summary. A report of the American College of Cardiology/American Heart Association Task Force on Practice Guidelines and the European Society of Cardiology Committee for Practice Guidelines and Policy Conferences. *Circulation.* 2001;104:2118-2150.
8. Hallevi H, Albright KC, Martin-Schild S, et al. Anticoagulation after cardioembolic stroke: to bridge or not to bridge? *Arch Neurol.* 2008;65(9):1169-1173.
9. deBruijn SFTM, Agema WRP, Lammers GJ, et al. Transesophageal echocardiography is superior to transthoracic echocardiography in management of patients of any age with transient ischemic attack or stroke. *Stroke.* 2006;37:2531-2534.
10. Block PC, Burstein S, Casale PN, et al. Percutaneous left atrial appendage occlusion for patients in atrial fibrillation suboptimal for warfarin therapy. 5-year results of the PLAATO (Percutaneous Left Atrial Appendage Transcatheter Occlusion) Study. *JACC Cardiovasc Interv.* 2009;2:594-600.
11. Becattini C, Vedovati MC, Agnelli G. Old and new oral anticoagulants for venous thromboembolism and atrial fibrillation: a review of the literature. *Thromb Res.* 2012;129:392-400.
12. Homma S, Thompson JLP, Pullicino PM, et al. Warfarin and aspirin in patients with heart failure and sinus rhythm. *N Engl J Med.* 2012;366:1859-1869.

9 ECHOCARDIOGRAPHY IN THE EVALUATION OF INTRACARDIAC MASSES

Saurabh Jha, MD, Teerapat Yingchoncharoen, MD, and Richard A. Grimm, DO

Echocardiography and in particular TEE is well suited to assess for the presence of intracardiac masses such as thrombus or tumor. Other imaging modalities, especially cardiac MRI, play an important complimentary role in characterization of the masses (eg, differentiating thrombus from tumor). In this chapter, Dr. Grimm and his colleagues from the Cleveland Clinic will highlight the value of echocardiography in the evaluation of patients with intracardiac masses, including cases of primary and metastatic cardiac tumors and intracardiac thrombus.

SECTION 1

Left Atrial Myxoma

CLINICAL CASE PRESENTATION

A 22-year-old woman who had been previously healthy, presented with acute right-sided paresthesias, expressive aphasia, and headache followed by weakness of all four extremities. The patient had an episode of tingling and numbness in the right lower extremity one month ago for which she did not seek medical care. The symptoms resolved spontaneously.

On physical examination she was hemodynamcially stable and had decreased motor strength in all four extremities. Cardiac exam revealed tachycardia without murmurs, gallops, or rubs. The initial CT scan of the head was negative; however, an MRI done later revealed acute infarcts in the territories of both middle cerebral and posterior inferior cerebellar arteries. An echocardiogram revealed depressed left ventricular systolic function (LVEF 25%) with wall motion abnormalities suggestive of Tako-tsubo cardiomyopathy, in addition to a left atrial (LA) mass attached to the fossa ovalis. Based on location, the echocardiographic appearance and the mobility of the left atrial mass, the presumptive diagnosis was an LA myxoma (Figures 9-1-1 to 9-1-5).

A diagnosis of multiple embolic events secondary to the left atrial mass was made, and the patient was urgently taken to the operating room for excision of the left atrial mass. The patient underwent successful excision of the left atrial mass, which was gelatinous in appearance with smooth surface in some areas and polypoid to irregular in others.

Her neurological status improved, and she regained normal strength in all four extremities except for some residual weakness in the right arm. Left ventricular systolic function improved significantly, and an echocardiogram done prior to discharge revealed LVEF of 45%.

A pathological assessment of the left atrial mass using Movat stain showed myxoid tumor with lipidic cells arranged in ring structures and cords confirming the diagnosis of left atrial myxoma.

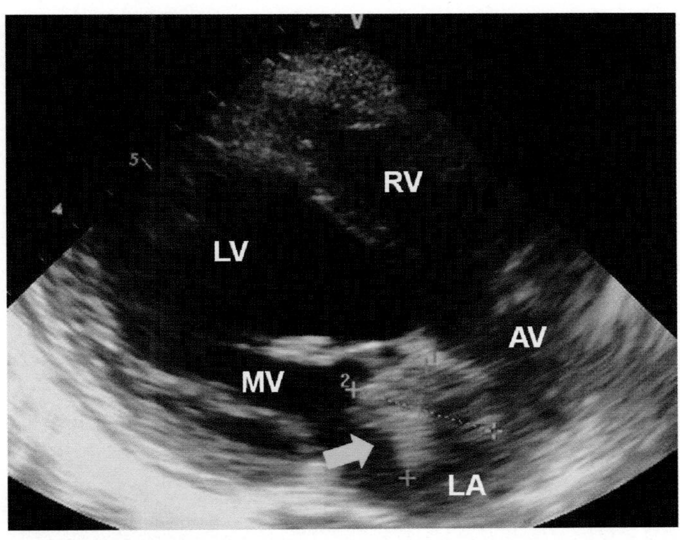

FIGURE 9-1-1 Parasternal long axis demonstrating a left atrial mass originating from the interatrial septum (arrow). RV = right ventricle, LV = left ventricle, LA = left atrium, MV = mitral valve, AV = aortic valve ► (see Video 9-1-1).

CLINICAL FEATURES

- Patients with cardiac myxoma mostly present with one or more features of the triad of embolism, intracardiac obstruction, and constitutional symptoms. However, sometimes myxomas are incidentally detected on noninvasive cardiac imaging done for unrelated reasons. Like other cardiac tumors, the clinical features of cardiac myxoma are determined primarily by its size, location, and mobility.[1]
- Most common symptoms include dyspnea (45%), constitutional symptoms (27%), thromboembolism (24%), chest pain (23%), incidental (22%), palpitations (21%), atrial fibrillation (14%), syncope (12%), and ventricular tachycardia (6%).[2]

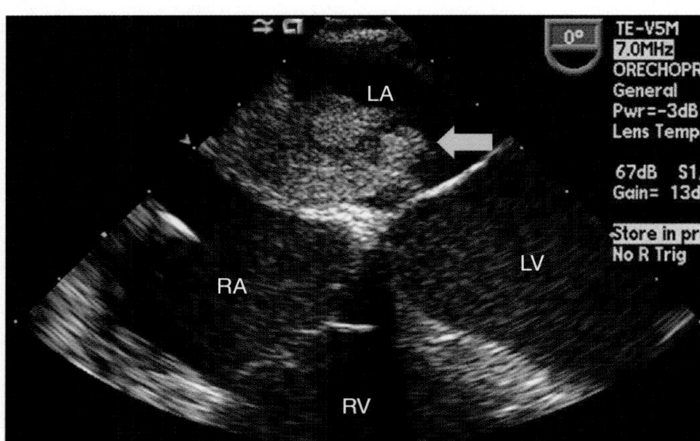

FIGURE 9-1-2 TEE midesophageal 4 chamber view showing a left atrial mass with irregular surface originating from the interatrial septum (arrow). RV = right ventricle, LV = left ventricle, RA = right atrium, LA = left atrium ► (see Video 9-1-2).

- Constitutional symptoms including fever, chills malaise, cachexia, and weight loss are attributable to secretion of inflammatory cytokines by the tumor or its release after tumor necrosis.
- Mechanical complications from myxoma commonly present as obstruction and/or regurgitation of the atrial ventricular valve (AV), as the tumor may prolapse through the AV valve especially when it is large and mobile. Severe obstruction may result in syncope, arrhythmia, and death.
- Symptoms related to the embolic event are primarily determined by location of the myxoma and may be the first presenting complaint in some patients. Emboli from a right sided myxoma results in pulmonary embolism. Embolism from a left sided myxoma may lead to stroke, TIA, myocardial infarction, limb and/or visceral ischemia. Systemic embolism from a right atrial myxoma in the presence of intracardiac shunt is rare.

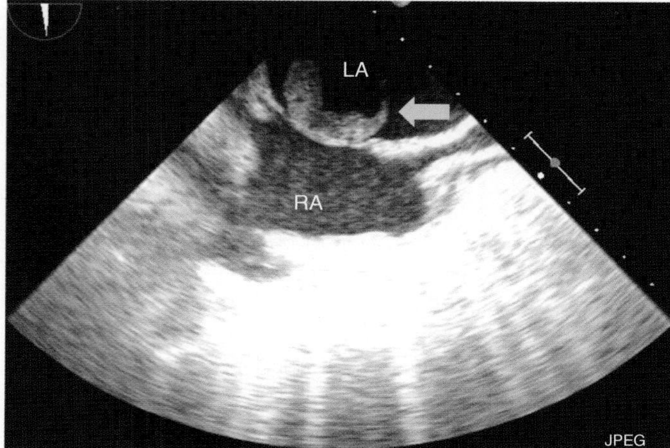

FIGURE 9-1-3 TEE bicaval view showing a left atrial mass originating from the fossa ovalis (arrow). RA = right atrium, LA = left atrium ► (see Video 9-1-3).

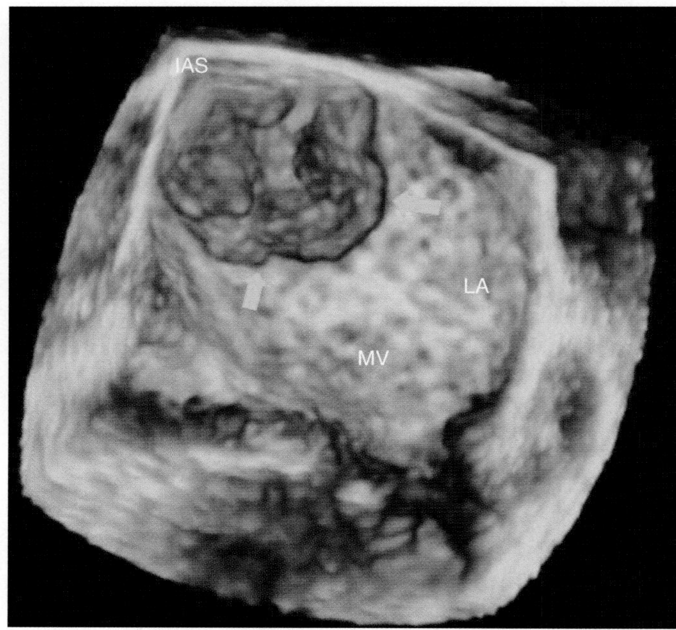

FIGURE 9-1-4 Three-dimensional TEE view of the left atrium showing a left atrial mass (arrows) originating from the interatrial septum. IAS = interatrial septum, LA = left atrium, MV = mitral valve ► (see Video 9-1-4).

- Myxoma can present as part of a familial syndrome known as the Carney complex, which is a multisystem tumorous disorder that features both cardiac and noncardiac myxomas (cutaneous myxoma and myxoid breast fibroadenomas), spotty skin pigmentation

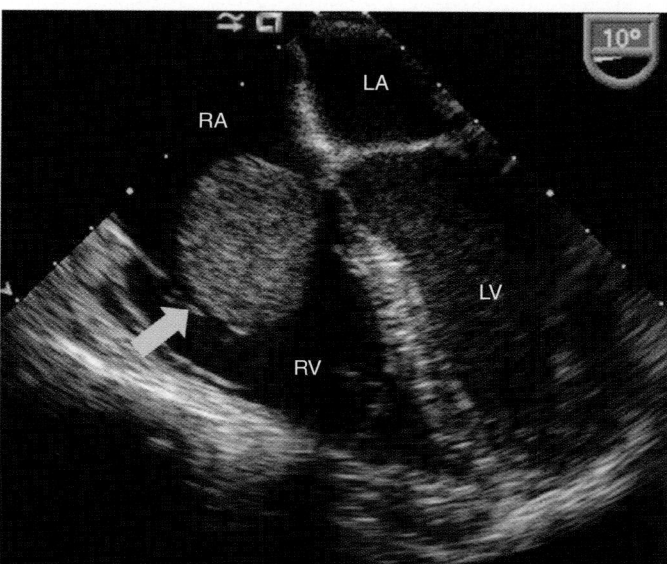

FIGURE 9-1-5 Midesophageal 4 chamber TEE view from different patient showing a right atrial mass with smooth surface, originating from the interatrial septum and prolapsing into the tricuspid valve (arrow). Pathology revealed findings consistent with a myxoma. RV = right ventricle, LV = left ventricle, RA = right atrium, LA = left atrium ► (see Video 9-1-5).

(lentigines and blue nevi), testicular tumors, endocrine hyperactivity (adrenocortical hyperplasia and pituitary hyperactivity), and peripheral nerve tumors (schwannomas).[3] The condition is inherited as autosomal dominant trait, so screening echocardiography is recommended for all first-degree relatives. The patients with familial myxoma syndrome present at a relatively younger age; the myxomas are more likely multiple and may be found in atypical locations.[1] There is a high rate of recurrence following resection. The cutaneous manifestations are a major clue to the diagnosis.

EPIDEMIOLOGY

- Primary cardiac tumors are rare with an autopsy frequency of 0.01% to 0.03%.[1] Myxomas are the most common cardiac tumors, accounting for 30% to 50% of all benign cardiac tumors.
- While the majority of the myxoma cases occur sporadically, approximately 7% of cases present as a familial syndrome with an autosomal dominant pattern of transmission.
- Myxomas are most commonly diagnosed between the third and sixth decades with a mean age of approximately 50 years at presentation.[4] Women are more commonly affected.
- Cardiac myxomas usually develop in the atria, with 75% originating in the left atrium and 15% to 20% originating in the right atrium.[1] Myxomas may be sessile or attached to the interatrial septum with a short peduncle.

PATHOPHYSIOLOGY AND ETIOLOGY

- Cardiac myxomas are either polypoid with a smooth, gently lobulated surface or papillary with friable, irregular appearing surface. Polypoid myxomas are usually well organized, and spontaneous fragmentation is rare, while papillary myxomas pose a higher risk of embolic complications. Myxomas internally may have areas of necrosis, cyst formation, and, rarely, calcification.[1]
- Characteristic histological finding of myxomas include the presence of lipidic cells in a stroma rich in glycosaminoglycans.
- Size may range from 1 to 15 cm; typical diameter at presentation is 4 to 8 cm.

ECHOCARDIOGRAPHY

- Echocardiography is the diagnostic modality of choice for detection of cardiac myxoma as it can not only accurately define the location and morphology, but also provide key information about mobility and hemodynamic effects. Transthoracic echocardiography is usually sufficient to make a diagnosis; however, transesophageal echocardiogram may also be employed in cases with suboptimal images.
- Cardiac myxomas typically appear as a mobile mass attached to the endocardial surface, usually the interatrial septum by a short peduncle.
- Myxomas usually have heterogeneous echogenicity due to areas of necrosis, cyst formation, and, rarely, calcification within primary tumor.
- Doppler echocardiography is used to demonstrate hemodynamic effects of myxoma, including valvular stenosis and/or regurgitation.
- Although not used routinely, contrast echocardiography can be used to demonstrate the vascularity of the cardiac mass and differentiate a vascular tumor from thrombus.

OTHER DIAGNOSTIC TESTING AND PROCEDURES

- Cardiac CT and MRI are complimentary techniques that can be used to obtain additional diagnostic information regarding tissue characterization of the cardiac mass and assessment of the extracardiac structures. A myxoma typically has heterogeneous contrast enhancement variably reflecting areas of necrosis. Areas of calcification can be best demonstrated by CT. Myxomas notably have increased signal intensity on T2 weighted images and has differential enhancement on perfusion sequences.
- Basic laboratory findings include anemia, leukocytosis, and elevated erythrocytic sedimentation rate.

DIFFERENTIAL DIAGNOSIS

- The differential diagnoses of cardiac masses is quite broad, as listed in Table 9-1-1.
- Metastatic disease of the heart is far more common than primary cardiac tumors and is discussed in detail in a later section of this chapter. The differential diagnosis of primary cardiac tumors can be categorized based on its potential of invasion and is summarized in Table 9-1-2.

DIAGNOSIS

- Noninvasive imaging, primarily echocardiography, is the mainstay of preoperative diagnosis. Final diagnosis is often made based on appearance and pathological analysis after surgical resection of the tumor.
- Symptoms and signs of cardiac myxoma are nonspecific. Cutaneous manifestations may help in the diagnosis of familial myxoma syndrome.

TABLE 9-1-1 Differential Diagnosis of Cardiac Mass

- Thrombus
- Vegetation
- Degenerative changes: Lambl's excrescences
- Calcification: caseous necrosis of mitral annulus
- Tumor: benign, malignant, and metastatic
- Normal structure/variant: prominent Chiari network, Eustachian valve, crista terminalis, lipomatous hypertrophy of interatrial septum
- Iatrogenic material

TABLE 9-1-2 Differential Diagnosis of the Primary Cardiac Tumors

Benign
• Myxoma
• Papillary fibroelastoma
• Rhabdomyoma
• Fibroma
• Lipoma
• Teratoma
• Hemangioma
• Lymphangioma
• Hemangiopericytoma
• Mesothelioma of AV node
• Pericardial cyst
Malignant
• Angiosarcoma
• Rhabdomyosarcoma
• Synovial sarcoma
• Liposarcoma
• Myxosarcoma
• Fibrosarcoma

MANAGEMENT

- Surgical en bloc resection of the myxoma with a margin of normal cardiac tissue is the treatment of choice and is curative in most cases. In addition to tumor resection, sometimes additional reconstruction may be warranted, eg, rare cases of myxoma arising from the mitral valve may further require valvular repair or replacement after resection of the tumor.
- After diagnosis of cardiac myxoma, surgical resection should be performed urgently to prevent embolic and/or mechanical complications like obstruction of the atrioventricular valves.[5]
- Surgical resection of cardiac myxomas carries low operative risk and affords excellent short and long term survival.[5] A single center study from the Mayo Clinic reported that survival after successful resection of myxoma is not significantly different from age- and gender-matched population.[2]

FOLLOW-UP

- There is an overall 13% risk of recurrence after surgical resection, which is much more frequent in patients with familial myxomas versus isolated, sporadic tumors (22% versus 3%).[1] The site of recurrence is most commonly at the location of the original tumor.[2]
- The cumulative incidence of recurrence increases steadily for 4 years following surgical resection, after which risk of recurrence is low. Semiannual follow-up with echocardiography has been recommended for the first 4 years following surgical resection to assess for recurrence.[1] Thereafter, annual follow-up with noninvasive cardiac imaging should be considered.

VIDEO LEGENDS

1. Video 9-1-1: Parasternal long axis demonstrating a left atrial mass originating from the inter-atrial septum.
2. Video 9-1-2: TEE mid-esophageal 4-chamber view showing a left atrial mass with irregular surface originating from the inter-atrial septum
3. Video 9-1-3: TEE bicaval view showing a left atrial mass originating from the fossa ovalis
4. Video 9-1-4: 3D TEE view of left atrium showing a left atrial mass originating from the interatrial septum.
5. Video 9-1-5: Mid-esophageal 4-chamber TEE view from a different patient showing a right atrial mass with smooth surface, originating from the inter-atrial septum and prolapsing into the tricuspid valve.

REFERENCES

1. Bruce CJ. Cardiac tumours: diagnosis and management. *Heart.* 2011;97(2):151-160.
2. Elbardissi AW, Dearani JA, Daly RC, et al. Survival after resection of primary cardiac tumors: a 48-year experience. *Circulation.* 2008;118(14 Suppl):S7-15.
3. Carney JA, Gordon H, Carpenter PC, et al. The complex of myxomas, spotty pigmentation, and endocrine overactivity. *Medicine (Baltimore).* 1985;64(4):270-283.
4. Burke AJ, Jeudy J Jr, Virmani R. Cardiac tumours: an update: Cardiac tumours. *Heart.* 2008;94(1):117-123.
5. Kuroczyński W, Peivandi AA, Ewald P, Pruefer D, Heinemann M, Vahl CF. Cardiac myxomas: short- and long-term follow-up. *Cardiol J.* 2009;16(5):447-454.

SECTION 2

Cardiac Papillary Fibroelastoma

CLINICAL CASE PRESENTATION

This patient is a 38-year-old woman who presented to the emergency department after she woke up with left arm numbness, which progressed rapidly to involve her left leg. She also has a history of hypertension and migraines. The patient denied any weakness or sensory symptoms anywhere else in the body.

On physical examination she was found to have diminished proprioception, two-point discrimination on the left upper and lower extremities. She had normal muscle strength in all four extremities. Cardiovascular examination was normal. A CT scan of the head revealed a small hypo density in the right temporal lobe and external capsule region suggesting acute infarction. MRI of the brain confirmed a right middle cerebral artery territory perisylvian acute nonhemorrhagic infarction. An echocardiogram, done to assess for intracardiac source of emboli, revealed an intracardiac mass, measuring 0.8 × 0.9 cm, attached to the ventricular side of the anterior mitral leaflet, suspicious for a cardiac papillary fibroelastoma (CPF) (Figures 9-2-1 to 9-2-4).

She was referred for surgical resection of the intracardiac mass. During cardiac surgery, a small mobile mass attached to the A_2 segment of the anterior mitral leaflet with a short peduncle was seen and successfully excised. The patient had an uneventful postoperative course and has had no recurrence so far after 3 years of follow-up.

Surgical pathology using Movat's pentachrome staining showed a papillary tumor with fibrous cords containing elastic fibers, which confirmed the preoperative diagnosis of cardiac papillary fibroelastoma.

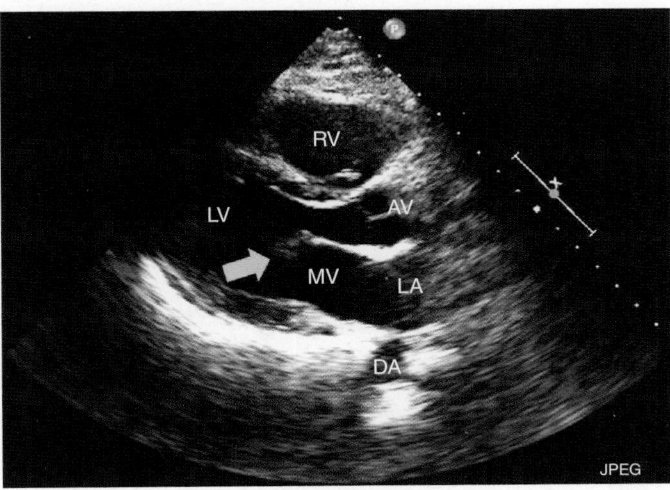

FIGURE 9-2-1 Parasternal long axis demonstrating a mass attached to ventricular side of the anterior mitral leaflet (arrow) consistent with a CPF. RV = right ventricle, LV = left ventricle, LA = left atrium, MV = mitral valve, AV = aortic valve, DA = descending aorta ▶ (see Video 9-2-1).

CLINICAL FEATURES

- Nearly 50% of cases are diagnosed incidentally on echocardiogram done for unrelated reasons or during assessment of a cardiac source of embolism.[1]
- Although frequently CPF is diagnosed incidentally, transient ischemic attack, stroke, myocardial infarction, sudden death, heart failure, presyncope, syncope, pulmonary embolism, blindness, and peripheral embolism related to CPF have been reported.[2]
- Tumor mobility is an independent predictor of death and nonfatal embolic event.[2]

EPIDEMIOLOGY

- CPF is the second most common primary cardiac tumor after myxoma. In a single center study based on postoperative surgical pathology, CPF accounted for 26% of benign cardiac tumors.[3] CPF accounts for approximately 75% of all cardiac valvular tumors.[4]
- The true prevalence of CPF is unknown, and reported data is likely an underestimation as a significant proportion of the patients remain asymptomatic. The frequency of detection of CPF has increased with improvements in echocardiographic resolution with advent of higher frequency transducers and more frequent use of TEE.[5]
- CPF has a wide range of age at presentation with a mean of 60 years. The highest prevalence is noted in the eighth decade followed by the fourth decade. Males comprise approximately 55% of cases.[2,5]
- There is a strong association between CPF and hypertrophic cardiomyopathy, cardiac surgery, hemodynamic trauma, and radiation exposure.[1]

PATHOPHYSIOLOGY AND ETIOLOGY

- CPF are mostly solitary, small (average 1.1 ± 0.5 cm), and originate from the valvular surface (80% versus 20% from atrial and ventricular surfaces).[5]
- CPF have a characteristic frond-like appearance that resembles a sea anemone on gross examination, especially when placed under saline. Histologically, the tumor is comprised of an inner avascular core of connective tissue containing collagen, smooth muscle, and elastic fibers that is surrounded by a layer of mucopolysaccharide, followed by an outermost layer on endothelium.
- CPF are considered to be slow-growing tumors, though the natural history has not been characterized.
- Embolic complications may occur due to embolization of attached thrombi or the tumor itself. CPF has been reported to prolaspe into the coronary ostium, which may lead to myocardial infarction.

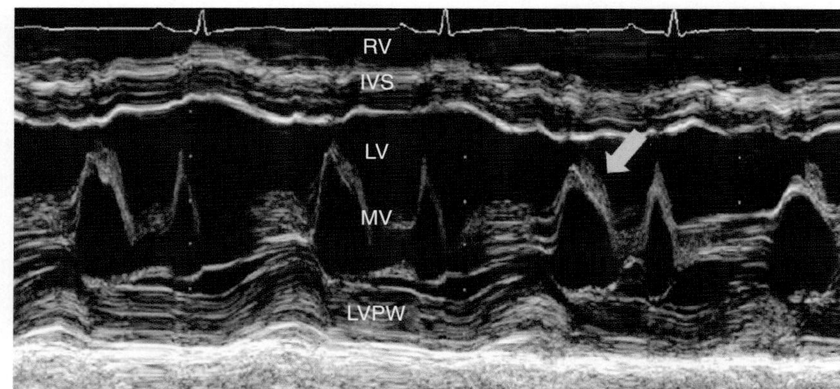

FIGURE 9-2-2 M-Mode imaging at the tip of mitral valve demonstrating the evidence of intracardiac mass (arrow).

ECHOCARDIOGRAPHY

- Due to superior spatial and temporal resolution, echocardiography is the principal imaging modality to diagnose and follow up CPF. TEE is an important diagnostic tool to define the extent and anatomic attachments of CPF.[5]
- CPF is traditionally described as a small and well-delineated mass with a predilection for valvular endocardium. Nearly 45% of CPF have a small stalk and are mobile. CPF has a characteristic echocardiograph appearance of a central homogeneous speckled pattern and a characteristic stippling along the edges with a "shimmer" or "vibration" at the tumor-blood interface.[1,4,5]
- CPF typically originates from the left sided cardiac valves, most commonly from the aortic valve, followed by mitral valve. CPF do not cause valvular dysfunction. The most common nonvalvular site of origin is the left ventricle.
- For CPF size more than 0.2 cm, the sensitivity, specificity, and accuracy of the transthoracic echocardiography is 88.9%, 87.8%, and 88.4%, respectively.[5]
- Figures 9-2-5 to 9-2-9 provide other examples of CPF.

OTHER DIAGNOSTIC TESTING AND PROCEDURES

- Even with technological advancements of cardiac CT and MRI, evaluation of small valvular tumors remains limited, and echocardiography is the diagnostic modality of choice. Cardiac CT plays an important role in the assessment of the coronary arteries and other extracardiac structures prior to surgical resection of CPF.

DIFFERENTIAL DIAGNOSIS

- Lambl's excrescences are comparatively smaller in size, often multiple, and frequently seen in the elderly patients.

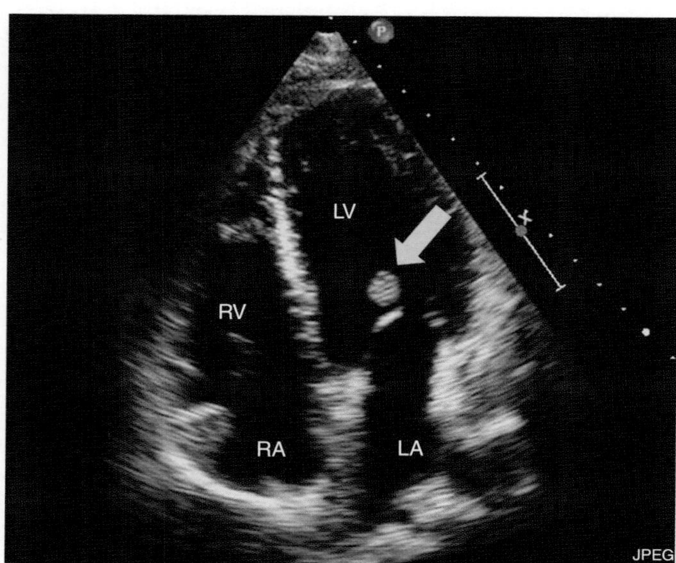

FIGURE 9-2-3 Apical 4 chamber view showing a mass attached to the ventricular side of the anterior mitral leaflet (arrow). RV = right ventricle, LV = left ventricle, LA = left atrium, RA = right atrium ▶ (see Video 9-2-3).

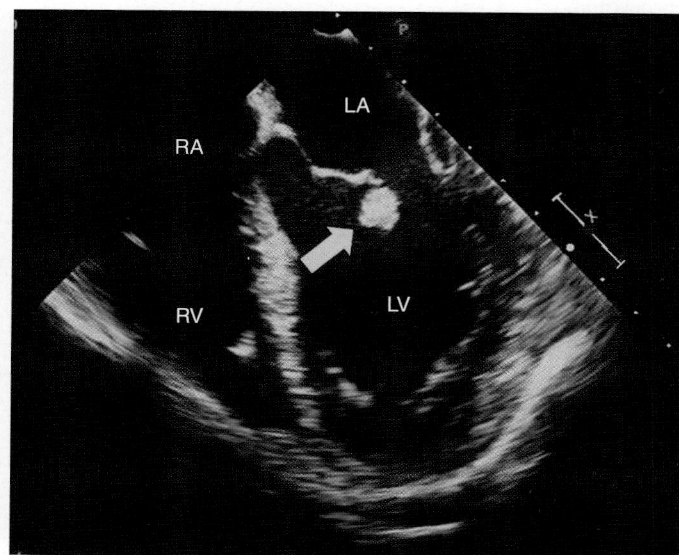

FIGURE 9-2-4 TEE midesophageal 4 chamber view demonstrating a mass attached to the ventricular side of the anterior mitral leaflet (arrow). RV = right ventricle, LV = left ventricle, LA = left atrium, RA = right atrium ▶ (see Video 9-2-4).

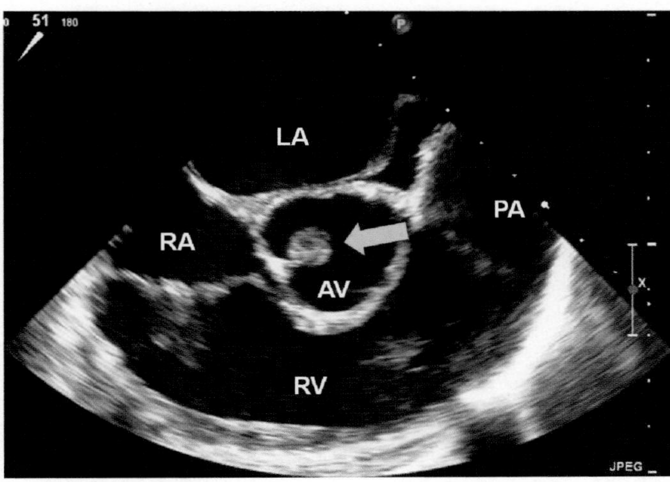

FIGURE 9-2-5 TEE midesophageal short axis aortic valve view demonstrating a mass attached to the noncoronary cusp of the aortic valve in a different patient with a CPF (arrow). RV = right ventricle, LA = left atrium, RA = right atrium, PA = pulmonary artery ▶ (see Video 9-2-5).

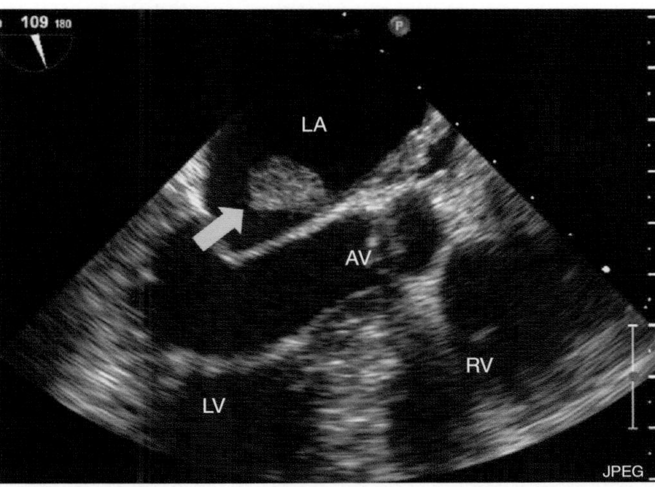

FIGURE 9-2-7 TEE midesophageal 3 chamber long axis view demonstrating a mass attached to interatrial septum in a different patient with CPF (arrow) confirmed with pathology. AV = aortic valve, LA = left atrium, RV = right ventricle, LV = left ventricle. ▶ (see Video 9-2-7).

- Vegetations may be of similar size; however, they are usually noted on upstream side of the valves and usually cause valvular dysfunction. In contrast, CPF is attached to the downstream side of the valves, and despite its attachment it does not cause valvular dysfunction. Clinical information, blood cultures, and other laboratory data may help in establishing the diagnosis.
- Cardiac myxoma, although rare, may originate from the valves. Likewise, CPF may develop in the left atrium, which is the most common location for cardiac myxoma. Differences in echocardiographic appearance of CPF (central homogenous specked pattern with stippled edges) and myxoma (heterogeneous) may occasionally help to establish a preoperative diagnosis.

DIAGNOSIS

- Noninvasive imaging, primarily echocardiography, is the mainstay of preoperative diagnosis of CPF. Final diagnosis is often made based on appearance and pathological analysis after surgical resection of the tumor.

MANAGEMENT

- Patients with embolic events that are not explained by other cardiac or neurological disorders should be referred for surgical resection, which is curative and has excellent long-term postoperative prognosis.

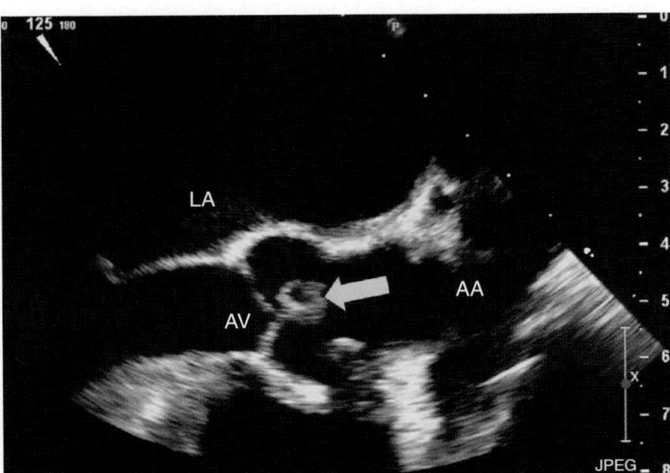

FIGURE 9-2-6 TEE midesophageal 3 chamber long axis view demonstrating a mass attached to the aortic valve in a different patient with CPF (arrow). AV = aortic valve, LA = left atrium, AA = ascending aorta. ▶ (see Video 9-2-6).

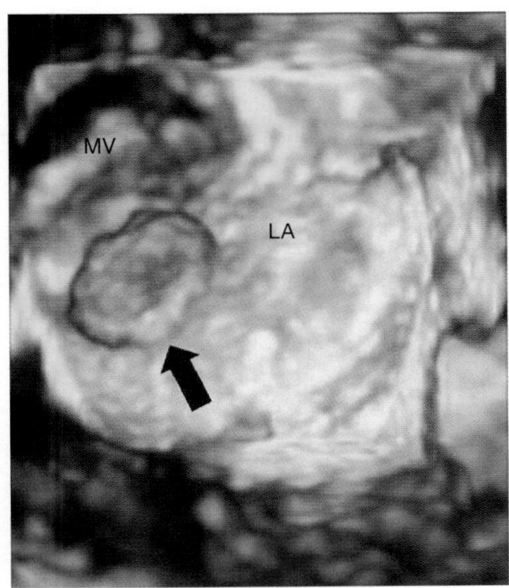

FIGURE 9-2-8 Three-dimensional view of the left atrium showing a left atrial mass originating from the interatrial septum in a different patient with CPF (arrow). LA = left atrium, MV = mitral valve ▶ (see Video 9-2-8).

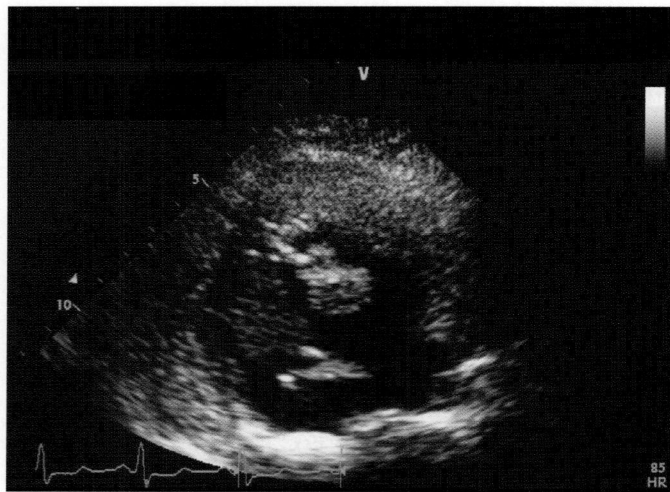

FIGURE 9-2-9 TTE apical 3 chamber view from another patient with a unique fibroelastoma ▶ (see Video 9-2-9). This patient had a large (asymptomatic) mass detected on TTE 5 years ago performed to evaluate a heart murmur. He was found to have moderate aortic stenosis (AS) at that time. He subsequently developed symptomatic severe AS and underwent aortic valve replacement. The mass appeared unchanged on echocardiography over the 5 years. At surgery, the mass was found attached to the LV wall and was excised. Pathology confirmed the diagnosis of a large CPF.

- Asymptomatic patients with large (>1 cm) or mobile CPF should be referred for consideration of surgical resection. In particular, young patients with low perioperative risk and a high cumulative risk of embolic event should be referred for surgical resection. Surgical resection should also be performed in patients requiring cardiac surgery for other reasons.
- Asymptomatic patients with small and sessile CPF should be observed and followed with periodic echocardiograms.

FOLLOW-UP

- Recurrences of CPF after surgical resection is uncommon.
- As noted above, CPF patients without definite indications for surgical resection should be monitored periodically with echocardiogram.

VIDEO LEGENDS

1. Video 9-2-1: Parasternal long axis demonstrating a mass attached to ventricular side of the anterior mitral leaflet consistent with a CPF.
2. Video 9-2-3: Apical 4-chamber view showing a mass attached to the ventricular side of the anterior mitral leaflet
3. Video 9-2-4: TEE mid-esophageal 4-chamber view demonstrating a mass attached to ventricular side of the anterior mitral leaflet
4. Video 9-2-5: TEE mid-esophageal short axis aortic valve view demonstrating a mass attached to the non-coronary cusp of the aortic in a different patient with a CPF
5. Video 9-2-6: TEE mid-esophageal 3-chamber long axis view demonstrating a mass attached to the aortic valve in a different patient with CPF
6. Video 9-2-7: TEE mid-esophageal 3-chamber long axis view demonstrating a mass attached to interatrial septum in a different patient with CPF confirmed with pathology
7. Video 9-2-8: 3D view of the left atrium showing a left atrial mass originating from the interatrial septum in a different patient with CPF
8. Video 9-2-9: TTE apical 3 chamber view from another patient with a unique fibroelastoma. This patient had a large (asymptomatic) mass detected on TTE 5 years ago performed to evaluate a heart murmur. He was found to have moderate aortic stenosis (AS) at that time. He subsequently developed symptomatic severe AS and underwent aortic valve replacement. The mass appeared unchanged on echocardiography over the 5 years. At surgery, the mass was found attached to the LV wall and was excised. Pathology confirmed the diagnosis of a large CPF.

REFERENCES

1. Bruce CJ. Cardiac tumours: diagnosis and management. *Heart.* 2011;97(2):151-160.
2. Gowda RM, Khan IA, Nair CK, Mehta NJ, Vasavada BC, Sacchi TJ. Cardiac papillary fibroelastoma: a comprehensive analysis of 725 cases. *Am Heart J.* 2003;146(3):404-410.
3. Elbardissi AW, Dearani JA, Daly RC, et al. Survival after resection of primary cardiac tumors: a 48-year experience. *Circulation.* 2008;118(14 Suppl):S7-15.
4. Klarich KW, Enriquez-Sarano M, Gura GM, Edwards WD, Tajik AJ, Seward JB. Papillary fibroelastoma: echocardiographic characteristics for diagnosis and pathologic correlation. *J Am Coll Cardiol.* 1997;30(3):784-790.
5. Sun JP, Asher CR, Yang XS, et al, Clinical and echocardiographic characteristics of papillary fibroelastomas: a retrospective and prospective study in 162 patients. *Circulation.* 2001;103(22):2687-2693.

SECTION 3

Metastatic Disease of The Heart

CLINICAL CASE PRESENTATION

A 71-year-old man was referred to our institution in September 2009 for evaluation of a right atrial (RA) mass detected by chest CT scan. His past medical history was notable for metastatic renal cell carcinoma (RCC) diagnosed in 2007. He presented initially with a right shin fracture, which led to the discovery of 1 × 3 cm soft tissue mass at the distal tibia. Pathology was renal cell carcinoma. Further investigation revealed evidence of left RCC with lung metastases. He underwent cytoreductive radical left nephrectomy with removal of renal vein thrombus and regional lymphadenopathy in March 2007 and was started on Bevacizumab/IL-2. This chemotherapy regimen had to be discontinued due to acute myocardial infarction suffered in June 2007. A new regimen of IV temsirolimus was then given, but the patient developed pneumonitis and the medication was discontinued. Oral sorafenib was tried since February 2009 but then was stopped due to myocardial depression (LVEF dropped from 45% to 20%) with a heart failure exacerbation. In March 2009, all chemotherapy was stopped, and surveillance CT scans were then performed. Clinically, the patient was doing well, however, he has had two heart failure hospitalizations in the past 6 months with recurrent right pleural effusion.

On physical examination, the patient's vital signs were stable (BP 150/66 mm Hg and heart rate 73 beats/min), and his jugular venous pressure was not elevated. The patient's lungs were clear to auscultation. The cardiac examination showed regular rate and rhythm with occasional premature beat. Normal S_1 and S_2 with a 2/6 diastolic murmur with probable tumor plop appreciated along the left parasternal border. The abdomen was soft and nontender.

Transthoracic echocardiography was performed and revealed a large, round, echodense right atrial mass sitting immediately under the tricuspid valve that measured 3.1 cm in diameter. No clear stalk or site of attachment to the interatrial septum or free wall was seen. There was no suggestion of mass extension from the IVC (Figures 9-3-1 to 9-3-4).

Cardiac MRI was then performed for tissue characterization of the mass, which confirmed a 3.3 × 4.5 cm bilobed mass in the medial basal right atrium (Figure 9-3-5). Also noted were multiple lung nodules and bilateral hilar and mediastinal partially necrotic lymphadenopathy. The RA mass demonstrated perfusion with perfusion imaging and mild evidence of delayed enhancement. The signal characteristics of the RA mass were similar to the lung lesions, suggesting likely metastatic disease.

The patient underwent successful RA mass resection. The mass was 3 × 5 cm arising from the atrial septum that appeared to involve the fibrous skeleton of the heart and was extending to the origin of the coronary sinus and into the RA. The tumor was completely excised.

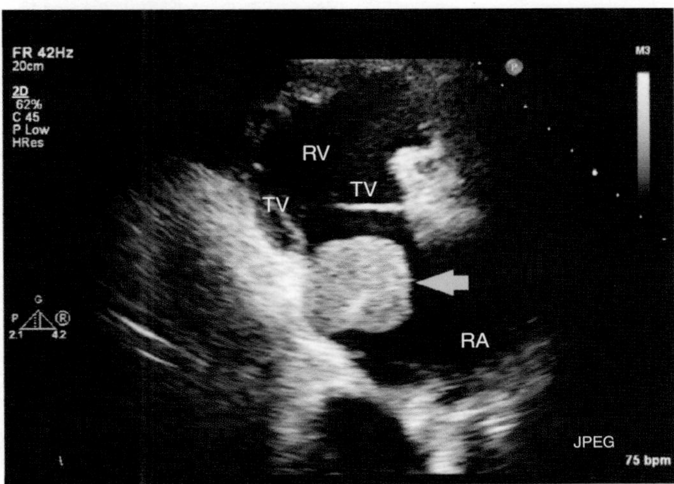

FIGURE 9-3-1 RV inflow view demonstrating a round, well circumscribed mass in the RA (arrow). RA = right atrium, RV = right ventricle, TV = tricuspid valve ▶ (see Video 9-3-1).

Pathological assessment of the tumor revealed metastatic carcinoma, consistent with the patient's known clear cell renal cell carcinoma. The patient tolerated all procedures well and was discharged without complications. He remained well without recurrence for 24 months since the procedure. Unfortunately, he developed progressive shortness of breath with massive right pleural effusion in 2011 and passed away comfortably at the local palliative medicine program.

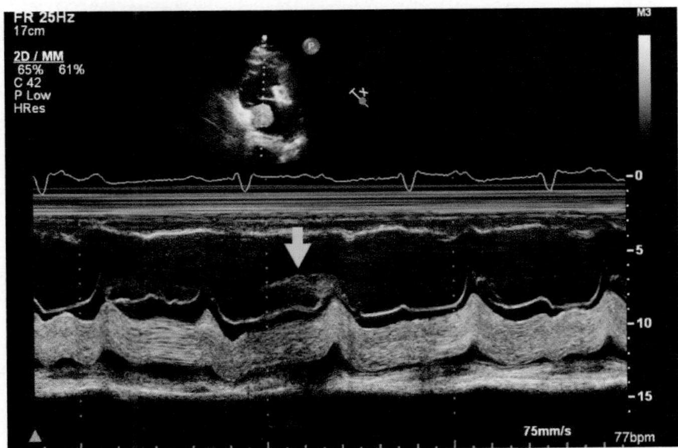

FIGURE 9-3-2 M-Mode imaging of the RV inflow showed the evidence of intracardiac mass (arrow).

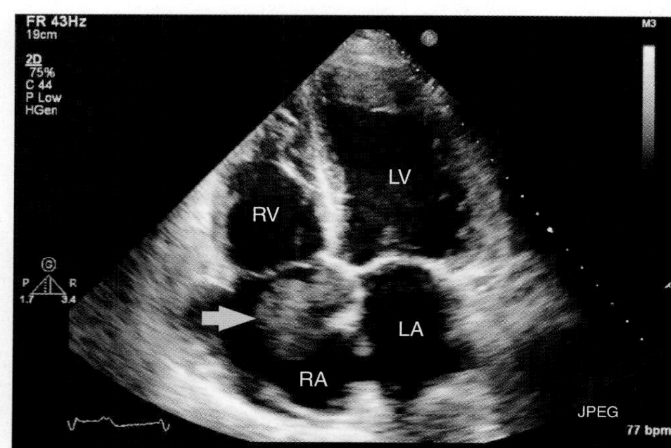

FIGURE 9-3-3 Apical 4 chamber view showed mass in the RA originating from the interatrial septum (arrow). RV = right ventricle, LV = left ventricle, RA = right atrium, LA = left atrium ► (see Video 9-3-3).

CLINICAL FEATURES

- The symptoms of cardiac metastases are extremely variable, depending on the location of the tumor, the extension of the involvement, and complications related to that particular tumor.
- The main presenting symptoms can be divided into three categories.
  - Cardiovascular-related symptoms (which result from valve obstruction, interference with valvular structures resulting in regurgitation, direct invasion of the myocardium with associated impaired contractility, arrhythmias and conduction disorders, pericardial effusion with or without cardiac tamponade or embolization).
  - Constitutional symptoms or symptoms related to the underlying malignancy.
  - Asymptomatic with the mass incidentally discovered during cardiac work-up.

EPIDEMIOLOGY

- The autopsy incidence of cardiac metastases ranges from 1.7% to 14% (average 7.1%) in cancer patients and 0.7% to 3.5% (average 2.3%) in the general population.[1]

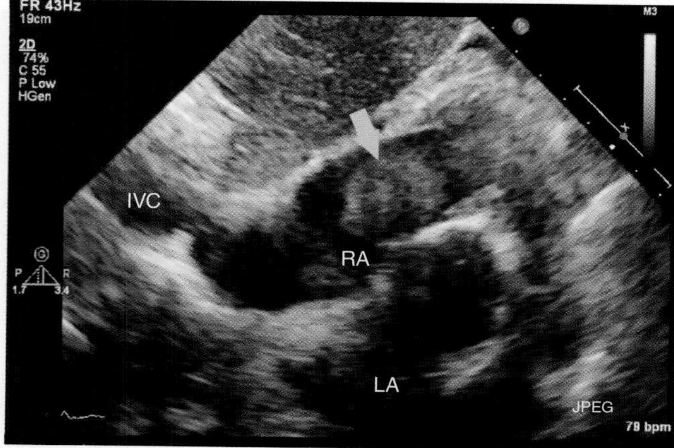

FIGURE 9-3-4 Subcostal view showing the RA mass without evidence of extension from the IVC. IVC = inferior vena cava, RA = right atrium, LA = left atrium ► (see Video 9-3-4).

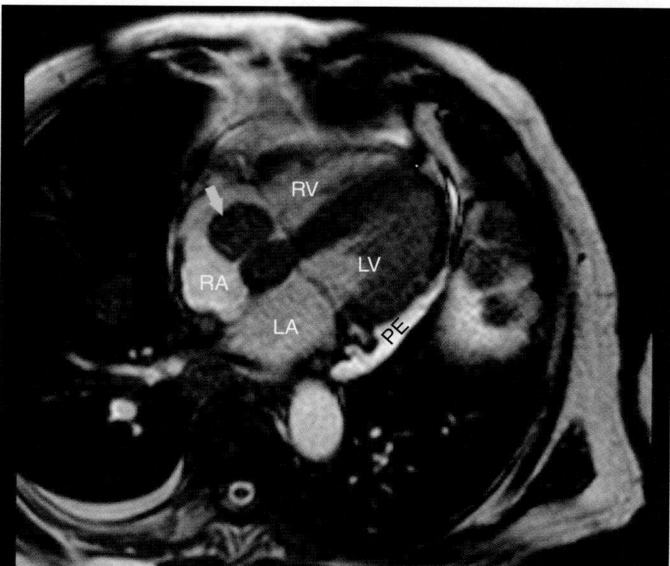

FIGURE 9-3-5 Cardiac MRI. Steady-state free precession (SSFP) imaging 4 chamber view demonstrating a lobulated RA mass originating from the interatrial septum (arrrow) with a small pericardial effusion. RV = right ventricle, LV = left ventricle, RA = right atrium, LA = left atrium, PE= pericardial effusion.

- In comparison to older series, there is a significant increase in the incidence of cardiac metastases in patients with cancers since 1970. This is likely due to improvement of imaging modalities and a greater detection rate.[2]

PATHOPHYSIOLOGY AND ETIOLOGY

- There are four general mechanisms responsible for the development of cardiac metastases.
  - Direct extension of a local tumor (eg, lung cancer)
  - Hematogenous spread
  - Lymphatic spread
  - Intracavitary spread through the inferior or superior vena cava or the pulmonary veins
- Pericardial metastasis (69%) are the most common type of cardiac metastasis, followed by epicardial metastisis (5%).[3]
- The epicardium is most often involved due to direct invasion by thoracic cancers. The myocardium or epicardium is most commonly involved through lymphatic spread and endocardial metastasis through hematogenous spread.
- Abdominal and pelvic tumors may reach the RA through the IVC. The most common tumor exhibiting this tendency is renal cell carcinoma.
- Most of the studies report that lung cancer is the most common cause of cardiac metastasis, followed by hematologic malignancy; however, one study from a tertiary care center hospital reported that the most common secondary cardiac tumor is renal cell carcinoma, followed by sarcoma.[2]
- Cardiac metastasis from RCC without vena cava involvement is rare.

- Zustovich and colleagues[2] reviewed 15 patients who were surgically treated for cardiac metastases from RCC without IVC involvement. They suggested that a venous hematogenous pathway is mainly the pathologic route of metastatic spread to the right side of the heart and a lymphatic pathway is the metastatic route to the lymph nodes, lungs, pericardium, and left side of the heart.

ECHOCARDIOGRAPHY

- Echocardiography is the initial test of choice to detect cardiac metastases and their complications.
- In pericardial metastases, malignant pericardial effusion is usually detected. Occasionally, intrapericardial masses, bands or fronds of soft tissue, and pericardial thickening may be seen.
- In myocardial metastases, a localized area of wall thickening may be seen.
- In intracavitary metastases, tumors may propagate within the blood vessels returning to the heart. These tumor usually appear as large elongated masses inside and extending from the inferior vena cava and entering right atrium, sometimes extending into the RV. These intraluminal tumors may be distinguished from simple thrombi which usually appear as thin, elongated venous casts.[4]

OTHER DIAGNOSTIC TESTING AND PROCEDURES

Electrocardiography (ECG)

- In isolation, the ECG provides little incremental clue to the diagnosis. However, changes in rhythm or voltage or development of new AV block on serial tracings may be the first sign of either extension of a primary cardiac tumor or development of cardiac metastasis.

Radionuclide Imaging

- Although gated blood pool scanning has been used to identify cardiac mass in the past, the inferior resolution and sensitivity has made this form of imaging obsolete.
- On the other hand, positron emission tomography (PET) scan is useful in identifying cardiac involvement in metastatic tumors as well as differentiating other cardiac mass mimickers such as sarcoidosis.

Computerized Tomography (CT)

- CT provides better soft-tissue contrast than echocardiography. It can depict calcification and may allow tissue characterization by measuring attenuation value (Hounsfield unit), although not as effectively as cardiac magnetic resonance (CMR). CT also allows the assessment of extracardiac structures that may be the primary tumors that metastasized to the heart.

Cardiac Magnetic Resonance

- Unlike two-dimensional echocardiography, CMR has the potential for tissue characterization by comparing relaxation properties of the mass with a reference tissue.
- However, due to the widespread variability in water content of the tumor, the differences in tumor age and vascularity and the limited data on cardiac malignancies tissue characteristics, the reliability of CMR to differentiate subtypes of cardiac malignancies is limited.[5]
- Features that may suggest malignant tumors, include but are not limited to: high degree of vascularity, infiltration of adjacent tissue, inhomogeneous appearance, presence of necrosis or calcification, peritumorous edema, and the presence of an indeterminate mass with a known primary elsewhere.[6]

Endomyocardial Biopsy (EMB)

- Limited data exist on the utility of EMB in the management of cardiac tumors. Generally, the diagnosis is made from noninvasive imaging; however, EMB can be considered if imaging is equivocal or if a tissue sample is required prior to treatment decisions (ie, chemotherapy).

DIFFERENTIAL DIAGNOSIS

- The differential diagnosis of cardiac metastases are broad. Table 9-3-1 provides the common causes of cardiac metastases.

TABLE 9-3-1 Differential Diagnosis of Cardiac Metastases Categorized by Mode of Metastasis

Direct extension
Breast cancer
Lung cancer
Esophageal cancer
Mediastinal tumors
Hematogenous
Malignant melanoma
Lymphoma
Leukemia
Soft tissue and bone sarcoma
Lung cancer
Breast cancer
Genitourinary tract cancers
Gastrointestinal tract cancers
Venous
Renal cell carcinoma
Nephroblastoma (Wilm's tumor)
Leiomyoma of the uterus
Carcinoma of the adrenal cortex
Thyroid cancer
Lung cancer
Hepatocellular carcinoma
Lymphatic
Lymphoma
Leukemia

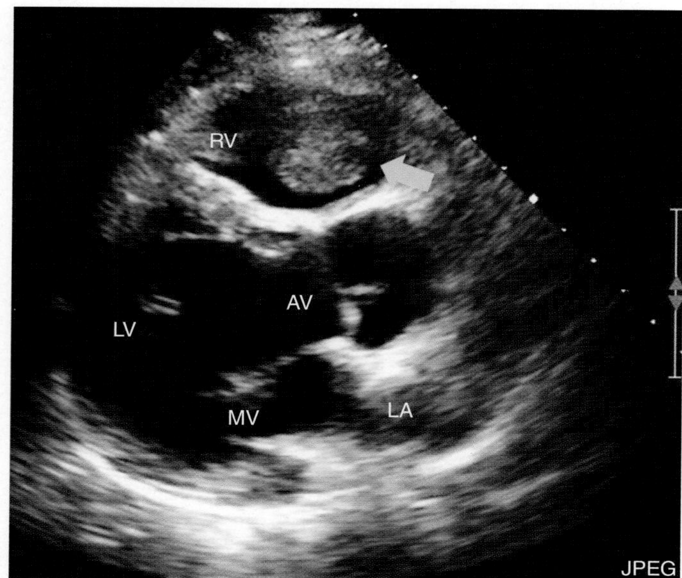

FIGURE 9-3-6 Parasternal long axis view image from a different patient showing metastatic fibrosarcoma in the right ventricle outflow tract (arrow). RV = right ventricle, LV = left ventricle, LA = left atrium, MV = mitral valve, AV = aortic valve ▶ (see Video 9-3-6).

- Establishing the correct diagnosis is imperative. A thorough differential diagnosis of nonmalignant conditions must be considered and ruled out. Figure 9-3-7 provides the differential diagnosis of RA mass and mass-like structures.

DIAGNOSIS

- The noninvasive imaging appearance of metastatic deposits seldom distinguishes the tumor type. Rather, a careful evaluation for the primary tumor or a detailed history of malignancy disease provides the strongest clue.[7] Unfortunately, the final diagnosis in many cases must still be made pathologically.

MANAGEMENT

- Treatment of metastatic cardiac tumors is usually palliative.
- Different series have shown that the median survival is 17 to 24 months for patients who can undergo complete resection and 6 to 10 months for patients unable to undergo complete resection.[8,9]
- Surgery with postoperative chemotherapy and/or radiotherapy to prevent local recurrence is indicated in patients with a better prognosis without disseminated disease.[1]
- Orthotopic heart transplantation is an option in selected patients, with improved survival.[10]
- In patients with disseminated disease, limited life expectancy and poor performance status make radiotherapy the treatment of choice
- Chemotherapy is recommended for chemo-sensitive tumors.
- In these patients, because of the grave prognosis, end-of-life care should be discussed, and all efforts should be made to improve the patients' quality of life.

FOLLOW-UP

- Regardless of the type of surgical resection or whether the tumor is sporadic, annual follow-up non-invasive imaging is recommended to detect the tumor recurrence or complications.
- Patients with cardiac metastases require thorough oncologic evaluation and follow-up for their underlying primary malignancy and its response to therapy.

VIDEO LEGENDS

1. Video 9-3-1: RV inflow view demonstrating a round, well circumscribed mass in the RA
2. Video 9-3-3: Apical four chamber view showed the mass in the RA originating from the interatrial septum
3. Video 9-3-4: Subcostal view showing the RA mass without evidence of extension from the IVC
4. Video 9-3-6: Parasternal long axis view image from a different patient showing metastatic fibrosarcoma in the right ventricular outflow tract

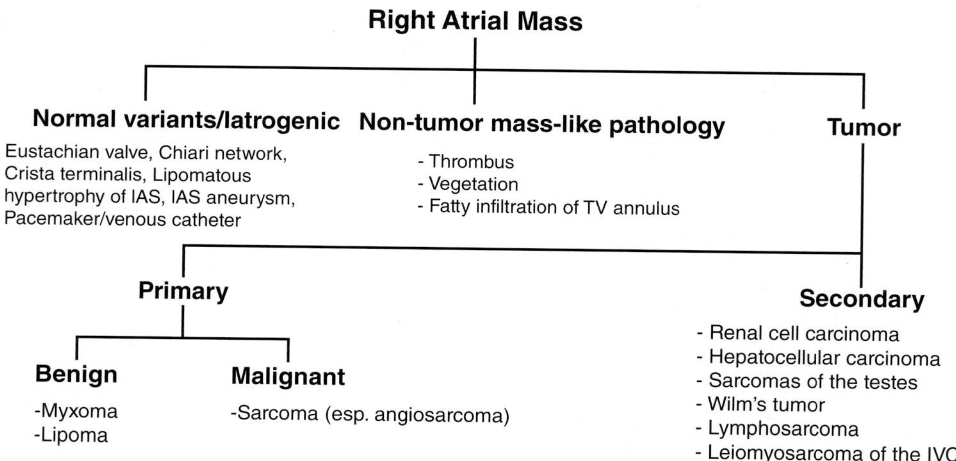

FIGURE 9-3-7 An algorithm to evaluate a right atrial mass.

REFERENCES

1. Al-Mamgani A, Baartman L, Baaijens M, de Pree I, Incrocci L, Levendag PC. Cardiac metastases. *Int J Clin Oncol.* 2008;13:369-372.
2. Yusuf SW, Bathina JD, Qureshi S, et al. Cardiac tumors in a tertiary care cancer hospital: clinical features, echocardiographic findings, treatment and outcomes. *Heart Int.* 2012;7:e4.
3. Bussani R, De-Giorgio F, Abbate A, Silvestri F. Cardiac metastases. *J Clin Pathol.* 2007;60:27-34.
4. Swenson JD, Hullander RM, Nolan JF, York JK. Renal cell carcinoma in the inferior vena cava demonstrated by transesophageal echocardiography. *J Cardiothorac Vasc Anesth.* 1993;7:335-336.
5. Dorsay TA, Ho VB, Rovira MJ, Armstrong MA, Brissette MD. Primary cardiac lymphoma: CT and MR findings. *J Comput Assist Tomogr.* 1993;17:978-981.
6. Tazelaar HD, Locke TJ, McGregor CG. Pathology of surgically excised primary cardiac tumors. *Mayo Clin Proc.* 1992;67:957-965.
7. Butany J, Nair V, Naseemuddin A, Nair GM, Catton C, Yau T. Cardiac tumours: diagnosis and management. *Lancet Oncol.* 2005;6:219-228.
8. Simpson L, Kumar SK, Okuno SH, et al. Malignant primary cardiac tumors: review of a single institution experience. *Cancer.* 2008;112:2440-2446.
9. Gross BH, Glazer GM, Francis IR. CT of intracardiac and intrapericardial masses. *AJR Am J Roentgenol.* 1983;140:903-907.
10. Winther C, Timmermans-Wielenga V, Daugaard S, Mortensen SA, Sander K, Andersen CB. Primary cardiac tumors: a clinicopathologic evaluation of four cases. *Cardiovasc Pathol.* 2011;20:63-67.

SECTION 4

Left Ventricular Thrombus

CLINICAL CASE PRESENTATION

An 88-year-old man with past medical history of hypertension, diabetes mellitus, and ischemic cardiomyopathy was referred to our institute for the treatment of stage IV diffuse large B-cell lymphoma involving multiple areas of the GI tract. He denies any recent history of dyspnea on exertion, paroxysmal nocturnal dyspnea, or orthopnea. The 12-lead ECG showed normal sinus rhythm with Q waves in V_1 to V_4. Echocardiography revealed a dilated left ventricle (LV diastolic internal diameter 6 cm) with severely depressed LV systolic function (LVEF 35%). The entire apex was akinetic. The mid anteroseptal, inferoseptal, and anterior segments were severely hypokinetic. The basal anteroseptal segment and midanterolateral segment were mildly hypokinetic. There was a mural left ventricular thrombus seen in the apex, which was clearly demonstrated with LV contrast opacification (Figures 9-4-1 to 9-4-4). He was anticoagulated with warfarin with an INR goal 2.0 to 3.0 for 1 month. On repeat echocardiography after 1 month of treatment, the LV mural apical thrombus had resolved. The LV size and systolic function were stable. The patient experienced no embolic phenomenon or significant bleeding.

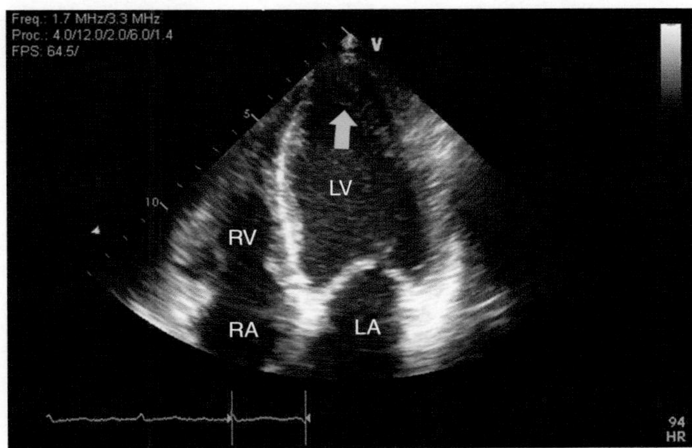

FIGURE 9-4-1 Apical 4 chamber view revealed a probable LV apical thrombus (arrow) in the area of apical akinesia ▶ (see Video 9-4-1). LA = left atrium, LV = left ventricle, RA = right atrium, RV= right ventricle.

CLINICAL FEATURES

- The presence of an LV thrombus increases the risk of peripheral embolization. Data from a meta-analysis including 11 studies of 865 patients who had had an anterior wall acute myocardial infarction (AMI) with documented LV thrombus showed that the odds ratio for an embolic event was 5.5 (95% CI 3.0-9.8) compared to those without an LV mural thrombus.[1]
- The patients with a peripheral embolic event had a significantly higher mortality (38.9%) when compared to those with severe systolic dysfunction but had no embolic event (10.3%) ($p<0.0001$).[2]

EPIDEMIOLOGY

- The incidence of LV thrombi in patients with AMI in the prereperfusion era was reported to be as high as 40% in patients with anterior infarction.[3] Most thrombi developed within the first 2 weeks (median 5 to 6 days) after AMI. In a series of 30 patients with LV thrombus after an anterior AMI, 27% were present at less than

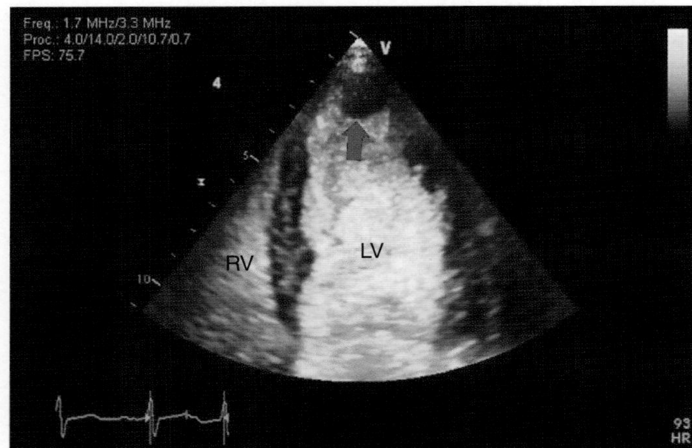

FIGURE 9-4-2 Apical 4 chamber view with IV contrast for LV opacification. The use of contrast more clearly defined the LV apical thrombus (arrow) ▶ (see Video 9-4-2). LV = left ventricle, RV = right ventricle.

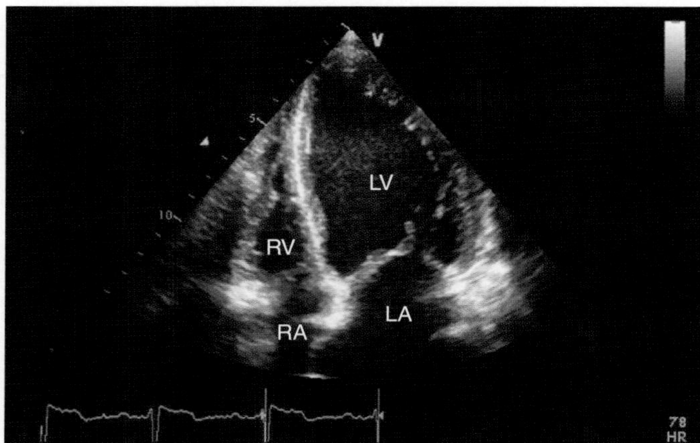

FIGURE 9-4-3 Repeat echo after 1 month of anticoagulation. Apical 4 chamber view showed no clear thrombus in the LV apex ▶ (see Video 9-4-3). LV = left ventricle, RV = right ventricle.

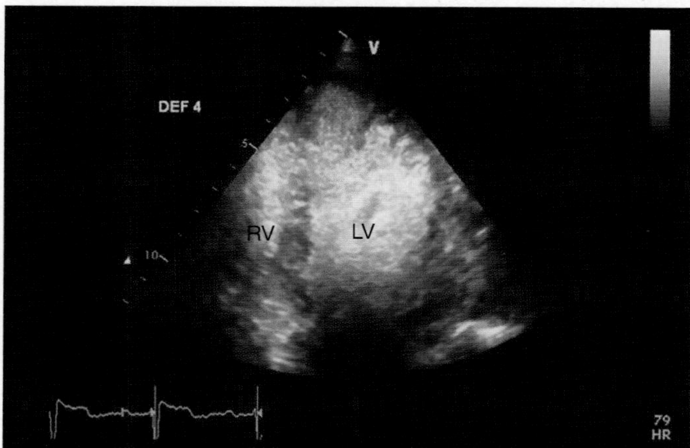

FIGURE 9-4-4 Apical 4 chamber view with contrast confirmed resolution of the LV thrombus after the treatment with anticoagulation. Note the swirling of contrast in the LV apex consistent with low flow, which provides a milieu for recurrent thrombus formation ▶ (see Video 9-4-4). LV = left ventricle, RV= right ventricle.

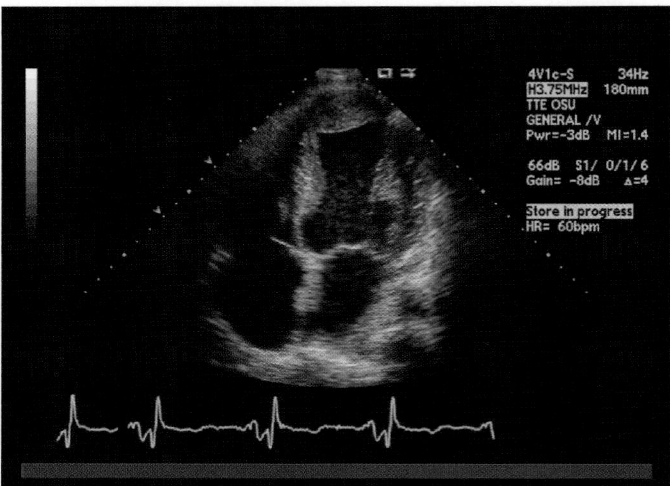

FIGURE 9-4-5 Transthoracic apical 4 chamber view from another patient who presented with symptoms of CHF. Based on his history, he had suffered a myocardial infarction 2 weeks prior, but did not seek medical advice. The TTE demonstrates an apical wall motion abnormality and a large apical mass consistent with a thrombus ▶ (see Video 9-4-5). History and laboratory data did not suggest evidence for endomyocardial fibroelastosis or hypereosinophilic syndrome. Catheterization demonstrated a total occluded LAD artery, and he was treated medically, including anticoagulation with warfarin.

24 hours, 57% at 48 to 72 hours, 75% at 1 week, and 96% at 2 weeks.[4]

- The rate of LV thrombi among anterior wall AMI in the postreperfusion era was reported to be about 6.2%. Predictors for LV thrombi included reduced ejection fraction and severe mitral regurgitation. The rate of thrombus formation was similar in patients who received rapid percutaneous coronary intervention (PCI) or thrombolytics.[5]

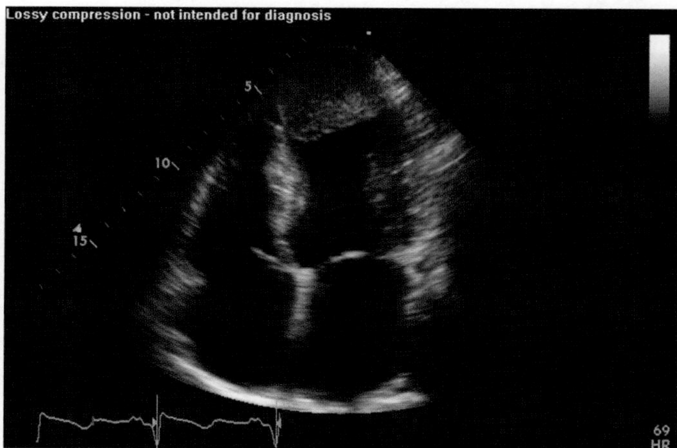

FIGURE 9-4-6 Repeat TTE when the patient in Figure 9-4-5 represented 3 months later with recurrent CHF. He had been noncompliant with medical therapy including his anticoagulation regimen. The apical thrombus was much larger as seen in this figure ▶ (see Video 9-4-6) and Figure 9-4-7. Therapy was reinstituted; however, he has been lost to follow-up.

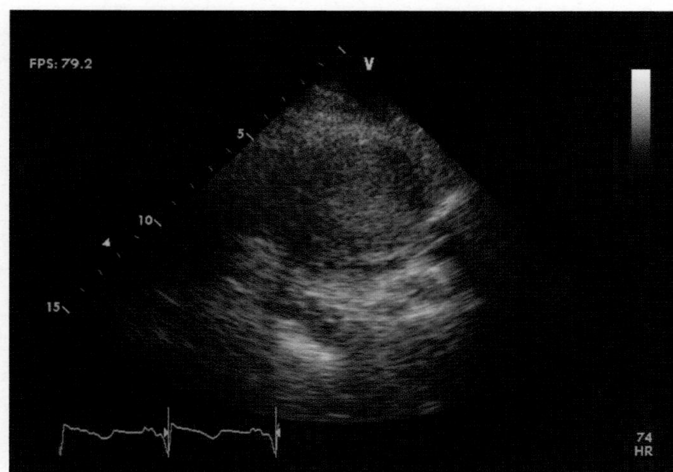

FIGURE 9-4-7 Apical short axis view demonstrated that the LV apex is filled with thrombus.

PATHOPHYSIOLOGY AND ETIOLOGY

- Left ventricular thrombi occur in conditions associated with blood stasis and/or regional wall motion abnormalities, including, but not limited to, acute myocardial infarction, left ventricular aneurysm/pseudoaneurysm, dilated cardiomyopathy, apical ballooning syndrome, as well as in patients with a hypercoagulable state.

ECHOCARDIOGRAPHY

- LV thrombi typically appear as a heterogeneous echo density superimposed on and interrupting the normal endocardial contour of the ventricle in the region of abnormal wall motion.
- LV thrombus formation is extremely rare in the absence of an akinetic or dyskinetic apex or diffuse LV dysfunction. When present, these thrombi are most commonly located in the apex (Figures 9-4-5 to 9-4-7).
- Thrombi may be laminated and parallel to the endocardial surface, spherical or pedunculated, and freely mobile. They may have a fixed base with mobile filaments extending from the base. An echo-lucent center may be present and suggests that the thrombus is relatively new and actively growing. When organized, thrombi may contain areas that are brighter than surrounding myocardium.
- The predictive accuracy of echocardiography for detecting LV thrombi is highly operator-dependent, but overall sensitivity and specificity were 92% to 95% and 86% to 88%, respectively.[6,7]
- To enhance sensitivity, a high-frequency (5- or 7.5-MHz) transducer with a short focal length should be used to improve near-field resolution. It is important to obtain the images from several apical views including standard and off-axis views of the apex.
- Use of an intravenous contrast agent to opacify the LV apex has been shown to improve the sensitivity and specificity of thrombus detection.[8] LV thrombi appear as a filling defect separated from the myocardium by contrast, while muscular structures are obscured.
- Real-time three-dimensional echocardiography provides more information about thrombus mobility, point of attachment, and identification of the presence of focal echolucent areas within thrombi indicative of the presence and extent of clot lysis.[9]

OTHER DIAGNOSTIC TESTING AND PROCEDURES

- Transesophageal echocardiography (TEE) is less sensitive than TTE and rarely helpful to detect LV thrombus due to the considerable distance of LV apex from the transducer.
- Cardiac computed tomography (CT) can differentiate the LV thrombus from myocardium. Thrombi are characterized by nonenhancement with contrast agent and appear as a filling defect within the LV. The attenuation (Hounsfield unit) within left ventricular thrombi is typically lower than the myocardium.
- Delayed-enhancement cardiac MRI (DE-CMR) appears to have a greater sensitivity than TTE and a similarly high specificity for the detection of LV thrombus. The absence of contrast enhancement can be used to distinguish thrombus from other masses such as neoplasm, which typically demonstrate contrast uptake due to tumor-associated vascularity. Thrombus appears black on long inversion time (ie, 600 msec) DE-CMR, which is a specific feature for thrombus identification on CMR.

DIFFERENTIAL DIAGNOSIS

The differential diagnosis of "masses" seen in the LV apex with echocardiography include:

- Near-field artifact
- Normal cardiac structures: papillary muscles, prominent trabeculations, false tendons
- Apical hypertrophy
- Endomyocardial fibroelastosis
- Hypereosinophilic syndrome
- Myocardial noncompaction
- Tumors
- Vegetations

DIAGNOSIS

- The diagnosis of LV thrombus is most secure when an echogenic mass is seen with a convex surface in the region of abnormal wall motion with echodensity that is clearly distinct from the endocardium.
- The diagnosis of laminated thrombus is often problematic unless a clear demarcation between the thrombus and the underlying myocardium is seen, but it can be suspected when the apex appears "rounded" and akinetic with apparent excessively thick apical myocardium.
- The use of transpulmonic contrast agents has clearly improved the diagnostic accuracy of TTE.[8]

MANAGEMENT

- For patients with documented LV thrombus by echocardiography, treatment with warfarin with a target international normalized ratio (INR) of 2.0 to 3.0 is recommended. Anticoagulation therapy should be lifelong in patients with atrial fibrillation—at least 3 months in patients with sinus rhythm. The continuation of treatment after 3 months should be decided based on follow-up echocardiographic findings (resolution or persistence of LV thrombus and the severity of LV dysfunction).[10]

FOLLOW-UP

- TTE can be used to monitor resolution of thrombus with anticoagulation. The use of contrast in the follow-up studies is critical in order to detect small residual thrombus.
- Thrombus resolution was seen in 69% at 1-year and 76% at 2-year follow-up.[3]

VIDEO LEGENDS

1. Video 9-4-1: Apical four chamber view demonstrates a probable LV apical thrombus in the area of apical akinesia
2. Video 9-4-2: Apical four chamber view with IV contrast for LV opacification. The use of contrast more clearly defines the LV apical thrombus
3. Video 9-4-3: Repeat echo after 1 month of anticoagulation. Apical four chamber view showed no clear thrombus in the LV apex
4. Video 9-4-4: Apical four chamber view with contrast confirmed resolution of the LV thrombus after the treatment with anticoagulation. Note the swirling of contrast in the LV apex consistent with low flow which provides a milieu for recurrent thrombus formation
5. Video 9-4-5: Transthoracic apical 4 chamber view from another patient who presented with symptoms of CHF. The TTE demonstrates an apical wall motion abnormality and a large apical mass consistent with a thrombus. History and laboratory data did not suggest evidence for Endomyocardial fibroelastosis or Hypereosinophilic syndrome.
6. Video 9-4-6: Repeat TTE when the patient in Video 9-4-5 represented 3 months later with recurrent CHF. He had been non-compliant with medical therapy including his anticoagulation regimen. The apical thrombus was much larger as seen in this video.

REFERENCES

1. Vaitkus PT, Barnathan ES. Embolic potential, prevention and management of mural thrombus complicating anterior myocardial infarction: a meta-analysis. *J Am Coll Cardiol.* 1993;22:1004-1009.
2. Sharma ND, McCullough PA, Philbin EF, Weaver WD. Left ventricular thrombus and subsequent thromboembolism in patients with severe systolic dysfunction. *Chest.* 2000;117:314-320.
3. Nihoyannopoulos P, Smith GC, Maseri A, Foale RA. The natural history of left ventricular thrombus in myocardial infarction: a rationale in support of masterly inactivity. *J Am Coll Cardiol.* 1989;14:903-911.
4. Kupper AJ, Verheugt FW, Peels CH, Galema TW, Roos JP. Left ventricular thrombus incidence and behavior studied by serial two-dimensional echocardiography in acute anterior myocardial infarction: left ventricular wall motion, systemic embolism and oral anticoagulation. *J Am Coll Cardiol.* 1989;13:1514-1520.
5. Osherov AB, Borovik-Raz M, Aronson D, et al. Incidence of early left ventricular thrombus after acute anterior wall myocardial infarction in the primary coronary intervention era. *Am J Heart.* 2009;157:1074-1080.
6. Visser CA, Kan G, David GK, Lie KI, Durrer D. Two-dimensional echocardiography in the diagnosis of left ventricular thrombus. A prospective study of 67 patients with anatomic validation. *Chest.* 1983;83:228-232.
7. Stratton JR, Lighty GW Jr, Pearlman AS, Ritchie JL. Detection of left ventricular thrombus by two-dimensional echocardiography: sensitivity, specificity, and causes of uncertainty. *Circulation.* 1982;66:156-166.
8. Mansencal N, Nasr IA, Pilliere R, et al. Usefulness of contrast echocardiography for assessment of left ventricular thrombus after acute myocardial infarction. *Am J Cardiol.* 2007;99:1667-1670.
9. Duncan K, Nanda NC, Foster WA, Mehmood F, Patel V, Singh A. Incremental value of live/real time three-dimensional transthoracic echocardiography in the assessment of left ventricular thrombi. *Echocardiography.* 2006;23:68-72.
10. Antman EM, Anbe DT, Armstrong PW, et al. ACC/AHA guidelines for the management of patients with ST-elevation myocardial infarction; A report of the American College of Cardiology/American Heart Association Task Force on Practice Guidelines (Committee to revise the 1999 guidelines for the management of patients with acute myocardial infarction). *J Am Coll Cardiol.* 2004;44:E1-E211.

SECTION 5

Left Atrial Thrombus

CLINICAL CASE PRESENTATION

This patient is an 82-year-old woman with persistent atrial fibrillation and known rheumatic heart disease affecting both the mitral and aortic valves who presented to the outpatient clinic with progressive worsening of exertional chest pain, shortness of breath, orthopnea, and paroxysmal nocturnal dyspnea, as well as intermittent palpitations. She also had long history of persistent atrial fibrillation and failed attempts at cardioversion. She denied any history suggestive of CVA or TIA and reported compliance with her home medications that included warfarin, β-blockers, and loop diuretics.

On physical examination, the patient was tachycardic (heart rate 101 BPM) and her BP was 156/66 mm Hg. Her jugular venous pressure was not elevated. The patient's lungs were clear to auscultation, and no wheezing or rhonchi were heard. The cardiac examination

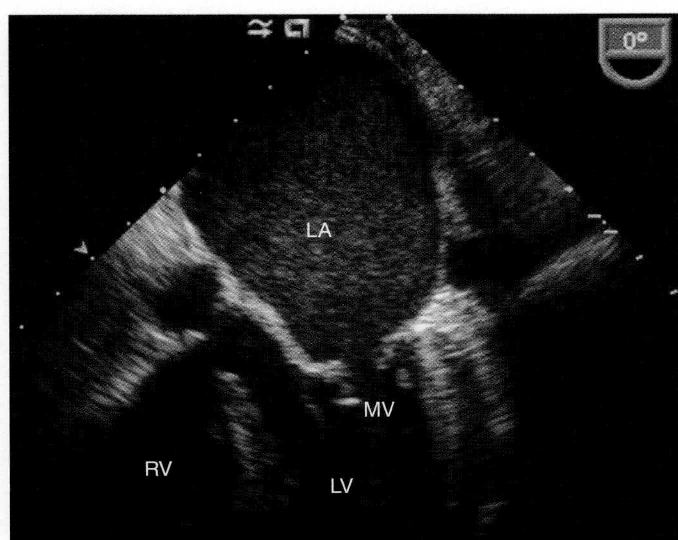

FIGURE 9-5-1 TEE midesophageal 4 chamber view showing the enlarged left atrium and rheumatic mitral stenosis. Spontaneous echo contrast is seen in the LA. LA = left atrium, LV = left ventricle, RV = right ventricle ► (see Video 9-5-1).

showed an irregularly irregular heart rhythm, an opening snap with a diastolic murmur heard best in the fourth left inter coastal space, and a holosystolic murmur best heart at apex and left lower sternal border. She was also found to have peripheral edema.

A transthoracic echocardiogram showed moderate mitral valve regurgitation and stenosis, moderate aortic stenosis with preserved biventricular systolic function, a severely dilated left atrium, and mild pulmonary hypertension (estimated RVSP 44 mm Hg). Given her symptoms, the patient was referred for replacement of the mitral and aortic valves.

Intraoperative TEE, in addition to confirming the valvular disease, also demonstrated severe spontaneous echocontrast in the left atrium and organized thrombus in the left atrial appendage (Figures 9-5-1 to 9-5-2).

The patient underwent successful mitral and aortic replacement with pericardial tissue valves, biatrial MAZE procedures, and resection of the left atrial appendage with extraction of the left atrial appendage clot. She was discharged home after 10 days of surgery and reported significant improvement in her symptoms on follow-up clinic visit.

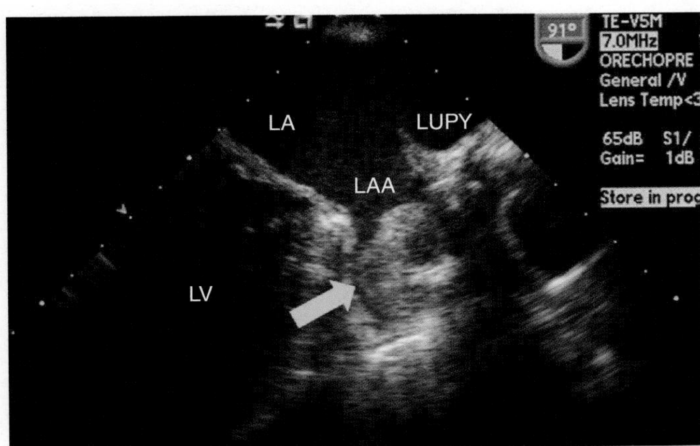

FIGURE 9-5-2 TEE midesophageal 2 chamber view showing thrombus in the left atrial appendage (arrow). LA = left atrium, LAA = left atrial appendage, LUPV = left upper pulmonary vein, LV = left ventricle ► (see Video 9-5-2).

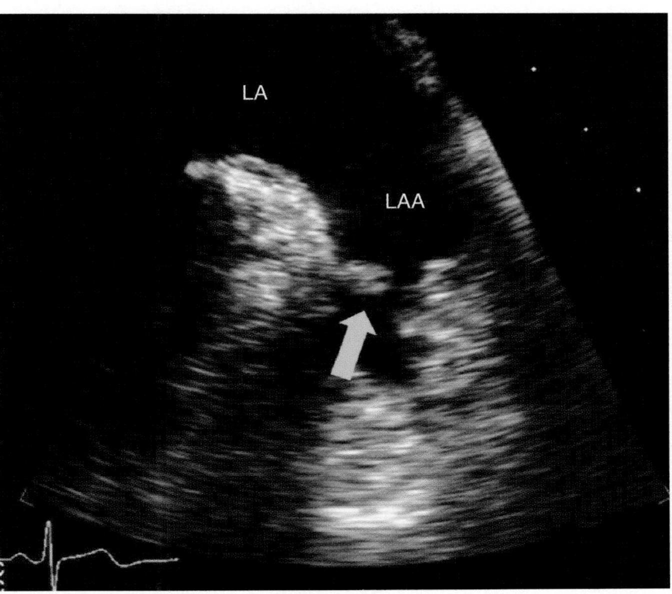

FIGURE 9-5-3 TEE midesophageal 2 chamber view from a different patient in sinus rhythm showing mobile thrombus in the left atrial appendage (arrow). LA = left atrium, LAA = left atrial appendage ► (see Video 9-5-3).

CLINICAL FEATURES

- Left atrial (LA) thrombus is usually detected in association with the atrial arrhythmias, most commonly atrial fibrillation (AF). The presence of an LA thrombus in patients with AF is a predictor of poor prognosis due to increased risk of thromboembolic complications and death.[1,2] The presence of LA thrombus is an absolute contraindication for elective cardioversion and catheter ablation procedures.

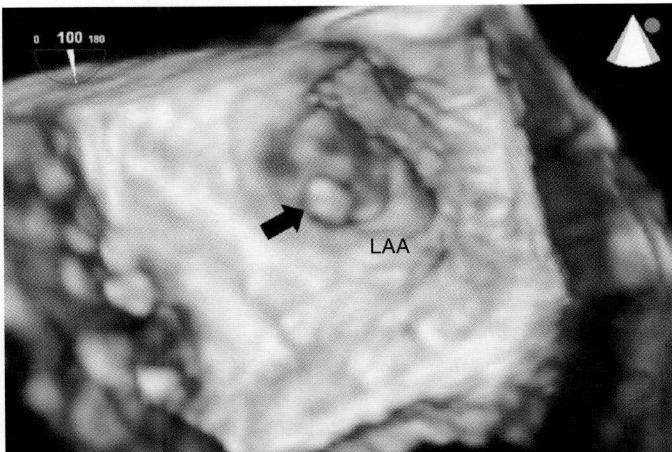

FIGURE 9-5-4 Three-dimensional view of the left atrial appendage from the patient in Figure 9-5-3 showing mobile thrombus in the left atrial appendage (arrow). LA = left atrium, LAA = left atrial appendage ► (see Video 9-5-4).

- LA thrombus is infrequently detected in the presence of sinus rhythm (Figures 9-5-3, 9-5-4). Patients in sinus rhythm with an LA thrombus usually have underlying organic heart disease including left ventricular dysfunction, valvular heart disease (mitral stenosis, aortic regurgitation, prosthetic valves) and/or a prior history of atrial fibrillation.[3]
- A hypercoagulability work-up should be performed in patients with LA thrombus in the presence of normal sinus rhythm and absence of underlying organic heart disease. Cardiac amyloidosis, particularly AL type, has been shown to be a risk factor of development of intracardiac thrombus.

EPIDEMIOLOGY

- The prevalence of LA thrombus in patients with AF referred for screening prior to catheter ablation is low (0.6%)[4] and has been shown to correlate with clinical risk factors including hypertension and cardiomyopathy.[5] In contrast, prior studies have reported a prevalence as high as 9.8% in patients with AF and subtherapeutic INR.[6]
- The left atrial appendage (LAA) is the most common site of thrombus formation (>90%) in patients with nonvalvular atrial fibrillation.[7]

PATHOPHYSIOLOGY AND ETIOLOGY

- AF results in chaotic contraction and loss of mechanical function of the atria resulting in stasis of blood. Coupled with endocardial damage and coexistent abnormalities of the coagulation cascade, AF results in a hypercoagulable milieu and thrombus formation.
- The anatomical structure of the left atrial appendage, a blind cul-de-sac, facilitates thrombus formation, especially after loss of contractile function.

ECHOCARDIOGRAPHY

- TEE is the principal imaging modality to detect LA thrombus with a sensitivity, specificity, and negative predictive value of 93% to 100%, 99% to 100%, and 98% to 100% respectively.[8,9]
- The LAA is multilobed in approximately 80% of cases and should be carefully interrogated with multiplanar TEE imaging.
- LA thrombus commonly appears as a well-circumscribed, echodense mass distinct from the underlying LA or LAA wall and pectinate muscles and should be seen in more than one imaging plane. In a fashion similar to the detection of LV thrombus (see Section IV), echo contrast agents can improve the visualization of thrombus, which appears as a filling defect. Echo contrast can also help in differentiating reverberation artifact from thrombus.
- Spontaneous echo contrast (SEC), a swirling haze of variable echodensity, is commonly seen in the LA/LAA in patients with atrial fibrillation. SEC signifies low blood flow velocity and non-laminar flow. The presence of SEC indicates an increased risk of thromboembolic complications.
- LAA filling and emptying velocities should be assessed using Doppler echocardiography. Low velocities suggest a low flow state and are predictive of future thrombus formation and embolic events.

OTHER DIAGNOSTIC TESTING AND PROCEDURES

- Cardiac CT can be reliably used as an alternative imaging modality for the detection of LA thrombus, which appears as a filling defect. The diagnostic accuracy of CT scan with contrast is 94%, which can be further increased to 99% with use of delayed contrast imaging.[10]
- Delayed-enhancement cardiac MRI can be used to differentiate between LA thrombus and neoplasm. Thrombus lacks contrast enhancement as opposed to other masses such as neoplasm, which typically demonstrate contrast uptake due to tumor-associated vascularity.

DIFFERENTIAL DIAGNOSIS

- Common differential diagnosis includes reverberation artifact, normal cardiac structures (pectinate muscle, ligament of Marshall/ "warfarin" ridge), tumors (commonly myxoma, fibroelastoma), and vegetations.

DIAGNOSIS

- The diagnosis of LA thrombus is mostly made on noninvasive imaging, particularly TEE performed to evaluate for cardiac source of embolus or as screening prior to cardioversion/catheter ablation procedures.

MANAGEMENT

- Patients with LA thrombus detected on screening TEE done prior to elective DC cardioversion or catheter ablation should be treated with warfarin (or one of the newer anticoagulant agents), with an INR goal of 2 to 3, for a period of 4 to 6 weeks. A repeat TEE should be performed to assess for thrombus resolution prior to attempts at cardioversion or ablation. Long-term anticoagulation therapy is indicated for primary or secondary prevention of thromboembolic complications in AF patients with LA thrombus.

FOLLOW-UP

- Follow-up is usually guided by the clinical condition. As noted above, TEE may be performed after 4 to 6 weeks of anticoagulation therapy to assess for resolution of the LA thrombus.

VIDEO LEGENDS

1. Video 9-5-1: TEE mid-esophageal 4 chamber view showing the enlarged left atrium and rheumatic mitral stenosis. Spontaneous echo contrast is seen in the LA
2. Video 9-5-2: TEE mid-esophageal 2 chamber view showing thrombus in the left atrial appendage
3. Video 9-5-3: TEE mid-esophageal 2 chamber view from a different patient in sinus rhythm showing a mobile thrombus in the left atrial appendage
4. Video 9-5-4: 3D view of the left atrial appendage from the patient in Video 9-5-3 showing mobile thrombus in the left atrial appendage

REFERENCES

1. Bernhardt P, Schmidt H, Hammerstingl C, et al. Atrial thrombi—a prospective follow-up study over 3 years with transesophageal echocardiography and cranial magnetic resonance imaging. *Echocardiography.* 2006;23(5):388-394.
2. Zabalgoitia M, Halperin JL, Pearce LA, Blackshear JL, Asinger RW, Hart RG. Transesophageal echocardiographic correlates of clinical risk of thromboembolism in nonvalvular atrial fibrillation. Stroke Prevention in Atrial Fibrillation III Investigators. *J Am Coll Cardiol.* 1998;31(7):1622-1626.
3. Agmon Y, Khandheria BK, Gentile F, Seward JB. Clinical and echocardiographic characteristics of patients with left atrial thrombus and sinus rhythm: experience in 20643 consecutive transesophageal echocardiographic examinations. *Circulation.* 2002:105(1):27-31.
4. Puwanant S, Varr BC, Shrestha K, et al. Role of the CHADS2 score in the evaluation of thromboembolic risk in patients with atrial fibrillation undergoing transesophageal echocardiography before pulmonary vein isolation. *J Am Coll Cardiol.* 2009;54(22):2032-2039.
5. McCready JW, Nunn L, Lumbiase PD, et al. Incidence of left atrial thrombus prior to atrial fibrillation ablation: is pre-procedural transoesophageal echocardiography mandatory? *Europace.* 2010;12(7):927-932.
6. Corrado G, Beretta S, Sormani L, et al. Prevalence of atrial thrombi in patients with atrial fibrillation/flutter and subtherapeutic anticoagulation prior to cardioversion. *Eur J Echocardiogr.* 2004;5(4):257-261.
7. Blackshear JL, Odell JA. Appendage obliteration to reduce stroke in cardiac surgical patients with atrial fibrillation. *Ann Thorac Surg.* 1996;61(2):755-759.
8. Fatkin D, Sacalia G, Jacobs N, et al. Accuracy of biplane transesophageal echocardiography in detecting left atrial thrombus. *Am J Cardiol.* 1996;77(4):321-323.
9. Manning WJ, Weintraub RM, Waksmonski CA, et al. Accuracy of transesophageal echocardiography for identifying left atrial thrombi. A prospective, intraoperative study. *Ann Intern Med.* 1995;123(11):817-822.
10. Romero J, Husain SA, Kelesidis I, Sanz J, Medina HM, Garcia MJ. Detection of left atrial appendage thrombus by cardiac computed tomography in patients with atrial fibrillation: a meta-analysis. *Circ Cardiovasc Imaging.* 2013;6(2):185-194.

10 ECHOCARDIOGRAPHY IN THE EVALUATION AND MANAGEMENT OF PATIENTS WITH ATRIAL DYSRHYTHMIAS

Demet Menekse Gerede, MD, and
Richard A. Grimm, DO, FACC

INTRODUCTION

Atrial fibrillation (AF) is the most common rhythm abnormality that is encountered in clinical practice. Echocardiography plays a critical role in the initial evaluation of these patients and in their ongoing management. Transesophageal echocardiography has emerged as an important imaging test in these patients. By virtue of its ability to assess for the presence of atrial thrombus, TEE now plays a pivotal role in the management of patients with atrial fibrillation and atrial flutter by screening for the presence of thrombus prior to cardioversion or ablation. In addition, new options for the prevention of thromboembolic events, such as the left atrial occluder device and the LARIAT procedure, employ TEE during the procedure to guide device placement. In this chapter, Dr. Grimm and his colleagues will explore the use of echocardiography in several of these clinical situations, including the assessment of the patient with atrial fibrillation and risk stratification for thromboembolic events, TEE-guided cardioversion, and intraprocedural TEE during LAA occluder device placement.

SECTION 1

Echocardiography in Atrial Dysrhythmias: Assessment of A Patient With Atrial Fibrillation/ Risk Stratification for Thromboembolic Events

CLINICAL CASE PRESENTATION

A 62-year-old man presented with lower extremity edema, shortness of breath, and atrial fibrillation. He had been seen in the past for coronary artery disease that was manifest by severe ischemic cardiomyopathy following an anterior myocardial infarction (MI) and a history of atrial fibrillation (AF). He had undergone coronary artery bypass surgery, mitral valve repair, pulmonary vein isolation (PVI), and stapling of left atrial appendage (LAA). His preoperative ejection fraction (EF) was 15%. Postoperatively, AF redeveloped, and he underwent radiofrequency ablation therapy (RFA) for AF. This procedure was complicated by high-grade atrioventricular (AV) block, and the following day, he underwent placement of a biventricular-pacing ICD. His EF substantially improved to 35%. He then developed gastrointestinal bleeding, which necessitated discontinuation of anticoagulation. Physical exam was unremarkable except for edema and an irregular rhythm. Prior to a planned cardioversion (CV) and in order to facilitate CV, the patient underwent TEE to assess for LA thrombus. Thrombus was identified, and the cardioversion was postponed (Figures 10-1-1 to 10-1-6). After 3 months of anticoagulant therapy, TEE was repeated and the thrombus resolved (Figure 10-1-7). He subsequently underwent CV and has done well.

CLINICAL FEATURES

- Patients may or may not have symptoms with AF.
- Commonly associated symptoms include palpitations, shortness of breath, fatigue, lightheadedness, decreasing exercise tolerance, or chest discomfort.
- An irregular pulse should raise suspicion for AF.
- Patients may present initially with transient ischemic attack (TIA) or ischemic stroke.

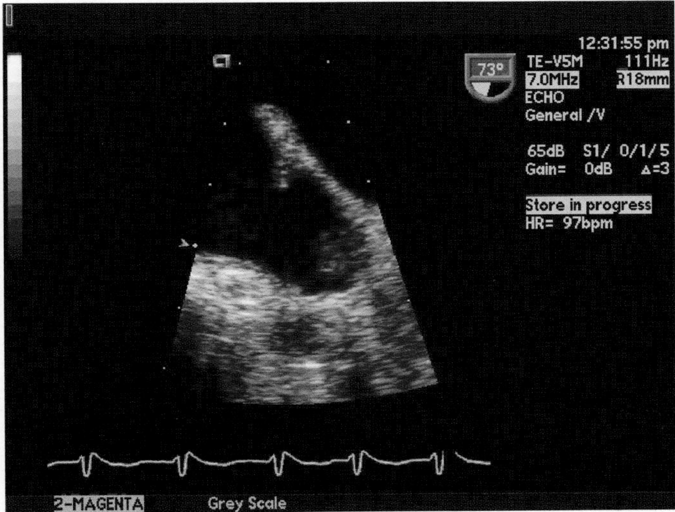

FIGURE 10-1-1 Two-dimensional TEE image at 73° in the mid-esophagus, showing the left atrial appendage LAA. This image shows thrombus attached near the apex of the LAA. The thrombus size was measured at 1.3 x 0.7 cm. The LAA is best visualized from midesophageal position. It is a complex anatomic structure and is multilobed in up to 80% of the general population. The presence of left atrial (LA) or LAA thrombus may preclude CV. The presence of LA and LAA thrombus is associated with a significantly increased risk of stroke. Following 3 weeks of therapeutic anticoagulation prior to, and at least 4 weeks of therapeutic anticoagulation after CV is recommended in the guidelines on the management of atrial fibrillation ▶ (see Video 10-1-1).

- Most patients experience asymptomatic episodes of arrhythmias before being diagnosed.
- Patients with mitral valve disease and heart failure often have a higher incidence of AF.
- Intermittent episodes of AF may progress in duration and frequency, and over time many patients will develop sustained AF.

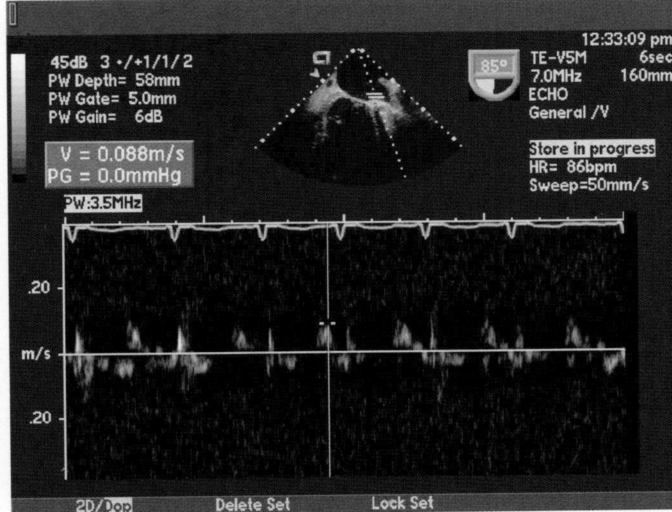

FIGURE 10-1-2 The left atrial appendage pulse wave Doppler pattern showing markedly diminished peak LAA emptying velocity. Multiple studies have found an association between low peak LAA emptying velocity (<20 cm/s) and incidence of stroke in patients with AF.

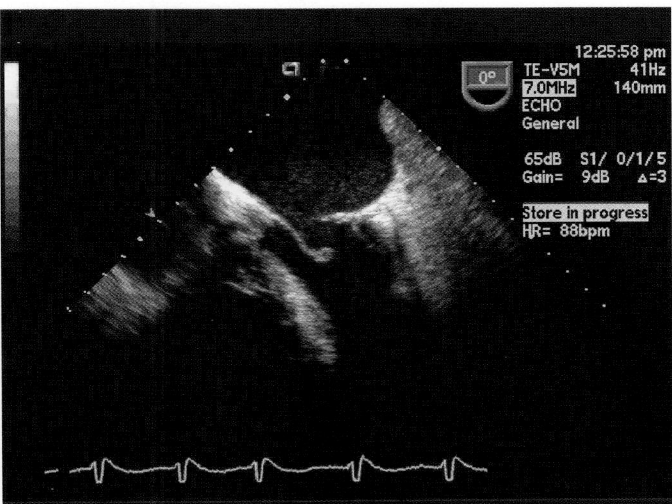

FIGURE 10-1-3 Two-dimensional TEE image at 0° in the mid-esophageous, showing the left atrium, the left ventricle, and the mitral valve. This image shows mitral ring and valve function ▶ (see Video 10-1-3).

- For a newly diagnosed patient with AF, reversible causes such as pulmonary embolism, hyperthyroidism, pericarditis, and MI should be investigated.

EPIDEMIOLOGY[1,2]

- Atrial fibrillation is the most common cardiac arrhythmia in clinical practice, accounting for approximately one-third of hospitalizations for cardiac rhythm disturbances.
- The estimated prevalence of AF is 0.4% to 1% in the general population, increasing with age.
- The age-adjusted prevalence of AF is higher in men.
- The median age of AF patients is about 75 years. Approximately 70% are between 65 and 85 years old.

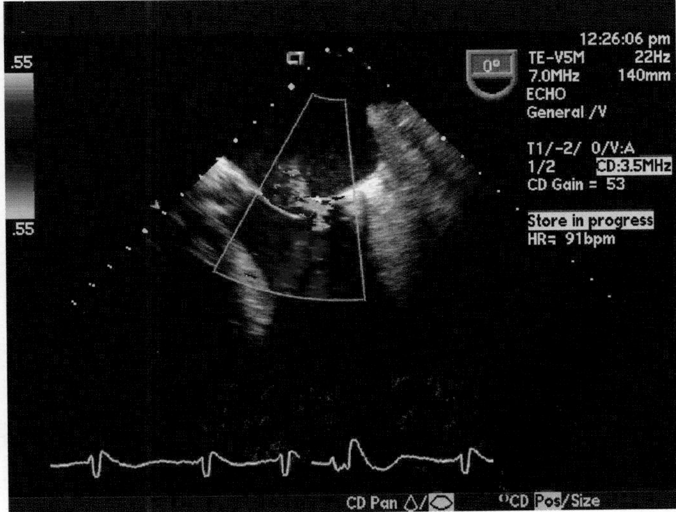

FIGURE 10-1-4 This image shows mild (1+) mitral regurgitation on the color Doppler echocardiography ▶ (see Video 1-1-4).

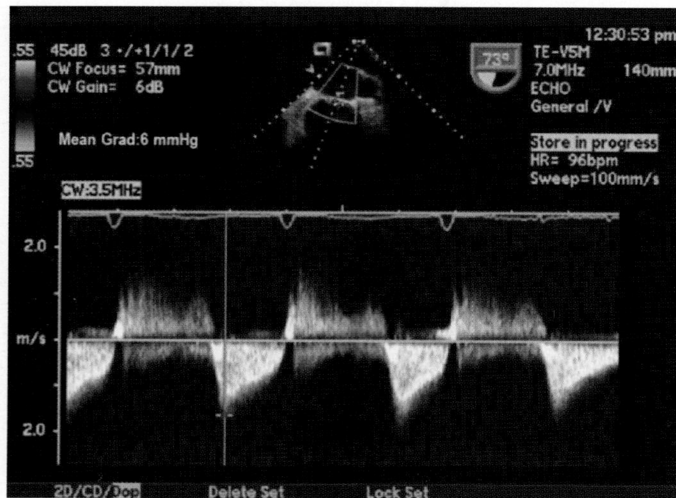

FIGURE 10-1-5 Continuous wave Doppler demonstrating mitral valve gradient (mean gradient 6 mm Hg).

- AF frequently accompanies common conditions such as hypertension, chronic heart failure, and valvular or ischemic heart disease, and is a common sequela of cardiothoracic surgery, especially in patients with valvular heart disease.
- The arrhythmia is associated with a five-fold risk of thromboembolic stroke and a three-fold incidence of congestive heart failure, and higher mortality.
- The risk of stroke is greater in the elderly and with concomitant valvular (particularly rheumatic) heart disease.

PATHOPHYSIOLOGY AND ETIOLOGY

- The etiology of AF is complex.
- AF is often an electrical manifestation of underlying cardiac disease. Nonetheless, approximately 30% to 45% of cases of paroxysmal AF and 20% to 25% of cases of persistent AF occur in younger patients without demonstrable underlying disease ("lone AF").[1]

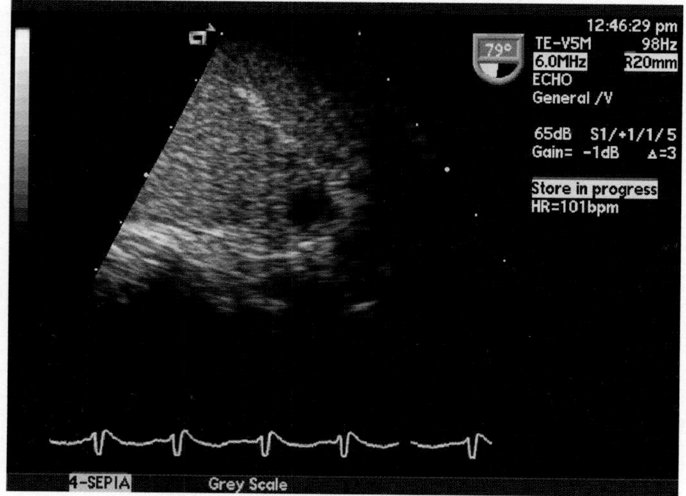

FIGURE 10-1-6 Postcontrast agent administration image demonstrating a filling defect representing an LAA thrombus ▶ (see Video 10-1-6).

- Any kind of structural heart disease may trigger remodeling of both the atria and ventricles. Structural remodeling facilitates initiation and perpetuation of AF.
- The arrhythmia is characterized by disorganized electrical activity with multiple re-entrant circuits in the atria that can lead to electrical and structural remodeling of the atria, which in turn reinforces the establishment of AF.
- The most frequent pathoanatomic changes in AF are atrial fibrosis and loss of atrial muscle mass.
- Perhaps most significant is the discovery that a proportion of AF cases caused by triggering from foci within the pulmonary veins can be successfully ablated with radiofrequency treatment.
- AF is associated with delayed emptying from left atrial appendage resulting in reduced LAA flow velocities that are implicated in thrombus formation.
- Additionally, the left atrial appendage has become a focus of attention for surgical and percutaneous closure techniques that are becoming available.

ECHOCARDIOGRAPHY

- Almost all patients presenting with their first episode of AF will benefit from transthoracic echocardiography (TTE) evaluation of left atrial size, left ventricular systolic function, and mitral valve morphology and function.
- TTE provides detailed information about cardiac anatomy and function, but it is less useful for the detection of thrombus in the LA or LAA.
- Echocardiography has an increasingly important therapeutic role in guiding these ablation and LAA closure procedures.[3]
- The management of AF can be divided into rhythm versus rate control strategies, combined with a risk assessment for prevention of thromboembolism. Echocardiography plays a critical role in defining the clinical context of the arrhythmia and therefore informs the clinician regarding the key issues of anticoagulation and overall cardiac management.
- Transesophageal echocardiography (TEE) is not part of the standard initial investigation of patients with AF, but it is a sensitive and specific technique for detection of LA and LAA thrombus, compared to TTE. This modality also permits superior evaluation for other causes of cardiogenic embolism, as well as a means of measuring LAA function.
- This technology has been used to stratify stroke risk in patients with AF and to guide cardioversion.
- Several TEE findings have been associated with thromboembolism, including thrombus, reduced LAA flow velocity (≤20 cm/s), spontaneous echo contrast in the LA or LAA, and atheromatous disease of aorta.[4]
- Detection of LA/LAA thrombus stands as a contraindication to elective cardioversion (CV) of AF.

OTHER DIAGNOSTIC TESTING AND PROCEDURES

- Electrocardiogram (ECG) is the principal testing modality for the diagnosis and follow-up of AF.

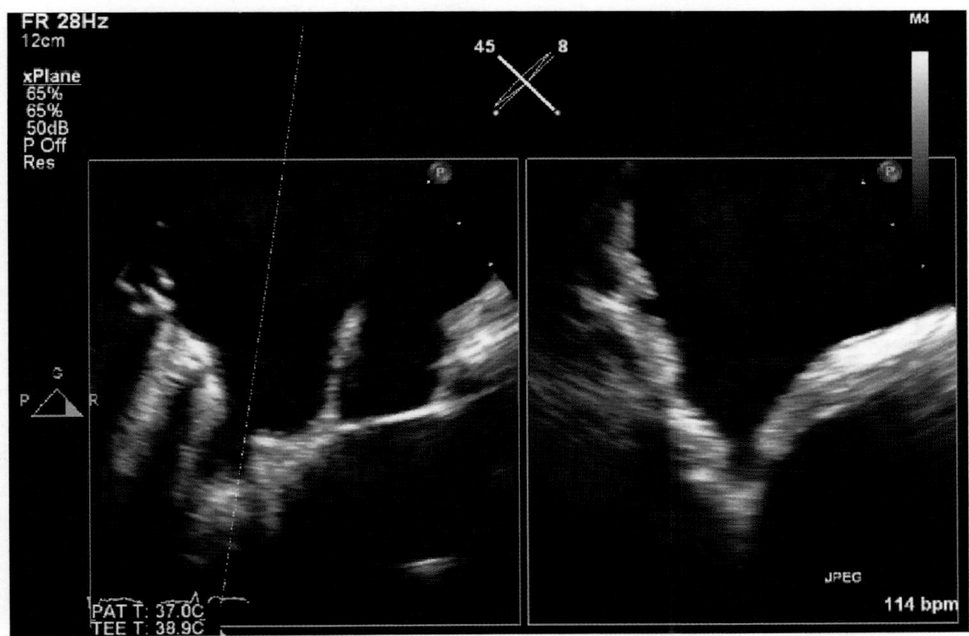

FIGURE 10-1-7 This image shows disappearance of thrombus following treatment. X-plane used to more comprehensively view orthogonal planes and hence more confidently demonstrate absence of thrombus ► (see Video 10-1-7).

- If the patient has normal sinus rhythm on ECG, but has suspected paroxysmal AF, Holter monitoring should be performed.
- An EP study can be helpful when AF is a consequence of reentrant tachycardia such as atrial flutter, intra-atrial reentry, or AV reentry involving an accessory pathway.

DIFFERENTIAL DIAGNOSIS

- Arrhythmias that can mimic AF include atrial tachycardia, atrial flutter with variable AV block, frequent atrial ectopies, and antegrade atrioventricular nodal conduction.
- Any episode of suspected AF should be recorded by a 12-lead ECG. An ECG recording will help in differentiating AF from rare supraventricular arrhythmias with irregular RR intervals.
- Occasionally, use of atrioventricular nodal blocking drugs, using Valsalva maneuver, carotid massage, or intravenous adenosine may be necessary to establish the diagnosis.

DIAGNOSIS

- An irregular pulse can increase the suspicion of AF, but ECG remains essential in diagnosing AF. AF is defined with the following characteristics:
  - Irregular RR intervals.
  - No distinct P waves on ECG.
  - Atrial cycle length (interval between two atrial activations) is usually variable and <200 ms (>300 BPM).
- Symptom-activated event recorders (30 day), Holter monitoring (24 h to 7 days), and implantable loop recorders can be used for AF diagnosis.
- AF may be categorized as paroxysmal (self-terminating), persistent (requiring electrical or pharmacological termination), or permanent (cardioversion impossible or futile).[1]

MANAGEMENT

- Management of patients with AF is directed at reducing symptoms by rate control, correction of rhythm disturbances, and prevention of thromboembolism. The management strategy should be discussed with the patient and should consider several factors:
- type and duration of AF
- severity and type of symptoms
- associated cardiovascular disease
- patient age
- associated medical conditions
- short-term and long-term treatment goals
- pharmacological and nonpharmacological therapeutic options.
- In a patient with asymptomatic persistent AF, attempts to restore sinus rhythm may not be needed.
- Prospective studies such as Rate Control Versus Electrical Cardioversion for persistent atrial fibrillation (RACE) and Atrial Fibrillation Follow-up Investigation of Rhythm Management (AFFIRM) showed that patients who tolerated rate-controlled AF had outcomes similar to those randomized to rhythm control.[5,6]
- None of the major trials demonstrated any significant difference in the quality of life with ventricular rate control compared to rhythm control.
- Drugs and ablation are effective for both rate and rhythm control, and in special circumstances, surgery may be the preferred option.
- For rhythm control, drugs are typically the first choice, and radiofrequency ablation is a second-line choice. In some patients, especially the young with very symptomatic lone AF who need sinus rhythm, radiofrequency ablation may be preferred over drug therapy.[2]

- Patients with preoperative AF undergoing cardiac surgery face a unique opportunity. While few patients are candidates for a standalone surgical procedure to cure AF using the MAZE procedure or LA ablation techniques, these approaches can be an effective adjunct to coronary bypass or valve surgery to prevent recurrent postoperative AF.
- Because the LAA is the site of over 95% of detected thrombi, this structure is often excluded from the circulation when possible during cardiac surgery in patients at risk of developing postoperative AF, although this has not been proven to prevent stroke.[1]
- Risk stratification for patients with nonvalvular AF is performed using the CHADS2 (Congestive heart failure, Hypertension, Age ≥75, Diabetes, Stroke [doubled]) risk assessment tool[1] (Table 10-1-1).
- Another risk stratification schema is the CHA2DS2-VASc (Congestive heart failure/left ventricular dysfunction, Hypertension, Age ≥75 [doubled], Diabetes, Stroke [doubled]-Vascular disease, Age 65-74, and Sex category [female]) risk assessment tool.[2]

TABLE 10-1-1 Stroke Risk in Patients with Nonvalvular AF Not Treated with Anticoagulation According to the CHADS2 Index

CHADS2 Risk Criteria	Score
Prior stroke or TIA	2
Age >75 y	1
Hypertension	1
Diabetes mellitus	1
Heart failure	1

Patients (N = 1733)	Adjusted Stroke Rate (%/y)* (95% CI)	CHADS2 Score
120	1.9 (1.2 to 3.0)	0
463	2.8 (2.0 to 3.8)	1
523	4.0 (3.1 to 5.1)	2
337	5.9 (4.6 to 7.3)	3
220	8.5 (6.3 to 11.1)	4
65	12.5 (8.2 to 17.5)	5
5	18.2 (10.5 to 27.4)	6

*The adjusted stroke rate was derived from multivariate analysis assuming no aspirin usage.

Adapted with permisison from Fuster V, Ryden LE, Cannom DS, et al. 2011 ACCF/AHA/HRS focused updates incorporated into the ACC/AHA/ESC 2006 Guidelines for the management of patients with atrial fibrillation: a report of the American College of Cardiology Foundation/American Heart Association Task Force on Practice Guidelines developed in partnership with the European Society of Cardiology and in collaboration with the European Society of Cardiology and in collaboration with the European Heart Rhythm Association and Heart Rhythm Society. J Am Coll Cardiol 2011 Mar 15;57(11):e101-98.[1]

- Major risk factors are prior stroke, TIA, and older age (>75 years).
- Clinically relevant nonmajor risk factors include heart failure, moderate to severe systolic LV dysfunction (LVEF <40%), hypertension, age 65 to 74 years, diabetes, female sex, and vascular disease (MI, peripheral artery disease, complex aortic plaque).
- There is a clear relationship between the CHA2DS2-VASc score and stroke rate.
- In patients with a CHA2DS2-VASc score of 2 or more, chronic anticoagulation therapy is recommended unless contraindicated.
- An assessment of bleeding risk should be a part of the patient assessment before starting anticoagulation. It is reasonable to use the HAS-BLED score (Hypertension, Abnormal renal/liver function, Stroke, Bleeding history or predisposition, Labile INR, Elderly (more than 65-years old), Drugs or alcohol use) to assess the bleeding risk in atrial fibrillation patients.

FOLLOW-UP

- Frequency of follow-up with AF patients depends upon anticoagulant and antiarrhythmic drug therapy use.
- When using warfarin, the target INR is in the range of 2.0 to 3.0.

VIDEO LEGENDS

1. Video 10-1-1: Two-dimensional TEE image at 73° in the mid-esophagus, showing the left atrial appendage (LAA). This image shows thrombus attached near the apex of the left atrial appendage (LAA). The thrombus size measured 1.3 × 0.7 cm.
2. Video 10-1-3: Two-dimensional TEE image at 0° in the mid-esophagus, showing the left atrium, the left ventricle, the mitral valve. This image shows the mitral ring and valve function.
3. Video 10-1-4: This image shows mild (1+) mitral regurgitation on the color Doppler echocardiography.
4. Video 10-1-6: Post-contrast agent administration image demonstrating a filling defect representing an LAA thrombus.
5. Video 10-1-7: This video demonstrates resolution of the thrombus following treatment. X plane was used to more comprehensively view orthogonal planes and hence more confidently demonstrate the absence of thrombus.

REFERENCES

1. Fuster V, Ryden LE, Cannom DS, et al. 2011 ACCF/AHA/HRS focused updates incorporated into the ACC/AHA/ESC 2006 Guidelines for the management of patients with atrial fibrillation: a report of the American College of Cardiology Foundation/American Heart Association Task Force on Practice Guidelines developed in partnership with the European Society of Cardiology and in collaboration with the European Society of Cardiology and in collaboration with the European Heart Rhythm Association and Heart Rhythm Society. *J Am Coll Cardiol.* 2011; 57(11):e101-198.
2. Camm AJ, Lip GY, De Caterina, et al. 2012 focused update of the ESC Guidelines for the management of atrial fibrillation: an update of the 2010 ESC Guidelines for the management of atrial fibrillation. Developed with the special contribution

of the European Heart Rhythm Association. *Eur Heart J.* 2012;33:2719-2747.

3. Troughton RW, Asher CR, Klein AL. The role of echocardiography in atrial fibrillation and cardioversion. *Heart.* 2003;89(12):1447-1454.
4. Zabolgoitia M, Halperin JL, Pearce LA, et al. Transesophageal echocardiographic correlates of clinical risk of thromboembolism in nonvalvular atrial fibrillation. Stroke Prevention in Atrial Fibrillation III Investigators. *J Am Coll Cardiol.* 1998;31:1622.
5. Olshansky B, Rosenfeld LE, Warner AL, et al. The Atrial Fibrillation Follow-up Investigation of Rhythm Management (AFFIRM) study: approaches to control rate in atrial fibrillation. *J Am Coll Cardiol.* 2004;43:1201-1208.
6. Hagens VE, Crijins HJ, Veldhuisen DJ, et al. Rate control versus rhythm control for patients with persistent atrial fibrillation with mild to moderate heart failure: results from the Rate Control versus Electrical Cardioversion (RACE) study. *Am Heart J.* 2005;149(6):1106-1111.

SECTION 2

Echocardiography in Atrial Dysrhythmias: TEE-Guided Cardioversion

CLINICAL CASE PRESENTATION

The patient is a 52-year-old man with the past medical history of previous IV drug and tobacco abuse, hypertension, and nonischemic cardiomyopathy. The last EF was 25%. He was found to be in AF with rapid ventricular response, which was treated with rate control, and cardioversion; however, the patient has not been taking his medication due to financial issues.

He presented to the emergency department with worsening dyspnea for approximately 2 weeks, palpitations, and chest pressure. His ECG showed AF with rapid ventricular response and T-wave inversions in the lateral leads as well as right axis deviation. He had elevated troponin levels, but CKMB was negative. Coronary angiography was performed and demonstrated normal coronary arteries. An echocardiogram demonstrated moderately to severely decreased left ventricular systolic function (EF 25%). His CHADS2 score was 2 for hypertension and heart failure. On physical examination he was found to be tachycardic (130 BPM). Cardiac exam revealed no murmurs, gallops, or rubs. An attempt to maintain in sinus rhythm was thought to be worthwhile due to his poor compliance. A TEE-guided cardioversion (CV) was therefore scheduled in order to facilitate an early CV, which would minimize the pre-CV duration of AF. A large thrombus was seen on TEE in the LAA, and CV was cancelled (Figures 10-2-1 to 10-2-5). Repeat TEE on warfarin therapy was scheduled for approximately 1 month later. The repeat TEE showed a smaller yet persistent LAA thrombus (Figures 10-2-6 and 10-2-7). Anticoagulation was continued following the TEE, but he unfortunately was lost to follow-up.

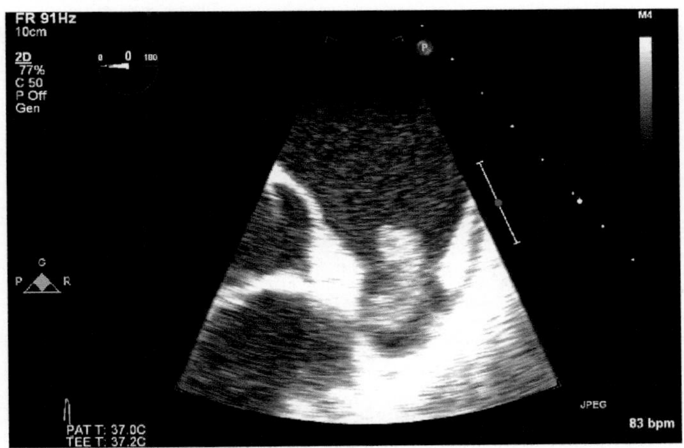

FIGURE 10-2-1 Two-dimensional TEE image at 0° at the midesophageal level showing the left atrium and the left atrial appendage. A large and mobile thrombus is seen in the LAA ▶(see Video 10-2-1).

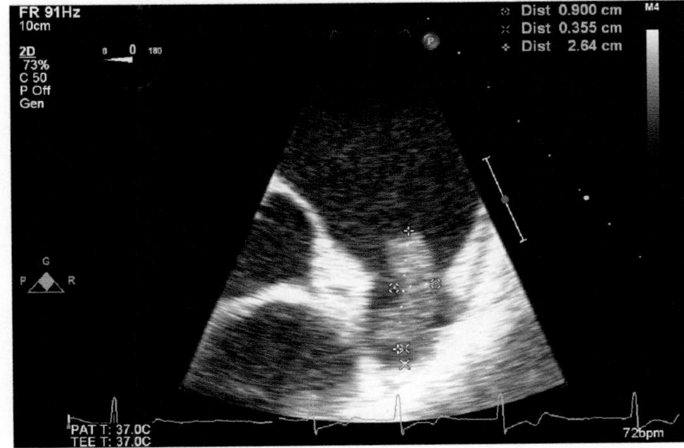

FIGURE 10-2-2 The thrombus size was measured at 2.6 x 0.9 cm.

CLINICAL FEATURES

- Cardioversion (CV) may be considered emergently or electively to restore the sinus rhythm in patients with AF.
- Immediate CV should be performed in patients who are hemodynamically unstable, even if they have not been anticoagulated; however, the patient should be anticoagulated as soon as possible.

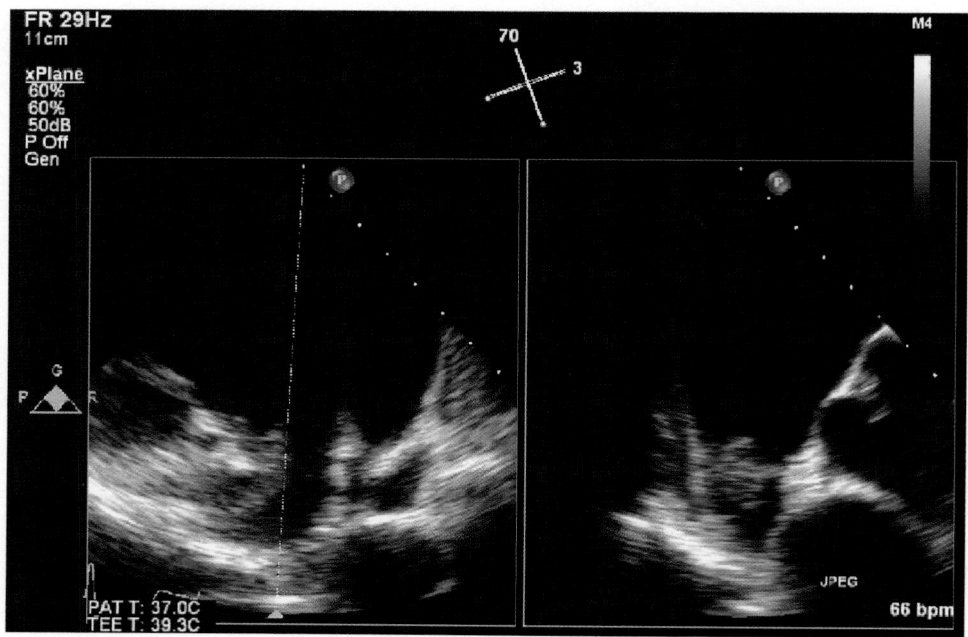

FIGURE 10-2-3 X-plane used to more comprehensively view orthogonal planes demonstrate size of thrombus ▶ (see Video 10-2-3).

- Anticoagulation is considered mandatory before elective cardioversion for atrial fibrillation of more than 48 hours or atrial fibrillation of unknown duration because of the increased risk of thromboembolic events following cardioversion.
- The current data suggest that patient needs to be anticoagulated for at least a 3-week duration before cardioversion. This is often referred to as the conventional strategy.[1]
- A transesophageal echo-guided cardioversion strategy can be employed as an alternative to precardioversion anticoagulation in order to facilitate more rapid cardioversion.
- CV can be performed with medications (pharmacologic CV) or electrical cardioversion (synchronized cardioversion).
- Pharmacologic CV is usually most effective within 7 days after the onset of an episode of AF.
- Conversion of AF to sinus rhythm often results in transient mechanical dysfunction of the LA and LAA known as "stunning," which can occur after spontaneous, pharmacological, or electrical conversion of AF or after radiofrequency catheter ablation of AF/atrial flutter (Aflt).
- This "stunning" phenomenon has been observed in patients undergoing TEE before and immediately post-CV and is thought to be one mechanism for post cardioversion stroke, especially in those patients who have had documentation of the absence of thrombus on a pre-CV TEE.

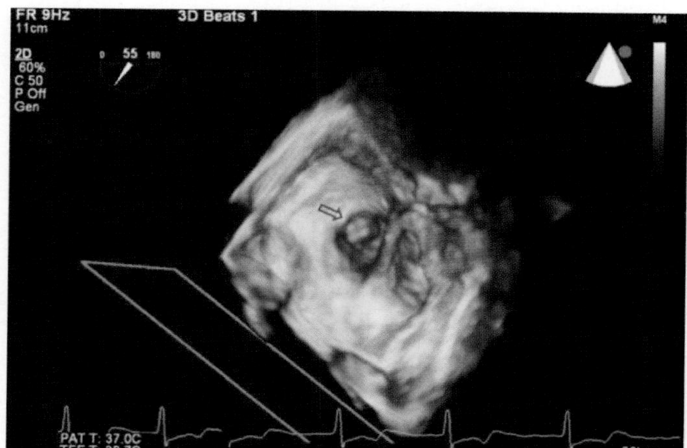

FIGURE 10-2-4 Real time three-dimensional zoomed transesophageal view of LAA from left atrial perspective obtained in a patient with large and mobile thrombus. The arrow shows LAA thrombus. To the right of the left atrial appendage is the left upper pulmonary vein.

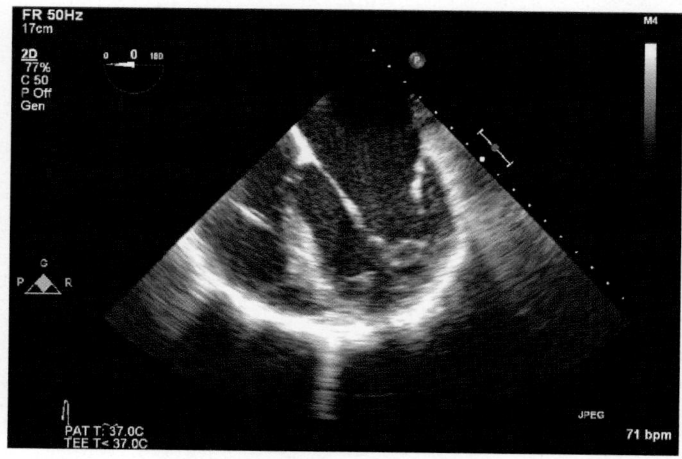

FIGURE 10-2-5 Two-dimensional TEE image at 0° in the mid-esophagus, showing the 4 chamber view. There was grade 1 to 2 SEC in the atrium ▶ (see Video 10-2-5).

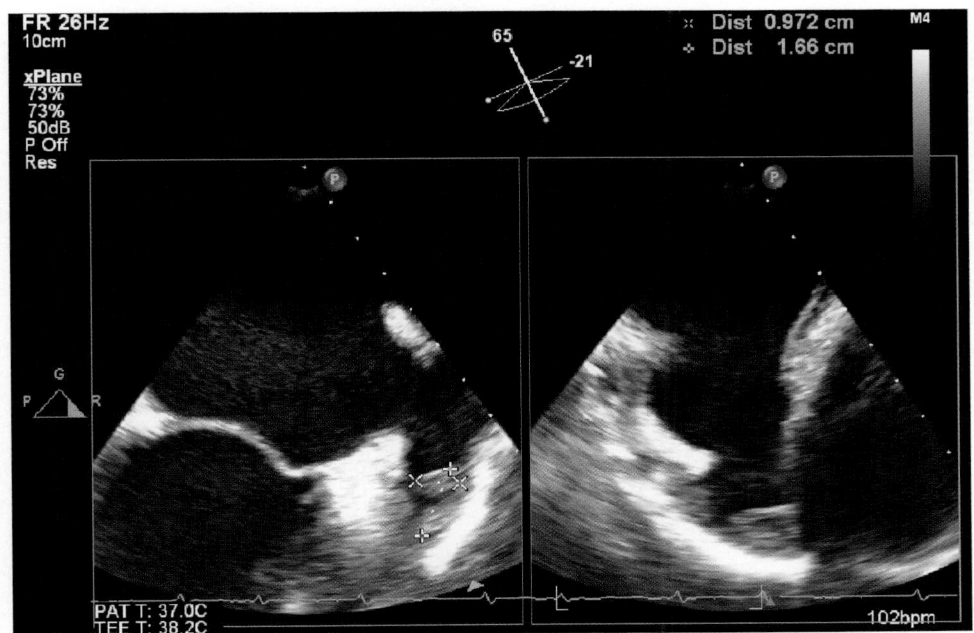

FIGURE 10-2-6 The pre-existent LAA thrombus was seen in two-dimensional X-plane midesophageal LAX and SAX views on repeat TEE, but size reduction of the thrombus was detected ▶ (see Video 10-2-6).

EPIDEMIOLOGY

- LA stunning has been reported with all modes of conversion of AFib/AFlt to sinus rhythm.
- The incidence of LA stunning is 38% to 80%.[2]
- The use of several weeks of anticoagulation before CV results in a reduction of CV-related thromboembolism from 6% to <1%.

PATHOPHYSIOLOGY AND ETIOLOGY

- Tachycardia-induced atrial cardiomyopathy and chronic atrial hibernation are the potential mechanisms underlying atrial stunning.
- The duration of atrial stunning is variable in individual cases, depending on the duration of preceding AFib/AFlt, atrial size, and underlying heart disease.

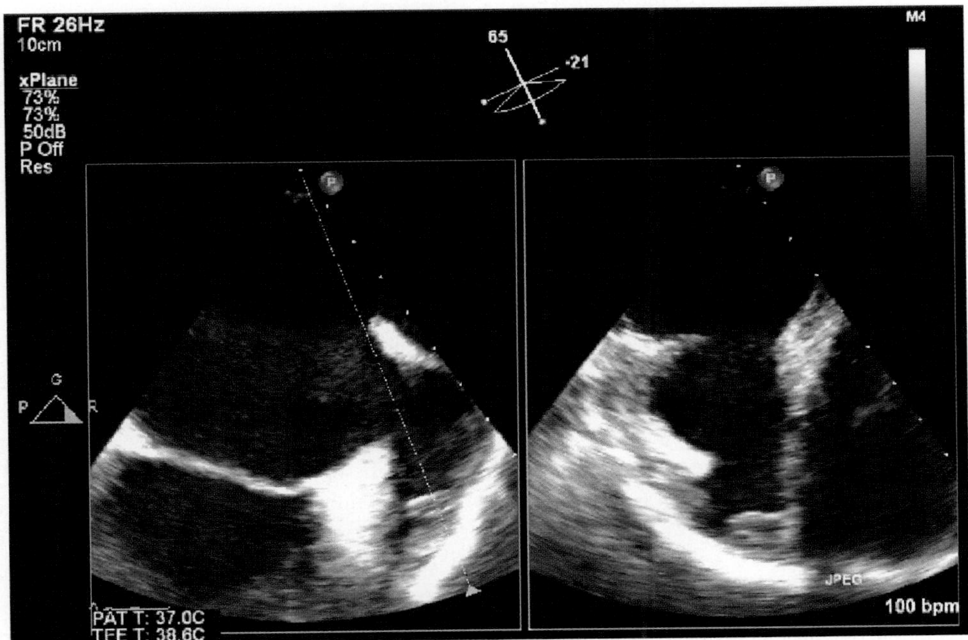

FIGURE 10-2-7 The thrombus size was measured at 1.6 x 0.9 cm on repeat TEE.

ECHOCARDIOGRAPHY

- TEE in patients with AF before cardioversion has shown LA or LAA thrombus in 5% to 15%, but thromboembolism after conversion to sinus rhythm has been reported even when TEE did not demonstrate thrombus.
- The "stunning" phenomenon may explain why some patients without demonstrable LA thrombus on TEE before cardioversion subsequently experience thromboembolic events.
- These events typically occur relatively (2-5 days) soon after CV in patients who were not treated with anticoagulation, reinforcing the need to maintain continuous therapeutic anticoagulation in patients with AF undergoing CV, even when no thrombus is identified.
- LA stunning has been determined by means of TTE and TEE studies, with parameters such as spontaneous echocardiographic contrast, LAA blood flow velocities, LAA emptying fraction, atrial contraction wave (A-wave) velocity, A-wave time-velocity integral, and atrial filling fraction.[2]
- For patients with AF for greater than 48 hours duration, a TEE-guided strategy can be used.
- CV can be performed with intravenous heparin if no thrombi are seen. This is followed by at least 1 month of warfarin therapy (or newer agents such as dabigatran or rivaroxaban) to prevent new thrombus formation after CV.
- In the ACUTE Trial, TEE-guided CV or the traditional (conventional) strategy of anticoagulation for 4 weeks before and 4 weeks after elective CV resulted in similar rates of thromboembolism (less than 1% during the 8 weeks).[3]
    - The clinical benefit of the TEE-guided approach in this trial was limited to saving time before cardioversion.
- An advantage of the TEE-guided approach is related to the lower incidence of hemorrhage. This difference is probably due to the longer duration of anticoagulant therapy required by the conventional strategy, which was almost double compared to the conventional approach, with higher incidence of bleeding.[3,4]

OTHER DIAGNOSTIC TESTING AND PROCEDURES

- Cardiac CT angiography can be used for diagnosis of atrial thrombus.

DIFFERENTIAL DIAGNOSIS

- Data for atrial flutter suggest that the incidences of atrial thrombi and thromboembolism are slightly reduced compared with AF, but that these patients should likely be treated with AF guidelines.

DIAGNOSIS

- The diagnosis of atrial fibrillation is made based on the ECG.
- TEE is increasingly used to guide interventional therapeutic procedures in the AF population, including pulmonary vein isolation and LAA exclusion.

MANAGEMENT

- After CV, LAA mechanical function may be even more depressed (stunning). Depression of LA and LAA mechanical function may persist for several weeks after CV, emphasizing the need for therapeutic warfarin (INR = 2.0-3.0) or the use of newer agents for at least 1 month after CV.

The decision regarding long-term maintenance of anticoagulation (after 1 month) should be based on the patients risk of thromboembolism and bleeding risk as detailed in Section I of this chapter, Echocardiography in Atrial Dysrhythmias: Assessment of a Patient with Atrial Fibrillation/Risk Stratification for Thromboembolic Events.

FOLLOW-UP

- The follow-up period should be set by the physician according to the patient's medication history.
    - In patients on warfarin, periodic assessment of the INR is warranted.
    - Monitoring for drug toxicity, renal function, and electrolytes should be performed in patients who have been placed on antiarrhythmic medications.
- Ongoing surveillance for the presence of symptomatic or asymptomatic AF is appropriate.

VIDEO LEGENDS

1. Video 10-2-1: Two-dimensional TEE image at 0° at the mid-esophageal level showing the left atrium and the left atrial appendage. A large and mobile thrombus is seen in the LAA.
2. Video 10-2-3: X plane was used to more comprehensively view orthogonal planes and demonstrate the size of the thrombus.
3. Video 10-2-5: Two-dimensional TEE image at 0° in the mid-esophagus, showing the four chamber view. There is grade 1-2 SEC in the left atrium
4. Video 10-2-6: The pre-existent LAA thrombus is seen in the two-dimensional X plane midesophageal LAX and SAX views on repeat TEE, but size reduction of the thrombus is demonstrated in this video.

REFERENCES

1. Fuster V, Ryden LE, Cannom DS, et al. 2011 ACCF/AHA/HRS focused updates incorporated into the ACC/AHA/ESC 2006 Guidelines for the management of patients with atrial fibrillation: a report of the American College of Cardiology Foundation/American Heart Association Task Force on Practice Guidelines developed in partnership with the European Society of Cardiology and in collaboration with the European Society of Cardiology and in collaboration with the European Heart Rhythm Association and Heart Rhythm Society. *J Am Coll Cardiol.* 2011;57(11):e101-198.
2. Khan I. Transient atrial mechanical dysfunction (stunning) after cardioversion of atrial fibrillation and flutter. *Am Heart J.* 2002;144:11-22.
3. Klein AL, Grimm RA, Black IW, et al. Cardioversion guided by transesophageal echocardiography: the ACUTE Pilot Study. A randomized controlled trial. Assessment of Cardioversion Using Transesophageal Echocardiography. *Ann Intern Med.* 1997;126:200-209.
4. Klein AL, Grimm RA, Murray RD, et al. Use of transesophageal ecocardiography to guide cardioversion in patients with atrial fibrillation. *N Engl J Med.* 2001;10;344(19):1411-1420.

SECTION 3

Echocardiography in Atrial Dysrhythmias: LAA Occluder Device Applications

CLINICAL CASE PRESENTATION

An 83-year-old man was diagnosed with AF with rapid ventricular response, initially responsive to medical therapy and warfarin. One year prior to his current encounter, he developed symptoms of dyspnea and fatigue in the setting of AF with a rapid ventricular response. He was then started on rivaroxaban and amiodarone. He failed amiodarone therapy, and it was discontinued. While on the rivaroxaban therapy, he developed anemia, and his stool was heme positive. Endoscopy was performed, which did not find an active bleeding source. Rivaroxaban was discontinued. He was maintained on rate control but presented to discuss options for mitigation of his risk for recurrent stroke in the setting of permanent atrial fibrillation. His past medical history included a stroke while he was on warfarin therapy (subtherapeutic as he was off warfarin for 4 days for dental surgery). His CHADS2 score was 4 for age, hypertension, stroke, and diabetes. On physical examination he was found to be tachycardic. He did not have significant jugular venous distension. Cardiac exam revealed that he was tachycardic with no murmurs, gallops, or rubs. Medications for rate control were adjusted. He was concerned about the risk of bleeding with long-term systemic anticoagulation. Left atrial appendage (LAA) occluder device implantation was proposed to the patient, and he agreed to proceed. The patient underwent a successful Watchman LAA occlusion procedure. The implantation was performed under transesophageal echocardiography (TEE) and fluoroscopic guidance (Figures 10-3-1 to 10-3-5). He was subsequently discharged without complications and has done well with medical therapy to control his heart rate. He remains in atrial fibrillation.

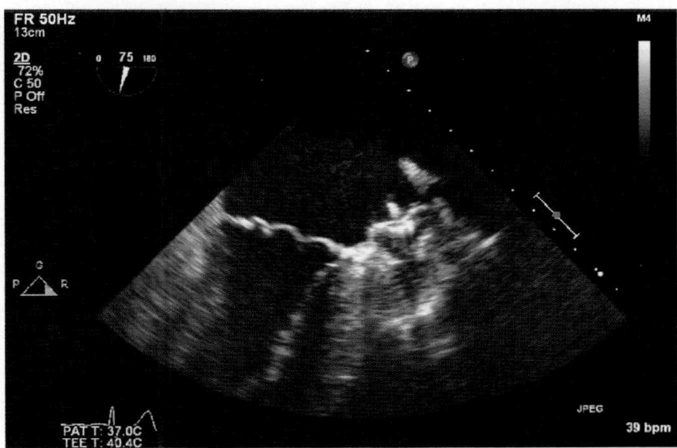

FIGURE 10-3-1 Two-dimensional multiplanar TEE image at 75° in the midesophagus, showing the left atrium (LA), left atrial appendage (LAA), left ventricle (LV), and left upper pulmonary vein (LUPV). This image demonstrates the placement of the Watchman device ▶ (see Video 10-3-1). This device is a self-expanding nickel titanium (nitinol) frame structure with fixation barbs and a permeable polyester fabric cover. The implantation is guided by fluoroscopy and TEE to verify proper positioning and stability. The device system is delivered via a transseptal sheath in the femoral vein through which the delivery catheter is deployed. A transseptal puncture is performed, and the device is introduced into the LA.

CLINICAL FEATURES

- Stroke is the third leading cause of death in several industrial countries and cardiogenic embolism accounts for 15% to 30 % of ischemic strokes.[1]
- The diagnosis of a cardioembolic source of stroke is frequently uncertain and relies on the identification of a potential cardiac source of embolism in the absence of significant cerebrovascular occlusive disease.
- Clinically, the most important cause of cardiogenic brain embolism is AF, both paroxysmal and chronic. Atrial fibrillation can result in the development of atrial thrombus, most frequently noted in the LAA.
- Other potential cardiac sources of embolism include LV thrombus, cardiac tumors such as myxomas, valvular vegetations (both bacterial and non-bacterial), and intracardiac shunts.

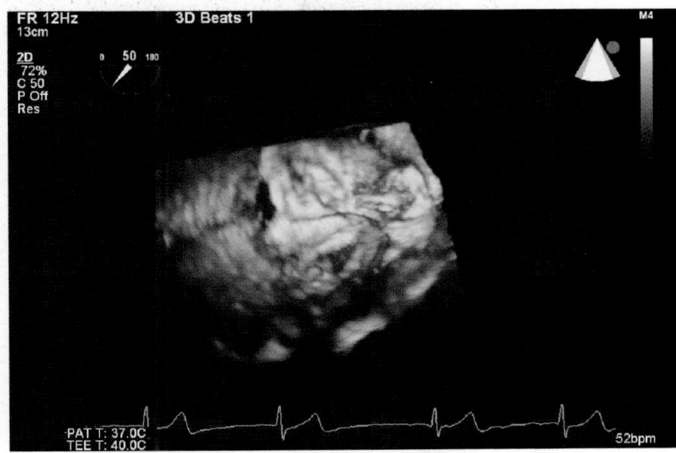

FIGURE 10-3-2 Three-dimensional full volume reconstruction demonstrating position of the Watchman device from the left atrial en face view. The occluder device covers the os of the left atrial appendage and can be seen to the right of the image.

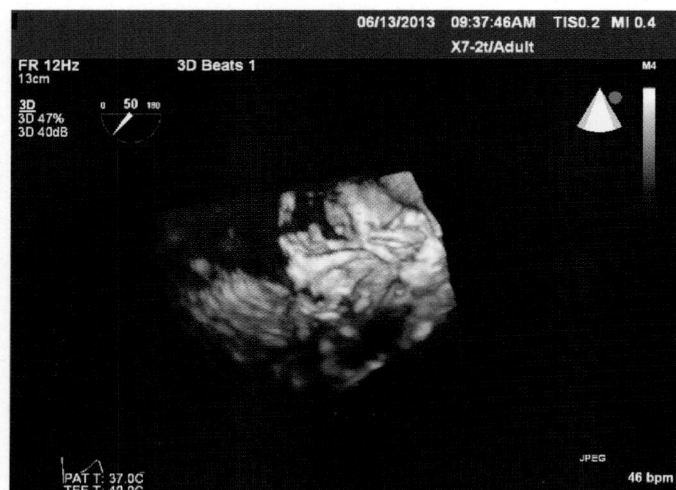

FIGURE 10-3-3 Three-dimensional live zoom image from the atrial perspective, showing the mitral valve (MV) and left atrial appendage (LAA) occluder device. This image shows the advantage of three-dimensional imaging in demonstrating the relationship and positioning of devices within the heart ►(see Video 10-3-3).

- The combination of patent foramen ovale (PFO) and atrial septal aneurysm seems especially important in young patients with cryptogenic stroke.[2]

EPIDEMIOLOGY

- Intracardiac sources of cerebrovascular ischemic events are increasingly being recognized and may account for 15% to 20% of the 500 000 strokes that occur annually in the United States.

PATHOPHYSIOLOGY AND ETIOLOGY

- The most frequent causes of cardiogenic stroke are AF, left ventricular (LV) dysfunction (congestive heart failure, LV aneurysm, apical thrombus), valve disease and prosthetic valves, intracardiac right-to-left shunts (PFO, particularly in conjunction with atrial septum aneurysm), cardiac masses (intracardiac tumours, fibroelastoma), and atheromatous thrombosis of the ascending aortic arch.
- The LAA plays a critical causal role in AF-related cardioembolic stroke.[3]
- Studies have shown that more than 90% of atrial thrombi in patients with nonrheumatic AF originate in the LAA.
- The LAA is a long, tubular, often multilobed and trabeculated blind spot and a remnant of the embryonic left atrium.[3]
- This accessory chamber extends over an area of 3 to 6 cm^2, is more compliant than the atrium, and is actively contractile in normal hearts, filling and emptying in response to both ventricular and atrial dynamics.[4]
- Receptors in the LAA influence heart rate, and granules secrete atrial natriuretic peptide, contributing to regulation of intravascular pressure and volume in response to stretch.[3,4]

ECHOCARDIOGRAPHY

- Echocardiography plays a key role in the initial evaluation and management of patients with AF as described in the prior two cases.
- Percutaneous device closure of the LAA has been used as a minimally invasive alternative treatment to long-term anticoagulation to reduce the risk of thromboembolism in patients with atrial fibrillation.
- Echocardiography is being more frequently employed to guide many interventional procedures and is an essential tool at all stages of the LAA device closure procedure.

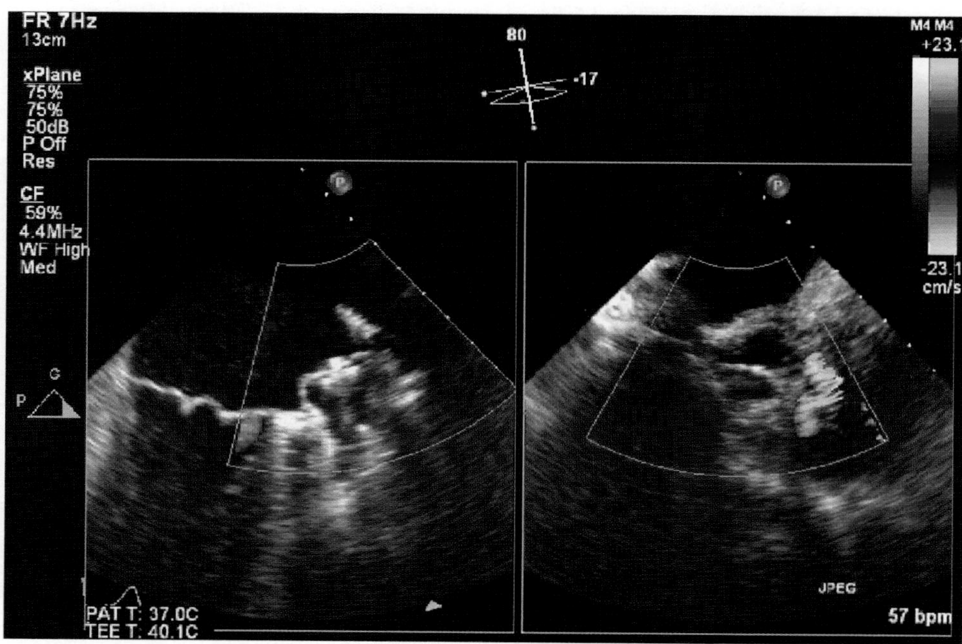

FIGURE 10-3-4 After deployment of the device, there is no residual peri-device flow as seen by X-plane, two-dimensional color Doppler TEE ► (see Video 10-3-4).

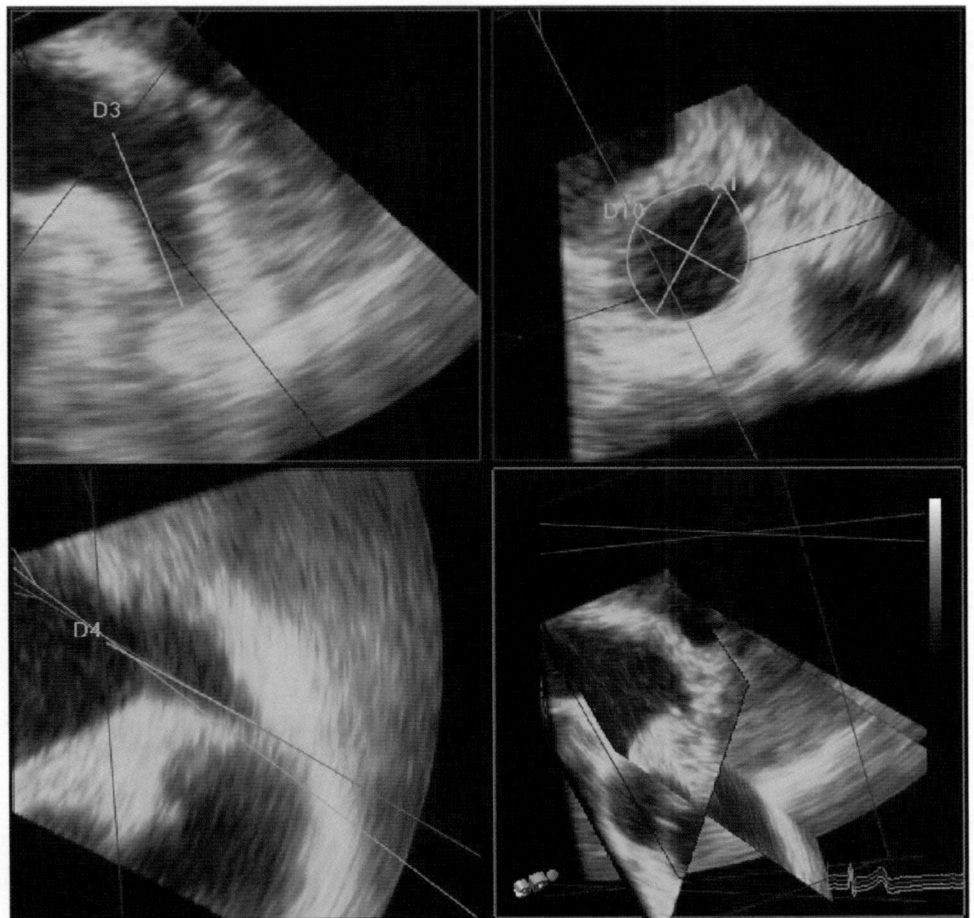

FIGURE 10-3-5 Three-dimensional full volume analysis using Q lab software showing the dimensions of LAA. The Watchman device ranges in diameter from 21 mm to 33 mm to accommodate varying LAA anatomy and size. Device size was chosen to be 10% to 20% larger than diameter of the LAA body to have sufficient compression for stable positioning of the device.[5] LAA anatomy tends to be highly variable, often with multiple lobes, and therefore no single device is likely to be suitable for all patients.

- Preprocedural TEE is used to identify suitable candidates and to describe LAA morphology and dimension.
- Periprocedural TEE or intracardiac echocardiography (ICE) has a major role in guiding catheter placement and the transseptal puncture as well as the delivery and deployment of the device, for screening of procedural complications and for assessing procedural success.
- TEE is used to evaluate LAA morphology, ostial dimension, and maximum length of the dominant lobe to provide a series of baseline measurements for procedural planning. Although multiplanar 2-D TEE measurements provide the main modality for preoperative assessment, the use of 3-D TEE gives useful additive information in identifying those with unusual morphology or irregular orifices.[5]

OTHER DIAGNOSTIC TESTING AND PROCEDURES

- The extension and site of the infarct on cranial computed tomography (CT) or magnetic resonance imaging (MRI) can deliver important clues towards a cardiogenic embolic stroke mechanism. This is the case if the infarct shows a cortical extension, multiplicity, or bilaterality.
- The presence of a suspected cardioembolic event on brain imaging in a patient with a stroke is often followed by echocardiography to ascertain potential sources of embolism.

DIFFERENTIAL DIAGNOSIS

- Multiplicity of lesions on cranial CT or MRI involving both the anterior and posterior circulation and/or both hemispheres is highly suggestive of cardiogenic embolism.[1]

DIAGNOSIS

- TTE and/or TEE serve as a cornerstone in the evaluation and diagnosis of cardiogenic embolism.
- TTE and TEE are recommended when symptoms potentially due to a suspected cardiac etiology, including syncope, TIA, and cerebrovascular events, are present.

MANAGEMENT

- Transesophageal echocardiography detects most thrombi in the LAA, and low stroke rates are reported in patients in whom the LAA has been surgically removed (although these patients were also reverted to sinus rhythm by various surgical techniques).[6]
- Surgical excision or stapling of the LAA is widely performed as a concomitant procedure during open-heart surgery. More recently, minimally invasive epicardial techniques and interventional transseptal techniques have been developed for occlusion of the LAA orifice to reduce the risk of stroke.
- Although clinically applied for decades, there is no conclusive evidence that surgical LAA excision or occlusion reduces stroke risk in AF patients, due to a lack of large, controlled trials with systematic follow-up.
    - In addition, no conclusive data are available on the best surgical technique for performing LAA closure.
    - Risks of surgical LAA excision include major bleeding and incomplete LAA occlusion with residual stroke risk.[7]
- Currently, two self-expanding percutaneous LAA occlusion devices, the WATCHMAN (Boston Scientific, Natick, MA, USA) and the Amplatzer Cardiac Plug (St. Jude Medical, St Paul, MN, USA), which are transseptally placed in the LAA, are available for clinical use.
- At present, interventional LAA closure is not indicated simply as an alternative to oral anticoagulation (OAC) therapy to reduce stroke risk.[8]
- Interventional, percutaneous LAA closure may be considered in patients with a high stroke risk and contraindications for long-term OAC (ESC guideline: class IIb).[9]
- Surgical excision of the LAA may be considered in patients undergoing open heart surgery (ESC guideline: class IIb).[9]
- Although the concept of LAA closure seems reasonable, the evidence of efficacy and safety is currently insufficient to recommend these approaches for any patients other than those in whom long-term OAC is contraindicated.[10]
- These devices/procedures may provide an alternative to OAC for AF patients at high risk for stroke but with contraindications for chronic OAC and if the efficiency of LAA closure can be conclusively shown to potentially replace long-term OAC.

FOLLOW-UP

- Patients are discharged from the hospital on aspirin 81 to 100 mg daily and warfarin for at least 45 days, with dosage of the latter adjusted to keep the INR between 2 and 3.
- If echocardiographic criteria for successful sealing of the LAA is fulfilled at 45 days, warfarin therapy may be discontinued while aspirin should be continued indefinitely.
- After the device is implanted, patients should be treated with warfarin for 45 days to facilitate device endothelialization.[11]
- Echocardiographic surveillance (TEE) is currently recommended at 1 month, 6 months, and annually postprocedure.[5]
- The need for lifelong aspirin treatment after placement of LAA closure devices, and the significant bleeding risk with aspirin, may weigh against preference for interventional LAA occlusion.

VIDEO LEGENDS

1. Video 10-3-1: Two-dimensional multiplanar TEE image at 75° in the mid-esophagus, showing the left atrium, left atrial appendage, left ventricle, and left upper pulmonary vein. This video demonstrates the placement of the Watchman device.
2. Video 10-3-3: Three-dimensional live zoom image from the atrial perspective, showing the mitral valve (MV) and left atrial appendage (LAA) occluder device. This image shows the advantage of three dimensional imaging in demonstrating the relationship and positioning of devices within the heart.
3. Video 10-3-4: After deployment of the Watchman device, there is no residual peri-device flow as seen by X-plane, two-dimensional color Doppler TEE.

REFERENCES

1. Pepi M, Evangelista A, Nihoyannopoulos P, et al. Recommendations for echocardiography use in the diagnosis and management of cardiac sources of embolism. *Eur J Echocardiogr.* 2010;11:461-476.
2. Cate FJ, Meijboom FJ, Michels M. Evaluation of cardiac emboli source. *Neth Heart J.* 2005;13:444-447.
3. Al Saady NM, Obel OA, Camm AJ. Left atrial appendage: structure, function, and role in thromboembolism. *Heart.* 1999;82:547-554.
4. Tabata T, Oki T, Yamada H, et al. Role of left atrial appendage in left atrial reservoir function as evaluated by left atrial appendage clamping during cardiac surgery. *Am J Cardiol.* 1998;81:327-332.
5. Chue CD, de Giovanni J, Steeds RP. The role of echocardiography in percutaneous left atrial appendage occlusion. *Eur J Echocardiogr.* 2011;12(10):i3-10.
6. Cox JL. Cardiac surgery for arrhythmias. *J Cardiovasc Electrophysiol.* 2004;15:250-262.
7. Dawson AG, Asopa S, Dunning J. Should patients undergoing cardiac surgery with atrial fibrillation have left atrial appendage exclusion? *Interact Cardiovasc Thorac Surg.* 2010;10:306-311,250-262.
8. Bayard YL, Omran H, Neuzil P, et al. PLAATO (Percutaneous Left Atrial Appendage Transcatheter Occlusion) for prevention of cardioembolic stroke in non-anticoagulation eligible atrial fibrillation patients: results from the European PLAATO study. *EuroIntervention.* 2010;6:220-226.

9. Camm AJ, Lip GY, De Caterina, et al. 2012 focused update of the ESC Guidelines for the management of atrial fibrillation: an update of the 2010 ESC Guidelines for the management of atrial fibrillation. Developed with the special contribution of the European Heart Rhythm Association. *Eur Heart J.* 2012;33:2719-2747.

10. Whitlock R, Healey J, Connolly S. Left atrial appendage occlusion does not eliminate the need for warfarin. *Circulation.* 2009;120:1927-1932.

11. Sick P, Schuler G, Hauptmann KE, et al. Initial worldwide experience with the WATCHMAN left atrial appendage system for stroke prevention in atrial fibrillation. *J Am Coll Cardiol.* 2007;49:1490-1495.

11 ECHOCARDIOGRAPHIC ASSESSMENT IN PULMONARY HYPERTENSION AND RIGHT HEART FAILURE

Gina G. Mentzer, MD, Karen Dugan, MD, and Sitaramesh Emani, MD

INTRODUCTION

The assessment of the right heart presents many challenges due to its unique anatomy and physiology.[1] In spite of these limitations, echocardiography remains the principal imaging method employed to assess patients with known or suspected right heart disease, especially in the acute setting. While other imaging techniques such as cardiac CT and MRI have provided additional tools to evaluate cardiac anatomy and function, they currently play a secondary role in most clinical settings. MRI is playing a larger role in the assessment of right ventricular size and function, especially in the congenital heart disease population.

The use of echocardiography is a class 1 indication for the evaluation of many clinical scenarios in which right heart disease is suspected.[2] In the recently revised appropriate use criteria for echocardiography,[3] echocardiography is deemed appropriate in a variety of such clinical scenarios.

In this chapter, we will demonstrate the utility of echocardiography in the assessment of acute right heart failure/pulmonary hypertension in a patient with pulmonary embolism and in a patient with chronic pulmonary hypertension and chronic right heart failure.

SECTION 1

Acute Pulmonary Embolism/Acute Pulmonary Hypertension

Karen Dugan, MD, and Gina G. Mentzer, MD

CLINICAL CASE PRESENTATION

A 73-year-old white man with a past medical history of coronary artery disease, status post 4-vessel coronary bypass surgery in 1997, Type 2 diabetes mellitus, hypertension, and diverticular disease presented to our hospital with a chief complaint of "shortness of breath." For 2 weeks, he had been complaining of dyspnea on exertion (DOE), a nonproductive cough, and chest heaviness that had progressively worsened. In the emergency department, he was hypoxic (requiring oxygen via a non-rebreather mask), tachycardic, and hypotensive with a systolic blood pressure (SBP) in the 80s that did not respond to intravenous (IV) fluids.

On examination, he was obese and appeared quite uncomfortable, only able to speak 4 to 5 words at a time. His cardiac exam showed significant tachycardia, a normal S_1 and S_2 with a prominent P_2 at the left sternal border at the 4th intercostal space and a right parasternal heave. Pulmonary examination revealed that he had decreased breath sounds at the bases bilaterally with poor chest expansion during inspiration. Extremity exam was significant for unilateral left lower leg 1+ pitting edema. Otherwise, the rest of the physical exam was unremarkable.

Laboratory results were significant for brain natriuretic peptide (BNP) 3382, troponin 5.3, and an arterial blood gas (ABG) of pH 7.2, Pco_2 30, Po_2 104, and HCO_3 11 on 100% oxygen. An electrocardiogram (ECG) showed an S wave in lead I, a Q wave in lead III, and an inverted T wave in lead III (Figure 11-1-1). A transthoracic echocardiogram (TTE) showed a large thrombus in the pulmonary arterial trunk that extended into the pulmonary arteries (PA) (Figure 11-1-2). The echocardiogram showed a moderately dilated right ventricle (RV) with severe systolic dysfunction, a flattened septum due to RV pressure overload, and a right ventricular systolic pressure (RVSP) of 51 mm Hg consistent with an acute pulmonary embolism (PE) (Figure 11-1-3). He underwent a computed tomography (CT) scan that confirmed large bilateral pulmonary emboli (PE) (Figure 11-1-4). Figure 11-1-5 demonstrates the thrombi removed at surgery.

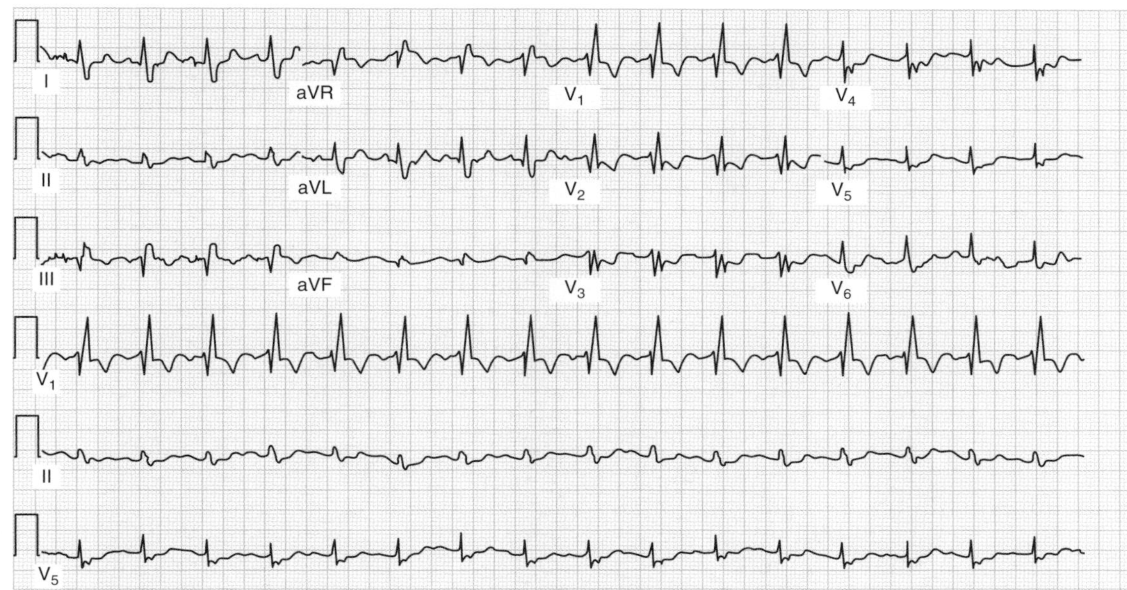

FIGURE 11-1-1 Classic ECG findings in acute PE with demonstration of sinus tachycardia, S wave in lead I, Q wave in lead III, and an inverted T wave in leads III and V3.

CLINICAL FEATURES

- Most patients with a pulmonary embolism (PE) present with dyspnea and/or chest pain. Less commonly, a patient may present with cyanosis, syncope, or hemoptysis.[4]
- Tachycardia is found in an average of 43% of patients diagnosed with PE.
- Typically, the remainder of the examination is normal, but in patients with massive or submassive PE, signs of RV dysfunction or failure such as hypotension, elevated jugular pressure, a RV S_3 gallop, a prominent P_2, and a left parasternal heave may be seen and can help narrow the diagnosis.[4]

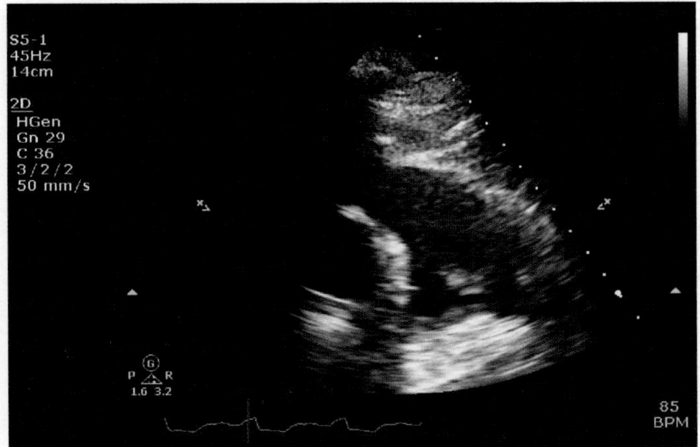

FIGURE 11-1-2 Two-dimensional image on TTE of a large embolism in the main pulmonary artery in the parasternal short-axis window ► (see Video 11-1-2).

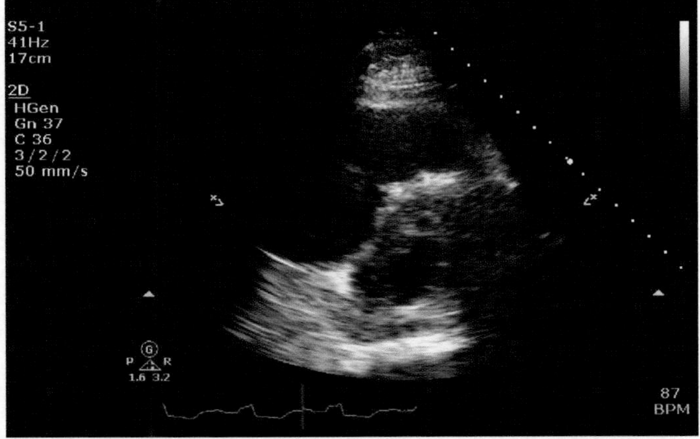

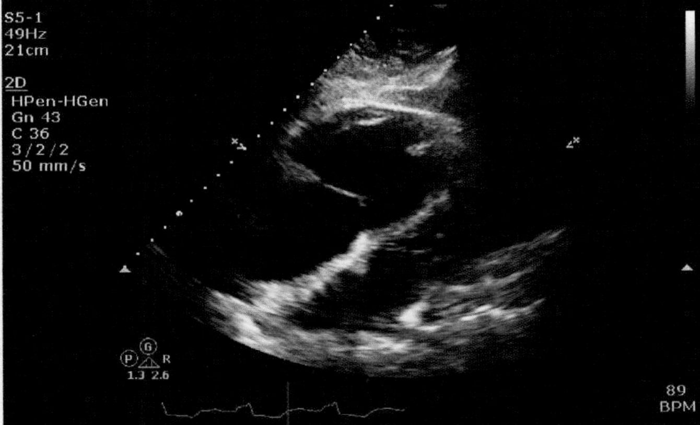

FIGURE 11-1-3 Two-dimensional image on TTE in the parasternal short-axis (upper panel) and subcostal views (lower panel). This demonstrates a dilated, hypokinetic right ventricle (RV) with signs of pressure overload (flattened septum in systole) ► (see Videos 11-1-3 A and B).

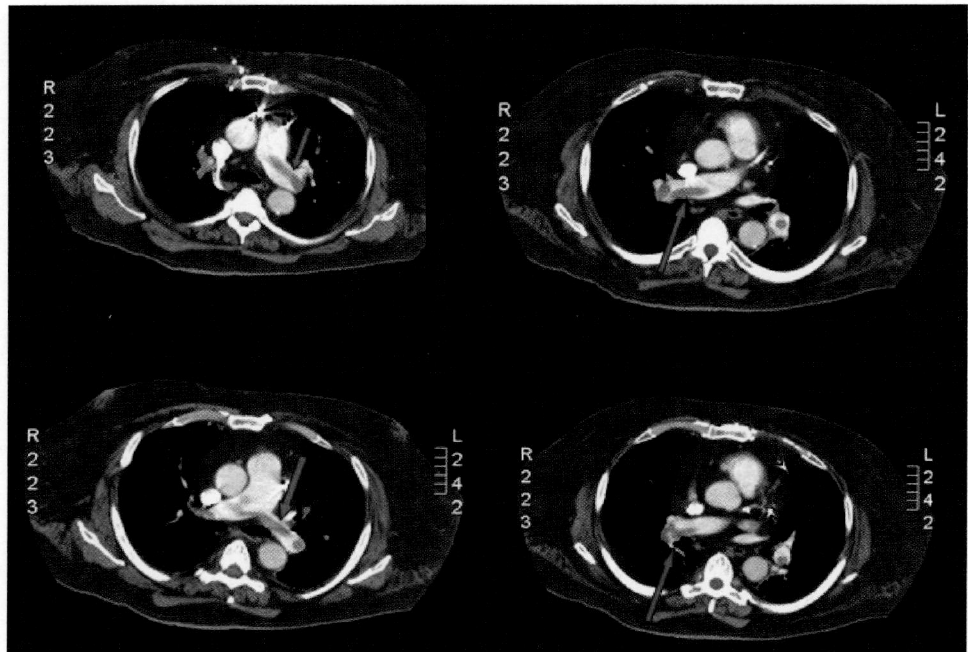

FIGURE 11-1-4 Computed tomography imaging of the massive bilateral PEs (arrows). The four images demonstrate the large thrombus in the main and left PA (upper left), in the right PA (upper right), in the main and both PAs (lower left), and in the more distal right PA (lower right).

EPIDEMIOLOGY

- The overall average incidence of acute PE is between 23 and 69 per 100 000.[4,5] Of these, 4.2% are massive PE, causing systemic hypotension or shock.[6] The mortality rate from PE is greater than 15% within the first 3 months after diagnosis in patients who are hemodynamically stable and up to 58% in those who present with hemodynamic instablility.[6]

ETIOLOGY AND PATHOPHYSIOLOGY

- Venous thrombi are typically formed in the deep veins of the calf, often arising in sites of venous stasis. From the deep veins of the calf, the thrombus will propagate to the proximal veins and, from there, embolize, traversing the inferior vena cava (IVC), right atrium (RA), RV, and finally dwelling in the pulmonary arteries (PA). Depending on the size of the embolus, it may cause obstruction in the main PA down to the subsegmental pulmonary arteries.
- Massive PE is defined as an embolism that causes shock, SBPs less than 90 mm Hg, or a drop in SBP greater than 40 mm Hg for greater than 15 minutes.[7] A submassive PE is an embolism that causes RV dysfunction without systemic arterial hypotension.
- In patients with either a submassive or massive PE, obstruction of the main PA or its branches along with increased pulmonary

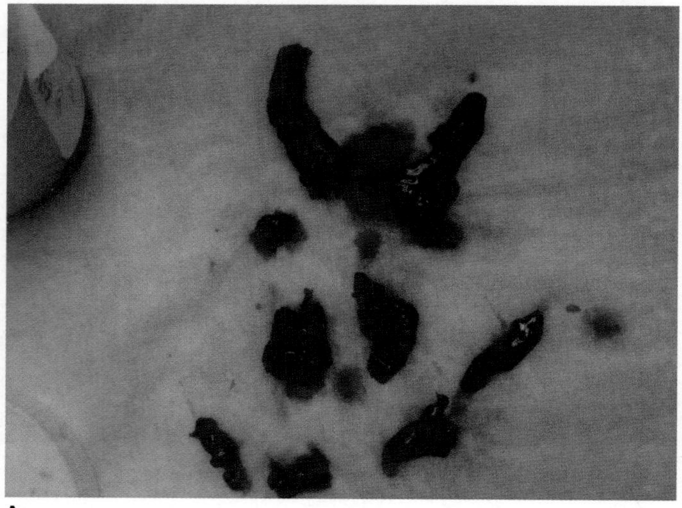

A

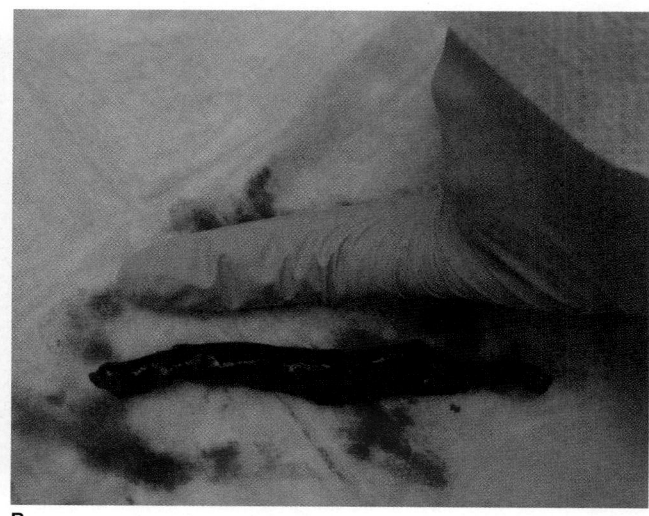

B

FIGURE 11-1-5 Demonstration of the pulmonary arterial clots in the operating room postembolectomy (A) and size comparison with a finger that measures 5 cm (B).

vascular resistance (PVR) from hypoxic vasoconstriction leads to increased pulmonary arterial pressure (PAP) and RV afterload.[8] The RV wall tension will rise, leading to RV enlargement, dysfunction, and failure. RV enlargement will cause a leftward shift of the interventricular septum and lead to reduced left ventricular (LV) filling. The combination of RV failure and decreased LV preload will ultimately lead to hemodynamic instability.[8]

- Inherited risk factors for PE include Factor V Leiden, prothrombin gene mutation, and deficiencies of antithrombin III, protein C, or protein S.[7] Acquired risk factors include conditions that cause alterations in Virchow's triad (endothelial injury, hypercoaguability, and venous stasis) such as cancer, congestive heart failure (CHF), chronic obstructive pulmonary disease (COPD), myocardial infarction (MI), obesity, aging smoking, stroke (CVA), oral contraceptive pills or hormone replacement, family history of venous thromboembolism, and recent surgery or trauma.[5]

ECHOCARDIOGRAPHY

- Patients presenting with symptoms and signs of PE do not typically undergo echocardiography for diagnosis. However, if a patient is hemodynamically unstable and/or is unable to undergo spiral CT, transthoracic echocardiography (TTE) should be performed if a PE is suspected, especially if the patient presents with unexplained dyspnea, syncope, or right ventricular failure.[9]
- Echocardiographic assessment, rather than being employed for diagnosis, is utilized to assess the hemodynamic consequences of PE and thus can further assist in guiding therapy. Figures 11-1-6 to 11-1-9 from other patients demonstrate additional echocardiographic images in patients with a PE.
- In addition, following therapy for acute PE, echocardiography is employed to evaluate RV function and PAP and in surveillance of cardiac function and pulmonary pressures following a PE for long-term effects.
- With echocardiography, a thrombus may be visualized in the main PA or in the proximal portions of the right or left PA. The presence of a RA or RV thrombus may also be seen. The sensitivity for detecting PA thrombus is improved with the use of transesophageal echocardiography (TEE).
- In addition to directly visualizing a PE on echocardiography, indirect signs of PE causing acute cor pulmonale may be seen as well. These will be detailed later in this section.
  - Pulmonary hypertension causing increased RV afterload. PAP is detected by Doppler flow velocity recording of the RV outflow tract. In a normal patient, peak ejection velocity is monophasic and occurs during midsystole. However, in patients with pulmonary hypertension, the ejection profile may be biphasic with a reduction in midsystolic velocity.[9]
  - RV enlargement on the apical 4 chamber view. Because the two ventricles are enclosed in the pericardial space, enlargement of the RV will cause a leftward shift of the interventricular septum. The RV end-diastolic to LV end-diastolic ratio will be increased

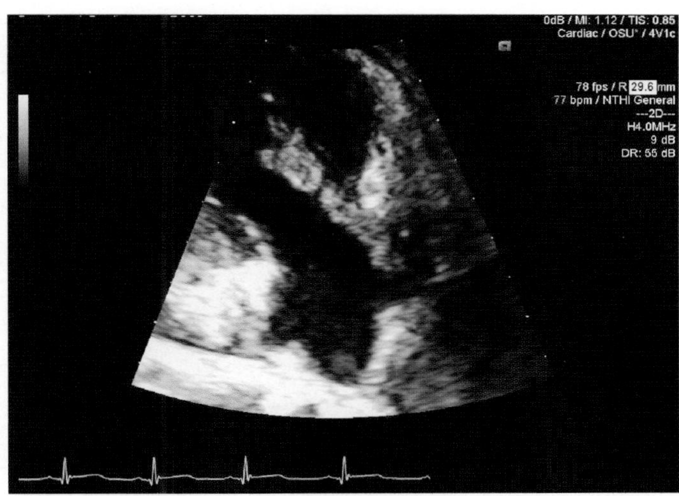

FIGURE 11-1-7 RV inflow view demonstrating a large thrombus in transit extending from the IVC into the RA and across the TV into the RV ▶ (see Video 11-1-7).

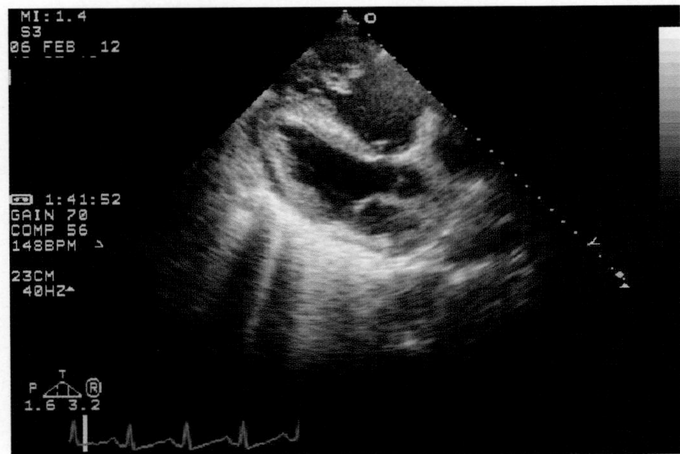

FIGURE 11-1-6 Parasternal long axis demonstrating a massively dilated RV that is severely hypokinetic from a patient presenting in shock from a massive PE ▶ (see Video 11-1-6)

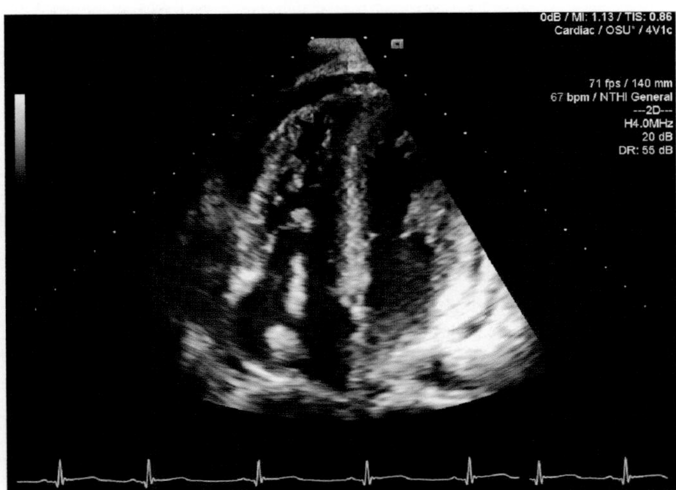

FIGURE 11-1-8 Apical 4 chamber view from the patient in Figure 11-1-7 again demonstrating a large thrombus in the RA and RV. The RV is dilated as well. There is a pericardial effusion present, most likely related to this patient's lung cancer ▶ (see Video 11-1-8).

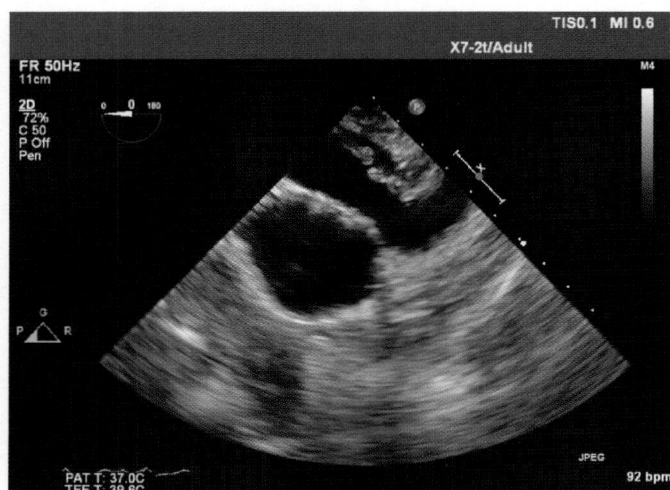

FIGURE 11-1-9 Intraoperative TEE from another patient who underwent pulmonary artery embolectomy for a massive PE. There is a saddle embolus seen at the bifurcation of the main PA extending into the RPA in this still frame ► (see Videos 11-1-9 A and B).

(greater than 0.6). A ratio ranging from 0.6 to 1 indicates mild RV dilatation, whereas a ratio from 1 to 2 indicates severe RV dilatation.[9]

- Septal flattening and paradoxical septal motion may be seen. Normally, the interventricular septum thickens during systole and moves toward the LV. In a patient with PE causing acute cor pulmonale, RV contraction is prolonged and the interventricular septum moves toward the LV during diastole.[9]
- McConnell sign. This occurs when there is appearance of normal wall motion of the apex of the RV accompanied by abnormal wall motion or hypokinesis of the RV free wall.[10]
- Diastolic LV impairment. Because the two ventricles are enclosed within the pericardium, the sum of diastolic ventricular dimensions remains constant. Therefore, with acute RV dilatation and failure, LV volume may be reduced and LV filling may be impaired resulting in a further reduction in LV dimension.[9]
- RV hypertrophy. In acute cor pulmonale, the RV should not demonstrate hypertrophy. However, in patients with chronic cor pulmonale, RV hypertrophy will be present. Therefore, a lack of RV hypertrophy can help differentiate acute cor pulmonale from chronic pulmonary hypertension.[9]

OTHER DIAGNOSTIC TESTING

- D-dimer ELISA should only be obtained in patients who present to the emergency department or outpatient office and are low or intermediate risk as determined by the Wells or Geneva critiera.[11] If the D-dimer is normal, PE can be excluded, and a different diagnosis should be sought. If positive, patients should undergo spiral CT or another imaging modality to detect PE.
- Spiral computed tomography (CT) has a 97% sensitivity and 99.6% negative predictive value for detecting pulmonary emboli.[12] Spiral CT is indicated in patients with a high risk for PE and in hospitalized patients in whom a PE is suspected. Spiral CT has limited utility in women who are pregnant, patients at risk for contrast induced nephropathy such as those with acute kidney injury or chronic kidney disease, and in those with contrast allergy.
- Lower extremity venous ultrasonography may identify a DVT. However, if a DVT has completely embolized to the lungs, venous ultrasonography will be negative. It should be noted, venous ultrasonography is insensitive for detecting DVT in asymptomatic patients.[12]
- Ventilation-perfusion scan is often nondiagnostic. One would use it only if unable to obtain spiral CT.[12]
- Pulmonary angiography is considered the gold standard for diagnosis of pulmonary embolism. However, it is invasive, costly, and rarely used.[12]
- ECG will typically show tachycardia as the most common finding. However, in patients with RV dysfunction, the ECG may show signs of RV strain, such as right axis deviation, inverted T waves in the precordial leads, a right bundle branch block, or the S1Q3T3 pattern (an S wave in lead I, a Q wave in lead III, and an inverted T wave in lead III or V3).[12]
- Chest radiograph is often normal in patients with PE. However, cardiomegaly may be seen in patients with massive PE.
- Arterial blood gas will typically show hypoxemia and hypocapnia. In many patients, an elevated alveolar-arterial oxygen gradient will be present.
- Elevations in brain natriuretic peptide (BNP) and troponins are used to help risk-stratify patients. Patients with elevated values are at high risk for acute mortality and morbidity.[13,14]

DIFFERENTIAL DIAGNOSIS

- For patients who present with signs of RV failure and concern for PE, the differential includes: PE, biventricular CHF, myocardial infarction (MI), constrictive pericarditis, pericardial tamponade, and valvular heart disease.
- In patients who present with dyspnea and/or chest pain but are hemodynamically stable, the differential diagnosis includes: PE, pneumonia, acute COPD exacerbation, MI, and pulmonary lymphangitic carcinomatosis in patients with cancer.

DIAGNOSIS

The diagnosis of PE is usually made based on a thorough history and physical exam, assessment of risk factors, and diagnostic tests such as D-dimer, spiral CT or ventilation-perfusion scans, and echocardiography.

- In the hemodynamically stable patient who presents to the office or emergency department and who is at low or intermediate risk as determined by either the Wells or Geneva criteria, a D-dimer should be obtained.[15] If the D-dimer is normal, a PE has been excluded, and another diagnosis should be sought. If the D-dimer is increased, the patient should undergo spiral CT scanning to confirm or exclude the diagnosis.
- If a patient is hospitalized or at high risk and hemodynamically stable, the patient should undergo spiral CT scanning without D-dimer testing. Since the D-dimer is often elevated in other inflammatory states, it is not useful in hospitalized patients.

- Some patients are unable to undergo spiral CT scanning due to pregnancy, kidney disease, or contrast allergy. In these cases, lower extremity Doppler ultrasonography should be done. This can be a useful strategy because the treatment for DVT and PE are often the same. If lower extremity Doppler ultrasonography is negative, that does not rule out PE, and the patient should either undergo ventilation-perfusion scanning or echocardiography.
- If a patient is hemodynamically unstable and is unable to be transferred to radiology for CT scanning, a bedside echocardiogram should be undertaken to look for RV dysfunction suggestive of PE as well as other conditions on the differential such as MI, aortic dissection, and pericardial tamponade.[9]

MANAGEMENT

- If hemodynamically stable, the patient should be started on intravenous unfractionated heparin, subcutaneous low molecular weight heparin, or subcutaneous fondaparinux in addition to warfarin. Once the INR is between 2 and 3 for 2 consecutive days, heparin or fondaparinux may be discontinued. The patient should remain on warfarin minimally for 3 months, and then the risks versus benefits should be evaluated for continued therapy. If the patient has risk factors or has had recurrent venous thromboembolism, anticoagulation may need to be continued indefinitely.
- If a patient is hemodynamically unstable, systemic or catheter directed thrombolysis should be considered. Contraindications for thrombolysis include history of intracranial hemorrhage, ischemic stroke in the past 6 months, intracranial neoplasm, recent head trauma or surgery in the past 3 weeks, or current/recent bleeding within 3 weeks. If thrombolysis is contraindicated, a cardiothoracic surgeon should be consulted for a pulmonary embolectomy.
- Poor prognostic indicators include marked dyspnea, anxiety and low oxygen saturation, RV dysfunction, elevated troponin indicating RV microinfarction, and RV enlargement.
- A TTE should be performed in follow-up to assess recovery of the RV, PAP, and LV function as determined by a cardiologist.

PATIENT EDUCATION

- Patients must be continued on warfarin or other systemic anticoagulants for at least 3 months following diagnosis of PE with total duration determined by their physician. Patients must be educated about the risks of bleeding while on warfarin.
- Even while on anticoagulation, patients are still at risk for recurrent thromboembolic at 1% per year.
- If anticoagulation is stopped, the risk of recurrent pulmonary embolism increases to 4% per year.[16]
- Chronic thromboembolic pulmonary hypertension occurs in 4% to 5% of patients after acute PE.[17]

FOLLOW-UP

The patient remained in the intensive care unit. He was weaned of pressor agents but remained hemodynamically guarded. Thrombolytics were contraindicated due to recent GI bleed from diverticulitis. Surgery was consulted, and he underwent successful bilateral pulmonary artery thrombectomy (Figure 11-1-5). Unfortunately, he did not survive due to complications with sepsis and extensive RV failure from the acute PE and underlying COPD.

VIDEO LEGENDS

1. Video 11-1-2: 2-D image on TTE of a large embolism in the main pulmonary artery in the parasternal short-axis view.
2. Video 11-1-3 A: 2-D image on TTE in the parasternal short-axis view. This demonstrates a dilated, hypokinetic right ventricle (RV) with signs of pressure overload (flattened septum in systole)
3. Video 11-1-3 B: 2-D image on TTE in the subcostal view. This demonstrates a dilated, hypokinetic right ventricle (RV).
4. Video 11-1-6 : Parasternal long axis demonstrating a massively dilated RV which is severely hypokinetic from a patient presenting in shock from a massive PE
5. Video 11-1-7: RV inflow view demonstrating a large thrombus in transit extending from the IVC into the RA and across the TV in to the RV.
6. Video 11-1-8: Apical 4 chamber view from the patient in Video 11-1-7 again demonstrating a large thrombus in the RA and RV. The RV is dilated as well. There is a pericardial effusion present as well, most likely related to this patient's lung cancer.
7. Video 11-1-9 A: Intraoperative TEE from another patient who underwent pulmonary artery embolectomy for a massive PE. There is a saddle embolus seen at the bifurcation of the main PA extending into the RPA
8. Video 11-1-9 B: Intraoperative TEE from the patient in Video 11-1-9 A who underwent pulmonary artery embolectomy for a massive PE. There is a saddle embolus seen at the bifurcation of the main PA extending into the LPA

REFERENCES

1. Rudski LG, Lai WW, Afilalo J, et al. Guidelines for the echocardiographic assessment of the right heart in adults: a report for the American Society of Echocardiography. *J Am Soc Echocardiogr.* 2010;23:685-713.
2. Cheitlin MD, Armstrong WF, Aurigemma GP, et al. ACC/AHA/ASE 2003 guideline update for the clinical application of echocardiography - summary article A report of the American College of Cardiology/American Heart Association Task Force on practice guidelines. (ACC/AHA/ASE 2003 Committee to Update the 1997 Guidelines for the Clinical Application of Echocardiography). *J Am Coll Cardiol.* 2003;42:954-970.
3. Douglas PS, Garcia MJ, Haines DE, et al. ACCF/ASE/AHA/ASNC/HFSA/HRS/SCAI/SCCM/SCCT/SCMR 2011 appropriate use criteria for echocardiography: a report of the American College of Cardiology Foundation Appropriate Use Criteria Task Force, American Society of Echocardiography, American Heart Association, American Society of Nuclear Cardiology, Heart Failure Society of America, Heart Rhythm Society, Society of Cardiovascular Angiography and Interventions, Society of Critical Care Medicine, Society of Cardiovascular Computed

Tomography, and Society of Cardiovascular Magnetic Resonance. *J Am Coll Cardiol.* 2011;57(9):1126-1166. doi: 10.1016/j.jacc.2010.11.002.

4. Anderson FA Jr, Wheeler HB, Goldberg RJ, et al. A population-based perspective of the hospital incidence and case-fatality rates of deep vein thrombosis and pulmonary embolism. The Worcester DVT study. *Arch Intern Med.* 1991;151(5):933-938.
5. Silverstein MD, Heit JA, Mohr DN, Petterson TM, O'Fallon WM, Melton LJ 3rd. Trends in the incidence of deep vein thrombosis and pulmonary embolism: a 25-year population-based study. *Arch Intern Med.* 1998;158(6):585-593.
6. Goldhaber SZ, Visani L, De Rosa M. Acute pulmonary embolism: clinical outcomes in the International Cooperative Pulmonary Embolism Registry (ICOPER). *Lancet.* 1999;353(9162):1386-1389.
7. Kasper W, Konstantinides S, Geibel A, et al. Management strategies and determinants of outcome in acute major pulmonary embolism: results of a multicenter registry. *J Am Coll Cardiol.* 1997;30(5):1165-1171.
8. Goldhaber SZ, Elliott CG. Acute pulmonary embolism: part I: epidemiology, pathophysiology, and diagnosis. *Circulation.* 2003;108(22):2726-2729.
9. Goldhaber SZ. Echocardiography in the management of pulmonary embolism. *Ann Intern Med.* 2002;136(9):691-700.
10. McConnell MV, Solomon SD, Rayan ME, Come PC, Goldhaber SZ, Lee RT. Regional right ventricular dysfunction detected by echocardiography in acute pulmonary embolism. *Am J Cardiol.* 1996;78(4):469-473.
11. Wells PS, Anderson DR, Rodger M, et al. Excluding pulmonary embolism at the bedside without diagnostic imaging: management of patients with suspected pulmonary embolism presenting to the emergency department by using a simple clinical model and d-dimer. *Ann Intern Med.* 2001;135(2):98-107.
12. Schoepf UJ, Kucher N, Kipfmueller F, Quiroz R, Costello P, Goldhaber SZ. Right ventricular enlargement on chest computed tomography: a predictor of early death in acute pulmonary embolism. *Circulation.* 2004;110(20):3276-3280.
13. Becattini C, Vedovati MC, Agnelli G. Prognostic value of troponins in acute pulmonary embolism: a meta-analysis. *Circulation.* 2007;116(4):427-433.
14. ten Wolde M, Tulevski II, Mulder JW, et al. Brain natriuretic peptide as a predictor of adverse outcome in patients with pulmonary embolism. *Circulation.* 2003;107(16):2082-2084.
15. Chagnon I, Bounameaux H, Aujesky D, et al. Comparison of two clinical prediction rules and implicit assessment among patients with suspected pulmonary embolism. *Am J Med.* 2002;113(4):269-275.
16. Agnelli G, Prandoni P, Becattini C, et al. Extended oral anticoagulant therapy after a first episode of pulmonary embolism. *Ann Intern Med.* 2003;139(1):19-25.
17. Torbicki A, Perrier A, Konstantinides S, et al. Guidelines on the diagnosis and management of acute pulmonary embolism: The Task Force for the Diagnosis and Management of Acute Pulmonary Embolism of the European Society of Cardiology (ESC). *Eur Heart J.* 2008;29(18):2276-2315.

SECTION 2

Chronic Pulmonary Hypertension

Sitaramesh Emani, MD

CLINICAL CASE PRESENTATION

A 54-year-old woman with a history of scleroderma presents as an outpatient for evaluation of worsening dyspnea. She has a long-standing history of scleroderma that has been intermittently treated with steroids. At presentation, she reports a significant decline in her functional status to the point that she becomes short of breath with approximately 50 feet of walking. She denies any orthopnea, chest pain, or syncope. She has occasional lower extremity edema. On exam her blood pressure is 120/64 mm Hg, her pulse is 88 beats/minute, and her oxygen saturation is 92% on room air. Pulmonary exam reveals clear lung fields bilaterally. Cardiac exam demonstrates a regular rate and rhythm with a loud P_2, a II/VI midsystolic murmur heard best at the sternal border and without radiation, and a right ventricular heave. An echocardiogram is ordered and shows a severely dilated and thickened right ventricle. Pulmonary arterial systolic pressures are estimated at 115 mm Hg. Left ventricular function and appearance are normal. A pericardial effusion is noted as well (Figure 11-2-1). A diagnosis of pulmonary hypertension is suspected. The patient is sent for confirmatory testing.

CLINICAL FEATURES[1,2]

- Pulmonary hypertension (PH) is defined by abnormally elevated pressures in the pulmonary arterial system.
- Patients with PH generally present with signs and symptoms of heart failure such as dyspnea on exertion (most common), fatigue, and sometimes edema or abdominal distention.
- Symptoms result from decreased cardiac output similar to systolic heart failure, but are attributed specifically to right ventricular dysfunction (see Pathophysiology).

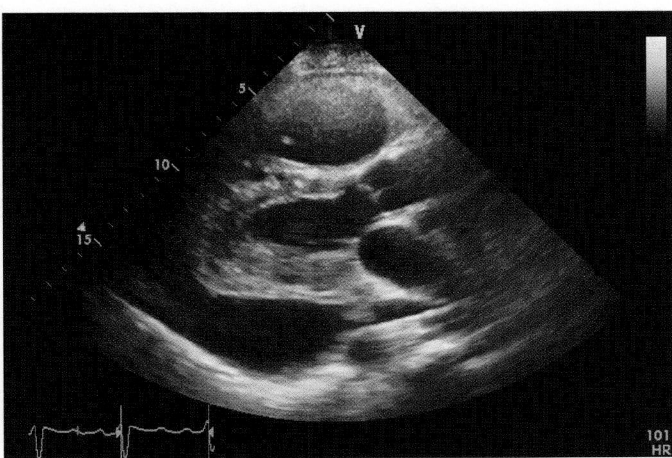

FIGURE 11-2-1 Parasternal long axis view. Note the enlarged right ventricle at the top of the image as well as the presence of a large pericardial effusion. The LV is relatively small and under-filled ▶ (see Video 11-2-1).

- Physical exam findings correlate with elevated pulmonary pressures and can include an accentuated pulmonic valve closure sound (loud P_2), a tricuspid valve regurgitation murmur, and signs of an elevated right atrial pressure (increased jugular venous distention).
- Other signs of venous congestion, such as lower extremity edema, can be found as well.
- Palpation of the cardiac impulse can reveal a right ventricular heave.
- Additional clinical signs that are associated with underlying and predisposing conditions can also be present.

EPIDEMIOLOGY[1,2]

The actual prevalence of pulmonary hypertension is unknown but may be around 10% based on observational data. Certain forms of PH, particularly those linked with autoimmune disorders, have a 2:1 female predominance.

DEFINITION, PATHOPHYSIOLOGY, AND ETIOLOGY[1,2]

- Pulmonary hypertension is defined by a mean pulmonary arterial (PA) pressure ≥25 mm Hg as directly measured by invasive hemodynamics.
- Specific nomenclature and classification of PH has evolved to standardize terminology. Current classification systems are well outlined in clinical practice guidelines.[1]
- Hemodynamically, PH is divided into two categories, pre- and postcapillary.
- In precapillary PH, increased vascular resistance of the pulmonary arterial bed causes increased pressures in prealveolar pulmonary circulation. Diagnostic criteria specify precapillary PH as a mean PA pressure ≥25 mm Hg with a PCWP ≤15 mm Hg.
- In postcapillary PH, elevated PA pressures result from congestion within the pulmonary circulation in the setting of abnormally elevated pulmonary venous pressures. Diagnostically, a right heart catheterization would reveal PA ≥25 mm Hg and PCWP ≥15 mm Hg.
- Underlying and associated causes of PH are numerous and are incorporated into the updated classification system. Among these causes are autoimmune disorders, rheumatic disorders, recurrent pulmonary emboli, and chronic lung disease for precapillary causes as well as left heart failure for postcapillary.

ECHOCARDIOGRAPHY[3-6]

Echocardiography can be used as both a screening tool for the diagnosis of PH as well as a monitoring tool in ongoing evaluation and management. However, the diagnosis must be confirmed by invasive hemodynamics prior to instituting specific therapy for PH.

- PA peak systolic pressures (PASP) can be estimated from Doppler interrogation of the tricuspid valve using the modified Bernoulli equation (Figure 11-2-2).
  - Maximum regurgitant velocity across the tricuspid valve, v, can estimate the right ventricular systolic pressure (RVSP) by the formula RVSP = $4v^2$+RAP (where RAP is the estimated right atrial pressure).
  - Assuming no significant gradient across the pulmonary valve, the RVSP is equal to the PASP.
- Recall that the diagnostic criteria for PH is a mean PA pressure ≥25 mm Hg. Echocardiography provides an estimate of peak PA pressures; however, correlation between mean and peak pressures is not completely understood. Previous reports have used a range of PASP as a screening cutoff for PH, most of which define elevated PASP as being greater than 30 to 40 mm Hg.
- Following the diagnosis of PH, echocardiography can be useful in evaluating cardiac function, particularly right ventricular function, which correlates to overall prognosis (see discussion in Section I, Acute Pulmonary Embolism) (Figure 11-2-3). Figures 11-2-4 to 11-2-7 demonstrate additional echocardiographic findings in patients with PH and chronic right heart failure.

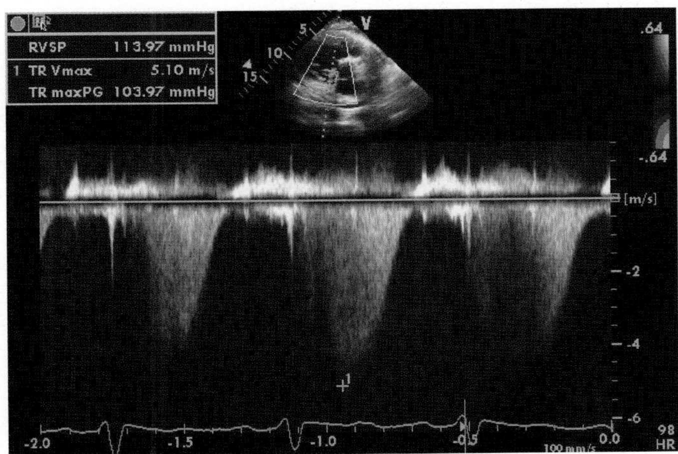

FIGURE 11-2-2 Doppler interrogation of tricuspid valve regurgitation. The maximum velocity is measured at 5.1 m/s, correlating to an estimated RVSP of 114 mm Hg using an estimated RA pressure of 10 mm Hg.

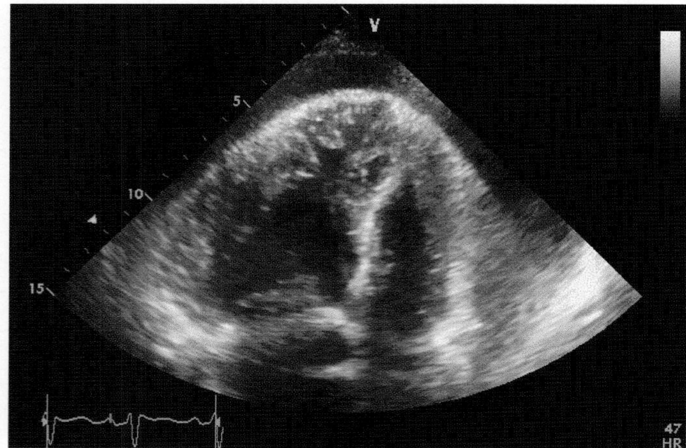

FIGURE 11-2-3 Apical 4 chamber from our patient showing RV enlargement as well as thickening of the RV signifying hypertrophy. This RV is dilated, hypertrophied, and hypokinetic ▶ (see Video 11-2-3).

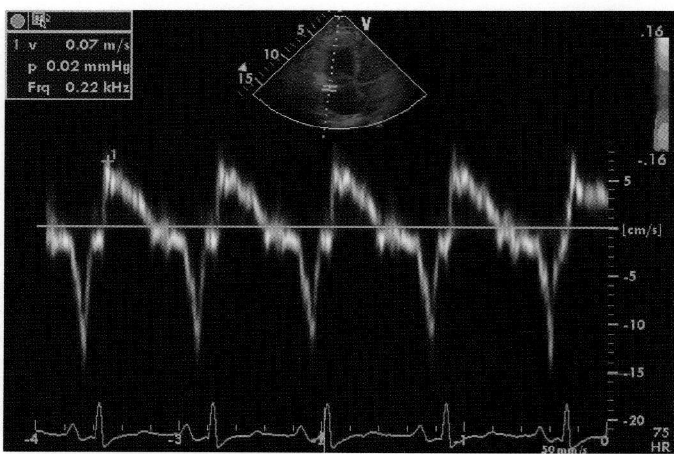

FIGURE 11-2-6 Tricuspid annular S′ from a patient with RV dysfunction due to severe COPD. In this patient, the S′ is 0.07 m/sec (7 cm/sec), which is abnormally low and consistent with RV dysfunction.

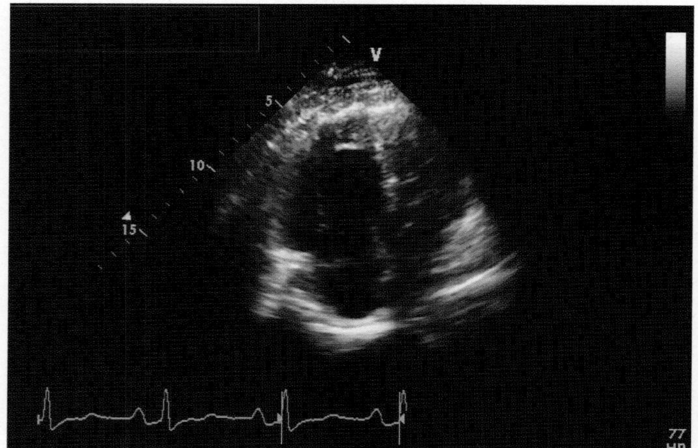

FIGURE 11-2-4 This is an apical 4 chamber view from another patient with idiopathic or primary PH. The RV is dilated and hypokinetic ▶ (see Video 11-2-4).

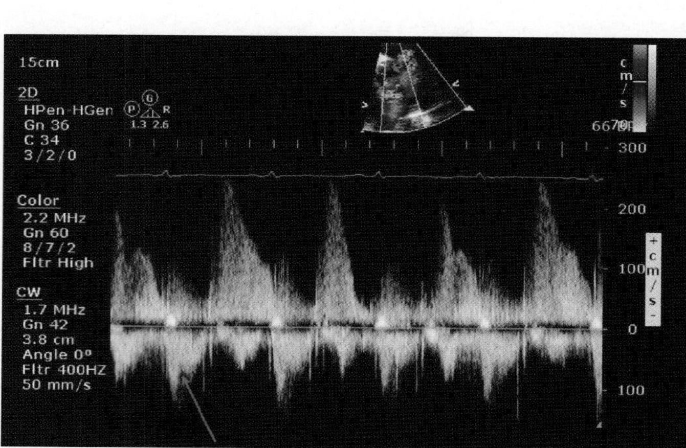

FIGURE 11-2-5 Pulsed wave Doppler of flow in the RVOT. This demonstrates a shortened acceleration time and midsystolic notching in a different patient with an estimated RVSP of 90 mm Hg. This is another Doppler-echocardiographic finding in pulmonary hypertension.

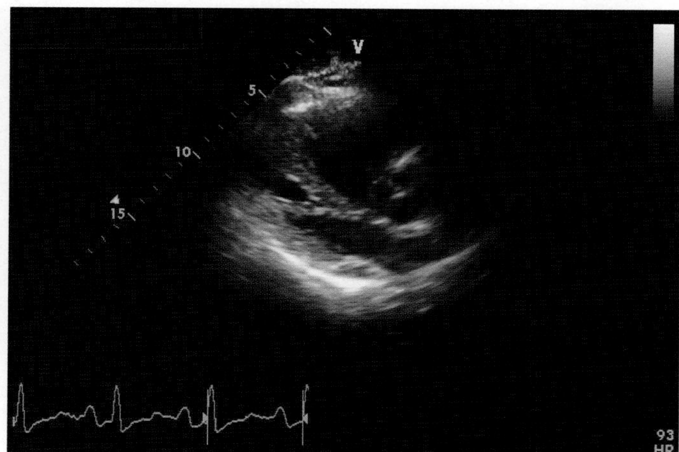

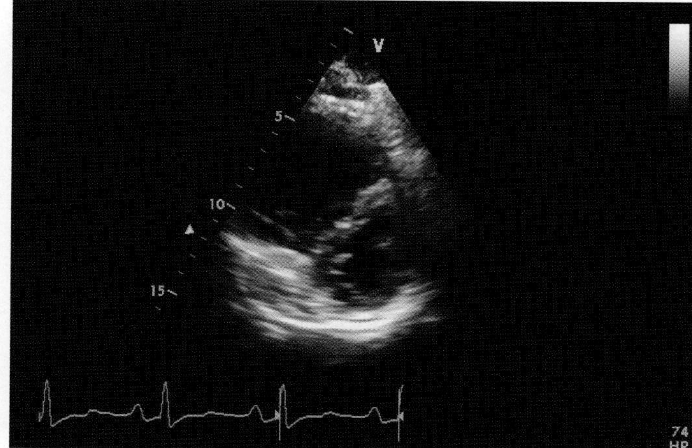

FIGURE 11-2-7 Parasternal long axis (top panel) and short axis (bottom panel) views demonstrating a dilated, hypokinetic RV and a relatively small LV cavity. In the short axis view, septal flattening in systole is noted ▶ (see Videos 11-2-7 L and R).

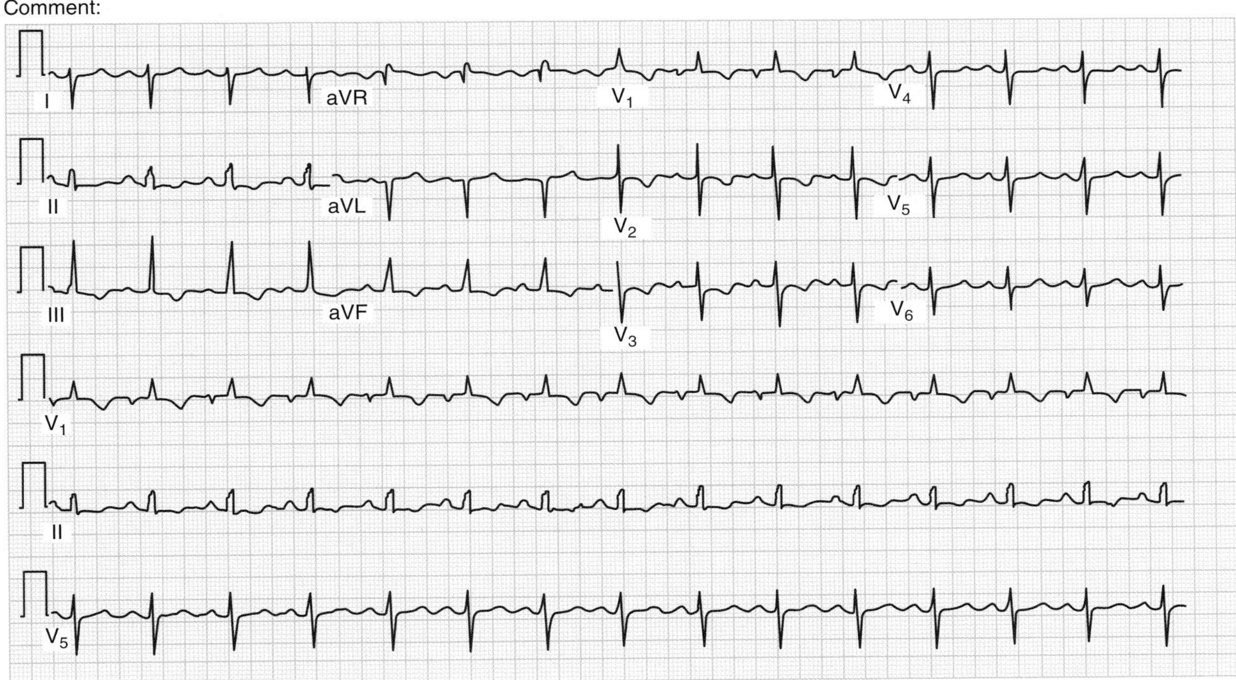

FIGURE 11-2-8 ECG showing right axis deviation, evidence of RVH, and atrial enlargement.

OTHER DIAGNOSTIC TESTS[3,7,8]

- Right heart catheterization is the gold standard for the diagnosis of PH and is required to differentiate between primary and secondary causes. Diagnostic criteria are mentioned previously.
- The electrocardiogram (ECG) in PH will often show a right axis deviation, signs of right ventricular hypertrophy, and right ventricular strain. Right atrial enlargement can also be noted on ECG (Figure 11-2-8).
- A chest x-ray (CXR) is often abnormal in patients with PH and may shows signs of RV enlargement or enlarged pulmonary arteries; however, a CXR is neither specific nor sensitive for the diagnosis of PH.
- Pulmonary function testing can help identify underlying pulmonary conditions associated with PH.
- When underlying lung pathology is suspected, high-resolution computed tomography (CT) scans can be ordered.
- If chronic thromboembolic pulmonary hypertension (CTEPH) is suspected, ventilation/perfusion scans can be ordered, which is a more sensitive test than a CT for this diagnosis.
- Diagnostic testing aimed at identifying associated causes and conditions should be conducted as clinically indicated.

TREATMENT[1,7]

Treatment options for PH are numerous and diverse. Therapeutic strategies aimed at underlying and associated conditions should be utilized as appropriate. Additional PH-specific treatment can include careful use of diuretics to help relieve venous congestion and volume overload. However, overdiuresis should be avoided as right-ventricular function is sensitive to preload, and aggressive volume depletion may result in a decline in cardiac output. Therapies targeting pathophysiological changes that occur in the pulmonary vascular bed can include the use of calcium channel blockers, phosphodiesterase inhibitors, endothelian antagonists, or prostacyclins. Oral anticoagulation with vitamin K antagonists is often a part of therapy. Typically, the diagnosis of PH warrants a referral to a specialist to help guide and monitor therapy.

FOLLOW-UP

The patient underwent an extensive work-up. No other etiology of her pulmonary hypertension was found, and she was felt to have pulmonary hypertension related to her underlying connective tissue disease. She had a minimal response to advanced therapies for her pulmonary hypertension and unfortunately died 3 months later from chronic right heart failure and her pulmonary hypertension.

VIDEO LEGENDS

1. Video 11-2-1: Parasternal long axis view. Note the enlarged right ventricle at the top of the image as well as the presence of a large pericardial effusion. The LV is relatively small and under-filled
2. Video 11-2-3: Apical four chamber from our patient showing RV enlargement as well as thickening of the RV signifying hypertrophy. This RV is dilated, hypertrophied and hypokinetic.
3. Video 11-2-4: This is an apical 4 chamber view from another patient with idiopathic or primary PH. The RV is dilated and hypokinetic.
4. Video 11-2-7 L: Parasternal long axis demonstrating a dilated, hypokinetic RV and a relatively small LV cavity.
5. Video 11-2-7 R: Parasternal short axis demonstrating a dilated, hypokinetic RV and a relatively small LV cavity. Septal flattening in systole is noted.

REFERENCES

1. Galie N, Hoeper MM, Humbert M, et al. Guidelines for the diagnosis and treatment of pulmonary hypertension: The Task Force for the Diagnosis and Treatment of Pulmonary Hypertension of the European Society of Cardiology (ESC) and the European Respiratory Society (ERS), endorsed by the International Society of Heart and Lung Transplantation (ISHLT). *Eur Heart J.* 2009;30:2493-2537.
2. Runo JR, Loyd JE. Primary pulmonary hypertension. *Lancet.* 2003;361:1533-1544.
3. Janda S, Shahidi N, Gin K, Swiston J. Diagnostic accuracy of echocardiography for pulmonary hypertension: a systematic review and meta-analysis. *Heart.* 2011;97:612-622.
4. Hatle L, Angelsen BA, Tromsdal A. Non-invasive estimation of pulmonary artery systolic pressure with Doppler ultrasound. *Br Heart J.* 1981;45:157-165.
5. Yock PG, Popp RL. Noninvasive estimation of right ventricular systolic pressure by Doppler ultrasound in patients with tricuspid regurgitation. *Circulation.* 1984;70:657-662.
6. Sciomer S, Magri D, Badagliacca R. Non-invasive assessment of pulmonary hypertension: Doppler-echocardiography. *Pulm Pharmacol Ther.* 2007;20:135-140.
7. Stringham R, Shah NR. Pulmonary arterial hypertension: an update on diagnosis and treatment. *Am Fam Physician.* 2010;82:370-377.
8. Tunariu N, Gibbs SJ, Win Z, et al. Ventilation-perfusion scintigraphy is more sensitive than multidetector CTPA in detecting chronic thromboembolic pulmonary disease as a treatable cause of pulmonary hypertension. *J Nucl Med.* 2007;48:680-684.

12 ECHOCARDIOGRAPHY IN SYSTEMIC DISEASE

Vincent Brinkman, MD, Kavita Sharma, MD, and
Jason Evanchan, DO

Many systemic diseases can involve the heart and result in cardiac dysfunction. In addition, treatment of some diseases, such as cancer, may adversely affect cardiac structure and function. Several of these conditions have been discussed in other sections of this atlas (eg, pericardial disease from malignancy, chemotherapy-related cardiomyopathy, cardiomyopathy related to muscular dystrophy, systemic amyloidosis).

In this chapter, Drs. Brinkman, Sharma, and Evanchan briefly present a few cases to highlight the role of echocardiography in other selected systemic disease states.

SECTION 1

Hypertensive Heart Disease

Vincent Brinkman, MD

CLINICAL CASE PRESENTATION

A 50-year-old man presented to the Ohio State University Medical Center for evaluation of elevated blood pressures noted at a routine eye appointment. He had been told of high blood pressures for at least the last 5 years, but he had not been established with a primary physician at the time and did not seek out medical attention. He recently became established with a primary physician and was noted to have a blood pressure greater than 170/110 mm Hg on repeat evaluations. He was on no medications at the time and otherwise denied any symptoms. His exam was normal other than the elevated blood pressure and a faint S_4 gallop heard on exam. His creatinine was mildly elevated (1.4 mg/dL), and an ECG showed borderline LVH by voltage criteria. He was reluctant to start any medications and was referred for an echocardiogram. This revealed moderate concentric hypertrophy of the left ventricle (Figures 12-1-1 and 12-1-2), a mildly dilated aortic root (Figure 12-1-3), left atrial enlargement (Figure 12-1-4), and grade II diastolic dysfunction (Figures 12-1-5 and 12-1-6). He agreed to start medical therapy and subsequent blood pressures have been normal at clinical visits.

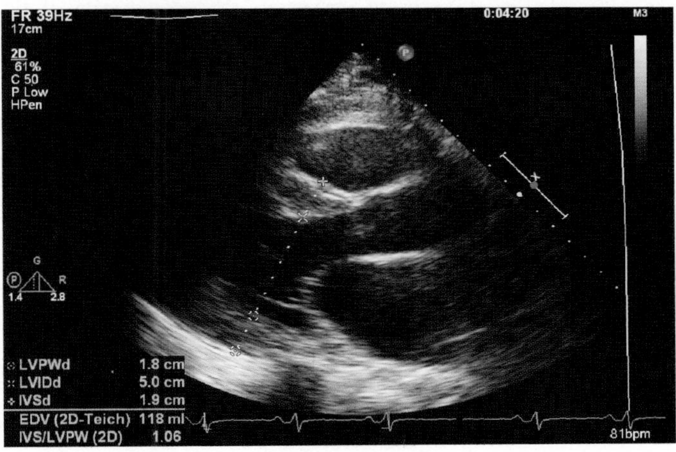

FIGURE 12-1-1 Parasternal long axis view of the left ventricle showing concentric hypertrophy of the left ventricle. The septal thickness measures 1.9 cm with a posterior wall thickness of 1.8 cm ▶ (see Video 12-1-1).

CLINICAL FEATURES

Hypertension, for the most part, is an asymptomatic disease in the early stages and is easily detected with routine screening. With prolonged hypertension, however, patients may show signs of end organ damage including renal failure, retinopathy, strokes, vascular disease, or progressive heart failure.

- In hypertensive heart disease, the early stages show signs of left ventricular hypertrophy including an S_4 gallop due to the noncompliant nature of the left ventricle (LV).
- As the disease progresses, signs of heart failure and volume overload can be present, including peripheral edema or pulmonary congestion.
- In some patients, the LV further remodels and dilates producing signs of systolic heart failure with an S_3 gallop and a laterally displaced apical impulse.
- Other signs of end-organ damage should be sought as well, including hypertensive retinopathy, neurologic defects, renal artery bruits, or an abdominal aneurysm.

EPIDEMIOLOGY

Hypertension is a common clinical entity and may be present in up to 28% of the population of North America and 44% in Europe.[1] Left ventricular hypertrophy (LVH) is also often seen during routine clinical echocardiograms (15%). Furthermore, an increase in blood pressure is associated with an increased prevalence of LVH—up to 60%

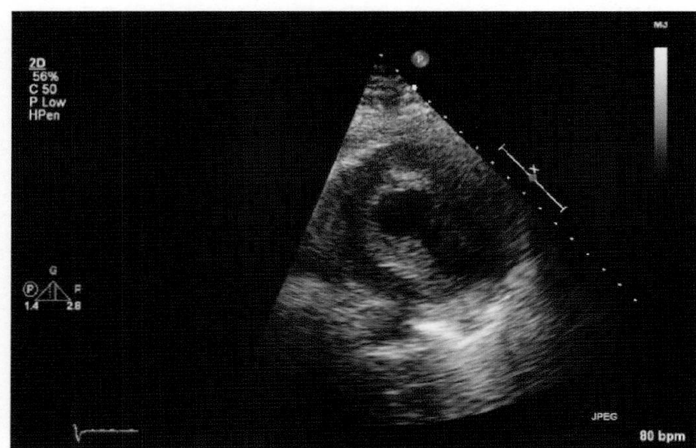

FIGURE 12-1-2 Parasternal short axis view demonstrating concentric left ventricular hypertrophy ▶ (see Video 12-1-2).

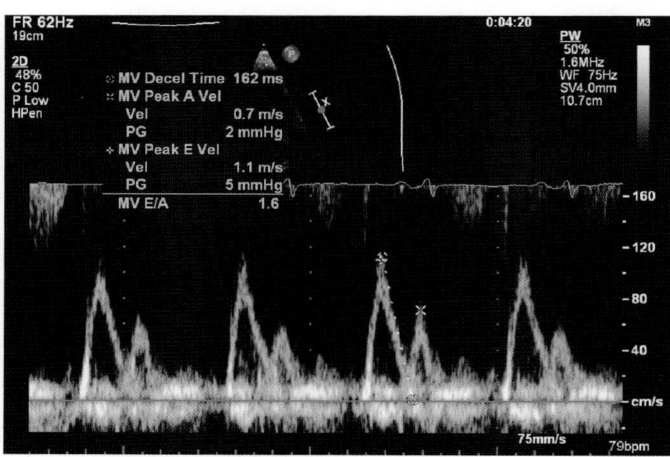

FIGURE 12-1-5 Mitral inflow velocity with a normal E/A ratio; however, the deceleration time is somewhat fast. This, in combination with the TDI (Figure 12-1-6) suggests moderate diastolic dysfunction.

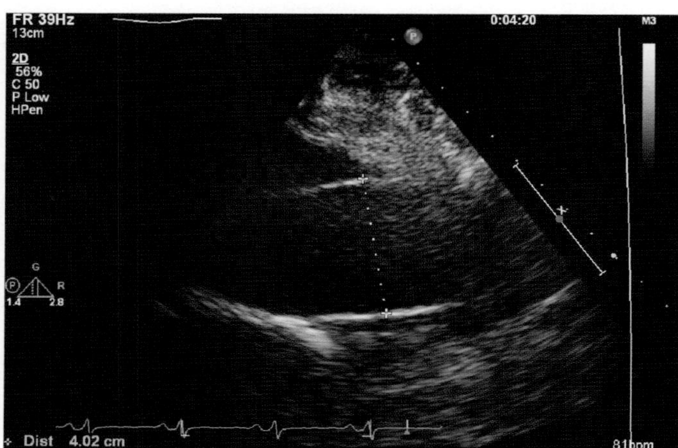

FIGURE 12-1-3 Parasternal view of the ascending aorta, which is mildly dilated (4.0 cm).

in patients with severe hypertension.[2] Hypertension is an independent risk factor for coronary disease, heart failure, renal failure, and stroke. LVH as well, is associated with an increase in cardiovascular morbidity including sudden death, heart failure, and mortality with a relative risk of 2.08 compared to patients with normal LV mass.[3]

PATHOPHYSIOLOGY AND ETIOLOGY

- LVH is at first an adaptive response to the load placed on the heart, in particular, increased afterload. Wall thickness and hypertrophy serve to decrease the overall LV wall stress and myocardial oxygen demand.
- Multiple hemodynamic, genetic, and neurohormonal factors likely contribute to the overall process of myocyte hypertrophy.
- Over time, however, this increase in left ventricular mass leads to diastolic dysfunction and increasing myocardial fibrosis.[4]
- In some patients, there is further remodeling, including cell apoptosis, eccentric remodeling, and eventually, systolic heart failure.
- In addition to the effects on the myocardium, hypertension affects endothelial function and vascular stiffness.

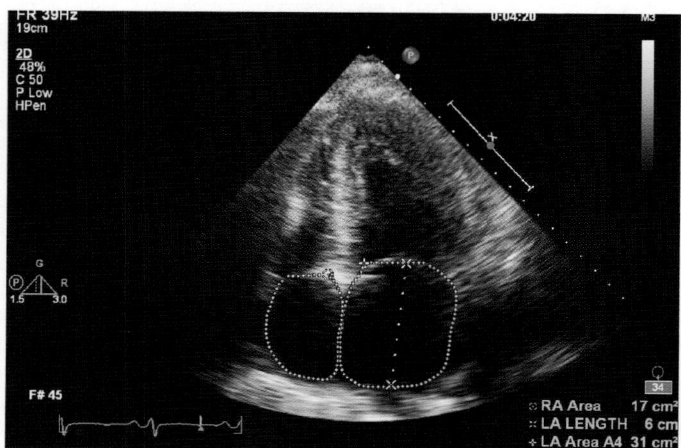

FIGURE 12-1-4 Apical 4 chamber view showing left atrial enlargement.

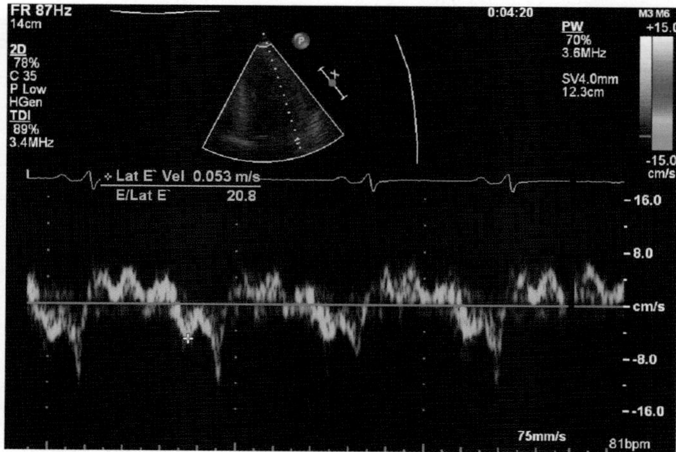

FIGURE 12-1-6 Tissue Doppler of the lateral mitral annulus with an elevated E/e' ratio, suggesting moderate diastolic dysfunction.

- Aortic dilation with or without aortic valve insufficiency can be a common consequence of hypertension.
- Hypertension can increase the risk of coronary vascular disease and myocardial ischemia with both macrovascular and microvascular consequences.
- All of these effects serve to increase the risk of overall cardiac morbidity and mortality[3] making this an important diagnosis to make at an early stage.

ECHOCARDIOGRAPHY

One of the earliest and most recognizable consequences of hypertensive heart disease is the increase in left ventricular mass.

- The American Society of Echocardiography (ASE) recommends calculating the LV mass based on the 2-D directed measurement of the septal wall thickness (SWTd), posterior wall thickness (PWTd), and the end diastolic cavity dimension (LVIDd).[5] The left ventricular cavity area is subtracted from the overall LV area using the equation:

$$\text{LV mass} = 0.8 \times \{1.04[(\text{LVIDd} + \text{PWTd} + \text{SWTd})^3 - (\text{LVIDd})^3]\} + 0.6\text{g}$$

- A left ventricular mass index (gm/M^2) greater than 95 in women and 115 in men suggests LV hypertrophy.
- The relative wall thickness (RWT), defined as $(2 \times \text{PWTd})/\text{LVIDd}$ helps to further classify the LV hypertrophy as either eccentric ($RWT<0.42$) or concentric ($RWT>0.42$). These two-dimensional (2-D) methods have the disadvantage of assuming a uniform shape to the heart. In the cases of uniform remodeling, this is typically accurate. However, with deformities in LV geometry, this assumption becomes less accurate.
- Some laboratories have begun to use three-dimensional echocardiographic techniques, which have been shown to correlate well with other techniques including cardiac MRI.

Diastolic dysfunction is another effect of ventricular hypertrophy and remodeling and can be evaluated by the combination of mitral inflow velocities, tissue Doppler, and secondary effects including left atrial enlargement, pulmonary vein flow patterns, and elevated right ventricular pressures.

- The ratio of the early to late mitral inflow velocities (E/A ratio) may be the first sign of hypertensive heart disease even in the absence of LVH.
- The ratio of the early mitral inflow velocity (E) to the early mitral annulus velocity (e') can be used to estimate LV filling pressures.[6]
- Newer techniques to evaluate strain and strain rate of the myocardium may in the future help better define this process as well.

In addition to abnormalities of the left ventricle, patients with hypertensive heart disease can show vascular changes including aortic aneurysms or dilation of the proximal ascending aorta. This may result in aortic insufficiency due to issues with valve coaptation.

Valve thickening or mitral annular calcification can also be seen, especially in patients with concomitant renal disease.

OTHER DIAGNOSTIC TESTING AND PROCEDURES

Secondary causes of hypertension should be sought in selected patients and may include renal disease (both as a cause and a consequence of hypertension), endocrine disorders, coarctation of the aorta, and drugs.

- Laboratory evaluations should be guided by the history and physical exam as well as clinical suspicion.
- An ECG is vital in screening patients with hypertension and can detect chamber enlargement and conduction system disease such as a left bundle branch block or atrial fibrillation.
- The chest x-ray can be helpful in patients presenting with shortness of breath and signs of pulmonary edema.
- If an echocardiogram is insufficient to estimate left ventricular function or dimensions, a cardiac MRI can accurately measure LV function and mass as well as provide evidence of myocardial fibrosis.
- With the prevalence of coronary disease in patients with long-standing hypertension, stress testing can also be used if the clinical scenario dictates.

DIFFERENTIAL DIAGNOSIS

Left ventricular hypertrophy due to hypertensive heart disease, especially in extreme cases, can be difficult to distinguish from other causes of LV hypertrophy including hypertrophic cardiomyopathy, Fabry disease, and athlete's heart. With progressive remodeling, thinning of the ventricle and chamber enlargement, the end stage of hypertensive heart disease can be difficult to distinguish from other cause of dilated cardiomyopathies.

DIAGNOSIS

- The diagnosis of hypertensive heart disease with echocardiography is made by demonstrating changes in the left ventricle, including increased LV mass or diastolic dysfunction with or without ECG changes consistent with LVH.
- Other potential causes of left ventricular hypertrophy should be ruled out as well before a presumptive diagnosis is made in patients with hypertension.
- Several symptoms can also be attributed to hypertensive heart disease, including exertional chest pain or shortness of breath, and are related to microvascular disease or increased myocardial oxygen demand. These should be distinguished from other causes, especially epicardial coronary disease, as these conditions share many of the same risk factors.

MANAGEMENT

The main treatment for hypertensive heart disease is aggressive lowering of the systemic blood pressure. The Joint National Committee (JNC 7) guidelines provide a framework for clinical control of blood pressure and selection of initial blood pressure agents.[7] Treating blood pressure in patients with left ventricular hypertrophy is particularly important as a reduction in left ventricular mass has been associated with reduction of cardiac events.[8] Selected medications, particularly ACE inhibitors, angiotensin receptor blockers, and calcium channel blockers—may have a faster effect on the rate at which left ventricular mass decreases; however, the clinical implications of this are not well established.[9] Patients should be followed to ensure that their resting blood pressures are within standard targets

(<130/80) as well as any age-appropriate screening or signs of other end organ damage. Echocardiograms can be performed as symptoms dictate. If heart failure develops, these patients should be treated with standard heart failure regimens.

VIDEO LEGENDS

1. Video 12-1-1: Parasternal long axis view showing concentric hypertrophy of the left ventricle. The septal thickness measures 1.9 cm with a posterior wall thickness of 1.8 cm.
2. Video 12-1-2: Parasternal short axis view demonstrating concentric left ventricular hypertrophy.

REFERENCES

1. Wolf-Maier K, Cooper RS, Banegas JR, et al. Hypertension prevalence and blood pressure levels in 6 European countries, Canada, and the United States. *JAMA.* 2003;289(18):2363-2369.
2. Levy D, Anderson KM, Savage DD, et al. Echocardiographically detected left ventricular hypertrophy: prevalence and risk factors. The Framingham Heart Study. *Ann Intern Med.* 1988;108(1):7-13.
3. Verdecchia P, Carini G, Circo A, et al. Left ventricular mass and cardiovascular morbidity in essential hypertension: the MAVI study. *J Am Coll Cardiol.* 2001;38(7):1829-1835.
4. Raman SV. The hypertensive heart. An integrated understanding informed by imaging. *J Am Coll Cardiol.* 2010;55(2):91-96.
5. Lang RM, Bierig M, Devereux RB, et al. Recommendations for chamber quantification. *Eur J Echocardiogr.* 2006;7:79-108.
6. Nagueh SF, Appelton CP, Gillebert TC, et al. Recommendations for the evaluation of left ventricular diastolic function by echocardiography. *Eur J Echocardiogr.* 2009;10:165-193.
7. Chobanian AV, Bakris GL, Black HR, et al. Seventh Report of the Joint National Committee on Prevention, Detection, Evaluation, and Treatment of High Blood Pressure. *Hypertension.* 2003;42(6):1206-1252.
8. Pierdomenico SD, Cuccurullo F. Risk reduction after regression of echocardiographic left ventricular hypertrophy in hypertension: a meta-analysis. *Am J Hypertens.* 2010;23(8):876-881.
9. Klingbeil AU, Schneider M, Martus P, Messerli FH, Schmieder RE. A meta-analysis of the effects of treatment on left ventricular mass in essential hypertension. *Am J Med.* 2003;115(1):41-46.

SECTION 2

Echocardiography In Renal Failure

Vincent Brinkman, MD

CLINICAL CASE PRESENTATION

A 45-year-old woman presented to the hospital with increasing shortness of breath. She had a longstanding history of diabetes and hypertension, which had resulted in renal failure, and had undergone a renal transplant 3 years prior to admission. Her renal function had gradually declined over the course of the last year, and over the last several weeks, she had been having dyspnea, fatigue, and worsening lower extremity edema. On admission, she was breathing comfortably while in bed. She was hypertensive with a blood pressure of 170/100 mm Hg. Her cardiac exam revealed a systolic ejection murmur with brisk carotid upstrokes. Jugular venous distension was noted to the angle of the jaw at 45°. She had rales in the bases of her lungs, and 2+ edema was noted in the lower extremities bilaterally. Her BUN was 90 mg/dL, and her creatinine was 4.80 mg/dL (her baseline had been approximately 2.0). Her chest x-ray showed mild pulmonary edema. Her echocardiogram showed mild left ventricular hypertrophy (LVH) (Figures 12-2-1 to 12-2-3) with calcification of the aortic and mitral leaflets without significant stenosis (Figures 12-2-4 and 12-2-5). She had mitral annular calcification as well as an enlarged left atrium (Figure 12-2-6). A small- to moderate-sized pericardial effusion was also noted without any signs of tamponade (there was no significant mitral inflow variation, no evidence of RA or RV collapse and 50% collapse of the IVC with respiration) (Figures 12-2-7 to Figure 12-2-9). She was initiated on dialysis with resolution of her symptoms and plans were made for permanent dialysis.

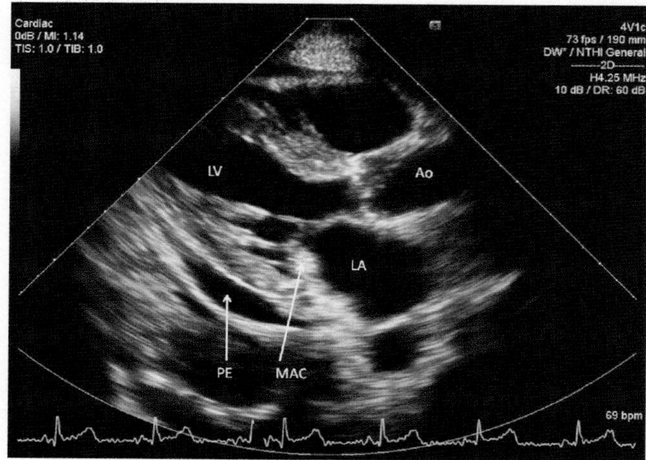

FIGURE 12-2-1 Parasternal long axis view of the heart. Note the mitral annular calcification (MAC) along with a small pericardial effusion (PE) ► (see Video 12-2-1).

CLINICAL FEATURES

- Renal disease can affect the heart in multiple ways, from valvular heart disease to myocardial infarction, heart failure, and

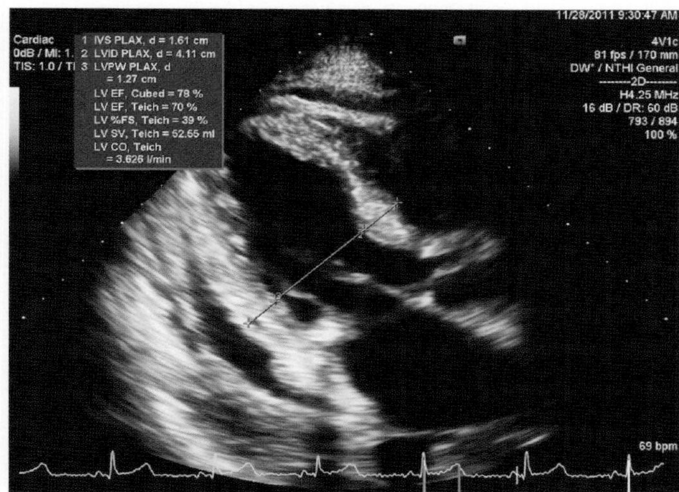

FIGURE 12-2-2 Concentric hypertrophy of the left ventricle is noted with normal LV chamber size. The septum measures 1.6 cm, and the posterior wall measures 1.3 cm.

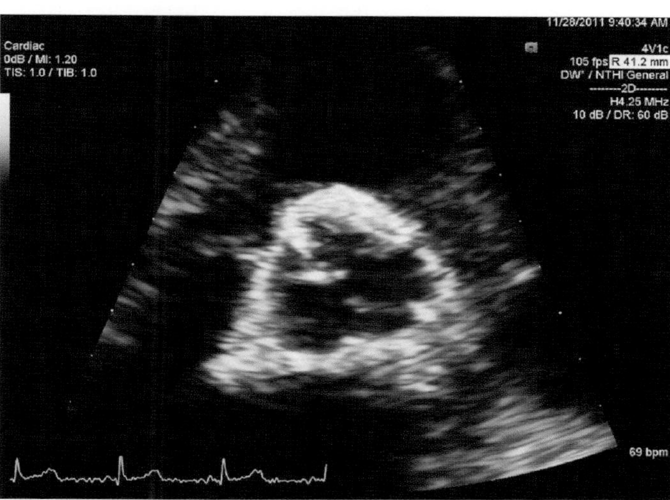

FIGURE 12-2-5 Parasternal short axis view of the aortic valve ▶ (see Video 12-2-5).

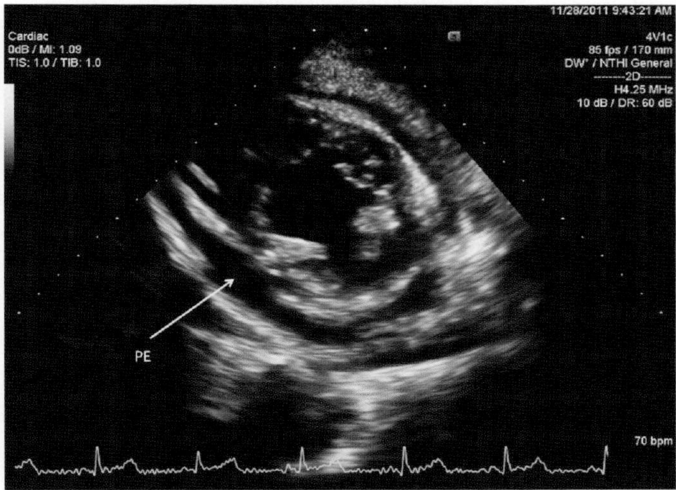

FIGURE 12-2-3 Parasternal short axis view showing LVH and a circumferential pericardial effusion (PE) ▶ (see Video 12-2-3).

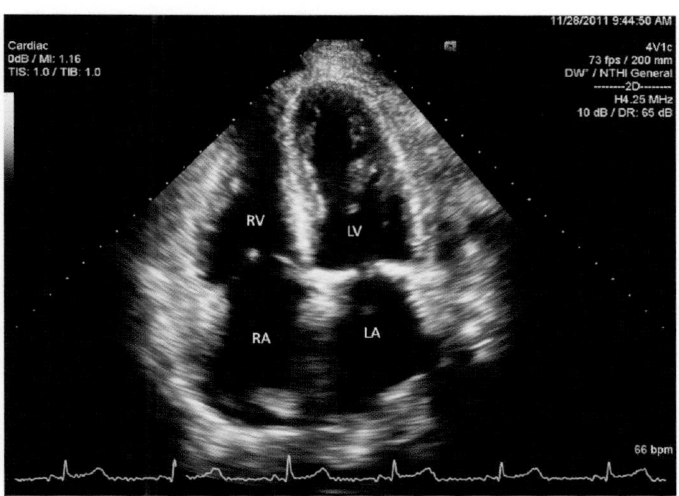

FIGURE 12-2-6 Apical 4 chamber view showing biatrial (LA and RA) enlargement ▶ (see Video 12-2-6).

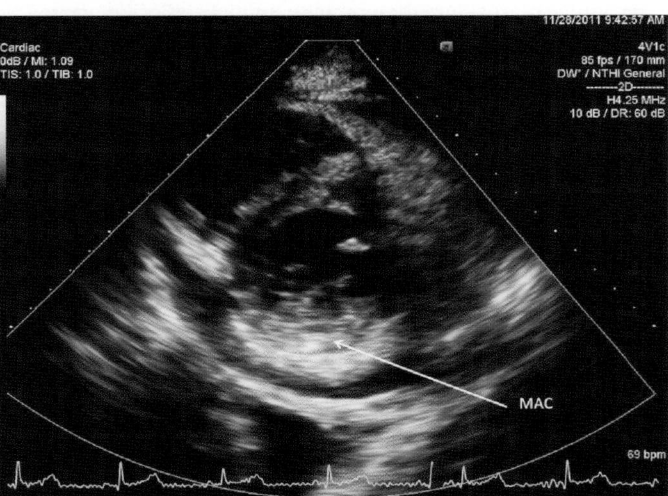

FIGURE 12-2-4 Parasternal short axis view of the mitral valve showing mitral annular calcification (MAC) ▶ (see Video 12-2-4).

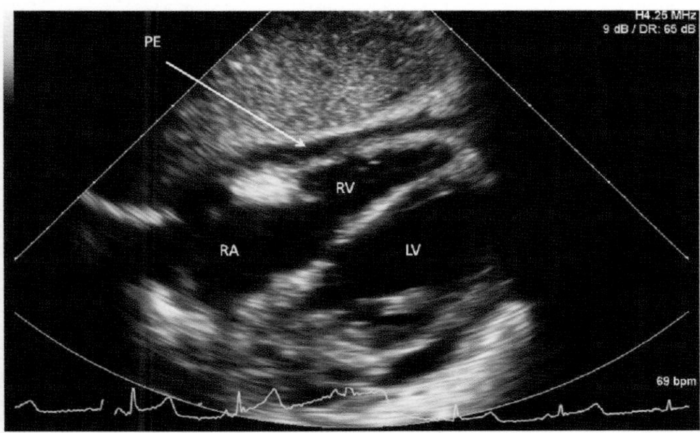

FIGURE 12-2-7 Subcostal 4 chamber view with a circumferential pericardial effusion (PE) and no evidence of RV or RA collapse ▶ (see Video 12-2-7).

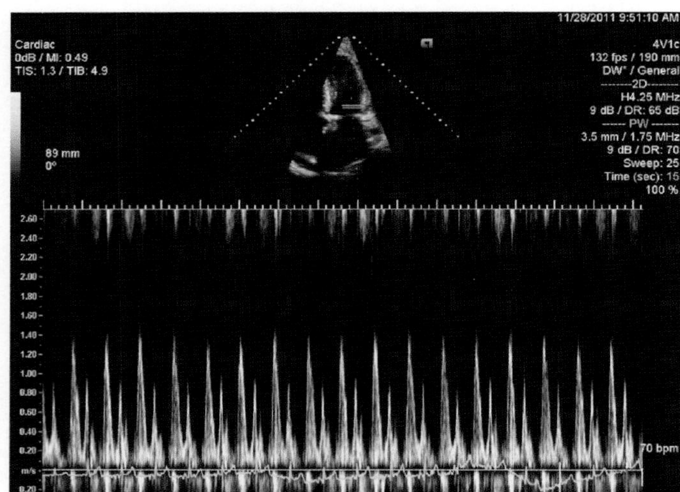

FIGURE 12-2-8 Mitral valve inflow showing no significant variation with respiration.

pericardial tamponade. There is significant overlap of risk factors for these conditions, and multiple issues can present in the same patient. Heart failure is one common presentation.

- Either dilated cardiomyopathies with low output heart failure or significant diastolic heart failure can be present with the latter often being difficult to distinguish from worsening renal function with volume retention.
- Ischemic heart disease is also common in this population with myocardial infarction and ischemic cardiomyopathy being some of the most frequent causes of morbidity and mortality in these patients.
- Valvular heart disease typically presents with increasing calcification of the valves leading to eventual valvular stenosis in some patients.
- Endocarditis is a particular concern in dialysis patients or patients with chronic indwelling catheters and can lead to further valve dysfunction.
- Finally, pericardial disease can present with a uremic pericarditis, including a friction rub or pericardial effusion of varying degrees.

EPIDEMIOLOGY

- Cardiac disease accounts for significant morbidity and mortality in patients with renal failure. In fact, renal patients are 30 times more likely to die from cardiovascular disease than the general population.[1]
- Coronary vascular disease is particularly common, but heart failure, valvular disease, and arrhythmias are also more common in this population, not to mention acute illnesses such as pericarditis and endocarditis. Valvular thickening and calcification can occur in up to 60% of patients on chronic dialysis with increased risk of valvular stenosis as well.[2]
- Given this high prevalence, aggressive risk factor modification and screening are important along with a heightened suspicion of cardiac disease.

PATHOPHYSIOLOGY AND ETIOLOGY

- Part of the pathophysiology of cardiac disease in this population certainly comes from the overlap of traditional cardiovascular disease risks factors and those for the development of renal disease. Chief among these are vascular disease, diabetes, and hypertension.[3]
- The accelerated nature of cardiovascular disease also accounts for an increased prevalence of heart failure and ischemic cardiomyopathy.
- These risk factors alone, however, do not account for all of the increased risk of cardiac diseases seen in this population.
  - Several potential etiologies have been proposed including abnormalities in calcium metabolism, inflammation, and uremia.
  - Increases in calcium levels and secondary hyperparathyroidism have been associated with early calcification of the mitral and aortic valves.[2]
  - Finally, the presence of indwelling catheters and vascular devices increase the risk of infections and endocarditis.

ECHOCARDIOGRAPHY

- Aside from diagnosing potential causes of renal failure (amyloidosis or systolic heart failure for example), multiple echocardiogram findings have been associated with patients on dialysis or with chronic kidney disease.

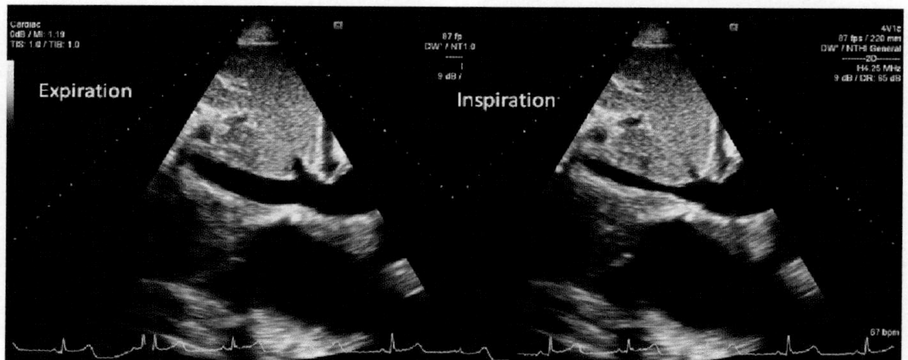

FIGURE 12-2-9 Subcostal view of the inferior vena cava during expiration (L) and inspiration (R). Overall, there is IVC dilation, but with >50% variation during inspiration ► (see Video 12-2-9).

- Abnormalities of left ventricular (LV) dimensions and function are seen with increasing frequency. In one study, 74% of patients starting dialysis had left ventricular hypertrophy with 35% also having left ventricular dilation and 15% with systolic dysfunction.[4] This results in increased prevalence of both systolic and diastolic abnormalities.
- As with hypertensive heart disease, attention should be given to determining LV mass and the Doppler diastolic parameters.
  - Due to the increasing frequency of mitral annular calcification (MAC), the early mitral annular velocity (e') is often not helpful for this purpose in renal failure patients.
  - Other signs of diastolic heart failure may include elevated right ventricular pressures and atrial enlargement, which are also more prevalent in renal disease.
- Valvular heart disease is also often present, with valve thickening and calcification most commonly seen.[2]
  - Mitral annular calcification is frequently present and in some cases can cause obstruction and mitral stenosis. Progressive valve thickening is also present and progresses to valvular stenosis with a greater frequency than in the general population.
  - Careful attention to the Doppler parameters of these valves—which is discussed elsewhere in this book (see Chapter 3, Echocardiographic Assessment of Valvular Heart Disease)—is important, and calcium deposits can sometimes make direct visualization of the valves difficult. Valvular regurgitation can also occur with increasing frequency either due to significant volume shifts or extreme systemic blood pressures along with endocarditis. In other cases, valvular calcification can result in decreased coaptation of the leaflets.
- Pericarditis and pericardial effusions can also be present in this population both with uremic pericarditis or simply seen with chronic hemodialysis. Tamponade is a potential complication, and echocardiography can play an important role along with the clinical assessment in diagnosing this condition (see Chapter 6, Echocardiographic Assessment of Pericardial Disease).

OTHER DIAGNOSTIC TESTING AND PROCEDURES

- The increased prevalence of cardiac disease in general with this population can lead to multiple cardiac tests.
- Stress testing plays a vital role given the increased risk of coronary artery disease with possible heart catheterization, depending on the clinical scenario.
  - In patients with renal failure not yet on dialysis, this is a particular concern given the possibility of contrast-induced nephropathy.
- Contrast-aided cardiac MRI (with gadolinium) is not recommended in patients with end stage renal disease given the risk of nephrogenic systemic sclerosis, although noncontrast MRI can be used.
- Transesophageal echocardiography is particularly useful in cases of suspected endocarditis or in patients with valvular heart disease that is inadequately evaluated with transthoracic echocardiography.

DIFFERENTIAL DIAGNOSIS

Heart failure in patients with concomitant renal failure is a difficult scenario as volume overload can be a result of either condition or, more likely, an interplay between the two. Given the prevalence and overlap of various risk factors and causes of heart disease in the renal failure population, cardiac symptoms should prompt consideration of multiple conditions in addition to the end organ effects that are seen in the heart. Hypertension, diabetes, ischemic cardiomyopathies, vascular disease, and valvular heart disease can all cause significant problems with overlapping symptoms. Systemic conditions can also contribute, including anemia and electrolyte abnormalities along with systemic causes of both cardiac and renal conditions (amyloidosis or Fabry disease, for example).

DIAGNOSIS

The diagnosis of cardiac disease in the renal failure population is typically made first with a good history and physical exam. As patients with renal failure can present with so many different cardiovascular complications, the echocardiogram plays a vital role in this population.

- All patients with renal failure should undergo an echocardiogram as part of the diagnostic workup as well as a screening tool for the various cardiac conditions associated with this disease.
- With one study, myocardial function and structure along with valvular or pericardial disease are evaluated without the risk of contrast material, which may damage the kidneys or causes further complications.
- An important point is again the prevalence of cardiac conditions in the renal failure population, which should always prompt increased suspicion.

MANAGEMENT

The management and treatment of the various end organ effects of renal failure—valvular heart disease, heart failure, ischemic heart disease, pericardial diseases—are discussed in detail elsewhere in this book and should be treated as per these guidelines. The main focus is on treating various risk factors, including control of the blood pressure, diabetes, and volume status. Optimal treatment of these conditions improves outcomes as with the general population. Renal transplant patients are a subset of this population who still carry a significantly increased risk of these cardiac conditions compared to the general population and should continually be evaluated for signs and symptoms.

VIDEO LEGENDS

1. Video 12-2-1: Parasternal long axis view. Note the mitral annular calcification (MAC) along with a small pericardial effusion (PE).
2. Video 12-2-3: Parasternal short axis view showing LVH and a circumferential pericardial effusion (PE).
3. Video 12-2-4: Parasternal short axis view of the mitral valve showing mitral annular calcification (MAC).
4. Video 12-2-5: Parasternal short axis view of the aortic valve.
5. Video 12-2-6: Apical 4 chamber view showing biatrial (LA and RA) enlargement.
6. Video 12-2-7: Subcostal 4 chamber view with a circumferential pericardial effusion (PE) and no evidence of RV or RA collapse.
7. Video 12-2-9: Subcostal view of the inferior vena cava demonstrating changes in the size of the IVC with respiration. There is IVC dilation, but with >50% variation (decrease in size) during inspiration.

REFERENCES

1. ML Schiffrin EL, Lipman, Mann, JFE. Chronic kidney disease effects on the cardiovascular system. *Circulation.* 2007;116(1);85-97.
2. Straumann E, Meyer B, Misteli M, Blumberg A, Jenzer HR. Aortic and mitral valve disease in patients with end stage renal failure on long-term haemodialysis. *Br Heart J.* 1992;67(3);236-239.
3. Sarnak MJ, Levey AS, Schoolwerth AC, et al. Kidney disease as a risk factor for development of cardiovascular disease: a statement from the American Heart Association Councils on Kidney in Cardiovascular Disease, High Blood Pressure Research, Clinical Cardiology, and Epidemiology and Prevention. *Circulation.* 2003;108(17):2154-2169.
4. Foley RN, Parfrey PS, Harnett JD, et al. Clinical and echocardiographic disease in patients starting end-stage renal disease therapy. *Kidney Int.* 1995;47(1):186-192.

SECTION 3

Carcinoid Syndrome and Tricuspid Regurgitation

Kavita Sharma, MD

CLINICAL CASE PRESENTATION

The patient is a 62-year-old man with a past medical history of hypertension. He presents with flushing, diarrhea, and dyspnea on exertion. These symptoms have been progressive over the past few months. He is on medication for hypertension. On exam, he was noted to have severe intermittent facial and arm swelling, lasting for a minute, then spontaneously resolving. His cardiovascular examination demonstrates a normal S_1 and S_2. He has a holosystolic murmur best heard at the left lower sternal border. Hepatomegaly was noted. His echocardiogram demonstrated mild global left ventricular dysfunction, moderate right ventricular dilation and dysfunction, and fixed tricuspid valve leaflets with severe tricuspid regurgitation and severe pulmonic regurgitation (Figures 12-3-1 to 12-3-5). He was found to have a very high serum chromogranin-A level and metastatic lesions on octreoscan and computed tomography. He was diagnosed

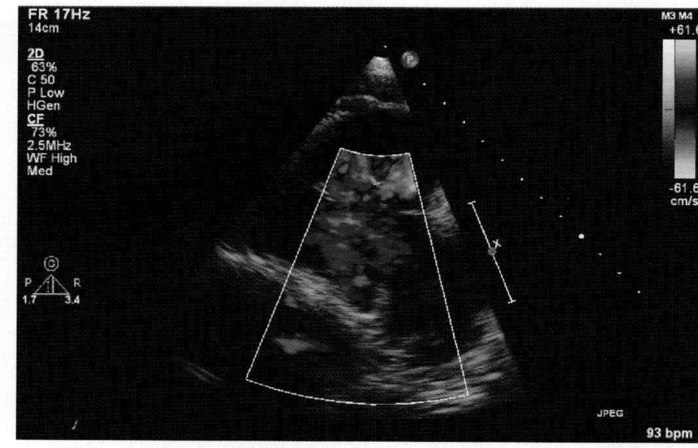

FIGURE 12-3-2 Tricuspid valve with color Doppler showing severe TR with no significant stenosis ► (see Video 12-3-2).

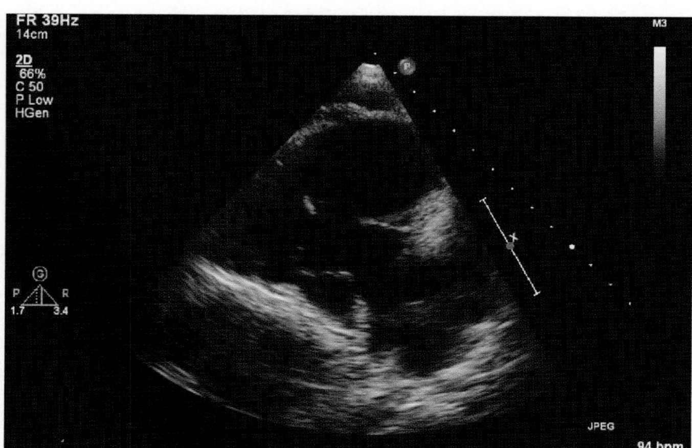

FIGURE 12-3-1 RV inflow view demonstrating thickened tricuspid valve leaflets with decreased mobility ► (see Video 12-3-1).

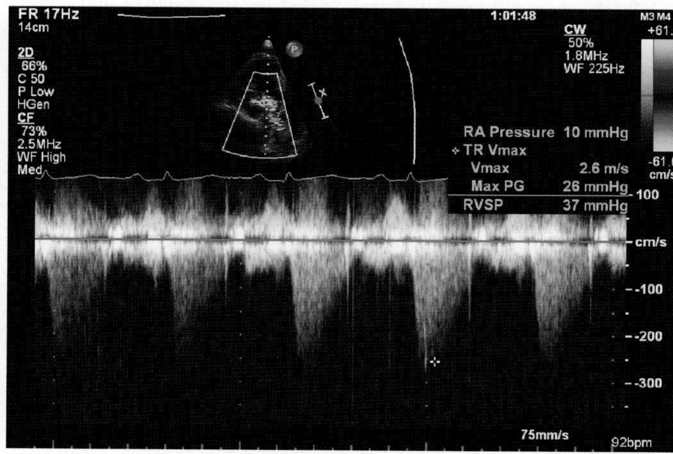

FIGURE 12-3-3 Continuous wave Doppler of the TV demonstrating severe TR.

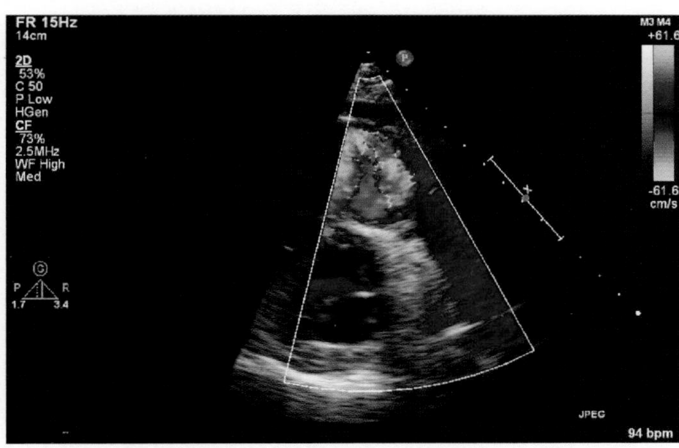

FIGURE 12-3-4 Color Doppler across the pulmonary valve demonstrating severe PR ▶ (see Video 12-3-4).

with severe metastatic carcinoid syndrome. He was begun on treatment with sandostatin. Due to his progressive triscuspid regurgitation, he was referred for consideration of tricuspid and pulmonic valve replacement.

CLINICAL FEATURES/NATURAL HISTORY

- Carcinoid tumors are most commonly found in the gastrointestinal tract and bronchus.
- The most common symptoms of carcinoid syndrome are flushing, diarrhea, hypotension, and bronchospasm.
- The symptoms are caused by the release of vasoactive substance, such as serotonin, histamine, bradykinin, and prostoglandins.
- Carcinoid heart disease eventually occurs in over 50% of patients with carcinoid syndrome.[1]

PATHOPHYSIOLOGY AND ETIOLOGY

- In carcinoid heart disease, plaque-like fibrous tissue deposits on the endocardium of valvular cusps and leaflets, as a result of an inflammatory response to circulating serotonin and its metabolites. It typically affects the right sided heart valves, most commonly the tricuspid valve, resulting in varying degrees of stenosis and regurgitation.[1]
- The fibrous deposits are uncommon on the left side of the heart due to inactivation of these vasoactive substances by the lungs.[1]
- Left sided valvular disease typically only occurs in patients with bronchial carcinoid, in patients with metastatic disease to the lungs from a primary tumor in the gastrointestinal tract, or in individuals with right-to-left shunts (eg, a patent foramen ovale or atrial septal defect with right to left shunting).
- The tricuspid leaflets become retracted and fixed, which results in reduced motion and lack of central coaptation, resulting in severe tricuspid regurgitation (TR). If the pulmonary valve is also affected, pulmonary regurgitation or stenosis can be seen.
- With progressive valve disease, patients develop peripheral edema, hepatomegaly, and ascites.

EPIDEMIOLOGY

- Carcinoid tumors are rare, arising in 1.2 to 2.1 per 100 000 people in the general population per year.[2]

ECHOCARDIOGRAPHY

- Echocardiography demonstrates thickened and retracted immobile tricuspid valve leaflets, with associated TR.[1]
- Immobile pulmonary valve leaflets with resultant pulmonic stenosis and regurgitation are also frequently present.[1]
- Severity of tricuspid regurgitation is assessed by color flow Doppler evaluation of the TR jet size, size of vena contracta, the presence of a dense spectral envelope on continuous wave Doppler, and systolic flow reversal of the hepatic vein flow.[3]

OTHER DIAGNOSTIC TESTING

- Carcinoid heart disease may be further visualized with cardiac MR and CT.[4]

MANAGEMENT

- Without treatment, survival with carcinoid syndrome is 12 to 38 months from the onset of systemic symptoms.[5]
- Somatostatin analogues are typically used to manage symptoms.
- Survival with carcinoid heart disease and advanced symptoms has a poor prognosis of only 11 months.[6]
- Cardiac surgery should be considered for symptomatic patients with carcinoid heart disease; tricuspid valve replacement is the surgery of choice.[6]
- Pulmonary valve replacement may be performed simultaneously if pulmonary valve disease is present.[7]
- The decision to proceed with surgical intervention in patients with carcinoid heart disease must factor in the patient's overall clinical situation/prognosis (noncardiac status) as well as the severity/symptomatology from the cardiac valvular heart disease.

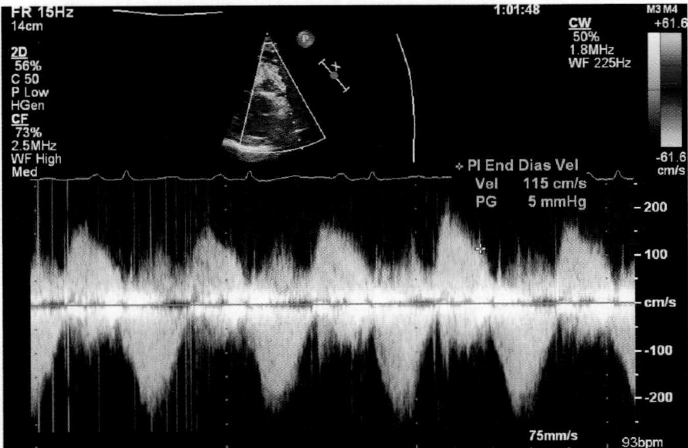

FIGURE 12-3-5 Continuous wave Doppler of the pulmonary valve showing severe PR and a small gradient.

FOLLOW-UP

- Patients with carcinoid heart disease require regular follow-up both for symptoms and serial echocardiography for severity of valve disease and right heart function.
- Patients who have undergone valve replacement require management with appropriate endocarditis prophylaxis, anticoagulation (depending on the type of valve), baseline echocardiography post-valve replacement, and follow-up echocardiography as described in Chapter 3, Echocardiograhic Assessment of Valvular Heart Disease.

VIDEO LEGENDS

1. Video 12-3-1: RV inflow view demonstrating thickened tricuspid valve leaflets with decreased mobility.
2. Video 12-3-2: Tricuspid valve with color Doppler showing severe TR with no significant stenosis.
3. Video 12-3-4: Color Doppler across the pulmonary valve demonstrating severe PR.

SUMMARY

- Carcinoid heart disease is characterized by plaque-like fibrous tissue deposition on the endocardium of valvular cusps and leaflets, most commonly on the right side of the heart.
- Echocardiography demonstrates thickened and retracted immobile tricuspid valve leaflets with associated TR.
- Survival with advanced carcinoid heart disease has a poor prognosis of only 11 months.
- Cardiac surgery should be considered for symptomatic patients with carcinoid heart disease; tricuspid valve replacement is the surgery of choice.

REFERENCES

1. Pellikka PA, Tajik AJ, Khandheria BK, et al. Carcinoid heart disease. Clinical and echocardiographic spectrum in 74 patients. *Circulation.* 1993;87:1188-1196.
2. Modlin IM, Sandor A. An analysis of 8305 cases of carcinoid tumors. *Cancer.* 1997;79:813-829.
3. Zoghbi WA, Enriquez-Sarano M, Foster E, et al. Recommendations for evaluation of the severity of native valvular regurgitation with two-dimensional and Doppler echocardiography. *J Am Soc Echocardiogr.* 2003;16:777-802.
4. Bastarrika G, Cao MG, Cano D, Barba J, de Buruaga JD. Magnetic resonance imaging diagnosis of carcinoid heart disease. *J Comput Assist Tomogr.* 2005;29:756-759.
5. Hajdu SI, Winawer SJ, Myers WP. Carcinoid tumors. A study of 204 cases. *Am J Clin Pathol.* 1974;61:521-528.
6. Connolly HM, Nishimura RA, Smith HC, Pellikka PA, Mullany CJ, Kvols LK. Outcome of cardiac surgery for carcinoid heart disease. *J Am Coll Cardiol.* 1995;25(2):410-416.
7. Voigt PG, Braun J, Teng OY, et al. Double bioprosthetic valve replacement in right-sided carcinoid heart disease. *Ann Thorac Surg.* 2005;79:2147-2149.

SECTION 4

Cardiac Sarcoidosis

Jason Evanchan, DO

CLINICAL CASE PRESENTATION

The patient is a 49-year-old man with a history of premature ventricular contractions (PVCs) who presents with palpitations and requests a second opinion. He has had frequent, symptomatic premature ventricular contractions (PVCs) for several years. He had been previously been managed on β-blockers and then a trial of sotalol without improvement. He had a negative electrophysiologic (EP) study 1 year prior to presentation. A Holter monitor revealed frequent PVCs, which comprised 18% of the total beats, with frequent nonsustained ventricular tachycardia (VT) (Figure 12-4-1).

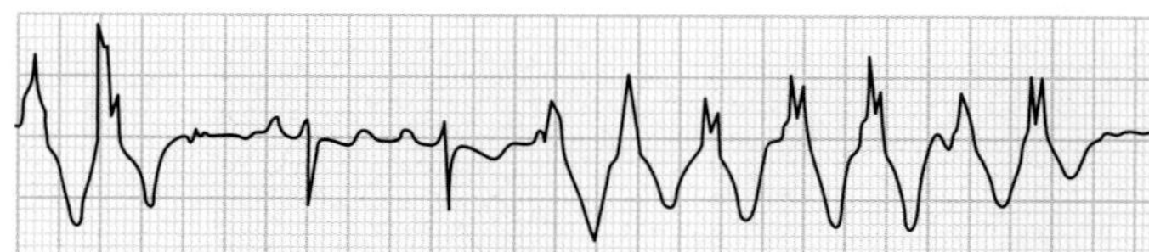

FIGURE 12-4-1 Rhythm strip from the Holter monitor showing runs of nonsustained ventricular tachycardia.

An echocardiogram was normal with an EF of 60%. A cardiac MRI, obtained to assess for structural heart disease showed late gadolinium enhancement of the basal anterior septum and inferolateral LV myocardium concerning for an infiltrating process such as cardiac sarcoidosis (Figure 12-4-2). This was further evaluated with PET-CT, which showed a focal region of intense FDG uptake in the basal anteroseptal region (Figure 12-4-3). These findings are consistent with cardiac sarcoidosis. Given the imaging findings, including the location of the uptake, biopsy was deferred given its likely low yield. He was treated empirically with prednisone and received a dual chamber ICD.

He had a dramatic improvement in his PVCs, essentially resolving at only 0.1% of his total beats with no episodes of NSVT

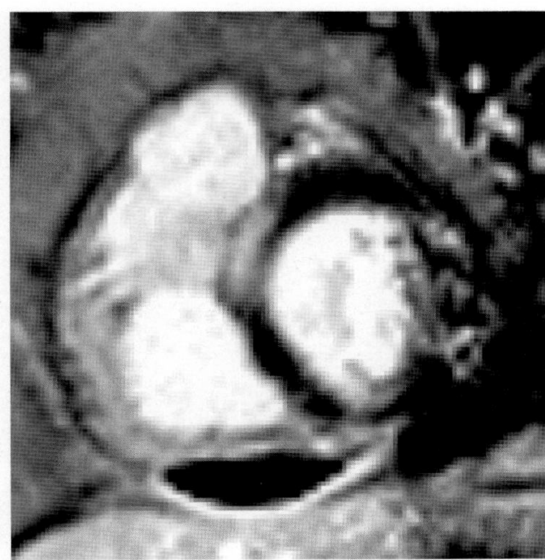

FIGURE 12-4-2 Cardiac MRI showing foci of delayed gadolinium enhancement involving the basal interventricular septum and inferolateral LV myocardium.

(Table 12-4-1). Follow-up PET-CT showed an improvement in the hypermetabolic activity in the basal anteroseptal region (Figure 12-4-4). His steroid dose was tapered, and he was started on methotrexate to minimize the long-term side effects of the steroids. He continues to be monitored via Holter monitors.

This case represents a "typical" presentation for cardiac sarcoid, including the fact that the echocardiogram was unremarkable. While it seems obvious in retrospect, it is rarely straightforward, and a high index of suspicion is needed in making the diagnosis, especially in patients without a known history of extra-cardiac sarcoidosis. PVCs and ventricular arrhythmias are common in patients with cardiac sarcoid. This, along with MRI and PET-CT findings consistent with sarcoidosis, and the fact that it improved with immunosuppressant therapy makes a diagnosis of cardiac sarcoid highly likely.

TABLE 12-4-1 Holter Monitor Results

Holter monitor	Ventricular ectopy (% of total beats)	Couplets	Runs of ventricular tachycardia (including nonsustained)
Pretreatment	18%	440	70
Posttreatment	<1%	2	0

CLINICAL FEATURES AND NATURAL HISTORY

- The clinical manifestations of cardiac sarcoidosis depend on the location and extent of granulomatous inflammation and myocardial fibrosis.
- While sarcoidosis can affect any part of the heart, there is predilection for involvement of the basal interventricular septum and the basal inferiolateral wall of the left ventricle.[1]
- Cardiac sarcoidosis (CS) can be clinically silent or can present as nonspecific constitutional symptoms, chest pain, heart failure, palpitations, syncope, or sudden cardiac death.[2]
- CS accounts for 25% of the disease-related deaths in sarcoidosis patients in the US, second only to respiratory complications.[3] Early detection and treatment is important because often the first manifestation of cardiac involvement in sarcoid patients is sudden cardiac death.
- Given the predilection for involvement of the basal interventricular septum, conduction system disease is an important and common cardiac manifestation of sarcoidosis.[4] Complete heart block has been found to be a strong predictor of sudden cardiac death.
- Congestive heart failure, as a result of systolic and/or diastolic dysfunction, is a marker for extensive myocardial involvement and portends a worse prognosis.[3]
- Ventricular arrhythmias, the most common cause of sudden cardiac death in CS patients, can range from frequent PVCs to sustained ventricular tachycardia. The mechanisms, and in turn its response to immunosuppressant therapy, depends on the stage of disease and

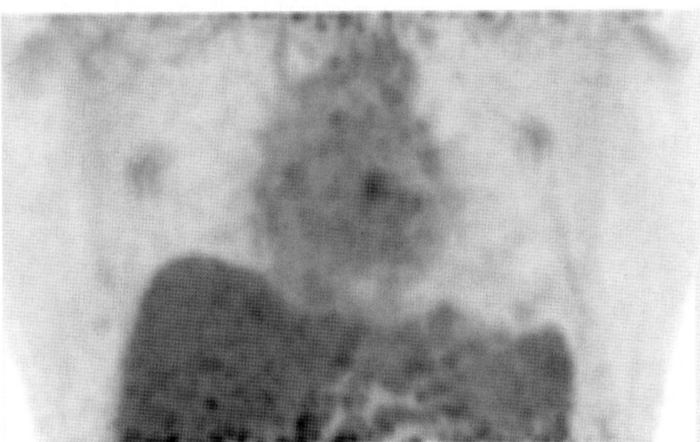

FIGURE 12-4-3 PET-CT at the time of the diagnosis demonstrating a focal region of FDG-18 uptake on the basal anteroseptal wall suspicious for cardiac sarcoidosis.

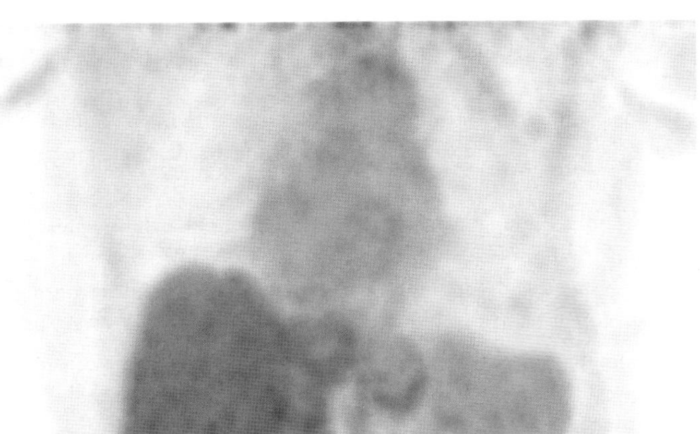

FIGURE 12-4-4 PET-CT after 3 months of prednisone therapy shows an interval improvement in the hypermetabolic activity.

extent of myocardial involvement. During the acute inflammatory phase, increased automaticity is the more likely mechanism. In the fibrotic or scar phase, reentry is the more frequent mechanism for ventricular arrhythmias.[5]

- Atrial fibrillation, and less commonly atrial tachycardia, occurs in approximately 20% of patients with CS.[1]

EPIDEMIOLOGY

- The overall prevalence of sarcoidosis is unknown, but has been estimated to be 15 per 100 000.[6]
- The incidence and prevalence varies according to race, age, and gender. According to an epidemiological study in the US, the annual incidence of sarcoidosis amongst white people and black people are 11 and 36 per 100 000 persons, respectively.[7] The peak incidence of diagnosis is between ages 20 and 49 years old. It is more common in women by a 1.3 to 1 ratio.
- The prevalence also varies widely by geographical location. In Columbus, Ohio, for example, a city that demographically closely matches the US population as a whole, a recent study found the prevalence in this region to be closer to 50 per 100 000.[8] The trend over the last 15 years shows an increase in incidence of sarcoidosis, either reflecting improved ability to diagnose the disease, an increase in a possible environmental exposure, or both.

PATHOPHYSIOLOGY AND ETIOLOGY

- Sarcoidosis is a multisystem disease characterized by the presence of noncaseating granulomas.
- Despite extensive research, the etiology remains unknown. It is thought to be caused by environmental stimuli in a genetically susceptible host.[9]
- Proposed environmental stimuli have ranged from airborne particles such as mold, pollens, and insecticides, to infectious organisms such as *Mycobacterium* and *Propionibacterium*.

ECHOCARDIOGRAPHY

- Echocardiography has an intermediate sensitivity and specificity as a screening tool in patients suspected of having cardiac sarcoidosis.[10] As was seen in the previously discussed case, the echocardiogram may be completely normal.
- Echo is a useful risk stratification tool, as CS patients with left and/or right ventricular dysfunction and pulmonary hypertension have a worse prognosis.
- Additional echo findings include abnormalities in wall thickness, regional wall motion abnormalities, pericardial effusions, ventricular aneurysms, and mitral regurgitation from papillary muscle involvement or from LV dilation (Figures 12-4-5 to 12-4-8).
- Asymmetric left ventricular hypertrophy can be present with acute myocardial granulomatous inflammation, which can markedly improve with immunosuppressant therapy. Alternatively, a thin and dysfunctional portion of the myocardium typically represents fibrosis and is unlikely to significantly recover with treatment.

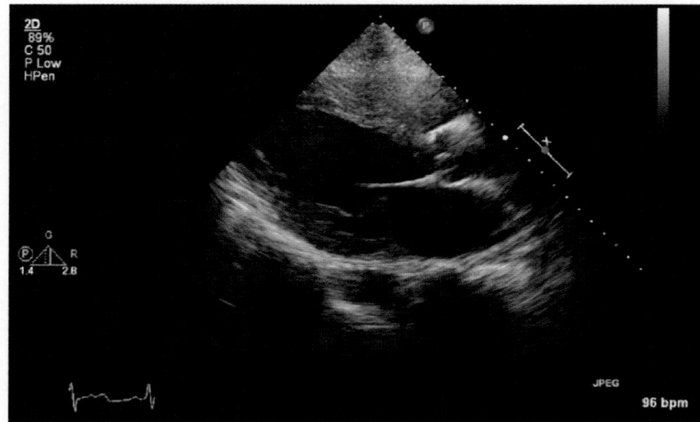

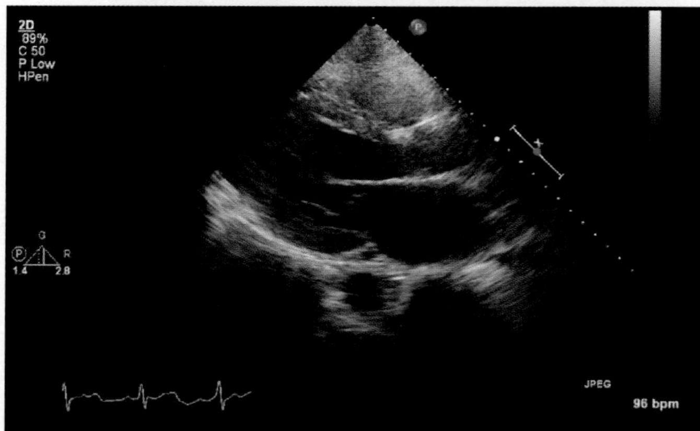

FIGURE 12-4-5 Parasternal long axis images at end-diastole (top panel) and end-systole (bottom panel) from a 41-year-old black man with a history of pulmonary sarcoidosis who presented with acute heart failure. The echo demonstrates global hypokinesis, with an EF of 30%. A cardiac MRI was consistent with cardiac involvement of his sarcoidosis.

- As opposed to MRI or PET-CT, typically cardiac involvement is more advanced when recognized on echocardiography. Myocardial strain is being evaluated as a tool for earlier detection of cardiac sarcoidosis.[11]
- Echo is not diagnostic for CS, and a confirmative test such as cardiac MRI, PET-CT, or, rarely, a myocardial biopsy is necessary.
- With the relatively inexpensive cost and wide availability of echo, however, it will continue to be heavily utilized in the care of CS patients.

OTHER DIAGNOSTIC TESTING AND PROCEDURES

- Cardiac MRI and PET-CT have become the gold standards in the diagnosis of cardiac sarcoidosis in most clinical situations.
- Cardiac MRI is very useful in establishing the diagnosis in patients with systemic sarcoidosis, and in differentiating sarcoid from other etiologies of heart failure, AV block, and ventricular arrhythmias in young to middle-aged patients. MRI is useful in determining the stage of the disease and thus can help predict its response to the treatment. An increase in signal intensity on T2-weighted imaging indicates the presence of edema. Cine imaging can determine LV function and chamber sizes, and delayed gadolinium enhancement is useful to determine prognosis and the degree of scar formation.[12]

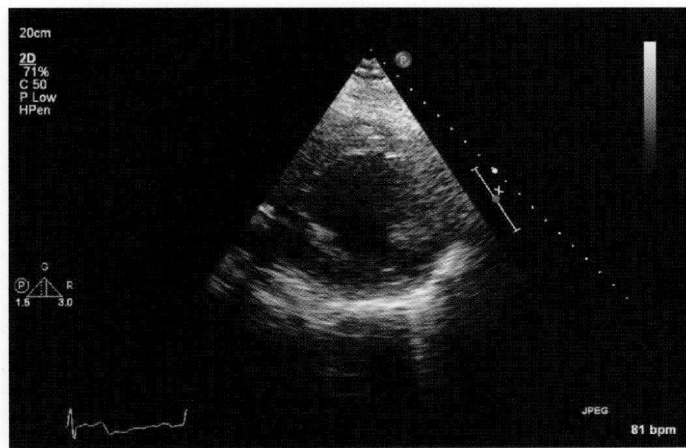

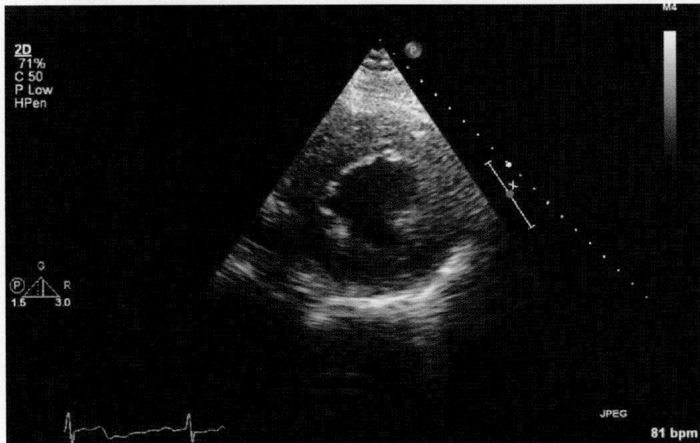

FIGURE 12-4-6 Short axis images at end-diastole (top panel) and end-systole (bottom panel) from the patient in Figure 12-4-5. There is global LV dysfunction with regional wall motion abnormalities as seen here in the short axis view in which the midseptum is more hypokinetic than the other walls.

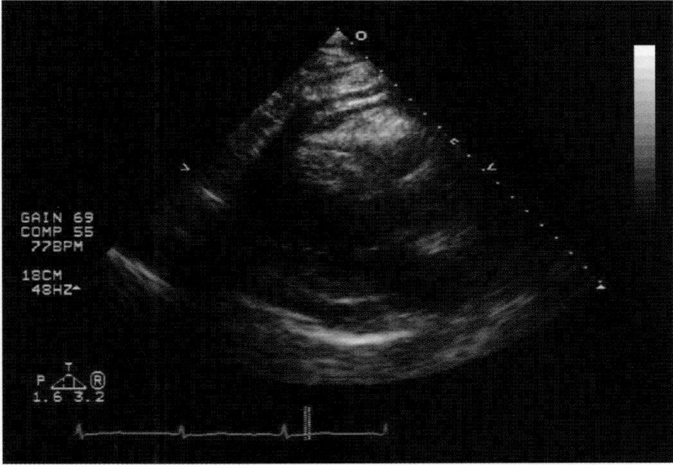

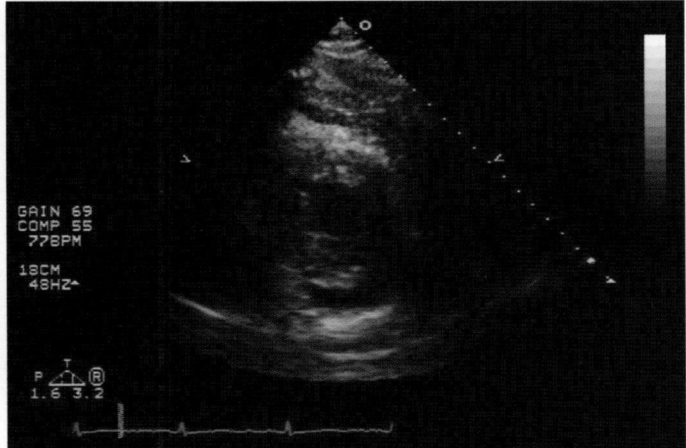

FIGURE 12-4-8 Images from a 57-year-old woman with a history of pulmonary sarcoidosis who presented with palpitations. A Holter monitor revealed frequent PVCs. Echocardiogram showed normal LV and RV size and function. A pericardial effusion, as well as pericardial thickening, was noted, demonstrated here in the long axis view (top panel) and short axis view (bottom panel). Since a pericardial effusion can indicate cardiac sarcoidosis, a cardiac MRI was obtained, which demonstrated delayed gadolinium enhancement in the basal anterior interventricular septum, consistent with CS.

- A main limitation to cardiac MRI is its limited availability outside tertiary medical centers, and that it cannot be used to follows CS patients with ICDs.
- PET-CT imaging using 18-FDG is highly sensitive for detecting CS.[13] The presence and amount of 18-FDG uptake has prognostic implications and has been shown to correlate with risk for VT. As opposed to MRI, PET scanning can be done in patients with ICDs and is very useful in monitoring response to therapy.[14]
- The main disadvantage of PET-CT, outside of cost, is that the protocol can be cumbersome and when done outside of experienced centers can yield variable results.
- The sensitivity for standard RV endomyocardial biopsies in diagnosing CS is very low at ~20%.[15] This is because of the patchy involvement of the granulomas and the predilection for areas that are not readily amenable to biopsies. In patients who have had a tissue diagnoses made in a noncardiac site, and with the improvements in advanced cardiac imaging, endomyocardial biopsies are rarely warranted. When isolated cardiac sarcoidosis is suspected and extracardiac tissue is not available, image-guided techniques can significantly improve the sensitivity of the biopsy.[16]

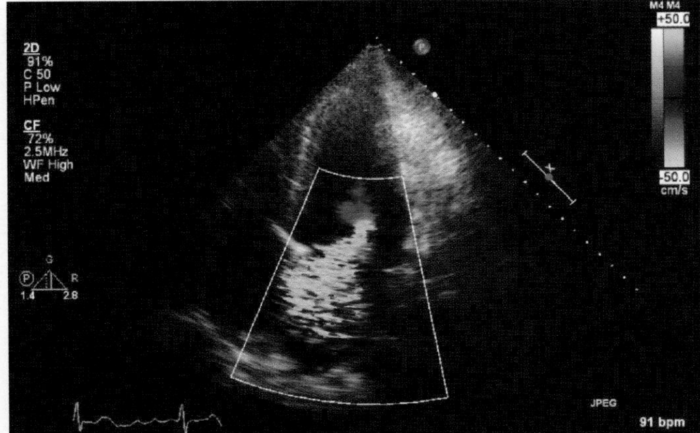

FIGURE 12-4-7 Apical 4 chamber view with color Doppler demonstrating significant mitral regurgitation in the patient described in Figure 12-4-5.

DIFFERENTIAL DIAGNOSIS

- Arrhythmogenic right ventricular dysplasia can be a mimicker of cardiac sarcoidosis. Although it is more likely for sarcoid to affect the left ventricle than the right ventricle, RV involvement can predominate in CS. MRI is helpful in differentiating these two, although sometimes tissue biopsy may be necessary.[17]
- Giant cell myocarditis can also be hard to distinguish from cardiac sarcoid. Clinically, patients with giant cell tend to present more acutely, whereas CS is more of a subacute presentation. AV block and syncope are more common with CS, and left sided heart failure is more common with giant cell myocarditis. The prognosis is generally worse with giant cell myocarditis. Still, CS and giant cell can be difficult to differentiate clinically, and a myocardial biopsy may be needed.[18]
- Cardiac sarcoidosis should be considered in young patients with a dilated cardiomyopathy (DCM). Features more common with CS than idiopathic DCM include abnormalities in regional wall motion, changes in wall thickness, and a higher prevalence of conduction system disease.[19] CS patients intend to have a worse prognosis and are treated differently, so making this diagnosis is important.
- Likewise, in young patients with AV block, CS should be highly considered. In patients less than 55 years old presenting with complete heart block, 19% were found to have CS.[20] These patients tend to have a worse prognosis and are best treated with an ICD as opposed to standard pacemaker therapy alone.

DIAGNOSIS

- The approach to the diagnosis of cardiac sarcoidosis is different based on the pretest probability of finding the disease.
- Roughly 30% of patients with systemic sarcoidosis have evidence of cardiac involvement on autopsy. Most of this, however, is subclinical, and the first manifestation of CS can be sudden cardiac death. Thus, when a patient is diagnosed with systemic (ie, pulmonary) sarcoidosis, it is prudent to screen these patients for cardiac involvement.
  - In addition to a detailed history and physical examination, a 12-lead ECG should be performed to look for atrial or ventricular arrhythmias or evidence of conduction system disease. Strong consideration can also be made for a screening Holter monitor and echocardiogram at this time as well. While individually the sensitivity may be low to intermediate, collectively ECG, Holter monitoring, and echocardiogram have an excellent negative predictive value.
  - These tests are not specific, however, and advanced cardiac imaging with cardiac MRI or cardiac PET-CT should be pursued if any of these screening tests are abnormal.
  - If the advanced cardiac imaging is suggestive of cardiac sarcoidosis, the diagnosis is highly probable, and a myocardial tissue biopsy is not necessary and potentially harmful.
- It can be more difficult to diagnose cardiac sarcoidosis in patients without a known history of sarcoid. When a patient between the ages of 20 to 50 years old presents with high grade AV block, ventricular tachycardia, or a dilated cardiomophathy, cardiac sarcoidosis should be in the differential diagnosis.
  - While ECGs, echocardiograms, and diagnostic heart catheterizations are often performed in these patients, cardiac MRI or PET-CT at an experienced center is suggested to look for cardiac sarcoidosis or an alternative explanation.
  - If these tests are suggestive of CS, a search for extracardiac involvement should be made so that a tissue diagnosis at these sites (ie, transbronchial biopsy) can be pursued.
  - If there is no evidence of extracardiac involvement, an endomyocardial biopsy or an empiric trial treatment of steroids while monitoring the response to treatment can be considered. An improvement on therapy, as in the previously discussed case presentation, is highly suggestive of CS.

MANAGEMENT

- Standard therapy for CS includes immunosuppressant medications and consideration of an implantable cardioverter defibrillator (ICD).
- Steroids are the mainstay of therapy for CS. They are most effective when administered early at reducing active inflammation.
- Steroids appear to prevent a decline in EF in patients with preserved ventricular function and help improved EF in those with up to a moderate decline in EF.[21]
- Likewise, in patients with ventricular arrhythmias and AV block and evidence of inflammation on cardiac testing, steroids can be an effective antiarrhythmic and can improve AV block.[22] They are less effective, however, when fibrosis predominates.
- The lowest effective dose of steroids is recommended due to the serious long-term consequences of its use.
- Steroid-sparing agents such as methotrexate and azathioprine are increasingly being used to treat CS. They are useful in patients who fail or are intolerant to steroids, but are also frequently used with steroids to minimize the steroid dose needed.
- Recently, a small study found that low-dose corticosteroids along with weekly methotrexate was an effective strategy at stabilizing the ejection fraction with minimal side effects.[23]
- The decision to place an ICD in CS patients can be a complicated one. According to ACC/AHA guidelines, cardiac sarcoid is a IIa indication for placement of an ICD for primary prevention of SCD.[24] That being said, these are often young patients, and exposing all patients with CS to device therapy could lead to inappropriate shocks, high costs, and potential complications to procedures.
- High-risk patients for SCD include patients with sustained VT (either spontaneous or induced on EP study), left or right ventricular dysfunction, and complete heart block. In these patients, an ICD is warranted.[25] Syncope and extensive myocardial involvement on MRI or PET-CT are also considered high-risk features.
- In patients without risk high features, EP testing can be useful to help risk stratify for SCD.[26] Those with normal ejection fractions and negative EP studies appear to have a low risk for SCD for the next several years and can likely be monitored without device therapy.
- In patients with refractory, end stage heart failure, transplantation should be a consideration, and these patients tend to do well post-transplant.[27]

FOLLOW-UP

- Consensus guidelines do not exist on the best way to follow CS patients.
- Patients started on immunosuppressant medications for CS should be monitored regularly to find the lowest effective dose in order to minimize long-term side effects of the medications.
- Whenever a decision is made to lower or stop immunosuppressant medications, the patient should be frequently reassessed for clinical symptoms. Objective evidence should be considered as well, either via arrhythmia burden on Holter monitoring/device interrogation/loop recorder, or via image studies using echocardiography, MRI, or PET-CT.
- In patients with ICDs, the devices should be regularly assessed for abnormal heart rhythms. An increased incidence of VT, for example, could represent an exacerbation of the underlying disease process, and treatment will need to be made accordingly, including an increased dose of immunosuppressant medications.
- Patients who do not receive an ICD also require frequent reassessments for worsening disease activity or the development of high-risk features that would indicate a benefit for ICD implantation.

REFERENCES

1. Roberts WC, McAllister HA Jr, Ferrans VJ. Sarcoidosis of the heart. A clinicopathologic study of 35 necropsy patients (group 1) and review of 78 previously described necropsy patients (group 11). *Am J Med.* 1977 Jul;63(1):86-108.
2. Chapelon-Abric C, de Zuttere D, Duhaut P, et al. Cardiac sarcoidosis: a retrospective study of 41 cases. *Medicine (Baltimore).* 2004 Nov;83(6):315-334.
3. Swigris JJ, Olson AL, Huie TJ, et al. Sarcoidosis-related mortality in the United States from 1988 to 2007. *Am Respir Crit Care Med.* 2011;183(11):1524-1530. Epub 2011 Feb 17.
4. Silverman KJ, Hutchins GM, Bulkley BH. Cardiac sarcoid: a clinicopathologic study of 84 unselected patients with systemic sarcoidosis. *Circulation.* 1978;58(6):1204-1211.
5. Furushima H, Chinushi M, Sugiura H, Kasai H, Washizuka T, Aizawa Y. Ventricular tachyarrhythmia associated with cardiac sarcoidosis: its mechanisms and outcome. *Clin Cardiol.* 2004;27(4):217-222.
6. www.orpha.net/orphacom/cahiers/docs/GB/Prevalence_of_rare_diseases_by_alphabetical_list.pdf.
7. Ryabicki BA, Major M, Popovich J Jr, Maliarik MJ, Iannuzzi MC. Racial differences in sarcoidosis incidence: a 5-year study in a health maintenance organization. *Am J Epidemiol.* 1997;145(3):234-241.
8. Erdal BS, Clymer BD, Yildiz VO, Julian MW, Crouser ED. Unexpectedly high prevalence of sarcoidosis in a representative U.S. Metropolitan population. *Respir Med.* 2012;106(6):893-899. Epub 2012 Mar 13.
9. Iannuzzi MC, Rybicki BA, Teirstein AS. Sarcoidosis. *N Engl J Med.* 2007;357:2153-2165.
10. Okura Y, Dec GW, Hare JM, et al. A clinical and histopathologic comparison of cardiac sarcoidosis and idiopathic giant cell myocarditis. *J Am Coll Cardiol.* 2003;41(2):322-329.
11. Lewin RF, Mor R, Spitzer S, et al. Echocardiographic evaluation of patients with systemic sarcoidosis. *Am Heart J.* 1985;110(1 pt 1):116-122.
12. Lo A, Foder K, Martin P, Younger JF. Response to steroid therapy in cardiac sarcoidosis: insights from myocardial strain. *Eur Heart J Cardiovasc Imaging.* 2012;13(2):E3. Epub 2011 Oct 11.
13. Vignaux O. Cardiac sarcoidosis: spectrum of MRI features. *AJR Am J Roentgenol.* 2005;184(1):249-254.
14. Youssef G, Leung E, Mylonas I, et al. The use of 18F-FDG PET in the diagnosis of cardiac sarcoidosis: a systematic review and meta analysis including the Ontario experience. *J Nucl Med.* 2012;53(2):241-248.
15. Treglia G, Taralli S, Giordano A. Emerging role of whole-body 18F-fluorodeoxyglucose positron emission tomography as a marker of disease activity in patients with sarcoidosis: a systematic review. *Sarcoidosis Vasc Diffuse Lung Dis.* 2011;28(2):87-94.
16. Uemura A, Morimoto S, Hiramitsu S, Kato Y, Ito T, Hishida H. Histologic diagnostic rate of cardiac sarcoidosis: evaluation of endomyocardial biopsies. *Am Heart J.* 1999(2 Pt 1);138:299-302.
17. Kandolin R, Lehtonen J, Graner M, et al. Diagnosing isolated cardiac sarcoidosis. *J Intern Med.* 2011;270(5):461-468.
18. Kaplan BA, Soejima K, Boughman K, Epstein LM, Stevenson WG. Refractory ventricular tachycardia secondary to cardiac sarcoid: electrophysiologic characteristics, mapping, and ablation. *Heart Rhythm.* 2006;3(8):924-929. Epub 2006 Mar 30.
19. Okura Y, Dec GW, Hare JM, et al. A clinical and histopathologic comparison of cardiac sarcoidosis and idiopathic giant cell myocarditis. *J Am Coll Cardiol.* 2003;41(2):322-329.
20. Yazaki Y, Isobe M, Hiramitsu S, et al. Comparison of clinical features and prognosis of cardiac sarcoidosis and idiopathic dilated cardiomyopathy. *Am J Cardiol.* 1998;82(4):537-540.
21. Kandolin R, Lehtonen J, Kupari M. Cardiac sarcoidosis and giant cell myocarditis as causes of atrioventricular block in young and middle-aged adults. *Circ Arrhythm Electrophysiol.* 2011;4(3):303-309.
22. Chiu CZ, N, Katani S, Zhang G, et al. Prevention of left ventricular remodeling by long-term corticosteroid therapy in patients with cardiac sarcoidosis. *Am J Cardiol.* 2005;95:143-146.
21. Banba K, Kusano KF, Nakamura K, et al. Relationship between arrhythmogenesis and disease activity in cardiac sarcoidosis. *Heart Rhythm.* 2007;4(10):1292-1299. Epub 2007 Jun 16.
22. Nagai S, Yokomatsu T, Tanizawa K, et al. Treatment with methotrexate and low-dose corticosteroids in sarcoidosis patients with cardiac lesions. *Intern Med.* 2014;53(5):427-433.
23. Epstein AE, DiMarco JP, Ellenbogen KA, et al. ACC/AHA/HRS 2008 Guidelines for Device-Based Therapy of Cardiac Rhythm Abnormalities: a report of the American College of Cardiology/American Heart Association Task Force on Practice Guidelines (Writing Committee to Revise the ACC/AHA/NASPE 2002 Guideline Update for Implantation of Cardiac Pacemakers and Antiarrhythmia Devices) developed

in collaboration with the American Association for Thoracic Surgery and Society of Thoracic Surgeons. *J Am Coll Cardiol.* 2008;51(21):e1-62.

24. Betensky BP, Tschabrunn CM, Zado ES, et al. Long-term follow-up of patients with cardiac sarcoidosis and implantable cardioverter-defibrillators. *Heart Rhythm.* 2012;9(6):884-891. Epub 2012 Feb 13.

25. Mehta D, Mori N, Goldbarg SH, et al. Primary prevention of sudden cardiac death in silent cardiac sarcoidosis role of programmed ventricular stimulation. *Circ Arrhythm Electrophysiol.* 2011;4(1):43-48. Epub 2010 Dec 30.

26. Zaidi AR, Zaidi A, Vaikus PT. Outcome of heart transplantation in patients with sarcoid cardiomyopathy. *J Heart Lung Transplant.* 2007;26(7):714-717.

13 ECHOCARDIOGRAPHY IN INTERVENTIONAL PROCEDURES

David A. Orsinelli, MD, FACC, FASE

INTRODUCTION

As we have explored in this atlas, echocardiography has assumed a primary role in the evaluation and management of patients with known or suspected cardiac disease.[1,2] Up until now, we have emphasized its role principally as a diagnostic test. Transesophageal echocardiography (TEE) has become an integral tool in the operating room for assessing and monitoring patients undergoing cardiac surgery. Its role in that setting is beyond the scope of this atlas. As new technologies and therapies have evolved, however, echocardiography is playing an increasingly important role in interventional procedures.[3,4] Echocardiography has demonstrated utility in a variety of such procedures, including pericardiocentesis, endomyocardial biopsy, transatrial septal catheterization, transcatheter closure of patent foramen ovale (PFO) and atrial septal defects (ASDs), percutaneous mitral and aortic balloon valvuloplasty, alcohol septal ablation for hypertrophic cardiomyopathy, some electrophysiologic procedures, as well as transcatheter mitral valve repair, left atrial appendage (LAA) occlusion procedures, and transcatheter aortic valve replacement procedures.[3,4] Many of these procedures have been described in prior chapters.

In this chapter, we will highlight the role of echocardiography, primarily TEE, as a tool to help guide interventional procedures performed in the cardiac catheterization lab and the operating room in several clinical settings from our institution that have not been addressed previously in this atlas.

SECTION 1

Echo-Guided Pericardiocentesis

CASE PRESENTATION

A 57-year-old man with a history of lung cancer and severe COPD presented to our institution with progressive dyspnea and dizziness. He denied any chest pain, recent febrile illness, cough or other constitutional symptoms other than anorexia. On arrival to the ED, he was noted to be tachypneic and tachycardic. His BP was 90/60 mm Hg. His lung exam revealed decreased breath sounds bilaterally, more prominent on the right. His neck veins were elevated. Cardiac exam revealed no murmurs; however, his heart sounds were distant. He had no edema. A chest x-ray revealed cardiomegaly and a right-sided pleural effusion. A stat bedside TTE revealed a large pericardial effusion with evidence of cardiac tamponade. He was taken to the cardiac catheterization lab where he underwent an echo-guided pericardiocentesis (Figures 13-1-1 to 13-1-3). Postprocedure echocardiography revealed resolution of the effusion. He was admitted to the oncology service. The pericardial drain was removed 2 days later after a limited echo revealed no reaccumulation of the fluid. He underwent further treatment of his lung cancer.

VIDEO LEGENDS

1. Video 13-1-1: Initial echocardiogram in the catheterization lab which confirmed the presence of a large pericardial effusion.
2. Video 13-1-2: Apical 4 chamber view from the procedure. Agitated saline was injected through the needle to confirm that the tip of the needle was indeed in the pericardial space and not in the right ventricle. The "hazy" echoes seen around LV apex are the saline contrast "bubbles" which are in the pericardial space and not the RV.
3. Video 13-1-3: Post tap echo demonstrating that the effusion is no longer present. The pericardium does appear thickened.

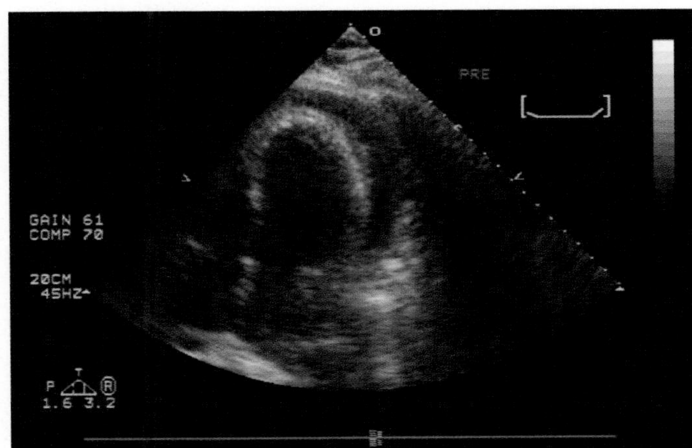

FIGURE 13-1-1 Initial echocardiogram in the catheterization lab which confirmed the presence of a large pericardial effusion ▶ (see Video 13-1-1).

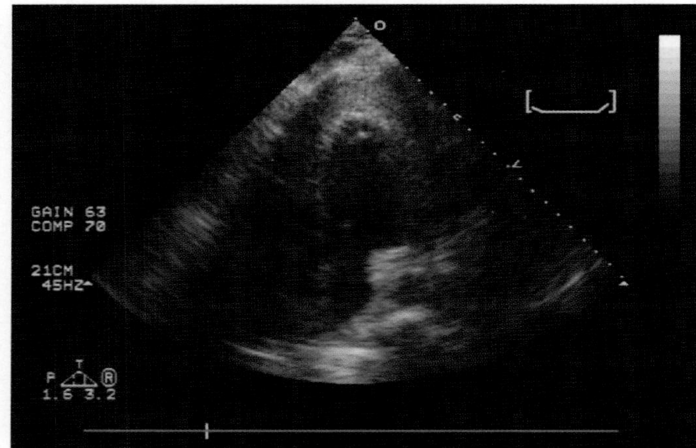

FIGURE 13-1-2 Apical 4 chamber view from the procedure. Agitated saline was injected through the needle to confirm that the tip of the needle was indeed in the pericardial space and not in the right ventricle. The "hazy" echoes at the LV apex are the saline contrast "bubbles" ▶ (see Video 13-1-2).

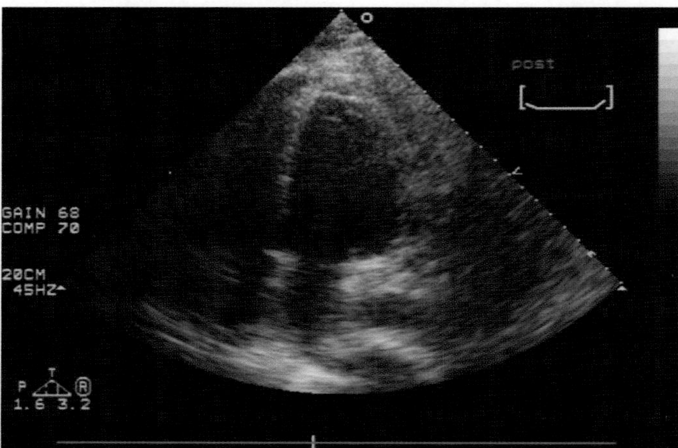

FIGURE 13-1-3 Post-tap echo demonstrating that the effusion is no longer present. The pericardium does appear thickened ▶ (see Video 13-1-3).

SECTION 2

Left Atrial Appendage Ligation

CASE PRESENTATION

A 72-year-old man with a history of permanent atrial fibrillation and a CHADS2 score of 3 has been maintained on chronic anticoagulation. He has a history of congestive heart failure, hypertension, Type 2 diabetes, and peripheral vascular disease. While on warfarin, with a therapeutic INR, he developed a spontaneous subdural hematoma. His coagulopathy was reversed with Vitamin K, and he underwent successful evacuation of the hematoma. He recovered with minimal neurologic sequelae. After discussion with the neurosurgical team and the patient, it was determined that systemic anticoagulation was not advisable. The patient was approached about LAA isolation with the LARIAT device, a new procedure that is performed to exclude the LAA from the body of the LA. The LAA is the site of thrombus formation in the majority of patients with atrial fibrillation. Exclusion of the LAA hopefully will decrease the patient's risk of stroke. The device was successfully placed with no residual communication between the LA and the LAA. He was discharged from the hospital on aspirin and his other cardiac medications and has done well with no systemic embolic events to date. The device is placed using a delivery system, which incorporates a guiding catheter system placed into the LAA via a transseptal puncture from the RA into the LA, and a delivery system for the LARIAT suture device placed externally around the LAA, which is delivered via the pericardial space.

TEE was used in this patient's procedure to exclude the presence of a preexisting thrombus (a contraindication to the procedure), to guide device placement, and exclude complications such as pericardial effusion. At the end of the procedure, TEE imaging confirmed that there was no residual communication between the LA and the LAA.

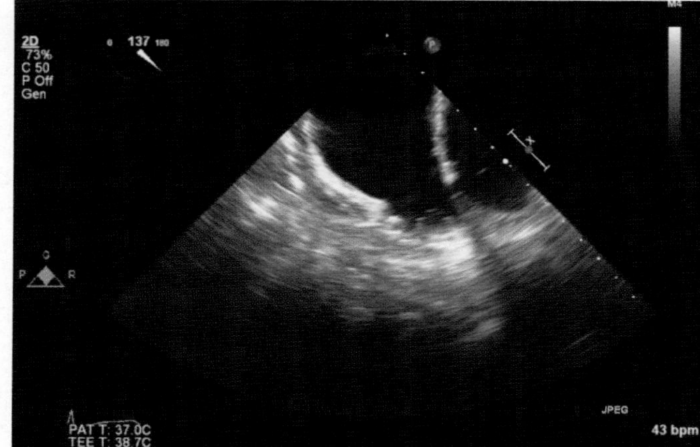

FIGURE 13-2-1 Initial TEE images of the LAA confirming the absence of an LAA thrombus. The ridges seen along the distal LAA wall are pectinate muscles, not thrombus ▶ (see Video 13-2-1).

Figures 13-2-1 to 13-2-6 are representative images from his procedure. He has done well with no neurologic events. A follow-up TEE subsequently confirmed that there was no communication between the occluded LAA and the LA, nor was there any thrombus at the site of the LAA closure.

VIDEO LEGENDS

1. Video 13-2-1: Initial TEE images of the LAA confirming the absence of a LAA thrombus. The ridges seen along the distal LAA wall are pectinate muscles, not thrombus.

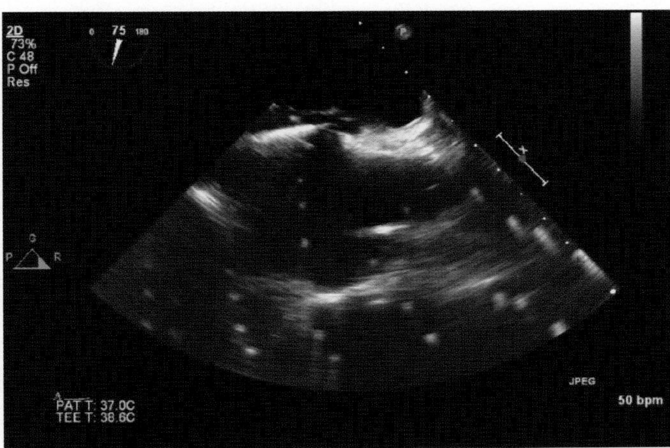

FIGURE 13-2-2 Transseptal Puncture. The catheter is being placed across the interatrial septum. The bright flashing signals are due to artifact from an intracardiac echo probe ► (see Video 13-2-2).

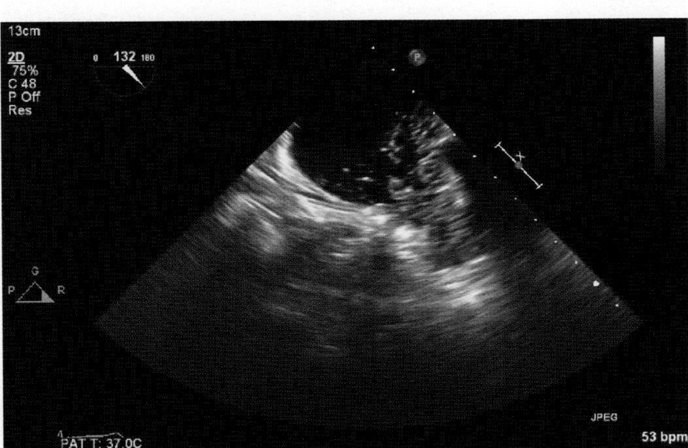

FIGURE 13-2-3 Contrast is injected into the LAA through the catheter in the LAA to define the LAA anatomy and confirm placement of the endocardial catheter ► (see Video 13-2-3).

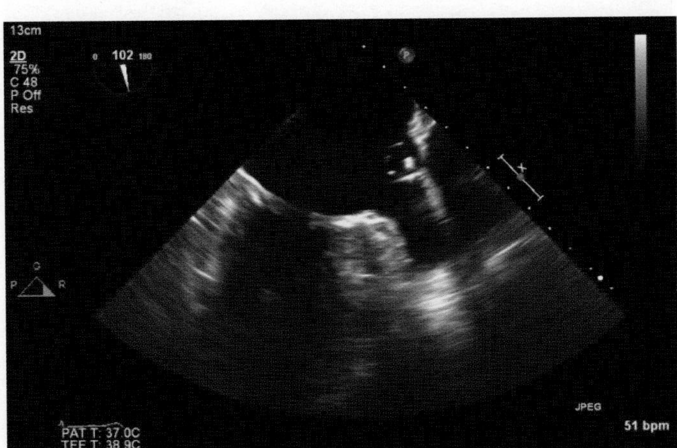

FIGURE 13-2-4 The catheter and balloon, used to help size the LAA and determine if the device will close the LAA, is seen in this image ► (see Video 13-2-4).

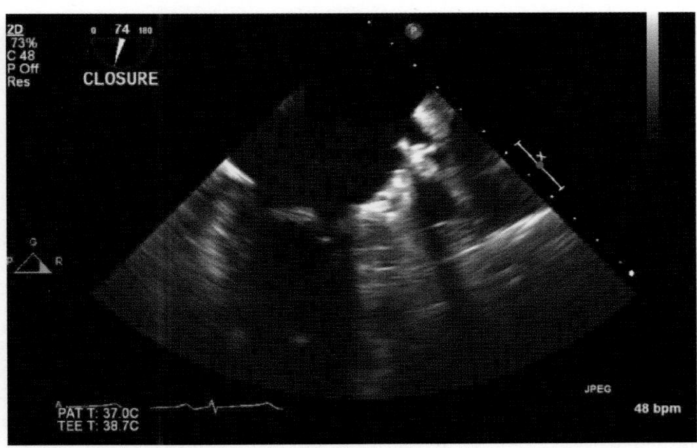

FIGURE 13-2-5 The LARIAT device has been placed, and the LAA is now closed from the LA ►(see Video 13-2-5).

2. Video 13-2-2: Trans-septal Puncture. The catheter is being placed across the interatrial septum. The bright flashing signals are due to artifact from an intra-cardiac echo probe.
3. Video 13-2-3: Contrast is injected into the LAA through the catheter in the LAA to define the LAA anatomy and confirm placement of the endocardial catheter
4. Video 13-2-4: The catheter and balloon, used to help size the LAA and determine if the device will close the LAA, are seen in this video.
5. Video 13-2-5: The LARIAT® device has been placed and the LAA is now closed from the LA
6. Video 13-2-6: Color Flow Doppler confirms that there is no flow from the LAA in to the LA. The color flow (red jet) seen in the upper portion of the sector is normal flow from the left upper pulmonary vein.

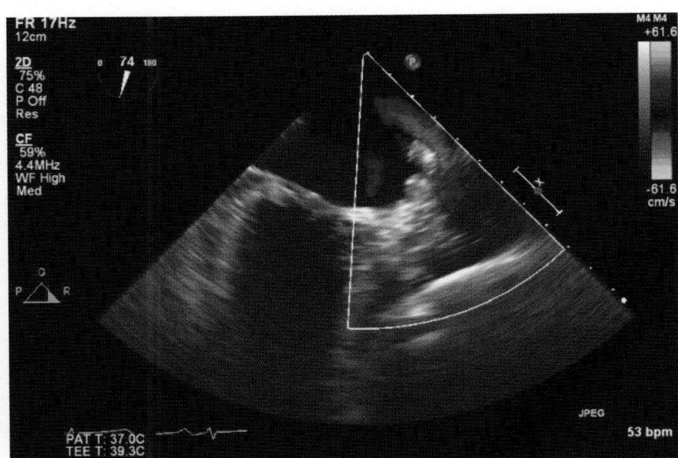

FIGURE 13-2-6 Color flow Doppler confirms that there is no flow from the LAA into the LA. The color flow (red jet) seen in the upper portion of the sector is normal flow from the left upper pulmonary vein ► (see Video 13-2-6).

SECTION 3

Transcatheter Aortic Valve Replacement (TAVR)

CASE PRESENTATION

An 82-year-old man presented with an acute episode of congestive heart failure. He had not seen his cardiologist for several years. He had a history of hypertension, COPD, hyperlipidemia, stage 3 chronic kidney disease, and coronary artery disease with previous coronary artery bypass surgery 13 years ago. He also had a prior stroke with mild impairment. On admission, his exam was remarkable for diffuse rales in both lung fields, a harsh, late-peaking grade 3/6 systolic ejection murmur that radiated to both carotids, and an absent aortic component of the second heart sound. He had 2+ pedal and pretibial edema. An echocardiogram confirmed the diagnosis of severe aortic stenosis with a peak gradient of 84 mm Hg and a mean gradient of 52 mm Hg. There was mild aortic regurgitation. He was treated with intravenous diuretics with improvement of his symptoms. He was evaluated by the structural heart disease team and was felt to be an extreme surgical risk due to his age and multiple comorbidities, as well as his previous bypass surgery. He was offered the option of TAVR and after extensive evaluation underwent placement of an Edwards SAPIEN transcatheter aortic valve, which is a balloon-expandable bovine pericardial valve. TEE was performed during the procedure prior to any intervention to establish a baseline and define the AV anatomy. During balloon valvuloplasty (performed prior to deployment of the new valve), TEE imaging was performed to help guide balloon placement and look for complications. TEE imaging was performed during and after valve deployment to assist in positioning the device and to assess valve function. He was discharged 3 days after the procedure. Postprocedure, his symptoms dramatically improved. Follow-up TTE revealed minimal aortic regurgitation and mean aortic valve gradient of 9 mm Hg. He will be followed with serial office visits and echocardiograms. Figures 13-3-1 to 13-3-7 are images from his procedure.

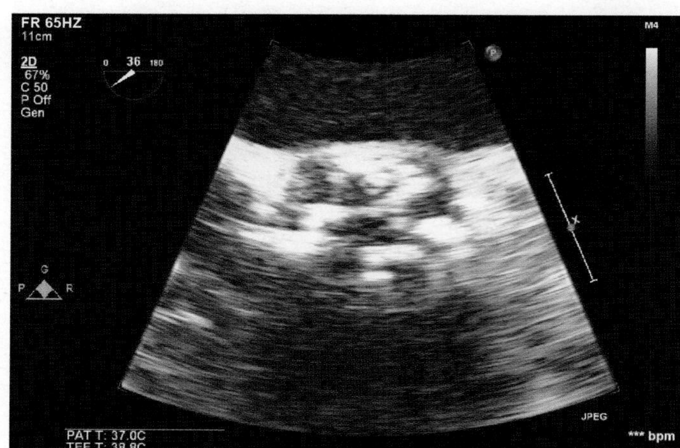

FIGURE 13-3-1 TEE short axis view of the AV prior to the balloon valvuloplasty. Note the heavily calcified valve ► (see Video 13-3-1).

VIDEO LEGENDS

1. Video 13-3-1: TEE short axis view of the AV prior to the balloon valvuloplasty. Note the heavily calcified valve.
2. Video 13-3-2 A: With the initial BAV attempt, the balloon "pops" out of the valve when it was inflated. This was due to loss of pacemaker capture (rapid ventricular pacing is performed to decrease LV contractility to prevent dislodgement of the balloon both during the BAV and during valve deployment).
3. Video 13-3-2 B: This video demonstrates a successful BAV in the long axis view. The balloon did not become dislodged with this inflation.
4. Video 13-3-2 C: A short axis view of the BAV is demonstrated in this video.
5. Video 13-3-3: Short axis view of the AV post BAV. There is minimal increase in leaflet mobility post BAV.
6. Video 13-3-4 L: Long axis view of the AV with color Doppler pre BAV demonstrating mild AR. An increase in the degree of aortic regurgitation (AR) post BAV is seen in the next video.

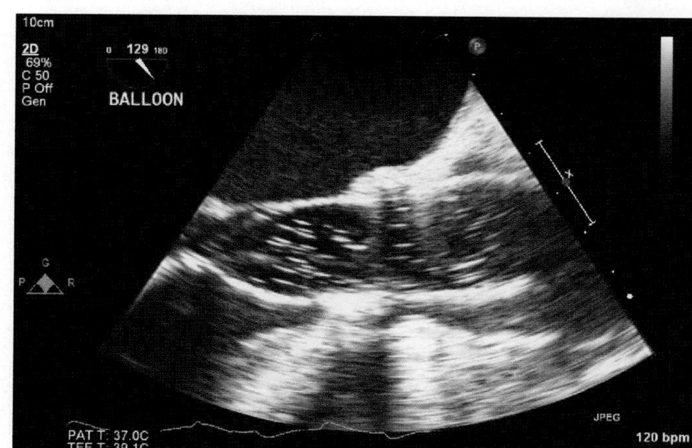

FIGURE 13-3-2 Imaging during the balloon aortic valvuloplasty (BAV). The balloon, filled with contrast, can be seen in this TEE long axis view. The accompanying 3 videos demonstrate the procedure. In the first video, the balloon "pops" out of the valve when it was inflated. This was due to loss of pacemaker capture (rapid ventricular pacing is performed to decrease LV contractility to prevent dislodgement of the balloon both during the BAV and during valve deployment). The second video demonstrates a successful BAV in the long axis view. A short axis view of the BAV is also demonstrated ► (see Videos 13-3-2 A-C).

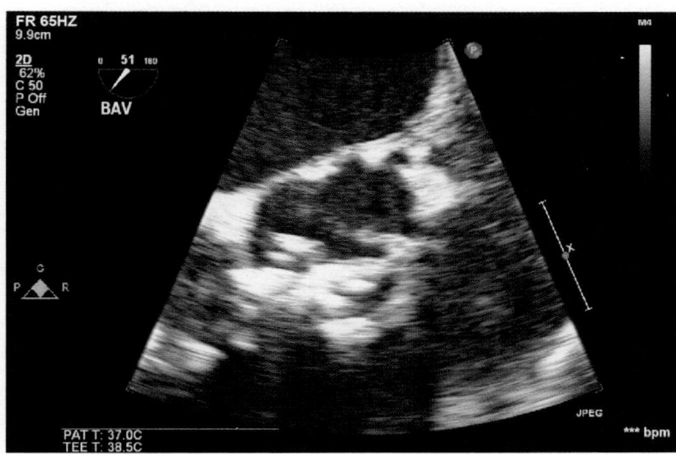

FIGURE 13-3-3 Short axis view of the AV post-BAV. There is minimal increase in leaflet mobility post-BAV ▶ (see Video 13-3-3).

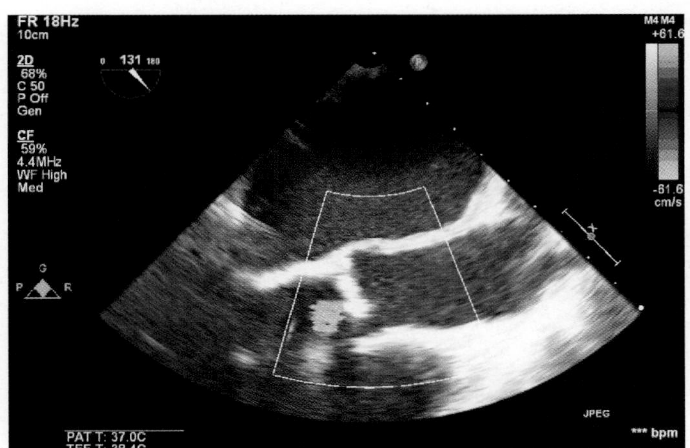

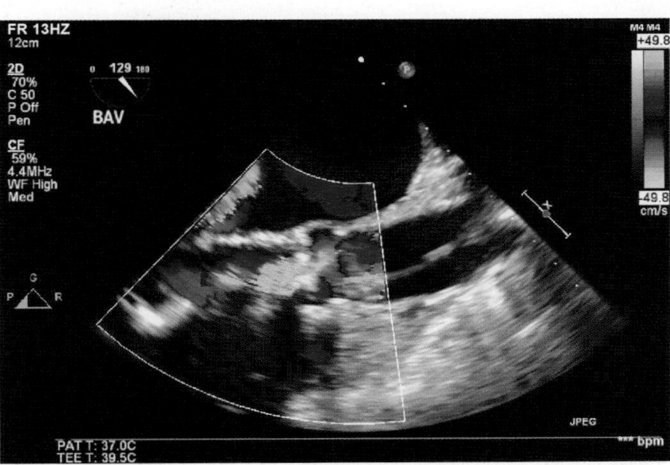

FIGURE 13-3-4 Long axis view of the AV with color Doppler pre- (top panel) and post- (bottom panel) BAV demonstrating an increase in the degree of aortic regurgitation (AR) post-BAV. Some of the AR is due to the presence of a catheter across the valve. Severe AR due to disruption of the AV is a potential complication of BAV ▶ (see Videos 13-3-4 L and R).

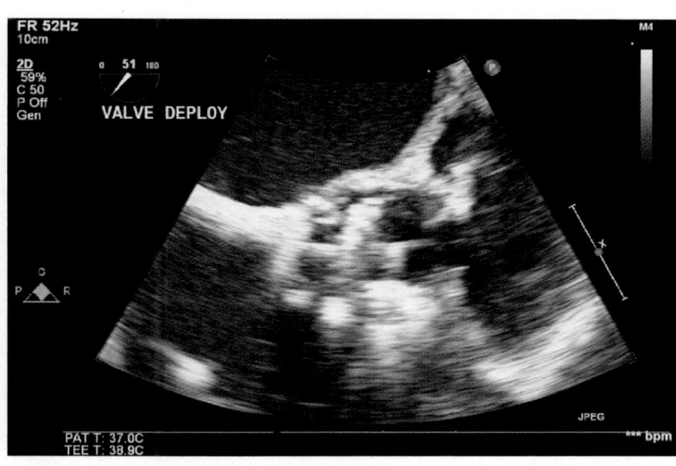

FIGURE 13-3-5 The SAPIEN valve is deployed under TEE guidance (see Video 13-3-5).

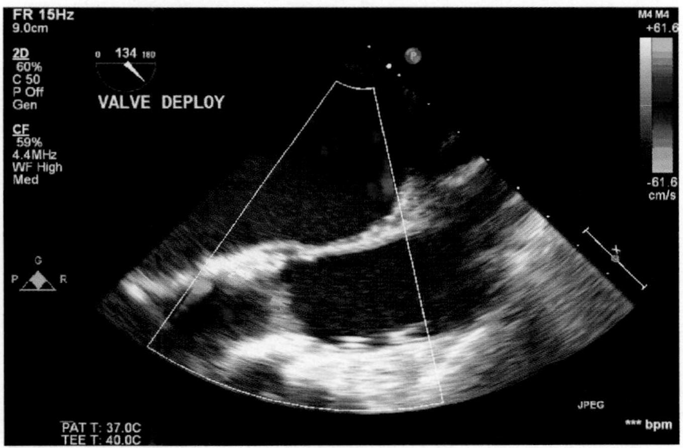

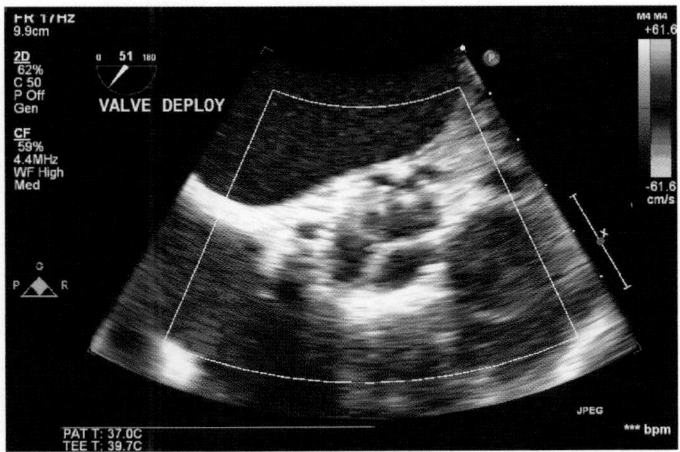

FIGURE 13-3-6 Long axis (top panel) and short axis (bottom panel) TEE views of the SAPIEN valve with color Doppler. There is minimal central AR and a small paravalvular leak. Paravalvular regurgitation is more common with TAVR than with surgical AVR and has been associated with a poorer outcome. In the short axis view, also note that there is color flow in the LMCA. Occlusion of the coronary artery by the new valve is also a potential complication of TAVR ▶ (see Videos 13-3-6 L and R).

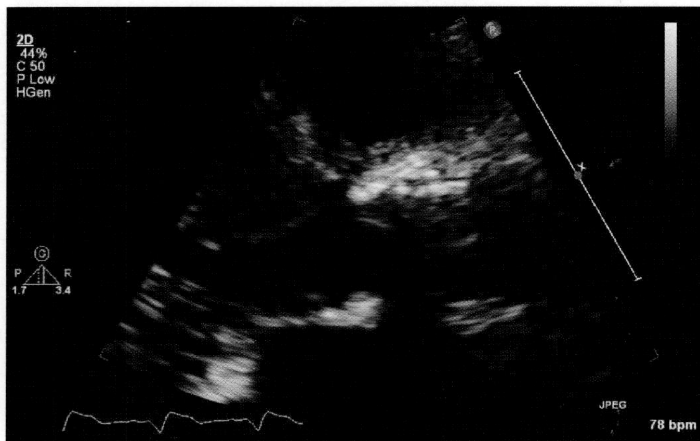

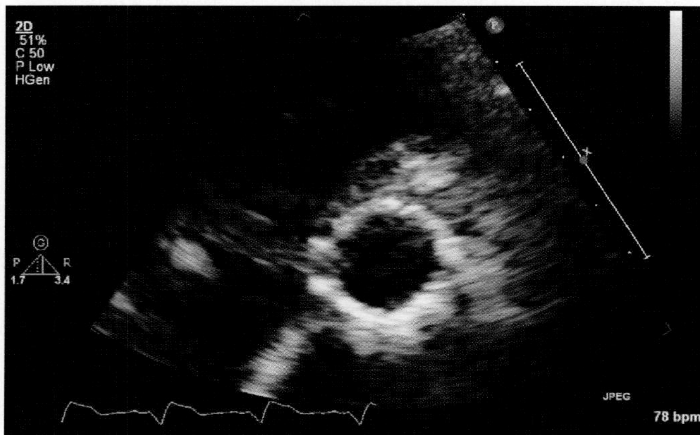

FIGURE 13-3-7 Subsequent TTE images (parasternal long axis view in the top panel and short axis view in the bottom panel) from a patient prior to discharge demonstrating a well-positioned SAPIEN valve. The accompanying 4 videos demonstrate good valve position and normal leaflet motion. Color Doppler demonstrates mild paravalvular AR ► (see Videos 13-3-7 A-D).

7. Video 13-3-4 R: Long axis view of the AV with color Doppler post BAV demonstrating an increase in the degree of aortic regurgitation (AR). Some of the AR is due to the presence of a catheter across the valve. Severe AR due to disruption of the AV is a potential complication of BAV.
8. Video 13-3-5: The SAPIEN valve is deployed under TEE guidance. Initially contrast is seen as the balloon expands. Once the balloon is deflated, the new prosthetic valve leaflets can be seen.
9. Video 13-3-6 L: Long axis TEE view of the SAPIEN valve with color Doppler. There is minimal central AR and a small paravalvular leak.
10. Video 13-3-6 R: Short axis TEE view of the SAPIEN valve with color Doppler. There is minimal central AR and a small paravalvular leak. In this short axis view, also note that there is color flow in the LMCA.
11. Video 13-3-7 A: TTE images from a patient prior to discharge demonstrating a well positioned SAPIEN valve. The valve is in good position and normal leaflet motion is seen in this long axis view.
12. Video 13-3-7 B: TTE images from a patient prior to discharge demonstrating a well positioned SAPIEN valve. The valve is in good position and normal leaflet motion is seen in this short axis view.
13. Video 13-3-7 C: TTE with color Doppler demonstrates mild paravalvular AR in this long axis view.
14. Video 13-3-7 D: TTE with color Doppler demonstrates mild paravalvular AR in this short axis view

SECTION 4

Transcatheter Occlusion of A Prosthetic Mitral Valve Paravalvular Leak

CASE PRESENTATION

A 62-year-old woman with multiple medical problems had undergone her second mitral valve replacement 6 months earlier. The procedure was complicated by a prolonged hospital course. She continued to exhibit symptoms of dyspnea and had evidence of hemolytic anemia. TTE and subsequent TEE imaging demonstrated the presence of significant paravalvular MR. She was not felt to be a good candidate for operative repair or replacement of the valve. After discussion with the structural heart disease team, she was offered the option of a transcatheter closure of the paravalvular leaks. Using an apical approach via a small anterior chest wall incision, two paravalvular leaks were successfully closed with Amplatzer occluder devices. Postprocedure, her anemia has improved, as have her symptoms. TEE, especially 3-D TEE, was instrumental in guiding the placement of the devices. Figures 13-4-1 to 13-4-4 are representative images from her procedure.

VIDEO LEGENDS

1. Video 13-4-1 L: TEE image with color flow Doppler demonstrating the smaller (posteromedial) paravalvular regurgitant jet.
2. Video 13-4-1 R: TEE images with color flow Doppler demonstrating the larger (anterolateral) paravalvular regurgitant jet.

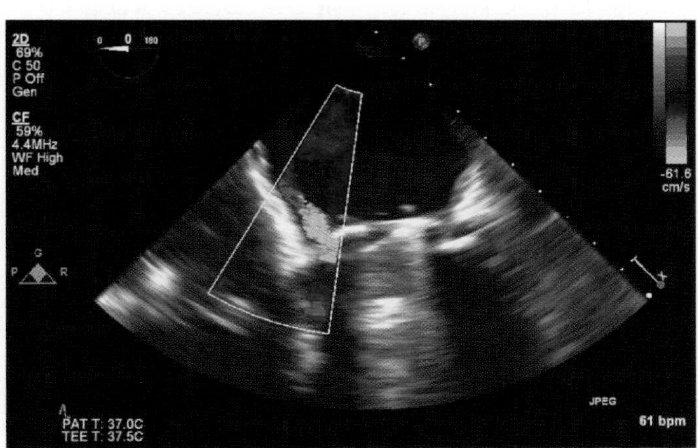

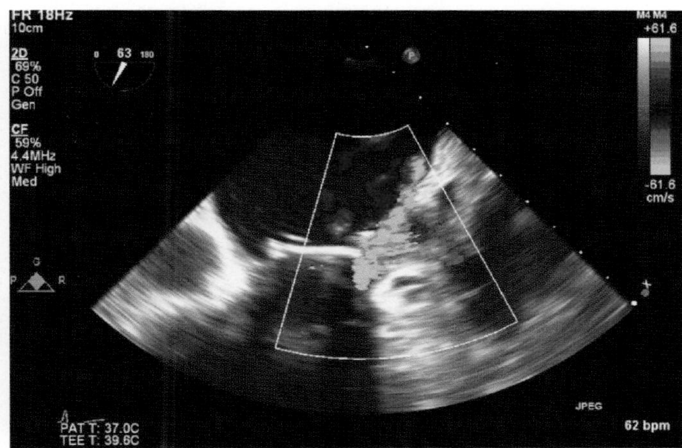

FIGURE 13-4-1 TEE images with color flow Doppler demonstrating the smaller posteromedial (L) and larger anterolateral (R) paravalvular regurgitant jets ▶ (see Videos 13-4-1L and R).

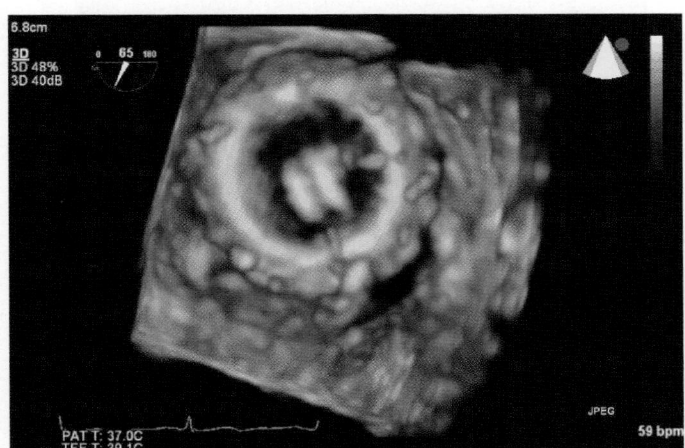

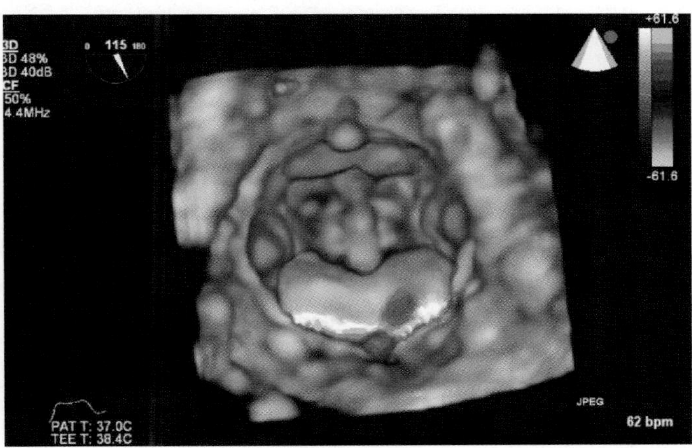

FIGURE 13-4-2 Three-dimensional TEE image (L) demonstrates a large echo-free space at the site of the large anterior paravalvular leak. The smaller defect is not seen well. Three-dimensional imaging with color flow Doppler (R) demonstrates the 2 regurgitant jets ▶ (see Videos 13-4-2 L and R).

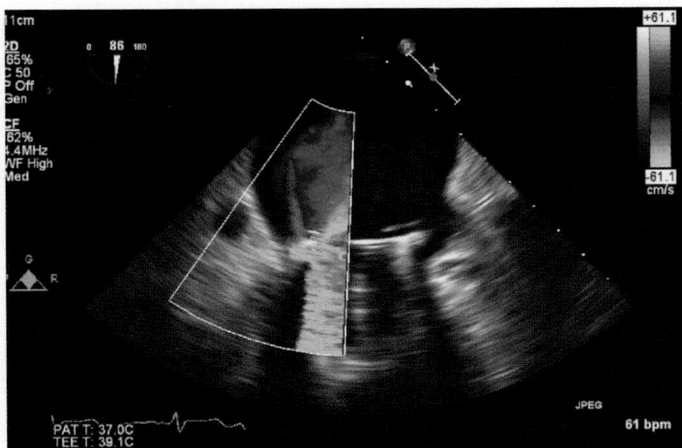

FIGURE 13-4-3 The guidewire used to position and deploy the Amplatzer closure device is seen in the posteromedial paravalvular leak. The catheter was placed via the LV apex and directed under TEE guidance into the LA ▶ (see Video 13-4-3). A similar approach was used to place 2 Amplatzer devices in the larger anterolateral defect.

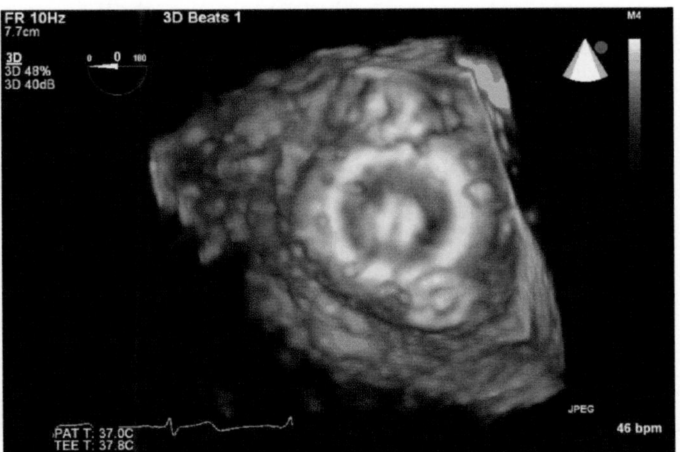

FIGURE 13-4-4 Three-dimensional TEE image demonstrating all 3 devices in place, 2 in the larger anterior defect (at ~12 o'clock in this image) and 1 in the posterior defect (at ~5 o'clock in this image) ▶ (see Video 13-4-4). Color flow Doppler confirmed successful closure of both defects with no residual paravalvular regurgitation.

3. Video 13-4-2 L: 3 D TEE image demonstrates a large echo free space at the site of the large anterior paravalvular leak. The smaller defect is not seen well.
4. Video 13-4-2 R: 3 D TEE imaging with color flow Doppler demonstrates the two regurgitant jets.
5. Video 13-4-3: The guide wire used to position and deploy the Amplatzer® closure device is seen in the posteromedial paravalvular leak. The catheter was placed via the LV apex and directed under TEE guidance into the LA.
6. Video 13-4-4: 3 D TEE image demonstrating all 3 closure devices in place, 2 in the larger anterior defect (at ~12 o'clock in this image) and one in the posterior defect (at ~5 o'clock in this image).

SECTION 5

Percutaneous Balloon Mitral Valvuloplasty

CASE PRESENTATION

A 39-year-old woman from Somalia presented with increasing dyspnea on exertion and palpitations. She denied any previous cardiac history and was on no medications. She did not recall a history of rheumatic fever. On examination, her BP was 98/70 mm Hg, pulse 110 beats/min and irregular, respiratory rate 20 breaths/min. She was in mild distress. Her neck veins were elevated, and she had rales approximately one-quarter of the way up bilaterally. Her cardiac exam was remarkable for an increased intensity of S_1, a loud opening snap, and an apical grade 3/6 diastolic murmur heard best in the left lateral decubitus position. Her abdominal examination was normal. She had 1+ pedal edema. A chest x-ray was consistent with CHF. Her ECG was consistent with atrial fibrillation with a rapid ventricular response. She was started on diltiazem for heart rate control, heparin, and given intravenous furosemide. She had a good diuresis and spontaneously converted to sinus rhythm. Her symptoms improved. A TTE (while in sinus rhythm, HR 78 BPM) revealed normal LV size and function, a thickened, rheumatic appearing mitral valve with minimal calcification and mild submitral thickening. There was minimal mitral regurgitation. The mean MV gradient in diastole was 10 mm Hg. She had mild TR, and the estimated RV systolic pressure was 52 mm Hg. She was placed on oral furosemide and diltiazem, as well as warfarin. She was discharged with follow-up with cardiology. At her follow-up appointment, she felt better but still complained of exertional dyspnea. Based on her valve anatomy, she was felt to be a good candidate for percutaneous balloon mitral valvuloplasty (BMV). The procedure was performed under general anesthesia with TEE guidance. Initial TEE imaging confirmed the MV anatomy and lack of LAA thrombus. The initial MV gradient was only 4 to 5 mm Hg, much lower than the gradient detected on the TTE. It was noted, however, that her HR was quite low, and she was also under anesthesia. A temporary pacemaker was placed, and she was paced at a HR of ~80 BPM. With this intervention, the MV gradient increased to nearly 10 mm Hg. Her pulmonary artery pressure also increased, confirming that she had significant mitral stenosis. Therefore, the team proceeded with the planned BMV. Figures 13-5-1 to 13-5-7 are representative images from her procedure. Following the procedure, she was discharged on oral anticoagulation and a β-blocker.

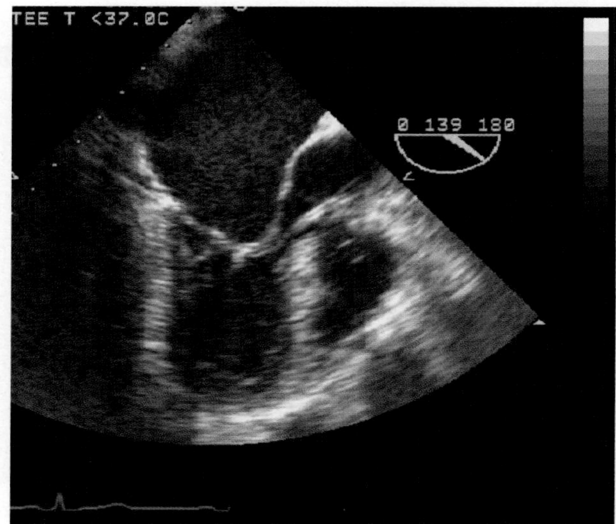

FIGURE 13-5-1 TEE long axis view demonstrating a typical rheumatic MV with good leaflet mobility and minimal calcification. The LA is enlarged ► (see Video 13-5-1).

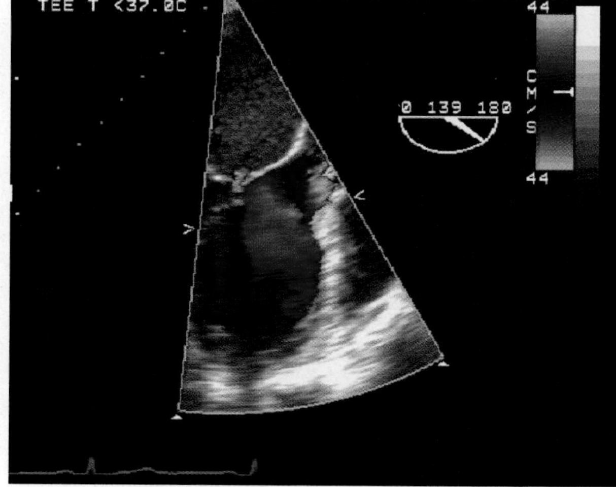

FIGURE 13-5-2 TEE long axis view with color Doppler that demonstrates minimal MR. There is AR present, in part due to the catheter, which has been placed across the AV ► (see Video 13-5-2).

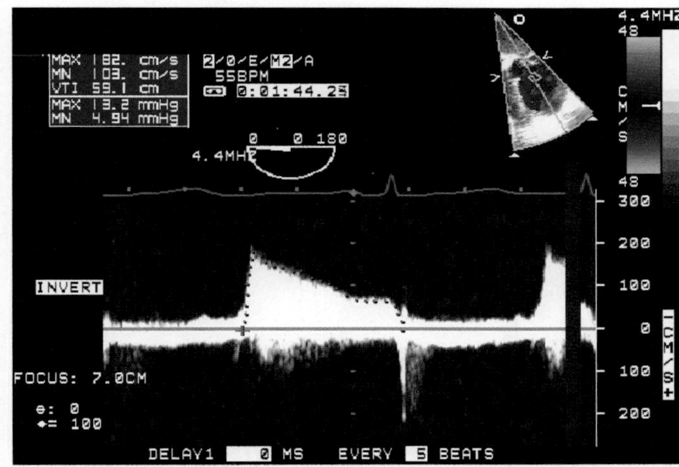

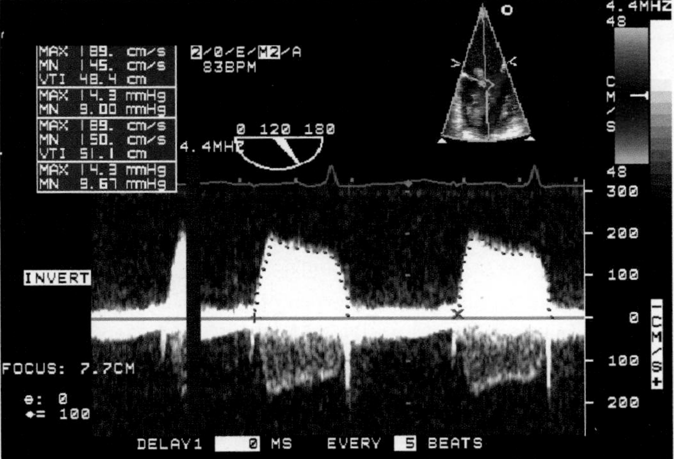

FIGURE 13-5-3 Continuous-wave Doppler demonstrating the initial (top panel) MV gradient (4-5 mm Hg). This was much lower than the gradient detected on the TTE. With pacing at a HR of ~80 BPM, the MV gradient increased to nearly 10 mm Hg (bottom panel). Her pulmonary artery pressure also increased.

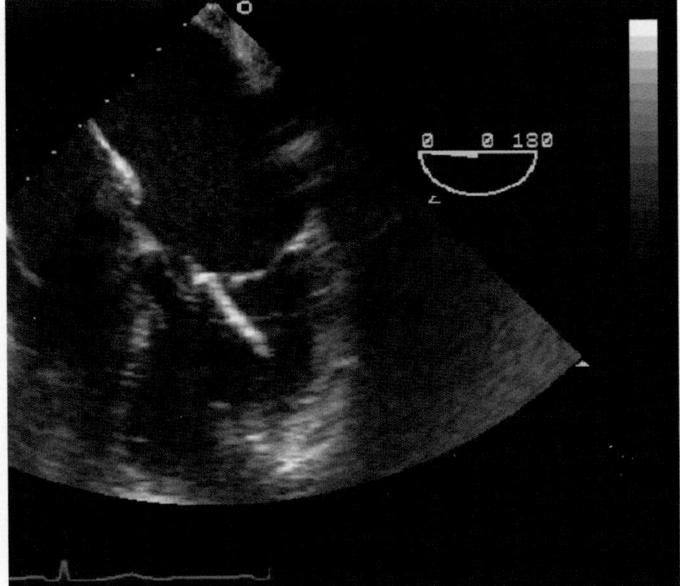

FIGURE 13-5-4 TEE 4 chamber view demonstrating the guide-wire across the MV ▶ (see Video 13-5-4).

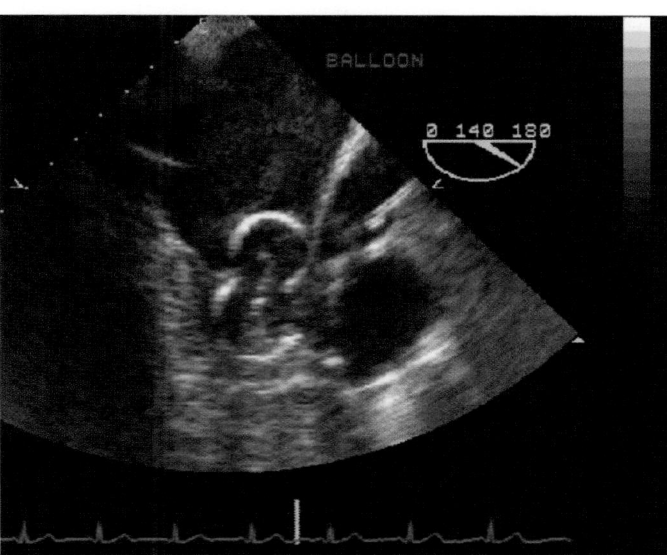

FIGURE 13-5-5 Imaging during the BMV. Note the "waist" on the balloon with this initial inflation ▶ (see Video 13-5-5). Note also the severe spontaneous contrast in the LA due to stagnation of blood flow with balloon inflation. A second balloon inflation was then performed.

She remained free of symptoms. A follow-up TTE demonstrated minimal MR and a mean MV gradient of 3 mm Hg.

VIDEO LEGENDS

1. Video 13-5-1: TEE long axis view demonstrating a typical rheumatic MV with good leaflet mobility and minimal calcification. The LA is enlarged.
2. Video 13-5-2: TEE long axis view with color Doppler which demonstrates minimal MR. There is AR present, in part due to the catheter which has been placed across the AV.

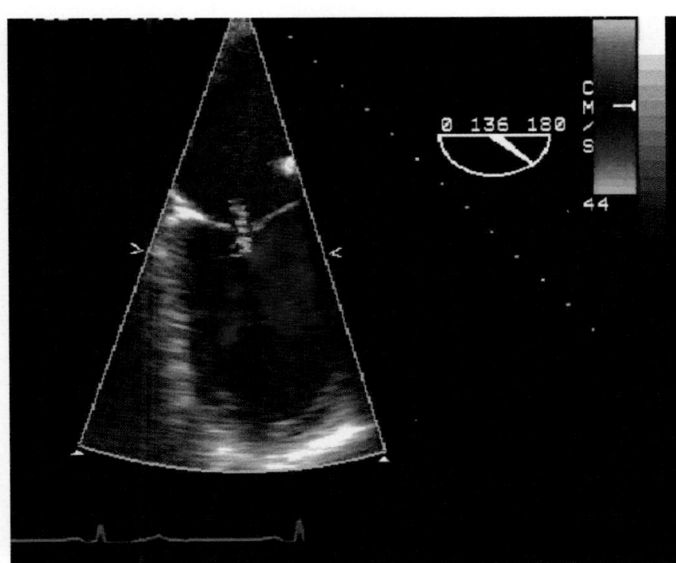

FIGURE 13-5-6 TEE with color Doppler after the second balloon inflation. There is minimal MR and no leaflet disruption ▶ (see Video 13-5-6).

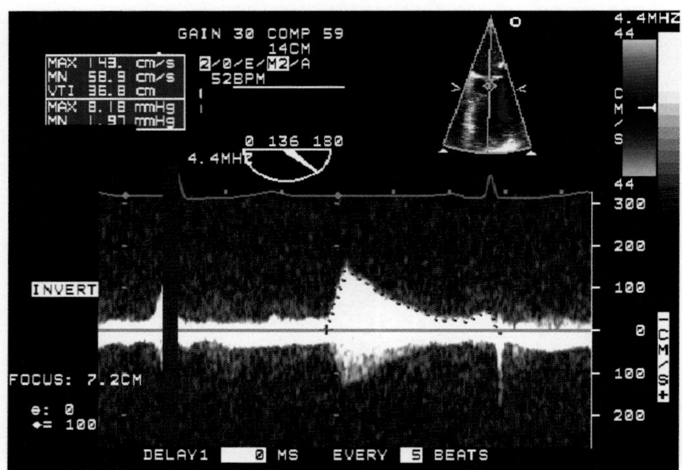

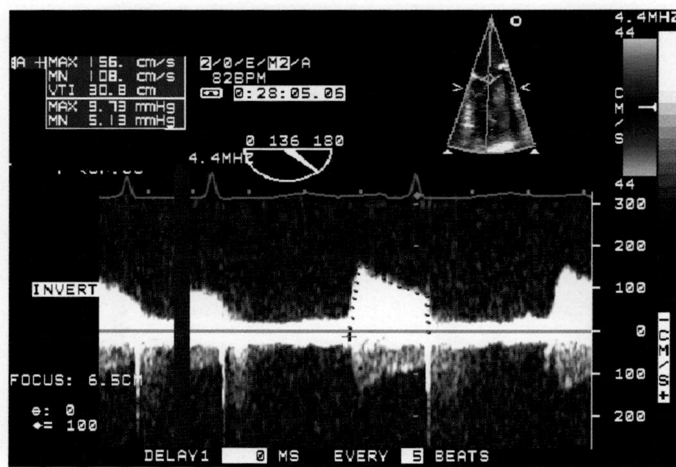

FIGURE 13-5-7 Continuous-wave Doppler at the end of the BMV procedure to reassess the hemodynamics. At baseline, the MV gradient was less than 2 mm Hg (L). The patient again was paced to a HR of ~80 BPM. There was an increase in the MV gradient to ~5 mm Hg; however, the pulmonary artery pressure did not increase (R). No further balloon inflations were performed.

3. Video 13-5-4: TEE four chamber view demonstrating the guidewire across the MV.
4. Video 13-5-5: Imaging during the BMV. Note the "waist" on the balloon with this initial inflation. Note also the severe spontaneous contrast in the LA due to stagnation of blood flow with balloon inflation. A second balloon inflation was then performed.
5. Video 13-5-6: TEE with color Doppler after the second balloon inflation. There is minimal MR and no leaflet disruption.

REFERENCES

1. Cheitlin MD, Armstrong WF, Aurigemma GP, et al. ACC/AHA/ASE 2003 guideline update for the clinical application of echocardiography - summary article A report of the American College of Cardiology/American Heart Association Task Force on practice guidelines. (ACC/AHA/ASE 2003 Committee to Update the 1997 Guidelines for the Clinical Application of Echocardiography). *J Am Coll Cardiol.* 2003;42:954-970.
2. Douglas PS, Garcia MJ, Haines DE, et al. ACCF/ASE/AHA/ASNC/HFSA/HRS/SCAI/SCCM/SCCT/SCMR 2011 appropriate US criteria for echocardiography: a report of the American College of Cardiology Foundation Appropriate Use Criteria Task Force, American Society of Echocardiography, American Heart Association, American Society of Nuclear Cardiology, Heart Failure Society of America, Heart Rhythm Society, Society of Cardiovascular Angiography and Interventions, Society of Critical Care Medicine, Society of Cardiovascular Computed Tomography, and Society of Cardiovascular Magnetic Resonance. *J Am Coll Cardiol.* 2011;57(9):1126-1166. doi: 10.1016/j.jacc.2010.11.002.
3. Silvestry FE, Kerber RE, Brook MM, et al. Echocardiography-guided interventions. *J Am Soc Echocardiogr.* 2009;22(3):213-231.
4. Zamorano JL, Badano LP, Bruce C, et al. EAE/ASE recommendations for the use of echocardiography in new transcatheter interventions for valvular heart disease. *J Am Soc Echocardiogr* 2011;24(9):937-965.

Page numbers followed by f and t refer to figures and tables, respectively.

R